PACS

PACS
BASIC PRINCIPLES AND APPLICATIONS

H. K. Huang, D.Sc., FRCR (Hon.)

Professor
Department of Radiology
University of California, San Francisco

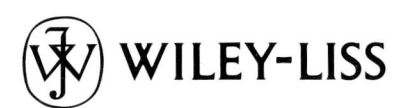

WILEY-LISS

A JOHN WILEY & SONS, INC., PUBLICATION

New York • Chichester • Weinheim • Brisbane • Singapore • Toronto

This book is printed on acid-free paper. ∞

Copyright © 1999 by Wiley-Liss, Inc. All rights reserved.

Published simultaneously in Canada.

While the authors, editor, and publisher believe that drug selection and dosage and the specification and usage of equipment and devices, as set forth in this book, are in accord with current recommendations and practice at the time of publication, they accept no legal responsibility for any errors or omissions, and make no warranty, express or implied, with respect to material contained herein. In view of ongoing research, equipment modifications, changes in governmental regulations and the constant flow of information relating to drug therapy, drug reactions, and the use of equipment and devices, the reader is urged to review and evaluate the information provided in the package insert or instructions for each drug, piece of equipment, or device for, among other things, any changes in the instructions or indication of dosage or usage and for added warnings and precautions.

No part of this publication may be reproduced, stored in a retrieval system or transmitted in any form or by any means, electronic, mechanical, photocopying, recording, scanning or otherwise, except as permitted under Sections 107 or 108 or the 1976 United States Copyright Act, without either the prior written permission of the Publisher, or authorization through payment of the appropriate per-copy fee to the Copyright Clearance Center, 222 Rosewood Drive, Danvers, MA 01923, (978) 750-8400, fax (978) 750-4744. Requests to the Publisher for permission should be addressed to the Permissions Department, John Wiley & Sons, Inc., 605 Third Avenue, New York, NY 10158-0012, (212) 850-6011, fax (212) 850-6008, E-Mail: PERMREQ@WILEY.COM.

Library of Congress Cataloging-in-Publication Data:

PACS : basic principles and applications / edited by H.K. Huang.
    p. cm.
  Includes index.
  ISBN 0-471-25393-6 (pbk. : alk. paper)
  1. Picture archiving and communication systems in medicine.
2. Diagnostic imaging. I. Huang, H.K., 1939– .
R857.P52P33 1999
616.07′54—dc21   98-23684
                                                          CIP

Printed in the United States of America.

10 9 8 7 6 5 4 3 2 1

To my wife, Fong, for her support and understanding and my daughter, Cammy, for her young wisdom.

Contents

Foreword	xix
Preface	xxiii
Acknowledgments	xxvii
List of Acronyms	xxix

1. Introduction   1

1.1	Introduction		1
1.2	History of Picture Archiving and Communication Systems (PACS)		2
1.3	What is PACS?		3
	1.3.1	PACS Design Concept	3
	1.3.2	PACS Infrastructure Design	3
1.4	PACS Implementation Strategies		4
	1.4.1	Background	4
	1.4.2	Four Methods of PACS Implementation	5
	1.4.3	PACS Evolution	6
	1.4.4	Large-Scale PACS and Some Examples	7
1.5	Organization of This Book		10

2. Digital Radiologic Image Fundamentals of Imaging   15

2.1	Terminology		15
2.2	Density Resolution, Spatial Resolution, and Signal-to-Noise Ratio		17
2.3	Radiologic Test Objects and Patterns		20
2.4	Spatial Domain and Frequency Domain		20
	2.4.1	Frequency Components of an Image	20
	2.4.2	The Fourier Transform Pair	21
	2.4.3	The Discrete Fourier Transform	25
2.5	Measurement of Image Quality		25
	2.5.1	Measurement of Sharpness	26
	2.5.2	Measurement of Noise	33

3. Projection Radiography   39

3.1	Principles of Conventional Projection Radiography		39

		3.1.1	Some Standard Procedures Used in Conventional Projection Radiography	39
		3.1.2	Image Receptor	43
	3.2	X-Ray Film Scanner		50
		3.2.1	Video Scanning System	50
		3.2.2	Laser Scanner	51
	3.3	Digitization		52
		3.3.1	Parameters Affecting the Quality of Digitization	52
		3.3.2	Aliasing Artifacts	57

4. Digital Radiography — 63

	4.1	Imaging Plate Technology		63
		4.1.1	Principle of the Laser-Stimulated Luminescence Phosphor Plate	64
		4.1.2	A Computed Radiography System Block Diagram and Its Principle of Operation	64
		4.1.3	Operating Characteristics of the CR System	67
		4.1.4	Imaging Plate Reader and Recorder	68
		4.1.5	Some Clinical Applications	69
		4.1.6	CR Background Removal	70
	4.2	Digital Fluorography		80
		4.2.1	Description of System Components	80
		4.2.2	Operational Procedure	82
	4.3	Low-Scattering Digital Radiographic System		83
		4.3.1	Line Scan Technique	83
		4.3.2	Flying-Spot Scan Technique	83
	4.4	Full-Field Digital Mammography		84
		4.4.1	Screen/Film and Digital Mammography	84
		4.4.2	Full Field Digital Mammography	86
	4.5	Recent Advances in Digital Radiography		89

5. Computed Tomography, Magnetic Resonance, Ultrasound, Nuclear Medicine, and Microscopic Imaging — 91

	5.1	Image Reconstruction from Projections		91
		5.1.1	The Fourier Projection Theorem	91
		5.1.2	The Algebraic Reconstruction Method	94
		5.1.3	The Filtered (Convolution) Back-Projection Method	95
	5.2	Transmission X-Ray Computed Tomography (XCT)		96
		5.2.1	Conventional XCT	96
		5.2.2	Spiral (Helical) XCT	98
		5.2.3	Cine XCT	99
		5.2.4	Operation Principle of an XCT Scanner	101

	5.3	Emission Computed Tomography	103
		5.3.1 Single Photon Emission CT (SPECT)	103
		5.3.2 Positron Emission CT (PET)	105
	5.4	Nuclear Medicine	106
		5.4.1 Principles of Nuclear Medicine Scanning	106
		5.4.2 The Gamma Camera and Associated Imaging System	107
	5.5	Ultrasound Imaging	109
		5.5.1 Principles of B-Mode Ultrasound Scanning	109
		5.5.2 System Block Diagram and Operational Procedure	109
		5.5.3 Sampling Modes and Image Display	112
		5.5.4 Color Doppler Ultrasound Imaging	113
		5.5.5 Cine Loop Ultrasound Imaging	113
	5.6	Magnetic Resonance Imaging	113
		5.6.1 MR Imaging Basics	113
		5.6.2 Magnetic Resonance Image Production	114
		5.6.3 Steps in Producing an MR Image	114
		5.6.4 Image Format, Resolution, and Contrast	116
	5.7	Microscopic Imaging	117
		5.7.1 Instrumentation	117
		5.7.2 Resolution	121
		5.7.3 Contrast	124
		5.7.4 Vidicon/CCD Camera and Scanning	124
		5.7.5 A/D Conversion	124
		5.7.6 Image Memory	125
		5.7.7 Computer	127

6. Image Compression — **129**

	6.1	Terminology	129
	6.2	Background	130
	6.3	Error-Free Compression	131
		6.3.1 Background Removal	131
		6.3.2 Run-Length Coding	132
		6.3.3 Huffman Coding	134
	6.4	Two-Dimensional Irreversible Image Compression	138
		6.4.1 Introduction	138
		6.4.2 Block Compression Technique	140
		6.4.3 Full-Frame Compression	143
	6.5	Measurement of the Difference Between the Original and the Reconstructed Image	151
		6.5.1 Quantitative Parameters	151
		6.5.2 Qualitative Measurement: Difference Image and Its Histogram	152

		6.5.3 Acceptable Compression Ratio	152
		6.5.4 Quality of the Reconstructed Image	155
		6.5.5 Receiver Operating Characteristic Analysis	156
	6.6	Three-Dimensional Image Compression	160
		6.6.1 Background	160
		6.6.2 Wavelet Theory and Multiresolution Analysis	161
		6.6.3 Three-Dimensional Image Compression with Wavelet Transform	164
	6.7	Color Image Compression	169
		6.7.1 Examples of Color Image in Radiology	169
		6.7.2 The Color Spaces	170
		6.7.3 Compression of Color Ultrasound Images	171
	6.8	Legal and Regulatory Issues	172
		6.8.1 Use of Irreversible Compression	172
		6.8.2 Measure of Image Compression	173
		6.8.3 Image Postprocessing	173
		6.8.4 Legal Standards for Compression	174
		6.8.5 Product Liability	174
	6.9	Summary and Research Directions	175
7.	**Picture Archiving and Communication System Components and Industrial Standards**		**177**
	7.1	PACS Components	177
		7.1.1 Data and Image Acquisition Component	177
		7.1.2 PACS Controller and Archive	178
		7.1.3 Display Workstations	179
		7.1.4 System Networking	180
	7.2	PACS Infrastructure Design Concept	181
		7.2.1 Industry Standards	181
		7.2.2 Connectivity and Open Architecture	182
		7.2.3 Reliability	182
		7.2.4 Security	182
	7.3	Two Health Care Industry Data and Image Standards	183
	7.4	The Health Level 7 (HL7) Standard	183
		7.4.1 Health Level 7	183
		7.4.2 An Example	184
	7.5	The ACR-NEMA Standard	186
		7.5.1 ACR-NEMA and DICOM	186
		7.5.2 The ACR-NEMA Standard	187
	7.6	The DICOM 3.0 Standard	188
		7.6.1 Object Class and Service Class	189
		7.6.2 DICOM Communication	192

	7.6.3	DICOM Conformance	192
	7.6.4	Examples of Using DICOM	194
7.7	Other Standards		197
	7.7.1	UNIX Operating System	197
	7.7.2	Windows NT Operating System	198
	7.7.3	C and C++ Programming Languages	198
	7.7.4	Structured Query Language (SQL)	198

8. Image Acquisition Gateway — 199

- 8.1 Background — 199
- 8.2 Automated Acquisition Interface Methods for Pre-DICOM Device — 200
  - 8.2.1 Sequential Chain Model — 201
  - 8.2.2 Direct Interface Model — 202
  - 8.2.3 Memory Access Model — 202
  - 8.2.4 Shared Disk Model — 204
  - 8.2.5 Interconnected Network Model — 204
- 8.3 Fault-Tolerance Methods for Automated Image Acquisition — 206
  - 8.3.1 Image Acquisition Software — 206
  - 8.3.2 Acquisition Process Recovery from Errors — 207
  - 8.3.3 Acquisition Process Recovery from Traps — 207
  - 8.3.4 Acquisition Computer Recovery from Downtime Occurrence — 208
  - 8.3.5 Handling Imaging System Shutdown — 209
- 8.4 Interface Using DICOM — 209
  - 8.4.1 Introduction — 209
  - 8.4.2 Concept of DICOM-Based PACS Image Acquisition — 210
- 8.5 Automatic Image Recovery Scheme for DICOM Conformance Device — 213
  - 8.5.1 Missing Images — 213
  - 8.5.2 Automatic Image Recovery Scheme — 213
- 8.6 Interface with a PACS Module — 216
- 8.7 Image Preprocessing — 219
  - 8.7.1 Computed Radiography (CR) — 219
  - 8.7.2 Digitized X-Ray Images — 223
  - 8.7.3 Digital Mammography — 223
  - 8.7.4 Sectional Images: CT, MR, and US — 224
- 8.8 Multilevel Adaptive Processing Control in the Image Acquisition Gateway — 224
  - 8.8.1 Concept of Multilevel Adaptive Processing Control — 224
  - 8.8.2 Data Flow of CR Images in PACS — 225
  - 8.8.3 Process Control Theory — 226

		8.8.4	Fault Tolerance Algorithm	227
		8.8.5	Combining the Control Theory and Fault Tolerance	228
		8.8.6	Event-Driven Multilevel Adaptive Process Control Structure	229
		8.8.7	Some Results	230

9. Communications and Networking — 233

- 9.1 Background in Communications and Networking — 233
  - 9.1.1 Terminology — 233
  - 9.1.2 Network Standards — 234
  - 9.1.3 Network Technology — 236
  - 9.1.4 Connecting Networks Together — 250
- 9.2 Cable Plan — 251
  - 9.2.1 Types of Network Cable — 251
  - 9.2.2 The Hub Room — 252
  - 9.2.3 Cables for Input Sources — 253
  - 9.2.4 Cables for Image Distribution — 254
- 9.3 Video Broadband Communication Technology — 255
  - 9.3.1 Broadband Technology — 255
  - 9.3.2 Fiber-Optic Broadband Video Communication System — 258
- 9.4 Digital Communication Networks — 262
  - 9.4.1 Background — 262
  - 9.4.2 Design Criteria — 262
- 9.5 PACS Network Design — 264
  - 9.5.1 External Networks — 264
  - 9.5.2 Internal Networks — 265
  - 9.5.3 An Example — 266

10. PACS Controller and Image Archive — 269

- 10.1 Image Management Design Concept — 269
  - 10.1.1 Local Storage Management Via PACS Intercomponent Communication — 269
  - 10.1.2 PACS Controller System Configuration — 270
- 10.2 PACS Controller System Software — 273
  - 10.2.1 Image Receiving — 274
  - 10.2.2 Image Stacking — 274
  - 10.2.3 Image Routing — 275
  - 10.2.4 Image Archiving — 275
  - 10.2.5 Studies Grouping — 275
  - 10.2.6 Platter/Tape Management — 275
  - 10.2.7 RIS and HIS Interfacing — 276
  - 10.2.8 PACS Database Updates — 277

		10.2.9	Image Retrieving	277

		10.2.9	Image Retrieving	277
		10.2.10	Image Prefetching	277
	10.3	Storage Media		278
		10.3.1	RAID	279
		10.3.2	Digital Optical Cartridge Tape	282
		10.3.3	DVD-ROM	282
	10.4	PACS Server System Operations		283
	10.5	Concept of DICOM-Compliant PACS Server		284
		10.5.1	Advantages of a DICOM-Compliant PACS Server	284
		10.5.2	DICOM Communications in a PACS Environment	284
		10.5.3	DICOM-Compliant Image Acquisition Gateways	285
		10.5.4	DICOM-Compliant PACS Server	287

11. HIS, RIS, and PACS Interface — 289

	11.1	Hospital Information System		289
	11.2	Radiology Information System		291
	11.3	Interface PACS with HIS and RIS		292
		11.3.1	Background	292
		11.3.2	Reasons for Interfacing PACS with HIS and RIS	294
		11.3.3	Some Common Rules	295
		11.3.4	Common Data in HIS, RIS, and PACS	296
		11.3.5	Implementation of RIS-PACS Interface	296
	11.4	Interface PACS with Other Medical Databases		299
		11.4.1	Multimedia Medical Data	299
		11.4.2	Multimedia in the Radiology Environment	300
		11.4.3	Integration of Heterogeneous Databases	301
	11.5	Electronic Medical Record		303

12. Display Workstation — 305

	12.1	Basics of a Display Workstation		305
		12.1.1	Image Display Board	305
		12.1.2	Video Monitor	308
		12.1.3	Color CRT	313
		12.1.4	Types of Image Workstation	314
	12.2	Ergonomics of Image Workstations		317
		12.2.1	Glare	317
		12.2.2	Ambient Illuminance	319
		12.2.3	Acoustic Noise Due to Hardware	319
	12.3	Image Processing and Display Functions		320
		12.3.1	Image Enhancement Functions	320
		12.3.2	Image Display and Measurement Functions	327
		12.3.3	Optimization of Image Perception in Soft Copy	330

	12.3.4	Montage	332
	12.3.5	Basic Software Functions in a Display Workstation	334
12.4	The Laser Film Imager		335
	12.4.1	The Block Diagram	336
	12.4.2	Performance Characteristics of a Laser Film Imager	337
12.5	DICOM-Based NT/PC Display Workstation		338
	12.5.1	Hardware Configuration	338
	12.5.2	Software System	338

13. PACS Data Management, Distribution, and Retrieval — 343

13.1	PACS Data Management		343
	13.1.1	Patient Folder Manager Concept: Preliminary	343
	13.1.2	Patient Folder Manager: Modules	344
13.2	Distributed Image File Server		351
	13.2.1	Concept of Distributed Image File Server	351
	13.2.2	Image Retrieval from Physician's Desktop	351
	13.2.3	Some Issues Related to Image and Information Retrieval	355
13.3	Web Server		359
	13.3.1	Web Technology	360
	13.3.2	Concept of Web Server in the PACS Environment	360
13.4	Medical Image Informatics Infrastructure		361
	13.4.1	Concept of MIII	361
	13.4.2	MIII Architecture and Components	361

14. Telemedicine and Teleradiology — 367

14.1	Introduction		367
14.2	Telemedicine		368
14.3	Teleradiology		369
	14.3.1	Background	369
	14.3.2	Teleradiology Components	372
	14.3.3	State-of-the-Art Technology	376
	14.3.4	Teleradiology Examples and Models	378
	14.3.5	Some Important Issues in Teleradiology	382
14.4	Telemammography		384
	14.4.1	Why Do We Need Telemammography?	384
	14.4.2	Concept of the Expert Center	384
	14.4.3	Technical Issues	385
14.5	Telemicroscopy		386
	14.5.1	Telemicroscopy and Teleradiology	386
	14.5.2	Telemicroscopy Applications	387
14.6	Trends in Telemedicine and Teleradiology		388

15. PACS Implementation and System Evaluation — 389

- 15.1 Planning to Install a PACS — 389
  - 15.1.1 Cost Analysis — 389
  - 15.1.2 Film-Based Operation — 391
  - 15.1.3 Digital-Based Operation — 395
- 15.2 Large-Scale PACS — 398
- 15.3 PACS Modules — 398
  - 15.3.1 ICU Module — 398
  - 15.3.2 Emergency Department Module — 399
  - 15.3.3 Ultrasound Module — 401
  - 15.3.4 Nuclear Medicine Module — 402
- 15.4 Integration of PACS Modules — 402
  - 15.4.1 Background — 402
  - 15.4.2 Integration of Existing PACS — 403
  - 15.4.3 Integration of PACS Modules — 406
- 15.5 Manufacturer's Implementation Strategy — 406
  - 15.5.1 System Architecture — 406
  - 15.5.2 Implementation Strategy — 406
- 15.6 Template for PACS RFP — 407
- 15.7 PACS System Evaluation — 408
  - 15.7.1 Subsystem Throughput Analysis — 408
  - 15.7.2 System Efficiency Analysis — 412
  - 15.7.3 Image Quality Evaluation — 415

16. PACS Clinical Experience, Pitfalls, and Bottlenecks — 419

- 16.1 Clinical Experience with PACS Modules — 419
  - 16.1.1 ICU PACS Module — 419
  - 16.1.2 Ultrasound PACS Module — 423
  - 16.1.3 Physician Desktop Access to PACS Images — 424
- 16.2 Neuroradiology — 426
  - 16.2.1 Neuroradiology Image Acquisition — 426
  - 16.2.2 Neuroradiology Examinations — 427
  - 16.2.3 Users' Reading Habits — 427
  - 16.2.4 Neuroradiology PACS Workstation System Utilization — 428
- 16.3 PACS Pitfalls — 436
  - 16.3.1 During Image Acquisition — 436
  - 16.3.2 At the Workstation — 439
- 16.4 PACS Bottlenecks — 441
  - 16.4.1 Network Contention — 442
  - 16.4.2 Slow Response at the Workstation — 444
  - 16.4.3 Slow Response from the Archive Server — 445

	16.5	Pitfalls in DICOM Conformance	447
		16.5.1 Incompatibility in a DICOM Conformance Statement	447
		16.5.2 Methods of Remedy	447

17. PACS Current Development Trends and Future Research Directions — 449

	17.1	Introduction	449
	17.2	Medical Image Informatics Infrastructure in a PACS Environment	449
		17.2.1 Hospital-Integrated (HI) PACS at UCSF	449
		17.2.2 MIII Based on the HI-PACS	450
		17.2.3 Some Research Using the MIII	452
	17.3	Computation and Three-Dimensional Rendering Node	454
	17.4	Image Content Indexing	455
	17.5	Distributed Computing	457
		17.5.1 Concept of Distributed Computing	457
		17.5.2 Distributed Computing in a PACS Environment	461
	17.6	Authenticity for PACS Images and Records	461
		17.6.1 Background	461
		17.6.2 Key-Based Cryptographic Algorithms	462
	17.7	Integration of Multiple PACS	464
	17.8	CAD in a PACS Environment	465
		17.8.1 Computer-Aided Detection or Diagnosis	465
		17.8.2 CAD without PACS	467
		17.8.3 Methods of Integrating CAD in a PACS Environment with DICOM	467

18. PACS Applications — 471

	18.1	Bone Age Assessment with a Digital Hand Atlas	471
		18.1.1 Background	471
		18.1.2 Methodology	472
		18.1.3 Operational Procedure	473
		18.1.4 Clinical Evaluation	474
	18.2	Outcome Analysis of a Lung Nodule with Temporal CT Image Database	475
		18.2.1 Background	475
		18.2.2 System Architecture	475
		18.2.3 Graphic User Interface	476
		18.2.4 An Example	476
		18.2.5 Temporal Image Database and the MIII	478
	18.3	Interactive Digital Breast Imaging Teaching File	479
		18.3.1 Background	479

	18.3.2	Computer-Aid Instruction Model	480
	18.3.3	The Teaching File Script and Data Collection	481
	18.3.4	Graphic User Interface	482
	18.3.5	Interactive Teaching File as a Training Tool	483
18.4	Real-Time Teleconsultation with High Resolution and Large-Volume Medical Images		484
	18.4.1	Background	484
	18.4.2	System Design	485
	18.4.3	Teleconsultation Procedure and Protocol	487
	18.4.4	Clinical Evaluation	489

References   **491**

Index   **511**

Foreword

THE MANUFACTURER'S POINT OF VIEW

William M. Angus, M.D., Ph.D.
Senior Vice President
Philips Medical Systems, Inc.
Shelton, Connecticut

Nearly two decades have passed since the first serious proposals were put forth for electronic systems which could manage the communication, display, and archiving of diagnostic image information, so-called PAC systems. Verification of these proposals progressed very slowly at first, primarily due to the lack of adequate and affordable enabling technologies.

This initial problem, although it will never be perfectly solved, was addressed steadily over time with pressure from the marketplace and under the guidance of early researchers in the fields of diagnostic imaging and medical informatics. Dr. H.K. Huang, one of the first and most prolific of these researchers, earned an industry-wide reputation as an insightful, enthusiastic, and competent cooperator in the development of technologies required for medical image management.

By the mid-to-late 1980s, the technology situation had greatly improved, and the focus of the problem shifted to the issue of proper application of technology. Early PAC systems supplied by industry were often marvels of technology which were for the most part incompatible with prevailing logistics of medical practice. The only PAC systems to actually serve some useful, clinical purpose were those comparatively low-tech systems developed in university departments through the interaction of medical specialists, imaging informatics scientists, and industrial suppliers.

Having anticipated this second problem early on, Dr. Huang had already begun a graduate program designed to produce scientists who could span the interdisciplinary gap between industry and medical imaging practice. At the same time he developed an informatics laboratory where informatics scientists, medical practitioners, and members of the industry could build-up new systems and subsystems, and observe both their technological functions and their impact on medical practice.

The knowledge and experience accumulated from all of these activities were presented in Dr. Huang's last book, *PACS: Picture Archiving and Communication Systems in Biomedical Imaging,* a text primarily directed to the training of medical informatics scientists urgently needed by both healthcare facilities and industry. Now, just two years after the publication of that text, Dr. Huang, anticipating the needs of other workers in the PACS field, comes to us again with an entirely new volume, *PACS (Picture Archiving and Communication Systems): Basic Principles and Applications.* This work, although it supplements its predecessor by including conceptual and technological advances which have surfaced in the intervening two years, is primarily intended for the training of those in industry and in the field of healthcare who deal with the everyday practical realities of planning, operating, and maintaining PAC systems.

For his early perception that this type of information is urgently needed, as well his willingness to compile and present it here in such a timely fashion, both industry and the medical profession again owe Dr. Huang a great deal of gratitude.

THE CAR (COMPUTER ASSISTED RADIOLOGY) ORGANIZER POINT OF VIEW

Professor Heinz U. Lemke, Ph.D.
Technical University of Berlin
Berlin, Germany

Since the first conferences on PACS at the beginning of the 1980s, we have experienced a speedy development of enabling technologics for the generation, management, and communication of digital medical images. Telematic technologies have now matured to be employed in PACS with improved cost effectiveness and clinical benefits. Additional motivation for PACS is expected to come from recent developments in direct digital radiography. Lower total cost of ownership (TCO) of medical workstations through NT PCs will further promote widespread acceptance of PACS. National and international conferences related to medical imaging give PACS increasing attention, and the number of presentations on this subject have more than doubled in recent years. PACS publications, however, are widely distributed over conference proceedings and technical/medical journals. A comprehensive book providing an in-depth coverage of PACS components and system integration is therefore urgently needed.

After reviewing the extensive list of topics covered in Dr. Huang's book, and knowing that they have been authored by one of the world's renowned experts on PACS, I am convinced that the book will become a prime source for teaching and for reference in many academic and healthcare settings. Some important parts of the content have been presented regularly in PACS tutorials given by Dr. Huang at CAR conferences. The tutorials have been very well received by attendees from all over the world.

As I have with Dr. Huang's previous book on PACS, I will use this new book in my own teaching at the Technical University of Berlin. It provides not only an understanding of the fundamentals of digital radiology and PACS, but also gives valuable references on current implementations and critical issues to be observed when building integrated healthcare systems. I am convinced that all those who face difficult decisions with regard to the allocation of limited resources in the health care sector will profit from the accumulated wisdom in this book.

The more general reader who is concerned about healthcare is likely to acknowledge the widespread changes now under way, induced by technology and other driving forces. Together with these developments, PACS will lead to a breakdown of traditional boundaries within and between primary, secondary, and tertiary care. Different infrastructures in health care will therefore evolve. New paradigms in thinking and workflow relating to PACS are emerging, and we have to thank Dr. Huang for effectively contributing towards this development.

THE ACADEMIC AND HEALTH CENTER POINT OF VIEW

Professor and Chairman
Edward V. Staab, M.D.
Department of Radiology
University of Florida
Gainesville, Florida

The initial publication of Bernie Huang's book *PACS in Biomedical Imaging* (Wiley-VCH, 1996) filled a need for a concise textbook dealing with the technology of PACS. Much has happened since the previous edition of this publication. The nihilists are mostly gone and the curent tune is not "should there be a conversion to the digital environment," but "when and for how much." Many partial and complete PACS installations have been undertaken. The partial PACS solutions are enthusiastically endorsed. The total PACS solutions are greeted with mixed reviews depending on the cost, process of installation, and subsequent reliability. As various information systems link, additional opportunities are recognized. Rather than the "have-nots" catching up with the "haves," it appears that the technological spread between them is widening. This is more related to local resources, politics, knowledge, and desire rather than to shortcomings in technology.

The practice of radiology will change dramatically in the next few years from the film-based system to PACS. It will be important for all of radiology to understand in some detail this new technology. Thus, we welcome this new edition of Dr. Huang's book.

PACS is no longer looked upon as a radiology-only system, but as a part of the entire enterprise global information system. The network and other infrastructure needs, such as handling the massive data that comes from modern radiology image studies, are taxing to health information systems. This has at times led to misunderstandings between various information teams. Those early birds who implemented PACS from a primary radiology perspective have sometimes encountered political difficulty integrating with the hospital information system team. This hurdle will and must be jumped to optimize the systems for patient care. Information that is provided in this book should help with this integration.

Industry is rapidly developing product lines that range from components to fully integrated PACS solutions. Film companies along with some of the instrument manufacturers have taken the initial lead in developing and marketing PACS products. More recently, some of the larger information system suppliers are entering this market. In my opinion, we will probably see some merging of talents and interests among these companies by the time that the next edition of this textbook is published.

DICOM is becoming the standard for the connectivity of various PACS components, but remains relatively immature. It is still necessary to validate and provide minor software changes for installations of equipment even when they come from the same manufacturer. More importantly, upgrades and minor software changes could, and have, caused problems for networks. Therefore, all changes, no matter how minor, to any component connected to the network must be validated prior to installation.

Most of the initial PACS development took place in academic environments. This was followed by the military, whose efforts were enhanced by significant financial resources. Now we see all aspects of our medical community involved. The role of major health care systems such as Kaiser and Tenet in the development of PACS is yet fully to be defined.

As radiology tries to provide expert subspecialty readings as well as good general on-site consultaton to an extended system, these digital solutions will become even more important. PACS is being recognized as a technology that can be used to solve some of the current problems.

Many issues remain. The integration with a comprehensive and robust enterprise information system has not taken place. The design of the new radiology reading areas to entice others to come for consultation will need considerable ingenuity. Image displays continue to improve but require much development. Displays with better spatial resolution will be needed to introduce digital mammography. Computer-aided diagnosis raises the whole question of how we can use these techniques to better assist radiologists. Maintenance of these systems will be increasingly integrated. Quality control of the various units will require a specialized expertise.

The radiologist of the future will still be the expert reader of images, but over time these will come together with physiological, biochemical, and other data. We will have to develop easy ways of communicating these interpretations to the busy clinicians.

Dr. Huang continues to be very active in the development of PACS and has included sections on many of the newest technologies and applications for using digital technology to assist with clinical care, education, and research in the current environment. His style of writing is direct and fluent. The book is organized to make quick reference possible to get at those frequently forgotten facts.

Dr. Huang's previous PACS book has become a reference for those of us who are enthusiasts in PACS. The index indicates that a very comprehensive look at PACS and related technologies is included in this new book. It is a very readable text with ample illustrations to assist those beginning to consider PACS in more detail. Many should find this text useful, including most of the radiology community, information service groups, and administrators, as well as individuals in service and industry.

Preface

Picture archiving and communication systems (PACS) is a concept that was perceived in the early 1980s by the radiology community as a future method of practicing radiology. PACS consists of image acquisition devices, storage archiving units, display workstations, computer processors, and databases. These components are integrated by a communications network and data management system. During the past ten years, technologies related to these components have matured, and their applications have gone beyond radiology to the entire health care delivery system. As a result, PACS for special clinical applications, as well as large-scale hospital-wide PACS, have been installed throughout the United States and the world.

Since the last book *PACS in Biomedical Imaging* was published by VCH in 1996, several important events have occurred related to PACS. First, many successful PACS installations, large and small, have documented the positive outcome in patient care using the system. Second, the health care administrators, through several years of continued education in PACS, have realized the importance of using PACS in streamlining their operations. The justification of purchasing PACS has not become the issue. Instead, the issue is the best mechanism for installing the PACS. Third, the U.S. military, due to its relative success in the MDIS project, has started a DIN/PACS II project, with an allocation of up to 800 million dollars for the next few years. The injection of new funds into PACS stimulates the further growth of the field. Fourth, digital imaging and communication in medicine (DICOM) has become the de facto standard, and is accepted by all major imaging manufacturers. The issue of connectivity has disappeared, and DICOM conformance components have become a commodity. Fifth, the NT PC hardware and software platform has advanced to the level that it can be used for high quality diagnostic workstations. The relatively inexpensive NT PC allows for affordable workstation installation throughout the health care enterprise.

Finally, in 1996, John Wiley & Sons took over the ownership of VCH and inherited the copyright of the last book. Mr. Shawn Morton, Senior Medical Editor, based on his experience in medical publishing, felt that a new book in PACS documenting the aforementioned changes in PACS was due. He suggested that I consider writing a new book reflecting the current trends in PACS and addressing a wider audience, rather than only engineers and medical physicists.

Through my interest in the field of PACS, I owe a debt of gratitude to Dr. Edmund Anthony Franken, Jr., past Chairman of the Department of Radiology, University of Iowa; and Drs. Gabriel Wilson, Robert Leslie Bennett, and Hooshang Kangarloo, past Chairmen of the Department of Radiological Sciences at UCLA for their encouragement and support.

During the past three years at UCSF, we have continued receiving support from the National Library of Medicine, National Institutes of Health, U.S. Army Medical Research and Material Command, California Breast Rescarch Program, and the Federal Technology Transfer Program, for future PACS R&D. This funding allows us to go beyond the boundaries of current PACS and open a new frontier research based on the PACS database. Examples are electronic patient records related to PACS, integration of multiple PACS, and large-scale longitudinal and horizontal basic and clinical research.

From our experience during the past fifteen years, we can identify some major contributions in advancing PACS development. Technologically, the first laser film digitizers developed for clinical use by Konica and Lumisys; the development of computed radiography (CR) was by Fuji and its introduction from Japan to the United States by Dr. William Angus of Philips Medical Systems; and the large-capacity optical disk storage developed by Kodak were all critical. Also highly significant were the redundant array of inexpensive disks (RAID); 2000-line and 72 Hz display monitors; the system integration methods developed by Siemens Gammasonics and Loral for large scale PACS; the DICOM Committee's efforts to standardize (especially Professor Steve Horii's unselfish and tireless educating the public on its importance); and the asynchronous transfer mode (ATM) technology for merging local area network and wide area network communications.

In terms of events, the annual SPIE PACS and Medical Imaging meeting, and the EuroPACS are the continuous driving force for PACS. In addition, the annual Computer Assisted Radiology (CAR) meeting organized by Professor Heinz Lemke, and the Image Management and Communication (IMAC) organized every other year by Professor Seong K. Mun, provide a forum for international PACS discussion. The InfoRAD Section at the RSNA since 1993 organized first by Dr. Laurens V. Ackerman, and then Dr. C. Carl Jaffe with the live demonstration of DICOM interface, set the tone for industrial PACS open architecture. The many refresher courses in PACS during RSNA organized first by Dr. C. Douglas Maynard and then Dr. Edward V. Staab, provided further education in PACS to the radiology community.

In 1992 *Second Generation PACS,* Professor Michel Osteaux's edited book, provided me with the inspiration that PACS is moving towards a hospital integrated approach. When Dr. Roger A. Bauman became Editor-in-Chief of the then-new *Journal of Digital Imaging* in 1998, the consolidation of PACS research and development publications became possible. Colonel Fred Goeringer orchestrated the Army MDIS project, resulting in several large-scale PACS installations which provided major stimuli and funding opportunities for the PACS industry.

All these contributions have profoundly influenced my thoughts on the direction of PACS research and development, as well as the contents of this book. This book summarizes our experiences in developing the concept of PACS, and its relationship to the electronic patient record, and more importantly, the potential of using PACS for better health care delivery and future research. Selected portions of the book have been used as lecture materials in graduate courses entitled *Medical Imaging and Advanced Instrumentation* at UCLA, UCSF, and UC Berkeley, and in the Biomedical Engineering Lectures in Taiwan, Republic of China, and the People's Republic of

China. We hope this book will provide a guideline for those contemplating a PACS installation, and inspire others using PACS as a tool to improve the future of health care delivery.

H.K. (BERNIE) HUANG

*San Francisco and
Agoura Hills, CA*

Acknowledgments

Many people provided assistance during the preparation of this book—in particular, many of my past graduate students, postdoctoral fellows, and colleagues from whom I have learned the most. Chapters 2, 3, 4, and 5 are revisions from my book, *PACS in Biomedical Imaging,* published in 1996. Some of the materials were originally contributed by K.S. Chuang, Ricky Taira, Brent Stewart, and Paul Cho. Many new sections were also added to these chapters. Chapter 6 on image compression was completely rewritten, and some of the figures are extracted from Ben Lo's Ph.D. dissertation. Chapters 7 to 18 are mostly new materials based on our research and development during the past three years.

Specifically, I am thankful for the contributions from Jun Wang (Sections 3.3.2.2, 6.6), Stephen Wong (Sections 6.8, 17.2.3.4, 17.6), Andrew Lou (Sections 4.4.2, 8.2–8.5, 12.3.4, 14.4, 15.7.2), Albert Wong (Sections 7.6.4, 7.7, 10.5, 15.7.1, 16.5), Xiaoming Zhu (Sections 17.5, 18.2), David Hoogstrate (Sections 4.4.2, 8.4, 8.5, 9.1.3, 14.4.3), Mohan Ramaswamy (Section 13.2), Paul Cho (Sections 11.1 and 11.2), Jianguo Zhang (Sections 4.1.6, 8.8, 18.4), Johannes Stahl (18.4), Guang Pu Lei and Hong Zhang (Section 9.1.3, 12.5), Ewa Pietka (Section 18.1), and Fei Cao (Sections 18.1.2.4, 18.3).

I also thank Mr. Shawn Morton, Senior Medical Editor of John Wiley & Sons for providing me the opportunity to write this book and his continued interest and encouragement throughout the preparation; and Camille Carter, the production manager of my last book, for insisting on taking the production responsibility again. Lastly, a special thank you to my assistant, Laura Snarr, for editing the entire manuscript and contributing much original art work.

Other contributions are from K.S. Chuang, Ph.D.; David Hoogstrate, B.S.; Hong Zhang, M.S., Research Fellow; Guang Pu Lei, M.S., Research Fellow; Ewa Pietka, Ph.D.; Kent Soo Hoo, Ph.D. Candidate; Koun Sik Song, M.D., Visiting Fellow; Johannes Stahl, M.D., Visiting Fellow; Jun Wang, Ph.D.; Stephen Wong, Ph.D., and those who contributed some original materials in the last book, *PACS in Biomedical Imaging.*

This book was written with the assistance of the following staff members of the Laboratory for Radiological Informatics at UCSF:

Shyh-Liang (Andrew), Ph.D.
Assistant Professor

Albert W.K. Wong, B.S.
Research Laboratory Manager

Jianguo Zhang, Ph.D.
Visiting Research Fellow and Associate Professor
Changchun Institute of Optics, PR China

Fei Cao, Ph.D.
Research Fellow

Laura Snarr, B.S.
Administrative Assistant

List of Acronyms

1-D	one-dimensional
2-D	two-dimensional
3-D	three-dimensional
4-D	four-dimensional
ABF	air blown fiber
ACR-NEMA	American College of Radiology—National Electrical Manufacturer's Association
ACSII	American standard code for information interchange
A/D	analog to digital converter
ADT	admission, discharge, transfer
AL	aluminum
AMLCD	active matrix liquid crystal device
AMP	amplifier
AP	anterior-posterior
API	application program interface
ASI	NATO Advanced Study Institute
ATM	asynchronous transfer mode
A_z	area under the ROC curve
BDF	building distribution center
BERKOM	Berlin Communication Project
BNC	a type of connector for 10 Base2 cables
CAD	computer-aided detection, diagnosis
CAI	computer-aided instruction
CalREN	California Research and Education Network
CAR	computer assisted radiology
CCD	charge-coupled device
CCU	coronary care unit
CDDI	copper distributed data interface
CFR	contrast frequency response
CIE	Commission Internationale de L'Eclairage
CNA	campus network authority
CORBA	common object request broker architecture
CPU	central processing unit
CR	computed radiography
CRF	central retransmission facility—headend
CRT	cathode ray tube

CSMA/CD	carrier sense multiple access with collision detection
CSU/DSU	channel service unit/data service unit
CT	computed tomography
CTN	central test node
DASM	data acquisition system manager
DB	a unit to measure the signal loss
DCT	discrete cosine transform
DEC	digital equipment corporation
DECRAD	DEC radiology information system
DF	digital fluorography
DICOM	digital imaging and communication in medicine
DIFS	distributed image file server
DIMSE	DICOM message service element
DIN/PACS	Digital Imaging Network/PACS
DLT	digital linear tape
DOD	(U.S.) Department of Defense
DOM	distributed object manager
DR11-W	a parallel interface protocol
DS	digital service
DSA	digital subtraction angiography
DSC	digital scan converter
DSP	digital signal processing chip
ECT	emission computed tomography
EIA	Electronic Industries Association
EMR	electronic medical record
EPR	electronic patient record
ESF	edge spread function
EuroPACS	Picture Archiving and Communication Systems in Europe
FCR	Fuji CR
FDA	(U.S.) Food and Drug Administration
FDDI	fiber distributed data interface
FFBA	full-frame bit allocation algorithm
FFD	focus to film distance
FFDDM	full-field direct digital mammography
FFT	fast Fourier transform
FID	free induction decay
FM	folder manager
FP	false-positive
FRS	fast reconstruction system
FT	Fourier transform
FTE	full time equivalent
FTP	file transfer protocol
FWHM	full width at half maximum
GEMS	General Electric Medical System
GUI	graphic user interface

H and D curve	Hurter and Driffield characteristic curve
HI-PACS	hospital-integrated-PACS
HIS	hospital information system
HL7	Health Level 7
HOI	Health Outcomes Institute
HP	Hewlett-Packard
HPCC	high performance computing and communications
HTML	hypertext markup language
HTTL	hypertext transfer protocol
Hz	Hertz (cycle/sec)
IAG	image acquisition gateway
ICD-9	International Classification of Diseases, ninth revision
ICU	intensive care unit
ID	identification
IDF	intermediate distribution frame
IDNET	a GEMS imaging modality network
IFT	inverse Fourier transform
IMAC	a meeting devoted to image management and communication
INC	identifier names and codes
InfoRAD	radiology information exhibit
I/O	input/output
IP	imaging plate
ISDN	integrated service digital network
ISO	International Standards Organization
IUPAC	International Union of Pure and Applied Chemistry
JAMIT	Japan Association of Medical Imaging Technology
Java	just another vague acronym
JND	just noticeable differences
JPEG	Joint Photographic Experts Group
kV(p)	kilovolt potential difference
LAN	local area network
LOINC	Logical Observation Inc.
lp	line pair
LRI	Laboratory for Radiological Informatics
LSF	line spread function
LUT	lookup table
mA	milliampere
MAN	metropolitan area network
Mbyte	megabyte
MDIS	medical diagnostic imaging support systems
MGH	Massachusetts General Hospital
MHS	message header segment—a segment used in HL7
MIDS	medical image database server
MIII	medical image informatics infrastructure

LIST OF ACRONYMS

MIMP	mediware information message processor—a computer software language for HIS used by the IBM computer
MITRE	a non-profit defense contractor
MODEM	modulator/demodulator
MP	multi-processors
MPEG	motion picture expert groups
mR	milliRoentgen
MRI	magnetic resonance imaging
MTF	modulation transfer function
MUMPS	Massachusetts General Hospital Utility Multi-Programming System—a computer software language
MZH	Mount Zion Hospital
NATO ASI	North Atlantic Treaty Organization-Advanced Science Institutes
NDC	national drug codes
NDC	network distribution center
NEC	Nippon Electronic Corporation
NFS	network file system
NGI	next generation Internet
NIE	network interface equipment
NIH	National Institutes of Health
NINT	nearest integer function
NLM	National Library of Medicine
NM	nuclear medicine
NMSE	normalized mean square error
NTSC	national television system committee
OC	optical carrier
OD	optical density
OSI	open system interconnection
PA	posterior-anterior
PACS	picture archiving and communication system
PC	personal computer
PET	positron emission tomography
PHD	personal health data
PICT	Macintosh picture format
PL	plastic
PMT	photomultiplier tube
PPI	parallel peripheral interface
ppm	parts per million
PRF	pulse repetition frequency
PSF	point spread function
PSL	photo-stimulable luminescence
PSNR	peak signal to noise ratio
PTD	parallel transfer disk
PVM	parallel virtual machine system

RAID	redundant array of inexpensive disks
RAM	random access memory
RETMA	Radio-Electronics-Television Manufacturers Association
RF	radio frequence
RFP	request for proposal
RGB	red green and blue
RIS	radiology information system
ROC	receiver operating characteristic
ROI	region of interest
S-bus	a computer bus used by SPARC
SCSI	small computer systems interface
SFVAMC	San Francisco VA Medical Center
SMPTE	Society of Motion Picture and Television Engineers
SMZO	Social and Medical Center East
SNOMED	systemized nomenclature of medicine
SNR	signal-to-noise ratio
Solaris 2.x	a computer operating system version 2.x used in a SUN SPARC workstation
SONET	synchronous optical network
SOP	service object pair—a functional unit of DICOM
SPARC	a computer system manufactured by Sun Microsystems
SPECT	single photon emission computed tomography
SPIE	International Society for Optical Engineering
SQL	structured query language
ST	a special connector for optical fibers
SUN OP	Sun computer operating system
T1	DS-1 private line
TCP/IP	transport control protocol/internet protocol
TDS	tube distribution system for optical fibers
TFS	teaching file script
TGC	time gain compensation
TIFF	tagged image file format
TP	true-positive
UCLA	University of California at Los Angeles
UCSF	University of California at San Francisco
UID	DICOM unique identifier
UMDNS	universal medical device nomenclature system
UMLS	unified medical language system
UNIX	a computer operating system software used by Sun and other computers
UPS	uninterruptible power supply
US	ultrasound
USAVRE	United States Army Virtual Radiology Environment
UTP	unshielded twisted pair
VA	Veterans Administration

VAX	a computer system manufactured by Digital Equipment Corporation
VM	a computer operating system software used by IBM computers
VME	a computer bus used by older Sun and other computers
VMS	a computer operating system software used by DEC computers
VRAM	video RAM
VRE	virtual radiology environment
WAN	wide area network
WORM	write once read many
WS	workstation
WSU	working storage unit
WWW	world wide web
XCT	x-ray transmission computed tomography
YCbCr	luminance and two chrominance coordinates used in color digital imaging
YIQ	luminance—in-phase and quadrature chrominance color coordinates

CHAPTER 1

Introduction

1.1 INTRODUCTION

There are many advantages of introducing digital and communication technologies to the conventional paper and film-based operation in radiology and medicine. For example, through the computer, it is possible to manipulate a digital image for value-added diagnosis, and through imaging plate technology and other imaging modalities it is possible to improve the diagnostic value while at the same time reducing the radiation exposure to the patient. Also, insofar as they promote a more efficient operating environment, digital and communication technologies can speed up health care delivery and reduce operation costs.

With all these benefits, the digital and communication technologies are gradually changing the method of acquiring, storing, viewing, and communicating diagnostic images and related information. One natural development along this line is the emergence of a digital radiology department and a digital hospital environment. A digital radiology department has two components: a radiology information management system (RIS) and a digital imaging system. The radiology information system is a subset of the hospital information system (HIS) or the electronic patient (or medical) record (EPR or EMR) system, which entails data management with respect to the patient (as opposed to images). The digital imaging system, sometimes referred to as picture archiving and communication system (PACS) or image management and communication system (IMAC), involves image acquisition, archiving, communication, retrieval, processing, distribution, and display. A digital hospital environment consists of the HIS or EPR, PACS, and other digital clinical systems. The combination of HIS or EPR and PACS is referred to as hospital-integrated PACS (HI-PACS). Up-to-date information on these topics can be found in multidisciplinary literature, research laboratories of university hospitals, and medical imaging manufacturers, but not in a coordinated way. Therefore, it is difficult for a radiologist, hospital administrator, medical imaging researcher, radiological technician, or trainee in diagnostic radiology to collect and assimilate this information.

The purpose of this book is to consolidate in a single text discussions of PACS-related topics and the integration of PACS systems with HIS or EPR. The emphasis is on basic principles, augmented with current technological developments and examples for each topic.

1.2 HISTORY OF PICTURE ARCHIVING AND COMMUNICATION SYSTEMS (PACS)

The term "digital radiology" was introduced by Dr. Paul Capp in the early 1970s. Lack of technological development to support the requirements of digital radiology, however, prevented the concept from becoming popular until the early 1980s. The concept of digital image communication and display was initiated by Professor Heinz U. Lemke, of the Technical University of Berlin, in one of his original papers.

The First International Conference and Workshop on Picture Archiving and Communication Systems (PACS), held in Newport Beach, California, in January 1982, was sponsored by SPIE (the International Society for Optical Engineering). Thereafter, the PACS conference has been combined with the Medical Imaging Conference. The joint meeting has become an annual event, always held in February in southern California.

In Japan, the First International Symposium on PACS and PHD (Personal Health Data) was held in July 1982, sponsored by the Japan Association of Medical Imaging Technology (JAMIT). This conference, combined with the Medical Imaging Technology meeting, also became an annual event. In Europe, the EuroPACS (Picture Archiving and Communication Systems in Europe) has held annual meetings since 1983 and is the driving force for European PACS information exchange.

One of the earliest research projects related to PACS in the United States was a teleradiology project sponsored by the U.S. Army in 1983. A follow-up project was the Installation Site for Digital Imaging Network and Picture Archiving and Communication System (DIN/PACS) funded by the U.S. Army and administered by the MITRE Corporation in 1985. Two university sites were selected for the implementation, the University of Washington in Seattle, and Georgetown University/George Washington University Consortium in Washington, D.C., with participation of Philips Medical Systems and AT&T. The U.S. National Cancer Institute funded UCLA one of its first PACS-related research projects in 1985 under the title Multiple Viewing Stations for Diagnostic Radiology.

A meeting dedicated to PACS sponsored by NATO ASI (Advanced Study Institute) was PACS in Medicine held in Evian, France, in October 1990. Approximately 100 scientists from over 17 countries participated. The ASI proceedings summarized international efforts in PACS research and development at that time. This meeting stimulated the Diagnostic Imaging Support Systems (MDIS) project sponsored by the U.S. Army Medical Command, which has been responsible for large-scale military PACS installations in the United States.

Other well-organized scheduled conferences dedicated to PACS and related topics are the CAR (computer assisted radiology) and IMAC (image management and communication) meetings. CAR is an annual event first organized by Lemke in 1985. IMAC is a biannual conference started in 1989 and organized by Professor Seong K. Mun of Georgetown University.

1.3 WHAT IS PACS?

1.3.1 PACS Design Concept

A picture archiving and communication system consists of image and data acquisition, storage, and display subsystems integrated by various digital networks. It can be as simple as a film digitizer connected to a display workstation with a small image data base, or as complex as a total hospital image management system. PACS developed in the late 1980s, designed mainly on an ad hoc basis to serve small subsets of the total operations of many radiology departments. Each of these PACS modules functioned as an independent island, unable to communicate with other modules. Although this piecemeal approach demonstrated the PACS concept and worked adequately for each of the different radiology and clinical services, it did not address all the intricacies of connectivity and cooperation between modules. This weakness surfaced as more PACS modules were added to hospital networks. Maintenance, routing decisions, coordination of machines, fault tolerance, and the expandability of the system became sources of increasingly difficult problems. The inadequacy of the early design concept was due partially to a lack of understanding of the complexity of a large-scale PACS and to the unavailability at that time of certain PACS-related technologies.

PACS design should emphasize system connectivity. A general multimedia data management system that is easily expandable, flexible, and versatile in its operation calls for both top-down management to integrate various hospital information systems and a bottom-up engineering approach to build a foundation (i.e., PACS infrastructure). From the management point of view, a hospital-wide PACS is attractive to administrators because it provides economic justification for implementing the system. Proponents of PACS are convinced that its ultimately favorable cost–benefit ratio should not be evaluated as a resource of the radiology department alone but should extend to the entire hospital operation. This concept has gained momentum. Several hospitals around the world have implemented large-scale PACS and have provided solid evidence that PACS improves the efficiency of health care delivery and at the same time saves hospital operational costs. From the engineering point of view, the PACS infrastructure is the basic design concept to ensure that PACS includes features such as standardization, open architecture, expandability for future growth, connectivity, and reliability. This design philosophy can be constructed in a modular fashion with an infrastructure design described in the next section.

1.3.2 PACS Infrastructure Design

The PACS infrastructure design provides the necessary framework for the integration of distributed and heterogeneous imaging devices and makes possible intelligent database management of all patient-related information. Moreover, it offers an efficient means of viewing, analyzing, and documenting study results, and furnishes a method for effectively communicating study results to the referring physicians. The

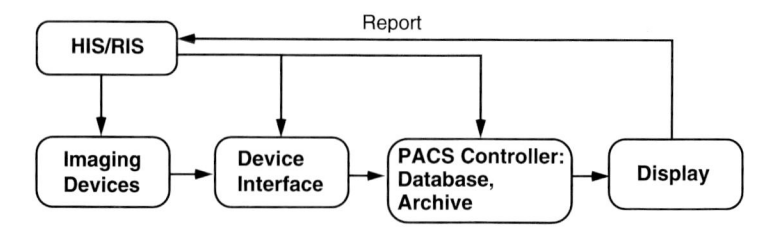

Figure 1.1 PACS basic components and data flow: HIS, hospital information system; RIS, radiology information system. System integration and clinical implementation are two necessary phases of implementation that occur after the system has been physically connected.

PACS infrastructure consists of a basic skeleton of hardware components (imaging device interfaces, storage devices, host computers, communication networks, display systems) integrated by standardized, flexible software subsystems for communication, database management, storage management, job scheduling, interprocessor communication, error handling, and network monitoring. The infrastructure as a whole is versatile and can incorporate rules to reliably perform not only basic PACS management operations but also more complex research job and clinical service requests. The software modules of the infrastructure embody sufficient understanding and cooperation at a system level to permit the components to work together as a system rather than as individual networked computers.

The PACS infrastructure is physically composed of several classes of computer systems connected by various networks. These include radiologic imaging devices, device interfaces, the PACS controller with database and archive, and display workstations. Figure 1.1 shows the PACS basic components and data flow. This diagram will be expanded to present additional detail in later chapters.

1.4 PACS IMPLEMENTATION STRATEGIES

1.4.1 Background

A PACS integrates many components related to medical imaging for clinical practice. Depending on the application, a PACS can be simple, consisting of just a few components, or it can be a complex hospital-integrated system. For example, a PACS for an intensive care unit may comprise no more than a scanner adjacent to the film developer for digitization of radiographs, a base-band communication system to transmit, and a video monitor in the intensive care unit (ICU) to receive and display images. On the other hand, implementing a comprehensive hospital-integrated PACS is major undertaking that requires careful planning and millions of dollars in investment.

During the past 15 years, many hospitals and manufacturers in the United States and abroad have researched and developed PACS of varying complexity. Many of these systems are in daily clinical use. These systems can be loosely categorized into four groups according to methods of implementation. The first category is the home-grown system, developed within the department or hospital because of clinical needs. The second category is a team effort between the hospital and manufacturers. This category emerged when the U.S. military services initiated the Medical Diagnostic Imaging Support System (MDIS) concept in the late 1980s. The MDIS adopted the military procurement procedures in acquiring PACS for military hospitals and clinics. This required a team to write the detailed specifications, followed by the selection of a manufacturer to implement the system. The third category is market driven. Some manufacturers see potential profit in developing a specialized turnkey PACS to promote the sale of other imaging equipment. The last category is partnership between a hospital and a manufacturer, which is the most recent trend in large-scale PACS implementation.

1.4.2 Four Methods of PACS Implementation

1.4.2.1 The Three Original Methods

Most early PACS implementation efforts were initiated by university hospitals and academic departments and by research laboratories of major imaging manufacturers. Consider the first three methods.

1. *Home-grown system:* a multidisciplinary team with technical know-how is assembled by the radiology department or the hospital. The team becomes a system integrator, selecting PACS components from various manufacturers. The team develops system interfaces and writes the PACS software according to the clinical requirements of the hospital.
2. *Two team effort:* from both outside and inside the hospital act as a team to write detailed specifications for the PACS for a certain clinical environment. A manufacturer is contracted to implement the system.
3. *Turnkey approach:* a manufacturer develops a completely operational PACS and installs it in a department for clinical use.

Each approach has advantages and disadvantages. The home-grown system integration approach, for example, allows the research team to continuously upgrade the system with state-of-the-art components. The system so designed is tailored to the clinical environment and can be upgraded without depending on the schedule of the manufacturer: it will not become obsolete. On the other hand, the assembly of a multidisciplinary team calls for a substantial commitment from the hospital. In addition, since the system developed will be one of a kind, consisting of components from different manufacturers, service and maintenance will be difficult.

The primary advantage of the two-team effort is that the PACS specifications are tailored to a certain clinical environment, yet the responsibility for implementation is delegated to the manufacturer. The department acts as a purchase agent and does not have to be concerned with the installation. The specifications tend to be overambitious, however, because of the potential for experts not familiar with the clinical environment to underestimate the technical and operational difficulty of certain clinical functions. The designated manufacturer, who may lack experience with some components in a clinical environment, may in turn overestimate the performance of each component. As a result, the completed PACS may not meet the overall specifications. The cost of contracting the manufacturer to develop a specified PACS is also high because when only one system is built, the narrow profit margin will not always permit the realization of economies of scale.

The advantage of the third or turnkey approach is that in a generalized production system, the cost tends to be lower. In this approach, the manufacturer needs a couple of years to complete the production cycle. By the time the system is commercially available, however, some components from the fast-moving computer and communication fields may have become obsolete. Also, it is doubtful whether a generalized PACS can be used for every specialty in a single department and for every radiology department.

1.4.2.2 The Fourth Method

During the past five years, because of the availability of PACS clinical data, health centers have learned to take advantages of the good and discard the bad features of each method during their implementation. As a result, the boundaries between the three original approaches have gradually fused. Thus a fourth implementation strategy emerges, which is partnership between a health center and a manufacturer. In this case, the health center contracts with a selected manufacturer, which is responsible for PACS implementation, maintenance, service, training, and upgrading. The arrangement can be a long-term purchase and maintenance contract, or a lease of the system. Table 1.1 summarizes the advantages and disadvantages of all four approaches.

1.4.3 PACS Evolution

Because of different operating conditions and environment, PACS has evolved differently in North America, Europe, and Asia. In the early date, PACS research and development in North America was mostly supported by government agencies and manufacturers. In the European countries, it was supported through either a multinational consortium, a country, or a regional resource. European research teams tended to work with a single major manufacturer, and, since most PACS components were developed in the United States and Japan, they were not as readily available to the Europeans. European research teams emphasized PACS modeling and simulation, as well as the investigation of the image processing component of PACS. In Asia, Japan led the early PACS research and development and treated it as a national project. The national resources were distributed to various manufacturers and university hospitals. A manufacturer or a joint venture from several companies integrated a PACS system

TABLE 1.1 Advantages and Disadvantages of Four Methods of PACS Implementation

Method	Advantages	Disadvantages
Home-grown system	Built to specifications State-of-the-art technology Continuously upgrading Not dependent on a single manufacturer	Difficult to assemble a team One-of-a-kind system Difficult to service and maintain
Two team effort	Specifications written for a certain clinical environment Implementation delegated to the manufacturer	Specifications overambitious Technical and operational difficulty underestimated Manufacturer lacks clinical experience Expensive
Turnkey approach	Lower cost Easier maintenance	Too general Not State-of-the-art technology
Partnership	System will keep up with technology advancement Health center does not have to worry if the system becomes obsolete Manufacturer has long-term contract to plan ahead	Expensive to the health center, Manufacturer may not want to sign a partnership contract with a center of lesser prominence Center must consider the longevity and stability of the manufacturer Legal issue when partnership dissolves

and installed it in a hospital for clinical evaluation. The manufacturer's PACS specifications tended to be rigid and left little room for the hospital research team to modify the technical specifications.

During the fifth IMAC meeting in Seoul, South Korea, in October 1997, three invited lecturers described the evolution of PACS in Europe, North America, and Japan. The early paths of varied PACS research and development gradually merged, eventually leading to many successful PACS implementations in these three regions. This trend can be traced to four major reasons: (1) the information exchange from the aforementioned conferences (SPIE, CAR, and IMAC), (2) the introduction of the image and data format standards and their gradual acceptance by the private industry, (3) the globalization of the imaging manufacturers, and (4) the resolution of the most difficult technical and clinical problems in PACS.

1.4.4 Large-Scale PACS and Some Examples

There are now many PAC systems, large and small, in daily clinical operation. In this section we describe four large PAC systems in the United States, Europe, and Asia to illustrate the capability of PACS. Roger Bauman and colleagues, in two 1996 recent papers in the *Journal of Digital Imaging,* defined a large-scale PACS as satisfying the following conditions:

1. System is in daily clinical operation.
2. At least three or four imaging modalities are connected to the system.
3. System contains workstations inside and outside the radiology department.
4. System is able to handle at least 20,000 procedures per year.

The first three systems described were implemented based on the second implementation strategy and have been used for primary diagnosis for at least two years. The fourth system was implemented using the first approach and is moving to partner with a manufacturer (fourth strategy).

1.4.4.1 Baltimore Veterans Administration Medical Center

The Baltimore VA Medical Center, operating with approximately 200 beds, has been totally digital except in mammography since its opening in 1994. All examinations are 100% archived in PACS with bidirectional HIS/RIS (hospital information system/ radiology information system) interface. Currently the system serves three other institutions in the region: the VA Medical Center Fort Howard Hospital (259 beds), the Perry Point Hospital (677 beds), and the Baltimore Rehabilitation and Extended Care Facility. Surveys of clinicians have consistently indicated a preference for the filmless system versus conventional films. An economic analysis also indicates that filmless operations are offset by the equipment depreciation and maintenance costs. The general statistics are as follows: radiology department volumes increased 58%, lost examinations decreased from 8% to 1%, productivity increased 71%, repeated examination decreased 60%, and image reading time decreased 15%. These results suggest that the medical center and the networked hospitals as a whole increased health care efficiency and reduced operational cost as a result of PACS implementation.

1.4.4.2 Hammersmith Hospital

When the Hammersmith Hospital in London, England, built a new radiology department, a committee chaired by the hospital director of finance and information planned a top-down, whole-hospital PACS project. The hypothesis of the project was that cost savings arising from PACS will contribute to increased efficiency in the hospital. Hammersmith Hospital includes the Royal Postgraduate Medical School and the Institute of Obstetrics and Gynecology. It consists of 500 beds and serves 100,000 people. The justification of the project was based on the direct cost/saving and the indirect cost/saving components. In direct cost/saving, the following components were considered: archive material and film use, labor, maintenance, operation and supplies, space and capital equipment, and buildings. Indirect cost/saving comprised junior medical staff time, reductions in unnecessary investigations, savings in radiologist, technologist, and clinician time, redesignation and change of use of a number of acute beds, and reduction in the length of stay.

Currently the system consists of a 10-terabyte long-term archive, and a 256-gigabyte short-term storage servicing 168 workstations.* Since the start of system operation in 1993, the PACS has improved hospital-wide efficiency, the number of filing clerks has been reduced from 8 to 1, 3.3 radiologists have been eliminated, physicist/information technology personnel has increased 1.5, and no films are stored on site.

1.4.4.3 Samsung Medical Center

Samsung Medical Center, a 1100-bed general teaching hospital, started a PACS implementation plan with gradual expansion beginning in 1994. The medical center has over 4000 outpatient clinic visits per day and performed about 340,000 examinations per year. The PACS in Samsung serves the following functions: primary and clinical diagnosis, conference, slide making, generation of teaching materials, and printing hard copies for referring physicians. The system started with 35 workstations and now has expanded to 145 workstations supported by a 4.5 Tbyte long-term archive and 256 gbyte short-term storage. It fetches an average of 600–900 examinations/day. All examinations and diagnoses are performed digitally except mammography.

Like the Baltimore VA Medical Center and Hammersmith Hospital, this PACS operation has the following characteristics:

1. It is totally digital and uses workstations as the primary diagnosis tool.
2. It was implemented using the second implementation strategy (i.e., two-team effort).
3. The Medical Center administration made the initial commitment of total PACS implementation, and has continued to support the system upgrade.
4. There is excellent leadership from the top down.

Since, however, these three systems were implemented using method 2, they now face problems during expansion of system upgrade and the extension of services to other affiliated hospitals. These problems are considered in Section 15.4.2.1.

1.4.4.4 University of California, San Francisco (UCSF)

The UCSF PACS was implemented in-house through a multidisciplinary team, many of whose members had participated in the implementation of the PACS at UCLA. The implementation started in October 1992 and the system was released for clinical use in February 1995. Since the system was designed in-house, the concept used was quite advanced compared with other manufacturers' systems. For example, it had open architecture, connectivity, integration with the hospital and radiology information

---

* Abbreviations throughout: Tbyte, terabyte ($= 10^{12}$ bytes); GByte, gigabyte ($= 10^9$ bytes); Mbyte, megabyte ($= 10^6$ bytes); Gbit, Mbit, Kbit, bits $\times 10^9$, 10^6, 10^3.

systems, system modularity, and asynchronous transfer mode (ATM) communication technology; it even distributed image data to physicians' desktop computers. Throughout this book these concepts are introduced and emphasized. The system architecture is shown in Figures 9.7, 9.8, 16.1, and 17.1, and its connection to imaging modalities and databases is given in Table 17.1. Because the system was built in-house, it is different from most other systems in two respects. First, it has great flexibility for future growth. Second, it can take full advantage of the system for PACS, applications including large-scale longitudinal and horizontal research and clinical service. Many applications described in later chapters stemmed from this architecture.

In April 1996 it was clear that the PACS technology had reached sufficient maturity to permit a manufacturer to take over the continued rudimentary implementation. For example, the system required the addition of more storage devices and workstations, and quality assurance of the daily clinical service. A clinical PACS team was assembled to take responsibility of the system's daily operation. In January 1997, UCSF partnered with a PACS manufacturer to continue its service to the expanding clinical enterprise.

1.5 ORGANIZATION OF THIS BOOK

PACS Principles and Applications consists of 18 chapters. Chapter 1 describes the history of PACS, tells what it is, discusses the implementation strategies used, and introduces some large-scale systems. Figure 1.1 presents the basic block diagram of PACS, and Figure 1.2, which charts the organization of this book, also gives the potential of PACS for large-scale research and clinical applications.

Chapter 2 describes the fundamentals of digital radiologic imaging. It is assumed that the reader has some basic knowledge in conventional radiographic physics. This chapter introduces the basic terminology used in digital radiologic imaging and gives some examples. Familiarizing oneself with this terminology will facilitate the reading of later chapters.

Chapters 3, 4, and 5 discuss radiologic image acquisition systems. Since conventional projection radiography is still responsible for 70% of radiological examinations in a typical radiology department, we consider methods of converting this imaging acquisition method from a film-based to a digital-based operation. For this reason, Chapter 3 includes a discussion on the principles and procedures of conventional projection radiographic acquisition systems and the laser film scanner and its accuracy.

Chapter 4 discusses some projection radiographic acquisition systems with direct digital image output. These include laser-stimulated luminescence phosphor plate, digital fluorography, and some emerging direct digital radiography technologies, such as full-field digital mammography. All these acquisition systems are digital-based and utilize electro-optical and solid state physics technologies.

Chapter 5 discusses sectional imaging. Section 5.1 introduces the concept of image reconstruction from projections. Sections 5.2, 5.3, 5.5, and 5.6 provide basic knowledge in transmission, emission computed tomography, ultrasound imaging, and

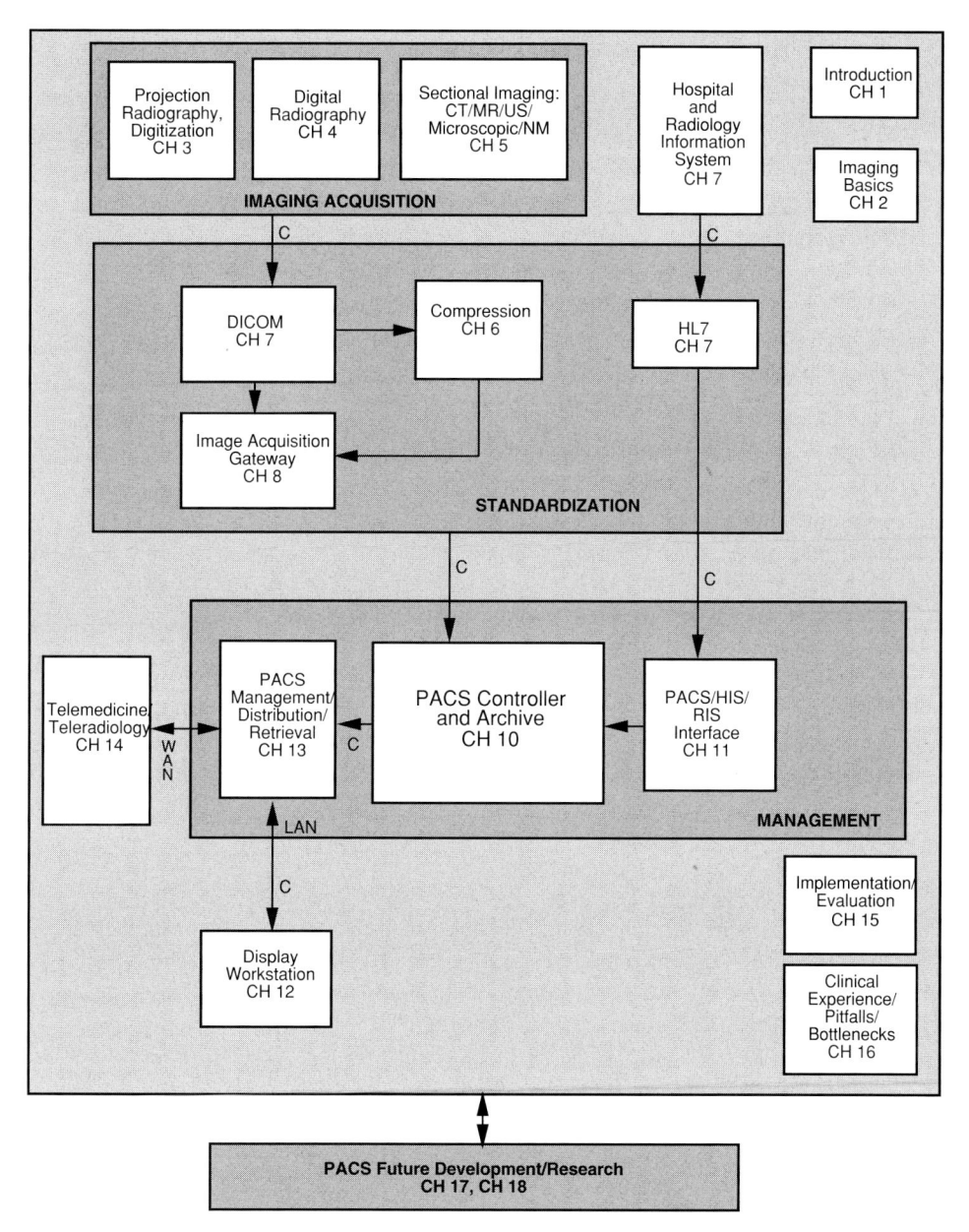

Figure 1.2 Organization of this book: C, communication, is covered in Chapter 9; LAN, local area network; WAN, wide area network.

magnetic resonance imaging, respectively. Section 5.4 discusses imaging in nuclear medicine. Section 5.7 deals with digital microscopy which is another imaging area requiring PACS integration.

Note that Chapters 3, 4, and 5 are not comprehensive treatises of projection and sectional imaging. Instead, they provide certain basic terminology of images encountered in diagnostic radiology and microscopic imaging, emphasizing the digital aspect, of these modalities, rather than the physics. The reader should grasp the digital procedure of these imaging modalities to facilitate his or her PACS design and implementation plan. This digital imaging basis is essential for a thorough understanding of interfacing these imaging modalities to a PACS.

Chapter 6 covers image compression. After an image has been captured in digital form from an acquisition device, it is transmitted to a storage device for long-term archiving. In general, a digital image file requires a large storage capacity for archival purposes. For example, an average computed tomography or two-view computed radiography study comprises about 20 Mbyte. Therefore, it is necessary to consider how to compress an image file into a compact form before storage or transmission. The concepts of reversible (lossless) and irreversible (lossy) compression are discussed in detail in Sections 6.1, 6.3, and 6.4. Section 6.5 describes methods of measuring the quality of the reconstructed image from compressed data. Three-dimensional image data sets occur very often in sectional imaging, and color images become important in Doppler ultrasound imaging. For these reasons, two current topics on three-dimensional and color image compression are given in Sections 6.6 and 6.7, respectively. Finally, image compression raises certain legal and regulatory issues, which are discussed in Section 6.8.

The rest of the book, Chapters 7 to 18, is devoted to topics in picture archiving and communication systems. In Chapter 7, we introduce the basic concept of PACS and its components. The industrial interface standard on medical data, Health Level 7 (HL7), is reviewed. There is also a detailed discussion of two image format and communication protocols, ACR-NEMA (American College of Radiology–National Electrical Manufacturers Association) and DICOM (Digital Imaging and Communication in Medicine) which have been adopted by the PACS community.

Chapter 8 presents the image acquisition gateway. It covers the systematic method of interfacing imaging acquisition devices using the HL7 and DICOM standards, and automatic error recovery schemes. Many image preprocessing functions used during the interface are described in Section 8.7. Section 8.8 is an advanced topic on using the multilevel adaptive processing control in the gateway as a means of fault tolerance design.

Chapter 9 discusses both digital and analog image communication methods. The latest technology in digital communication using asynchronous transfer mode and gigabit Ethernet is described.

Chapter 10 presents the PACS controller and image archive. Sections 10.1 and 10.2 describe the design concept and software for PACS image management. Three storage technologies essential for PACS operation are redundant array of inexpensive disks (RAID), digital optical cartridge tape, and DVD-ROM (digital versatile disk), discussed in Section 10.3. Section 10.5 introduces the concept of a DICOM-compliant PACS server.

Chapter 11 describes the PACS interface with the hospital information system (HIS), the radiology information system (RIS), and other medical databases. This chapter forms the cornerstone of extending the PACS in one department to a hospital-integrated system. Section 11.5 introduces the development of the electronic medical record and its potential interface with the PACS.

Chapter 12 discusses image display (both soft copy and hard copy output). Effective image display and processing functions, which are necessary to optimize the usefulness of the soft copy display method, are considered in Section 12.3. Section 12.5 introduces the DICOM-based NT/PC display workstation as the inexpensive PACS workstation.

Chapter 13 presents PACS data management, distribution, and retrieval. Two new concepts on Web-based server and medical image informatics infrastructure are introduced in Sections 13.3, and 13.4, respectively. The former delivers PACS image and related data to every desktop computer using Internet technology. The latter provides the foundation for large-scale research and clinical service based on the richness of the PACS database.

Chapter 14 describes telemedicine and teleradiology. State-of-the-art technologies and teleradiology service models are given in Section 14.3. Some important issues in teleradiology including cost, quality, and medical-legal issues are discussed in Section 14.3.5. A current view on telemammography and its technical requirements is given in Section 14.4. Telemicroscopy is introduced in Section 14.5.

Chapter 15 presents the PACS implementation and system evaluation. The points of view of both the institution and the manufacturer are discussed. Section 15.7 describes some standard methodologies in the PACS system evaluation.

Chapter 16 is about PACS clinical experience, pitfalls, and bottlenecks. In clinical experience, special interest is attached to the ICU PACS module, the neuroradiology workstation, and the ultrasound unit PACS module. Some commonly encountered situations are illustrated and remedies recommended.

Chapters 17 and 18 are devoted to the future and applications of PACS. Chapter 17 discusses PACS current development trends and future research directions. Topics on medical imaging informatics infrastructure in PACS environment, distributed computing, 3-D rendering node, and authenticity for PACS images and records are introduced. Chapter 18 discusses four current research topics based on the PACS infrastructure on bone age assessment with a digital hand atlas, outcome analysis of lung nodules with a temporal image database, the interactive digital breast imaging teaching file, and real-time teleconsultation with high resolution and large-volume images.

CHAPTER 2

Digital Radiologic Fundamentals of Imaging

2.1 TERMINOLOGY

This chapter discusses some fundamental concepts and tools in digital radiologic imaging that are used throughout the text. These concepts are derived from conventional radiographic imaging and digital image processing. For an extensive treatment of these subjects, see the following materials, which are listed in the References at the end of the book:

Barrett and Swindell (1981)
Benedetto, Huang, and Ragan (1990)
Bertram (1970)
Bracewell (1965)
Brigham (1974)
Cochran et al. (1967)
Curry, Dowdey, and Murry (1987)
Dainty and Shaw (1984)
Gonzalez and Wintz (1987)
Hendee and Wells (1997)
Huang (1996)
Robb (1995)
Rosenfeld and Kak (1976)
Rossman (1969)

Digital image. A digital image is a two-dimensional array of nonnegative integers $f(x,y)$, where $1 \leq x \leq M$ and $1 \leq y \leq N$ in which M and N are positive integers representing the number of rows and columns. For any given x and y, the small square in the image represented by the coordinates (x,y) is called a picture element, or a pixel, and $f(x,y)$ is its corresponding functional value. When $M = N$, f becomes a square image; most sectional images used in medicine are square images. If the image $f(x,y,z)$ is three-dimensional, its functional value at a given point (x,y,z) is called a voxel.

Digitization and digital capture. Digitization is a process that quantizes or samples analog signals into a range of digital values. Digitizing a picture means converting the continuous gray tones in the picture into a digital image. About 70% of all radiologic examinations, including skull, chest, breast, abdomen, and bone, are acquired and stored on X-ray films. This process, which compresses a three-dimensional object into a two-dimensional image, is called projection radiography. An X-ray film can be converted to digital numbers with a film digitizer. The laser scanning digitizer is the gold standard among digitizers because it can best preserve the resolutions of the original analog image. A laser film scanner can digitize a standard X-ray film (14 in. × 17 in.) to 2000 × 2500 pixels with 12 bits per pixel. Another method for acquiring digital projection radiography is computed radiography (CR), a technology that uses a laser-stimulated luminescence phosphor imaging plate as an X-ray detector. A laser beam is used to scan the exposed imaging plate, which contains the latent X-ray image. The latent image is excited and emits light photons, which are detected and converted to electronic signals. The electronic signals are converted to digital signals to form a digital X-ray image. Recently developed direct X-ray detectors can capture the X-ray image without going through an additional medium like the imaging plate. This method of image capture is sometimes called direct digital radiography.

Images obtained from the other 30% of radiology examinations, which include computed tomography (CT or XCT), nuclear medicine (NM), positron emission tomography (PET), single photon emission computed tomography (SPECT), ultrasonography (US), magnetic resonance imaging (MRI), digital fluorography (DF), and digital subtraction angiography (DSA) are already in digital format when they are generated.

Digital radiologic image. The aforementioned images are collectively called digitized or digital radiologic images: digitized if obtained through a digitizer, digital if generated digitally. The pixel value, (or gray level value, or gray level) can range from 0 to 255 (8-bit), 0 to 511 (9-bit), 0 to 1023 (10-bit), 0 to 2045 (11-bit), and 0 to 4095 (12-bit), depending on the digitization procedure or the radiologic procedure used. These gray levels represent physical or chemical properties of the anatomical structures in the object. For example, in an image obtained by digitizing an X-ray film, the gray level value of a pixel represents the optical density of the small square area of the film. In the case of X-ray computed tomography, the gray level value represents the relative linear attenuation coefficient of the tissue; in magnetic resonance imaging, it corresponds to the magnetic resonance signal response of the tissue.

Image size. The dimensions of an image are the ordered pair (M,N), and the size of the image is the product $M \times N \times k$ bits, where 2^k equals the gray level range. In sectional images, most of the time $M = N$. The exact dimensions of a digital image sometimes are difficult to specify because of the design constraints imposed on the detector system for various examination procedures. Therefore, for convenience, we call a 512 × 512 image a 512 image, a 1024 × 1024 a 1 K, and a 2048 × 2048 a 2K, even though the image itself may not be exactly 512, 1024, or 2048 pixels square. Also, in computers, 12 bits is an odd number for the computer memory and storage device to handle. For this reason, 16 bits or 2 bytes are normally allocated to store a 12-bit pixel. Table 2.1 lists sizes of some conventional medical images.

TABLE 2.1 Size of Some Common Medical Images

	One Image (bits)	# of Images/Exam	One Examination Mbyte
Nuclear Medicine (NM)	128×128×12	30–60	1–2
Magnetic Resonance Imaging (MRI)	256×256×12	60	8
Ultrasound (US)*	512×512×8(24)	20–230	5–60
Digital subt. Angiography (DSA)	512×512×8	15–40	4–10
Digitized Electonic Microscopy	512×512×8	1	0.26
Digitized Color Microscopy	512×512×24	1	0.79
Computed Tomography (CT)	512×512×12	40	20
Computed Radiography (CR)	2048×2048×12	2	16
Digitized X-Rays	2048×2048×12	2	16
Digital Mammography	4000×5000×12	4	160

*Doppler US with 24 bit color images.

Histogram. The histogram of an image is a plot of the gray level value (abscissa) against the frequency of occurrence of pixels of the gray level value in the entire image (ordinate). For an image with 256 possible gray levels, the abscissa of the histogram ranges from 0 to 255. The total pixel count under the histogram is equal to $M \times N$. The histogram represents gray level distribution, an important characteristic of an image.

Image Display. In visualizing a digital image, either of two methods may be used: the digital image may be printed on film or paper for a hard copy, or displayed on a video monitor or other electronic device as a soft copy (volatile). To display a digital radiologic image on a video monitor, the gray level values are converted to analog signals compatible with conventional video signals used in the television industry. This procedure is called digital-to-analog (D/A) conversion. Video display monitors can be used to display an image of 512-, 1024-, or 2048-pixel size. A new type of display device is called active matrix liquid crystal device (AMLCD) which has the potential to replace the cathode ray tube (CRT) technology.

Figure 2.1 shows the relationship between a radiologic image, the image size, the pixel, and the gray level value.

2.2 DENSITY RESOLUTION, SPATIAL RESOLUTION, AND SIGNAL-TO-NOISE RATIO

The quality of a digital image is characterized by three parameters: spatial resolution, density resolution, and signal-to-noise ratio. The spatial and density resolutions are related to the number of pixels and the range of gray levels per pixel used to represent the objects. In a square image $N \times N \times k$, it is clear that N and k are related to the spatial resolution and density resolution, respectively. A high signal-to-noise ratio means the image has little noise and is very pleasing to the eyes, hence is a better quality image.

Figure 2.2 demonstrates the concept of spatial and density resolutions of a digital image using a lymphocyte as an example. The left hand column in Figure 2.2 shows digitized images of the lymphocyte with a fixed spatial resolution (21 × 15) and variable density resolutions (from top to bottom: 16, 4, and 2 gray levels). The right hand

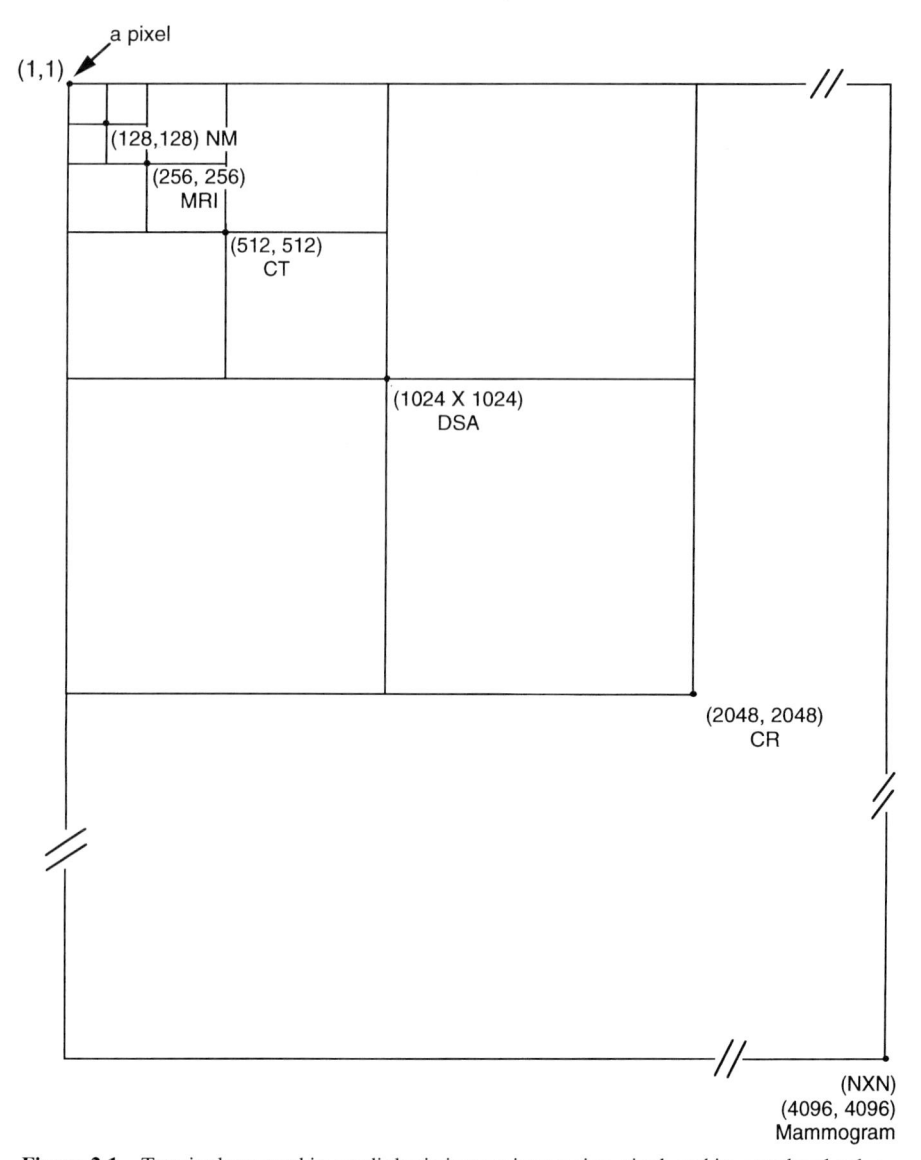

18   DIGITAL RADIOLOGIC FUNDAMENTALS OF IMAGING

Figure 2.1   Terminology used in a radiologic image: image size, pixel, and its gray level value.

Figure 2.2   Illustration of spatial and density resolutions using a lymphocyte image (L) as an example. The 16 levels are represented by: ●, 1, 2, 3, 4, 5, 6, 7, 8, 9, A, B, C, D, E, and F. (A) Fixed spatial resolution, variable density resolutions: 16, 4, and 2 gray levels. (B) Fixed density resolution (16 levels), variable spatial resolutions.

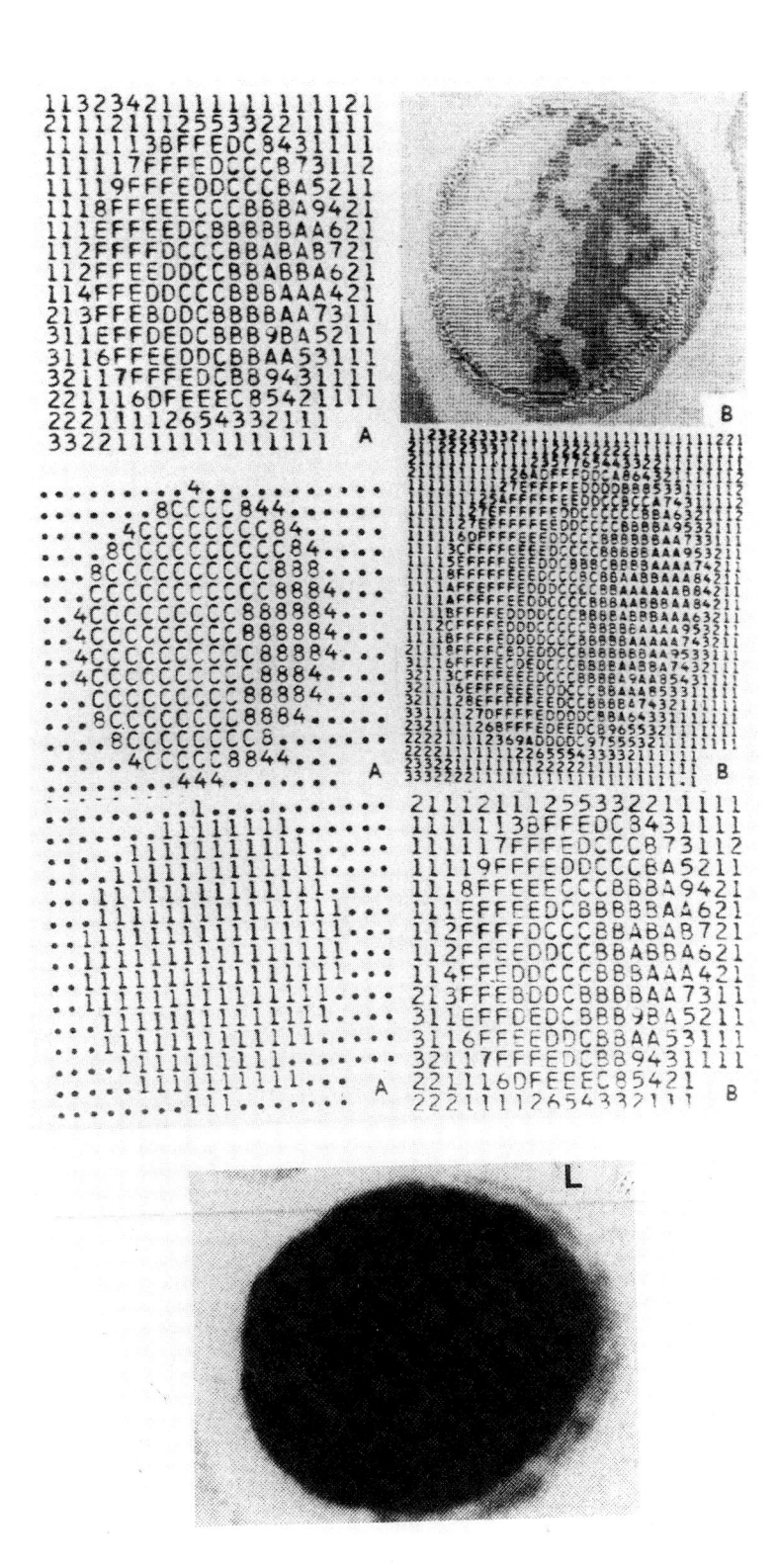

```
1132342111111111121
211121112553322111111
1111113BFFEDC8431111
111117FFFEDCCCB73112
11119FFFEDDCCCBA5211
1118FFEEECCCBBBA9421
111EFFFEEDCBBBBBAA621
112FFFFDCCCBBABAB721
112FFEEDDCCBBABBA621
114FFEDDCCCBBBAAA421
213FFEBDDCBBBBAA7311
311EFFFDEDCBBB9BA5211
3116FFEEDDCBBAA53111
32117FFFEDCB89431111
221116DFEEEC85421111
2221111126543332111   A
33221111111111111
```

```
. . . . . . . . . 4 . . . . . . . .
. . . . . . 8CCCC844 . . . . . . .
. . . . . 4CCCCCCCC84 . . . . . .
. . . . 8CCCCCCCCCC84 . . . . .
. . . 8CCCCCCCCCCC888 . . . . .
. . . CCCCCCCCCCC8884 . . . . .
. . 4CCCCCCCCCC888884 . . . .
. . 4CCCCCCCCCC888884 . . . .
. . 4CCCCCCCCCC888884 . . . .
. . 4CCCCCCCCCC88884 . . . .
. . . CCCCCCCCCC88884 . . . .
. . . 8CCCCCCCCC8884 . . . . .
. . . . 8CCCCCCCC8 . . . . . . .
. . . . 4CCCCC8844 . . . . .   A
. . . . . . .444. . . . . . . . .
```

B

```
8123223332111111111111121
111111234476543322111111
. . . 26AD FFFDC-AB6432111115
1111127EFFFEDDDDB88535111
. . 16AFFFFFEEDDCCBCCA74311112
1116DFFFFFEEDDCCCBBBBA9532111
1115EFFFFFEEDDCCCBBBBBAAA74311
1116FFFFFEEDCCCBBBBBBAAA9532111
1116FFFFFEEDCCCBBBBBAABBAA84211
111AFFFFFEDDDCCCCBBAAAAAB8421111
111BFFFFEDDDDCCCBBBBABBBAAA6321111
1112CFFFFEDDDCCCCBBBBBBEAAA49532111
112BFFFFEDDDDCCCBBBBBAAAA74321111
2118FFFFECBEDDCCBBBBBBBAA953211111
3216CFFFFEDCBBBBBBBAABBA7432111
3213CFFFFEDCCBBBBBBBA9AA8543111
3215EFFFFEEDCCCBBAAAAB85331111
3312BFFFEEDDCCBBA8743211111
331111270FFFEEDCBBA6433311111
2321111268FFFEDEEDC89655321111
2222111112369ADDDDC9955532111111
222211111122265554333321111111
22221111111122221111111111
3332222111111122221111111111
```

```
211121112553322111111
1111113BFFEDC8431111
111117FFFEDCCCB73112
11119FFFEDDCCCBA5211
1118FFEEECCCBBBA9421
111EFFFEEDCBBBBBAA621
112FFFFDCCCBBABAB721
112FFEEDDCCBBABBA621
114FFEDDCCCBBBAAA421
213FFEBDDCBBBBAA7311
311EFFFDEDCBBB9BA5211
3116FFEEDDCBBAA53111
32117FFFEDCB89431111
221116DFEEEC85421    B
2221111126543332111
```

```
. . . . . . . . . . . . . . . . . . . .
. . . . . . . . .1. . . . . . . . .
. . . . . . 11111111. . . . . . .
. . . . . 1111111111 . . . . . .
. . . 111111111111111 . . . . .
. . 1111111111111111 . . . . . .
. 11111111111111111 . . . . . .
. 111111111111111111 . . . . .
. 1111111111111111111 . . . .
. 1111111111111111111 . . . .
. .1111111111111111111 . . .
. 11111111111111111111 . . .
. . 111111111111111111 . . .
. . 1111111111111111 . . . .
. . 11111111111111 . . . .
. . . 1111111111 . . . . .
. . . . 111111111 . . . .  A
. . . . . .111. . . . . . .
```

L

column depicts the digital representation of the same analog image with a fixed density resolution (16) and variable spatial resolutions (from top to bottom: high, medium, low). Clearly, the digital image in the upper right-hand corner is the best representation of the original analog image, having the highest spatial and density resolutions. The image in the lower left-hand corner, which has the lowest spatial and density resolutions, is a binary image. For an example of an image with noise introduced, see Figure (12.12). Spatial resolution, density resolution, and signal-to-noise ratio of the image should be adjusted properly during image acquisition. A high resolution image requires a larger memory capacity for storage and longer time for image transmission and processing.

2.3 RADIOLOGIC TEST OBJECTS AND PATTERNS

Test objects or patterns (sometimes called phantoms), used to measure the density and spatial resolutions of radiologic imaging equipment, can be either physical phantoms or digitally generated patterns.

A physical phantom is used to measure the performance of a digital radiologic device. It is usually constructed with different materials shaped in various geometrical configurations that are then embedded in a uniform background material (e.g., water or plastic). The most commonly used geometrical configurations are circular cylinder, sphere, line pairs (alternating pattern of rectangular bar with background of the same width), step wedge, and star shape. Materials used to construct these configurations are lead, various plastics, air, and iodine solutions of various concentrations. The circular cylinder, sphere, and step-wedge configurations are commonly used to measure spatial and density resolutions. Thus, the statement that an X-ray device can detect a 1 mm cylindrical object with 0.5% density difference from the background means that this particular radiologic imaging device can produce an image of the cylindrical object made from material that has an X-ray attenuation difference from the background of 0.5%; thus the difference between the average gray level of the object and the average gray level of the background is measurable or detectable.

A digitally generated pattern, on the other hand, is used to measure the performance of the display component of a digital radiologic device. In this case, the various geometrical configurations are generated digitally. The gray level values of these configurations are input to the display component according to certain specifications. A digital phantom is an ideal digital image. Any distortion of these images observed from the display component is a measure of the imperfections of the display component. Figure 2.3 shows some commonly used physical phantoms, their corresponding X-ray images, and digitally generated patterns.

2.4 SPATIAL DOMAIN AND FREQUENCY DOMAIN

2.4.1 Frequency Components of an Image

If a digital radiologic image $f(x,y)$ is the gray level representation of anatomical structures in space, one can say that it is defined in the spatial domain. The image, $f(x,y)$, can also be represented as its spatial frequency components u,v through a mathematical transform (see next section). In this case, we use the symbol $F(u,v)$ to represent the transform of $f(x,y)$ and say that $F(u,v)$ is defined in the frequency domain. $F(u,v)$ is again a digital image, but it bears no visual resemblance to $f(x,y)$ (see Fig. 2.4). With proper training, however, one can use information appearing in the frequency domain, not easily visible in the spatial domain, to detect some inherent characteristics of each type of radiologic image.

The concept of using frequency components to represent anatomical structures might seem strange at first, and one might wonder why we even have to bother with this representation. To understand better, consider that a radiologic image is composed of many two-dimensional sinusoidal waves, each with individual amplitude and frequency. For example, a digitally generated "uniform image" has no frequency components, only a constant (dc) term. An X-ray image of the hand is composed of many high frequency components (edges of bones) and few low frequency components, while an abdominal X-ray image of the gall bladder filled with contrast material is composed of many low frequency components (the contrast medium inside the gall bladder) but very few high frequency components. Therefore, the frequency representation of a radiologic image gives a different perspective on the characteristics of the image under consideration.

Based on this frequency information in the image, we can selectively change the frequency components to enhance the image. To obtain a smoother appearing image, therefore, we can increase the amplitude of low frequency components, whereas to enhance the edges of bones in the hand X-ray image, we can magnify the amplitude of the high frequency components.

Manipulating an image in the frequency domain also yields many other advantages. If, for example, we can use the frequency representation of an image to measure its quality. We are led to the concepts of point spread function (PSF), line spread function (LSF), and modulation transfer function (MTF), to be discussed in Section 2.5.1. In addition, radiologic images obtained from image reconstruction principles are based on the frequency component representation. Utilization of frequency representation also gives an easier explanation of how an MRI image is formed. (This is discussed in Chapter 5.)

2.4.2 The Fourier Transform Pair

As discussed earlier, a radiologic image defined in the spatial domain (x,y) can be transformed to the frequency domain (u,v). The Fourier transform is one method for doing this. The Fourier transform of a two-dimensional image $f(x,y)$, denoted by $\mathcal{F}\{f(x,y)\}$, is given by:

$$\mathfrak{I}\{f(x,y)\} = F(u,v) = \int_{-\infty}^{\infty}\int f(x,y)\exp[-i2\pi(ux+vy)]dx\,dy$$
$$= \mathrm{Re}(u,v) + i\,\mathrm{Im}(u,v) \qquad (2.1)$$

where $i = \sqrt{-1}$, and $\mathrm{Re}(u,v)$ and $\mathrm{Im}(u,v)$ are the real and imaginary components, respectively, of $F(u,v)$.

A-1 A-2

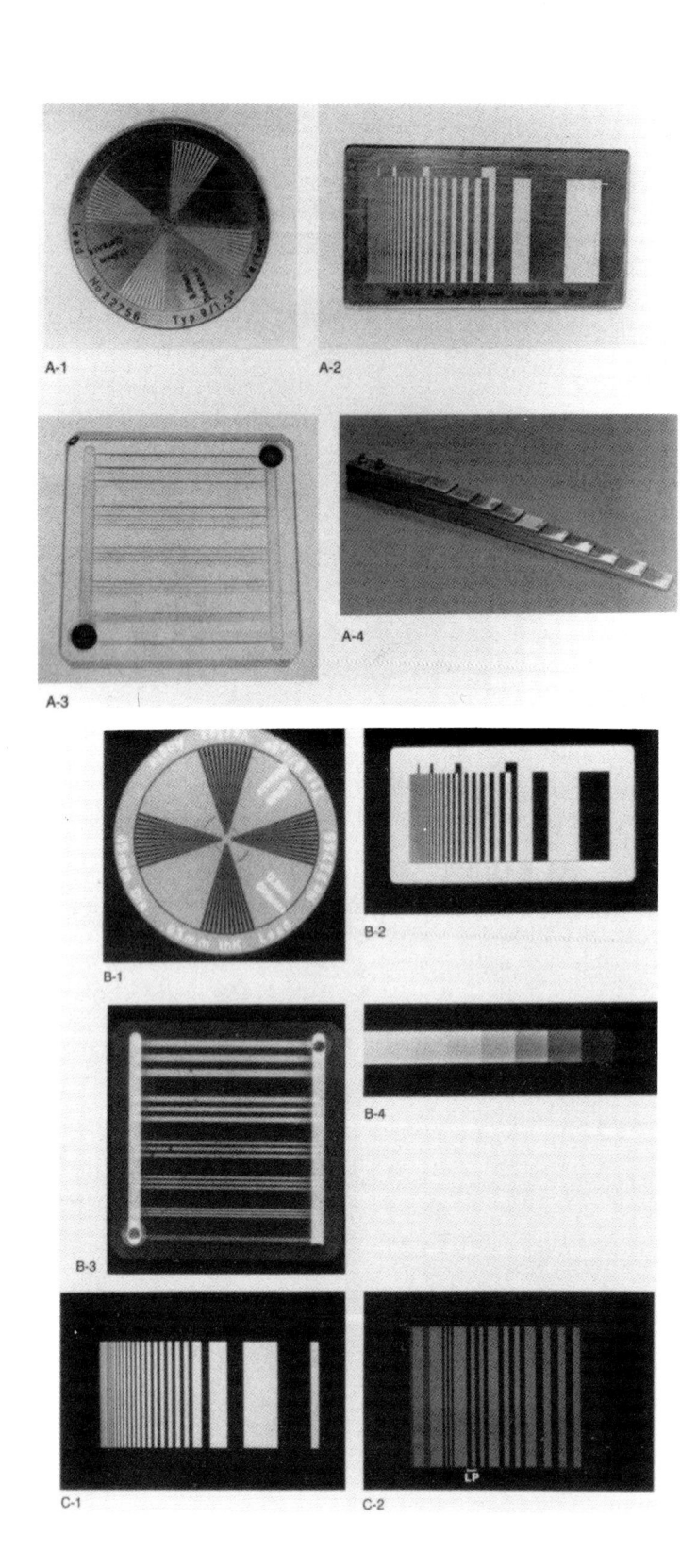

A-3 A-4

B-1 B-2

B-3 B-4

C-1 C-2

22

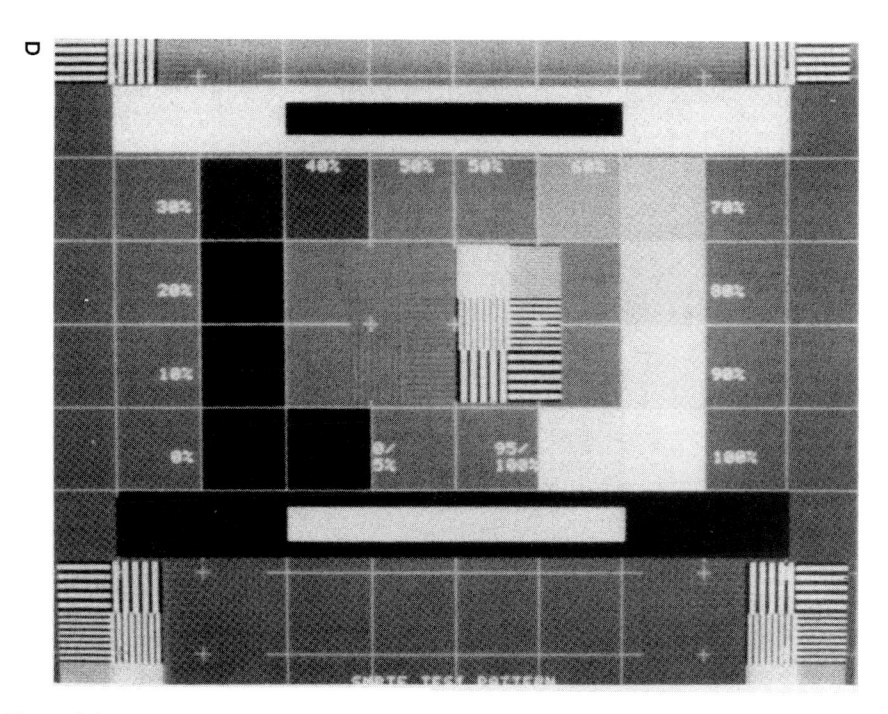

Figure 2.3 Some commonly used physical test objects and digitally generated test patterns. (A) Physical: A-1, star-shaped pattern embedded in water contained in a circular cylinder; A-2, high contrast line pair, A-3, low contrast line pair; A-4, step wedge. (B) Corresponding X-ray images. (C) Digitally generated 512 image: C-1, high contrast [gray level = 0, 140; width (in pixel) of each line pair = 2, 4, 6, 8, 10, 12, 14, 16, 32, 64, and 128 pixels]; C-2, low contrast line pair: [gray level = 0, 40; width (in pixel) of each line pair = 2, 4, 8, 16, 20 and 28 pixels]. The line pair (LP) indicated in the C-2 shows the width of 16 pixels. (D) SMPTE phantom (Society of Motion Picture and Television Engineers). (Courtesy of Dr. J. Gray.)

The magnitude function

$$|F(u,v)| = [Re^2\,(u,v) + Im^2\,(u,v)]^{1/2} \qquad (2.2)$$

is called the Fourier spectrum, and $|F(u,v)|^2$ the energy spectrum of $f(x,y)$, respectively. The function

$$\Phi(u,v) = \tan^{-1}\frac{Im(u,v)}{Re(u,v)} \qquad (2.3)$$

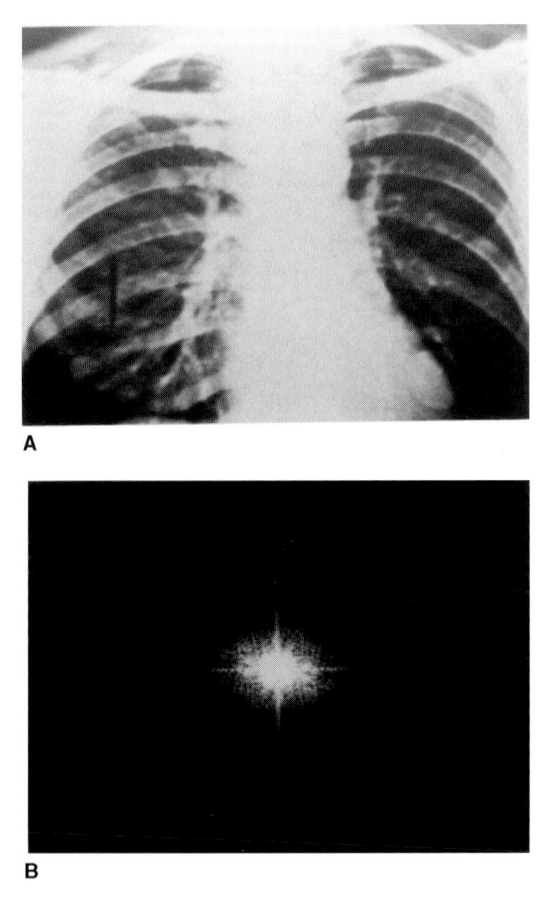

Figure 2.4 (A) A digital chest X-ray image represented in spatial domain. (B) The same digital chest X-ray image represented in the frequency domain. The low frequency components are in the center and the high frequency components are on the periphery.

is called the phase angle. The Fourier spectrum, the energy spectrum, and the phase angle are three parameters derived from the Fourier transform which can be used to represent the properties of an image in the frequency domain. Figure 2.4B shows the Fourier spectrum of the chest image in Figure 2.4A.

Given $F(u,v)$, $f(x,y)$ can be obtained by using the inverse Fourier transform

$$\mathfrak{I}^{-1}[F(u,v)] = f(x,y)$$
$$= \int_{-\infty}^{\infty}\int F(u,v)\exp[i2\pi(ux+vy)]du\ dv \qquad (2.4)$$

The two functions $f(x,y)$ and $F(u,v)$ are called the Fourier transform pair. The Fourier and the inverse transforms enable the transformation of a two-dimensional image from the spatial domain to the frequency domain, and vice versa. In digital imaging, we use the discrete Fourier transform for computation instead of using Eq. (2.1), which is continuous.

2.4.3 The Discrete Fourier Transform

The discrete Fourier transform is an approximation of the Fourier transform used to perform the transform on a digital image. For a square digital radiologic image, the integrals in the Fourier transform pair can be approximated by summations as follows:

$$F(u,v) = \frac{1}{N} \sum_{x=0}^{N-1} \sum_{y=0}^{N-1} f(x,y) \exp\left[\frac{-i\,2\pi(ux+vy)}{N}\right] \quad (2.5)$$

for $u, v = 0, 1, 2, \ldots, N-1$, and

$$f(x,y) = \frac{1}{N} \sum_{u=0}^{N-1} \sum_{v=0}^{N-1} F(u,v) \exp\left[\frac{-i\,2\pi(ux+vy)}{N}\right] \quad (2.6)$$

for $x, y = 0, 1, 2, \ldots, N-1$

The $f(x,y)$ and $F(u,v)$ shown in Eqs. (2.5) and (2.6) are called the discrete Fourier transform pair. It is apparent from these two equations that once the digital radiologic image $f(x,y)$ is known, its discrete Fourier transform can be computed with simple multiplication and addition, and vice verse.

2.5 MEASUREMENT OF IMAGE QUALITY

Image quality is a measure of the performance of an imaging system used for a specific radiologic examination. Although the process of making diagnoses from a radiologic image is often subjective, higher quality images provide better diagnostic information. We will describe some physical parameters for measuring image quality based on the concepts of density, spatial resolution, signal-to-noise level introduced earlier.

In general, the quality of an image can be measured from its sharpness and its noise level. Image unsharpness is inherited from the design of the instrumentation, while image noise arises from photon fluctuations from the energy source, and electronic noise is accumulated through the imaging chain. Even if there were no noise in the imaging system (a hypothetical case), the inherent optical properties of the imaging system used might well prevent the image of a line pair phantom from giving sharp edges between black and white areas. By the same token, if a perfect imaging system could be designed, the nature of random photon fluctuation would introduce noise into the image.

Sections 2.5.1 and 2.5.2 discuss the measurement of sharpness and noise. This treatment is based on the established theory of measuring image quality in diagnos-

26 DIGITAL RADIOLOGIC FUNDAMENTALS OF IMAGING

tic radiologic devices. Certain modifications are included to permit adjustment for digital imaging terminology.

2.5.1 Measurement of Sharpness

2.5.1.1 Point Spread Function (PSF)

Consider the following experiment. A small circular hole is drilled in the center of a lead plate, which is placed between an X-ray tube and an image receptor. An image of this plate is then obtained, which can be recorded by a film or by digital means and displayed on a TV monitor (see Fig. 2.5A). Upon measuring the gray level distribution of this image, we will see that the gray level (corresponding to the optical density) is comparatively high in the center of the image where the hole is located and decreases radially outward, becoming zero at a certain distance away from the center. Ideally, if the circular hole is small enough and the imaging system is a perfect system, we would expect to see a perfectly circular hole in the center of the image with identical gray level within the hole and zero everywhere outside. The size of the circle in the image would be equal to the size of the circular hole in the plate if no magnification was introduced during the experiment. However, in practice, such an ideal

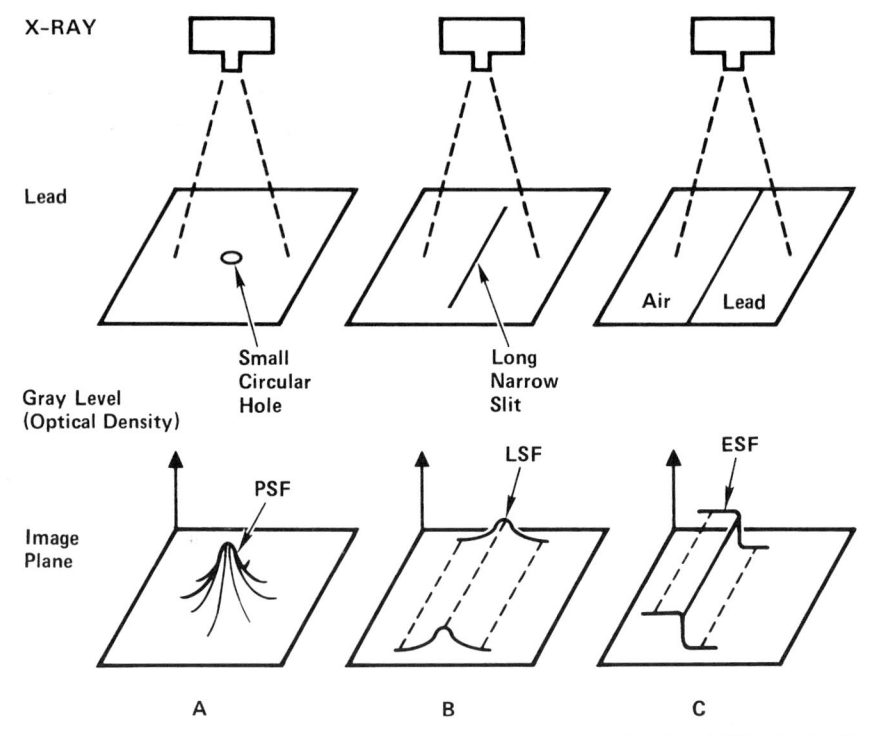

Figure 2.5 Experimental setup for defining (A) the point spread function (PSF), (B) the line spread function (LSF), and (C) the edge spread function (ESF).

image never exists. Instead, a distribution of the gray level, as described earlier, will be observed.

This experiment demonstrates that the image of a circular hole in the lead plate never has a well-defined sharp edge but has, instead, a certain *unsharpness*. If the circular hole is small enough, the shape of this gray level distribution is called the point spread function (PSF) of the imaging system (consisting of the X-ray source and the image receptor). The point spread function of the imaging system can be used as a measure of the unsharpness of an image produced by this imaging system. In practice, however, the point spread function of an imaging system is very difficult to measure. For the experiment described in Figure 2.5A, the size of the circular hole must be chosen very carefully. If the circular hole is too large, the picture formed in the detector becomes the image of the circular hole. On the other hand, if the circular hole is too small, the image formed becomes the image of the X-ray focal spot which does not represent the complete imaging system. In either case, the image cannot be used to measure the PSF of the imaging system.

Theoretically, the point spread function is a useful concept in estimating the sharpness of an image. Experimentally, the point spread function is difficult to measure because of constraints just noted. To circumvent this difficulty in determining the point spread function of an imaging system, the concept of the line spread function is introduced.

2.5.1.2 Line Spread Function (LSF)

Let us replace the circular hole with a long narrow slit in the lead plate and repeat the experiment. The image formed on the image receptor becomes a line of certain width with nonuniform gray level distribution. The gray level value is high in the center of the line, decreasing toward both sides until it assumes the gray level of the background. The shape of this gray level distribution is called the line spread function (LSF) of the imaging system. Theoretically, a line spread function can be considered as a line of continuous holes placed very close together. Experimentally, the line spread function is much easier to measure than the PSF. Figure 2.5B illustrates the concept of the line spread function of the system.

2.5.1.3 Edge Spread Function (ESF)

If the lead plate is replaced by a single step wedge such that half of the imaging area is lead and the other is air, then the gray level distribution of the image is the edge spread function (ESF) of the system. For an ideal imaging system, any trace perpendicular to the edge of this image would yield a step function

$$\begin{aligned} \text{ESF}(x) &= 0 \quad -B \leq x < x_0 \\ &= A \quad x_0 \leq x \leq B \end{aligned} \quad (2.7)$$

where x is the direction perpendicular to the edge, x_0 is the location of the edge, $-B$, and B are the left and right boundaries of the image, and A is a constant. Mathematically, the line spread function is the first derivative of the edge spread function given by the equation

$$\mathrm{LSF}(x) = \frac{d[\mathrm{ESF}(x)]}{dx} \qquad (2.8)$$

It should be observed that the edge spread function is easy to obtain experimentally, since only a sharp-edged lead plate is required to set up the experiment. Once the image has been obtained with the image receptor, a gray level trace perpendicular to the edge yields the edge spread function of the system. To compute the line spread function of the system, it is only necessary to take the first derivative of the edge spread function. Figure 2.5C depicts the experimental setup to obtain the edge spread function.

2.5.1.4 Modulation Transfer Function (MTF)

Let us now substitute for the lead plate a line pair phantom with different spatial frequencies, and repeat the preceding experiment. In the image receptor, an image of the line pair phantom will form. From this image, the output amplitude (or gray level) of each spatial frequency can be measured. The modulation transfer function (MTF) of the imaging system, along the line perpendicular to the line pairs, is defined as the ratio between the output amplitude and the input amplitude expressed as a function of spatial frequency

$$\mathrm{MTF}(u) = (\text{output amplitude} / \text{input amplitude})_u \qquad (2.9)$$

where u is the spatial frequency measured in the direction perpendicular to the line pairs. Mathematically, the MTF is the magnitude (see Eq. 2.2) of the Fourier transform of the line spread function of the system given by the following equation:

$$\mathrm{MTF}(u) = |\Im[\mathrm{LSF}(x)]| = \left| \int_{-\infty}^{\infty} [\mathrm{LSF}(x) \exp(-i2\pi xu)] dx \right| \qquad (2.10)$$

It is seen from Eq. (2.9) that the MTF measures the modulation of the amplitude (gray level) of the line pair pattern in the image. The amount of modulation determines the quality of the imaging system. The MTF of an imaging system, once known, can be used to predict the quality of the image produced by the imaging system. For a given frequency u, if $\mathrm{MTF}(v) = 0$ for all $v \geq u$, then the imaging system under consideration cannot resolve spatial frequency equal to or higher than u. The MTF so defined is a one-dimensional function; it measures the spatial resolution of the imaging system only in a certain direction. Extreme care must be exercised when the MTF is used to describe the spatial resolution of the system; the direction of the measurement must also be specified.

Notice that the MTF of a system is multiplicative; that is, if an image is obtained by an imaging system consisting of n components, each having its own MTF_i, then the total MTF of the imaging system is expressed by the following equation:

$$\text{MTF}(u) = \prod_{i=1}^{n} \text{MTF}_i(u) \tag{2.11}$$

where Π is the multiplication symbol. It is obvious that a low $\text{MTF}_i(u)$ value in any given component i will yield an overall low $\text{MTF}(u)$ of the complete system.

2.5.1.5 Relationship Between ESF, LSF, and MTF

The MTF obtained as described in Section 2.5.1.4 is sometimes called the high contrast response of the imaging system, because the line pair pattern or the edge source used is a high contrast phantom. By "high contrast" we mean that the object (lead) and the background (air) offers high radiographic contrast. On the other hand, MTF obtained with a low contrast phantom constitutes the low contrast response of the system. The MTF value obtained with a high contrast phantom is always larger than that obtained with a lower contrast phantom for a given spatial frequency.

With this background, we are ready to describe the relationship between the edge spread function, the line spread function, and the modulation transfer function. Let us set up an experiment to obtain the MTF of a digital imaging system composed of a light table, a television camera, and a digital chain that converts the video signals into digital signals and forms the digital image. The experimental steps are as follows:

1. Cover half the light table with a sharp-edged, black-painted metal sheet. Such an object is called an *edge source*.
2. Obtain a digital image of this edge source with the imaging system, as shown in Figure 2.6A. Then the ESF(x) has a gray level distribution (as shown in Fig. 2.6B arrows), which is obtained by taking the average value of several lines (a—a) perpendicular to the edges. Observe the noise characteristic of the ESF(x) in the figure.
3. The line spread function (LSF) of the system can be obtained by taking the first derivative numerically from the edge spread function (ESF) (Eq. 2.8), which is indicated by the arrows shown in Fig. 2.6B. The resulting LSF is depicted in Fig. 2.6C.
4. To obtain the MTF of the system in the direction perpendicular to the edge, a 1-D Fourier transform (Eq. 2.10) is applied to the line spread function shown in Fig. 2.6C. The magnitude of this 1-D Fourier transform is then the MTF of the imaging system in the direction perpendicular to the edge. The result is shown in Fig. 2.6D.

This completes the experiment to obtain the MTF from the ESF and the LSF. In practice, we can take 10% of the MTF values as the minimum resolving power of the imaging system. In this case, the MTF of this imaging system is about 1.0 cycle/mm.

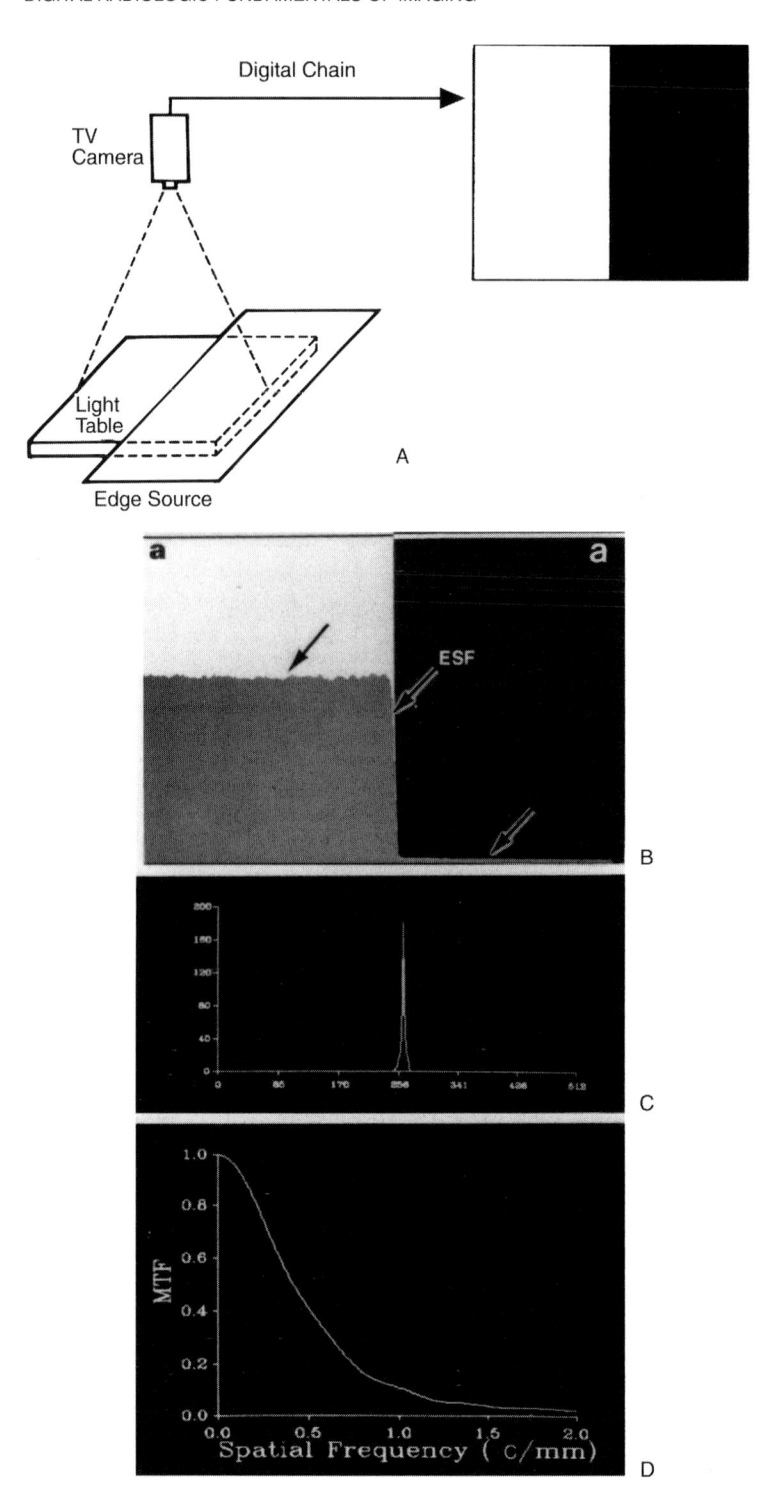

30 DIGITAL RADIOLOGIC FUNDAMENTALS OF IMAGING

2.5.1.6 Relationship Between the Input Image, the MTF, and the Output Image

Let $A = 1$, $B = \pi$, and $x_0 = 0$, and extend the edge spread function described in Eq. (2.7) to a periodic function with period 2π (Fig. 2.7A). This periodic function can be expressed as a Fourier series representation, or more explicitly, a sum of infinitely many sinusoidal functions, as follows:

$$\text{ESF}(x) = \frac{1}{2} + \frac{2}{\pi}\left[\sin + \frac{(\sin 3x)}{3} + \frac{(\sin 5x)}{5} + \frac{(\sin 7x)}{7} + \ldots\right] \quad (2.12)$$

The first term in this Fourier series, 1/2, is the dc- term. Subsequent terms are sinusoidal, and each is characterized by an amplitude and a frequency.

If the partial sum of Eq. (2.12) is plotted, it is apparent that the partial sum will approximate the periodic step function more closely as the number of terms increases (Fig. 2.7B). We can also plot the amplitude spectrum or the spatial frequency spectrum shown in Figure 2.7.C, which is a plot of the amplitude against the spatial frequency (Eq. 2.12). From this plot we can observe that the periodic step function ESF(x) can be decomposed into infinite components, each of which has an amplitude and frequency. To reproduce this periodic function ESF(x) exactly, it is necessary to include all the components. If some of the components are missing or have diminished amplitude values, the result is a diffused edge. A major concern in the design of an imaging system is ensure that there are no missing components or diminished amplitudes.

The MTF of a system can be used to predict the missing or modulated amplitudes. Consider the lateral view image of a plastic circular cylinder taken with a perfect X-ray imaging system. Figure 2.8A shows the optical density trace perpendicular to the edges of the circular cylinder in the image. How will this trace look if the X-ray image is digitized by the video camera digital system described in Section 2.5.1.5?

To answer this question, we first take the Fourier transform of this perfect trace, which gives its spatial frequency spectrum (Fig. 2.8B). If this frequency spectrum is multiplied by the MTF of the imaging system shown in Figure 2.6D, frequency by frequency, the result is the output frequency response of the trace (Fig. 2.8D) obtained with this digital imaging system. It is seen from Figures 2.8.B and 2.8.D that there is no phase shift; that is, all the zero crossings are identical between the input and the output spectra. The output frequency spectrum has been modulated to compensate for the imperfection of the video camera digital imaging system. Figure 2.8.E shows the expected trace. Figure 2.8F is the superposition of the perfect and the expected trace. It is seen that both corners in the expected trace (arrows) lose their sharpness.

Figure 2.6 Relationship between the ESF, the LSF, and the MTF. (A) Experimental setup. The imaging chain consists of a light table, a TV camera, and a digital chain. The object under consideration is a one-step wedge. (B) The ESF (arrows) by averaging several lines through a—a. (C) The LSF. (D) The MTF.

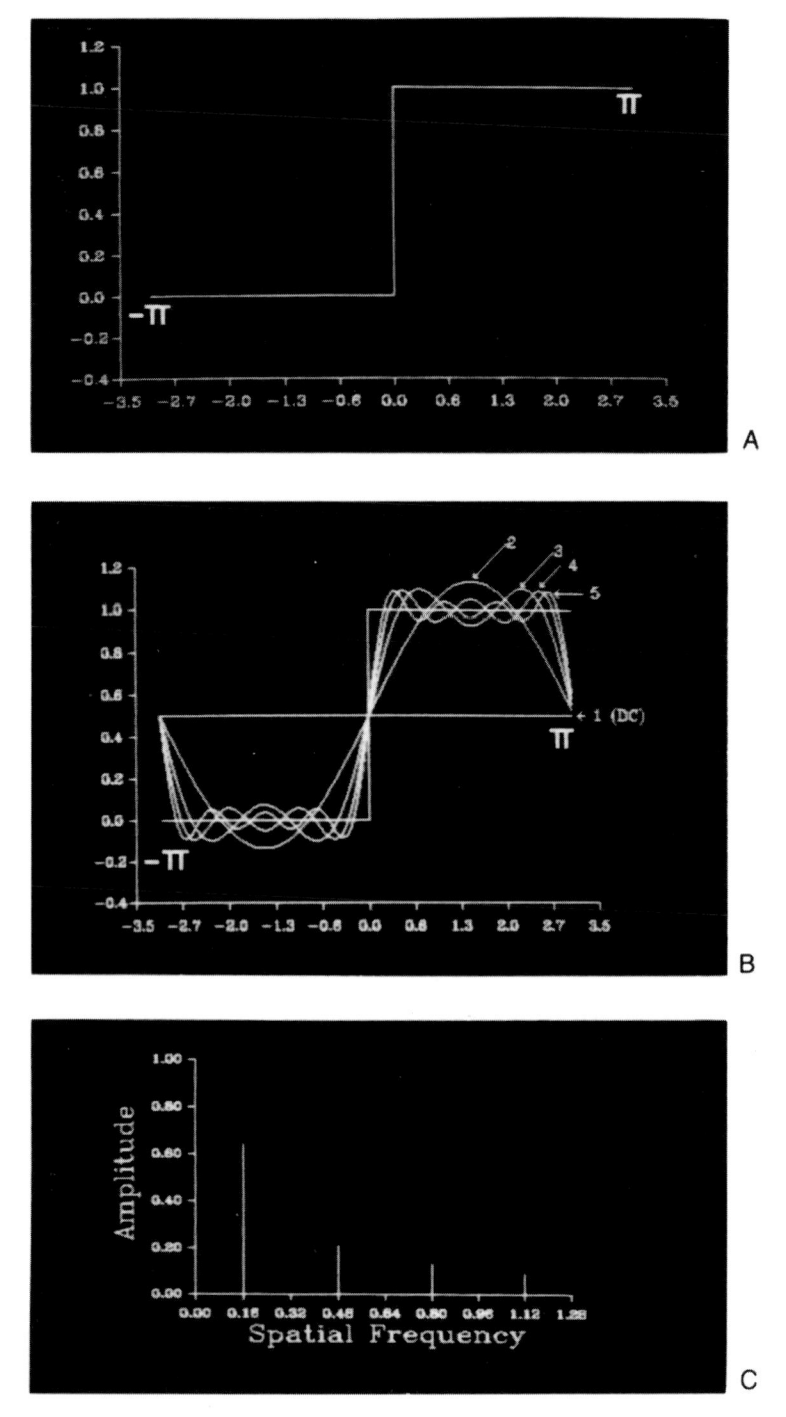

Figure 2.7 Sinusodial functions representation of an edge spread function. (A) The edge step function. (B) Partial sums of sinusodial functions, numerals correspond to the terms, described in Eq. (2.12). (C) Amplitude spectrum of the step function.

This completes the description of how the concepts of point spread function, line spread function, edge spread function, and modulation transfer function can be used to measure the unsharpness of an image. The concept of using the MTF to predict the unsharpness due to an imperfect system has also been introduced.

2.5.2 Measurement of Noise

MTF is often used as a measure of the quality of the imaging system. By definition, it is a measure of certain optical characteristics of an imaging system; namely, the ability to reproduce fine details. It provides no information regarding the effect of noise on the radiological contrast on the image. Since both unsharpness and noise can affect the image quality, an imaging system with large MTF values at high frequencies does not necessarily produce a high quality image if the noise level is high. Figure 2.9A shows a chest radiograph, and Figure 2.9B shows the same radiograph with random noise added. Upon comparing these two figures, it is clearly seen that noise degrades the quality of an image. The study of the noise that arises from quantum statistics, electronic noise, and film grain represents another measure of image quality. To study the noise, we need the concept of the power spectrum, or Wiener spectrum, of noise produced by an imaging system. Let us make the assumption that all the noise N is random in nature and does not correlate with the signals S that form the image. Then the signal-to-noise power ratio spectrum, or the signal-to-noise power ratio $P(x,y)$, of each pixel is defined by

$$P(x,y) = \frac{S^2(x,y)}{N^2(x,y)} \qquad (2.13)$$

Figure 2.10 illustrates signal and the associated random noise in a line trace on a uniform background image.

A high signal-to-noise ratio (SNR) means that the image is less noisy. A common method increasing the SNR (i.e., reducing the noise in the image) is to obtain many images of the same object under the same conditions and average them. This, in a sense, minimizes the contribution of the random noise to the image. If M images are averaged, the average signal-to-noise power ratio $P(x,y)$ becomes

$$\overline{P}(x,y) = \frac{M^2 S^2(x,y)}{M N^2(x,y)} = M\, P(x,y) \qquad (2.14)$$

The signal-to-noise ratio is the square root of the power ratio

$$SNR(x,y) = \sqrt{\overline{P}(x,y)} = \sqrt{M}\,\sqrt{P(x,y)} \qquad (2.15)$$

Therefore, the signal-to-noise ratio increases by the square root of the number of images averaged.

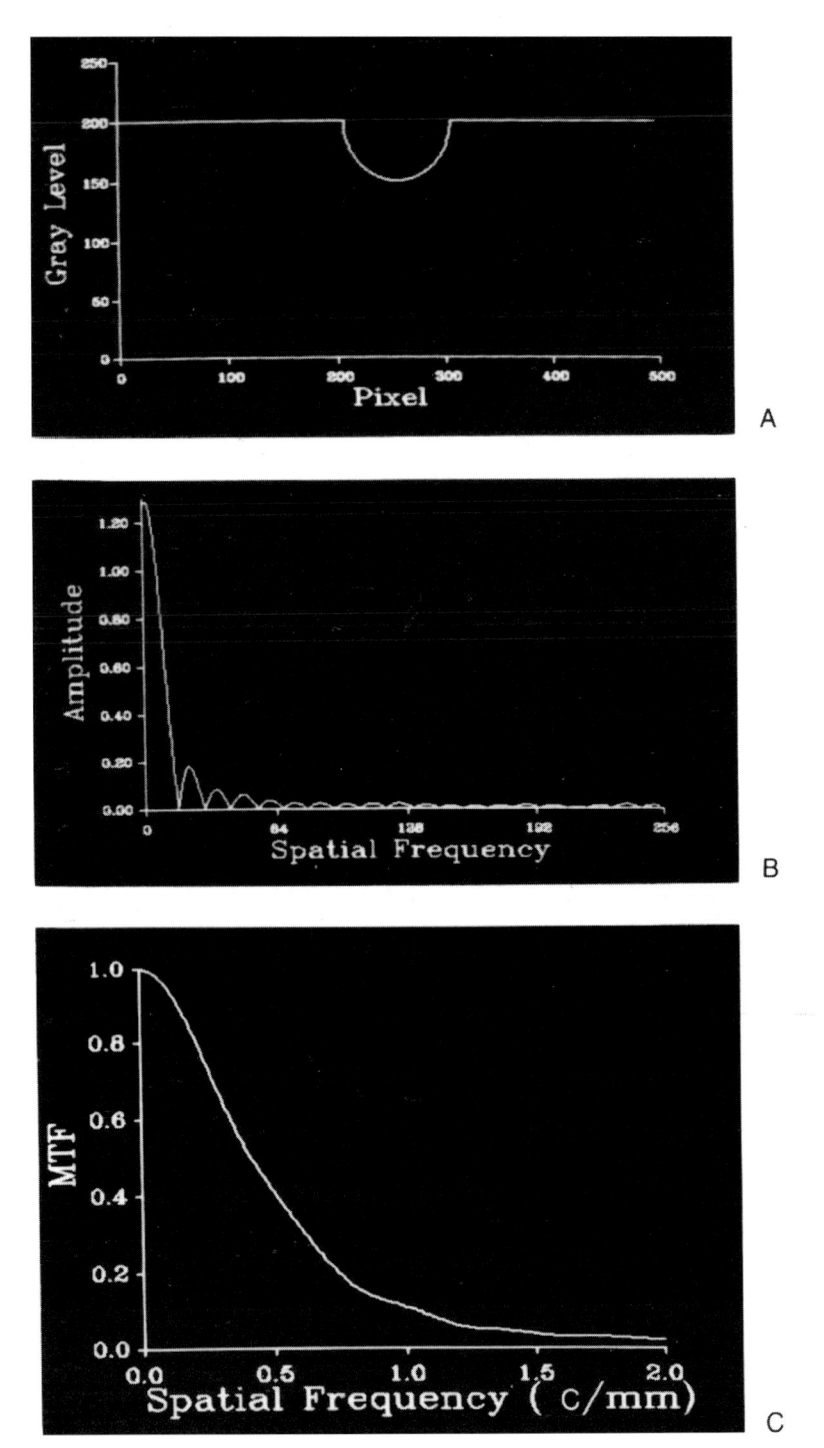

Figure 2.8 Relationship between the input, the MTF, and the output. (A) A line profile from a lateral view of a circular cylinder from a perfect imaging system. (B) The spatial frequency spectrum of A. (C) MTF of the imaging system described in Figure 2.6D. (D) The output fre-

quency response (B × C). (E) The predicted line trace from the imperfect imaging system obtained by an inverse Fourier transform of D. (F) Superposition of A and E showing the rounding of the edges (arrows) due to the imperfect imaging system.

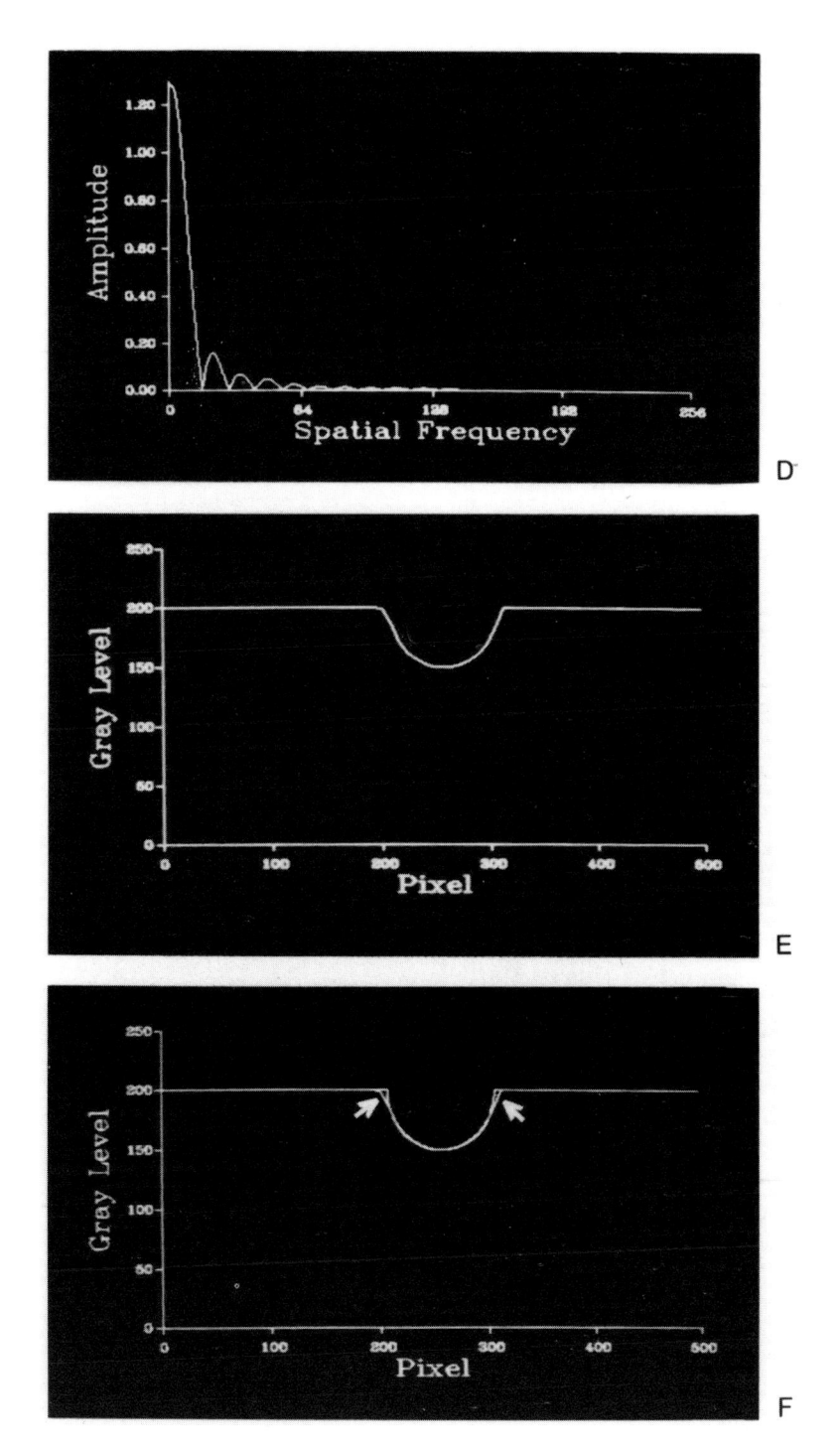

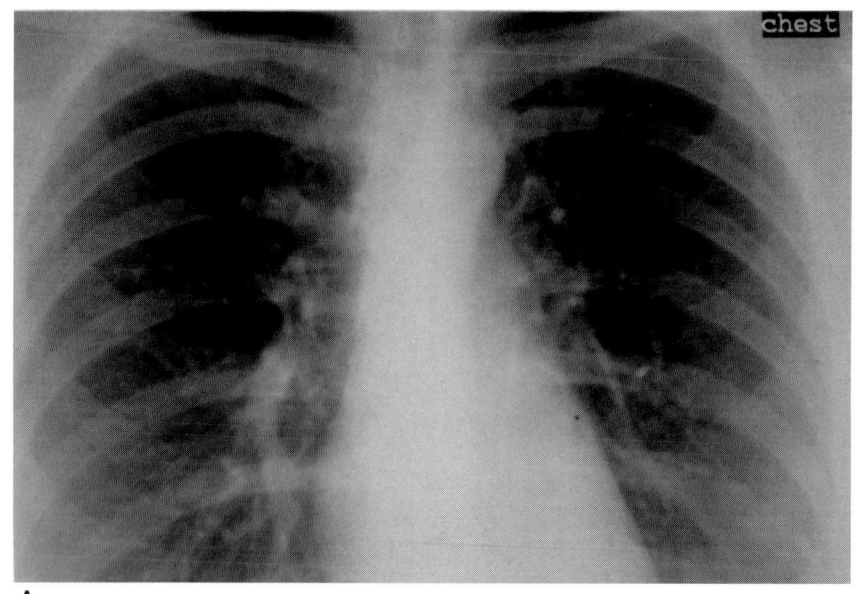

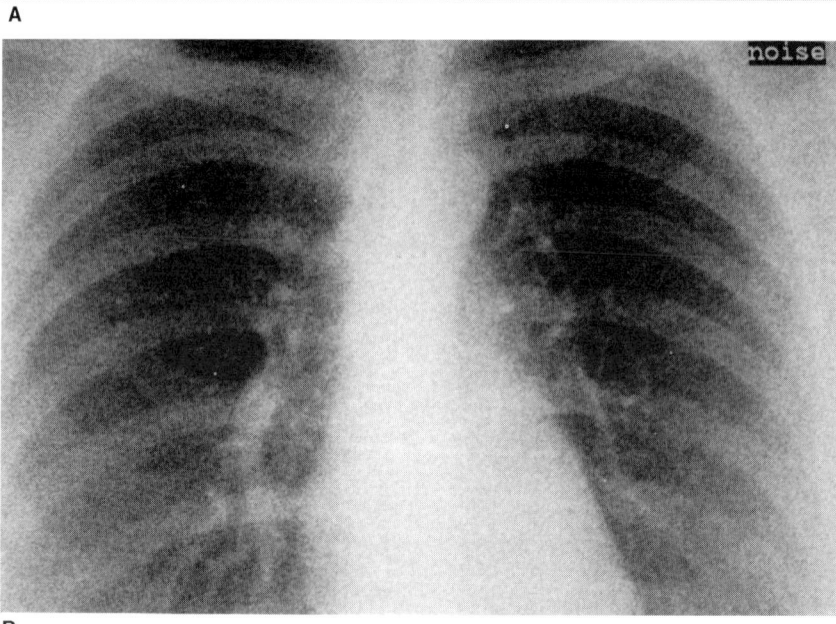

Figure 2.9 (A) A chest radiograph. (B) The same radiograph with random noise added. (Courtesy of K. S. Chuang.)

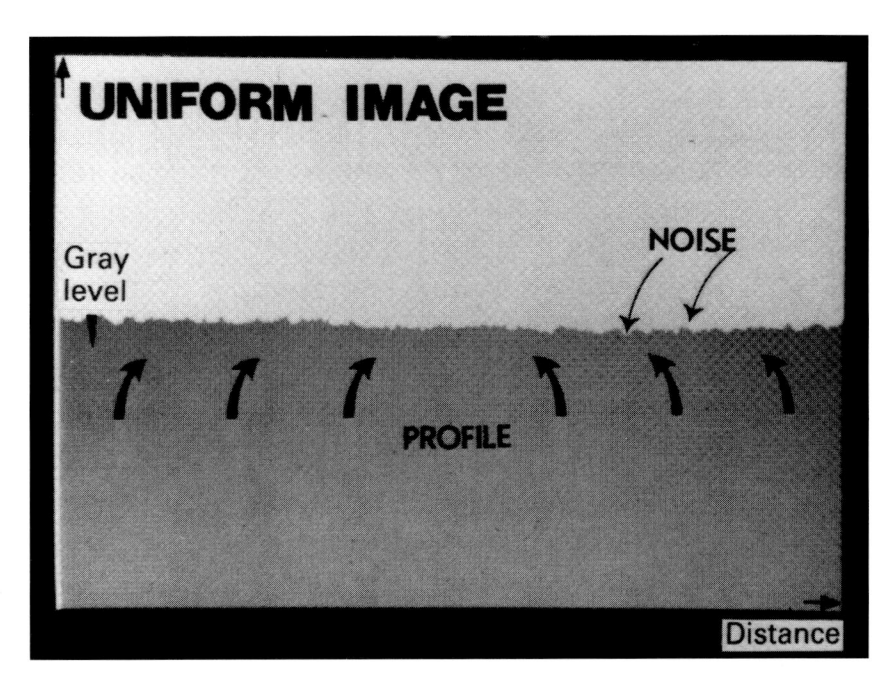

Figure 2.10 Example demonstrating the signal and the noise in a line trace on a uniform background image (white). The small variation along the profile is the noise. If there had been no noise, the line trace would be a straight line.

Equation (2.15) indicates that it is possible to increase the signal-to-noise ratio of the image by this averaging technique. The average image will have less random noise and a smoother visual appearance. For each pixel, the noise $N(x,y)$ defined in Eq. (2.13) can be approximated by using the standard deviation between the average image and the image under consideration.

Figure 2.11 illustrates how the signal-to-noise ratio of the imaging system is computed. Take a chest X-ray image, digitize it with an imaging system M times, and average the results pixel by pixel. If we assume the average image $f(x,y)$ is the signal (Fig. 2.11B), and the noise of each pixel (x,y) can be approximated by the standard deviation between f_i and f where f_i is a digitized image, and $1 \leq i \leq M$, then the signal-to-noise ratio for each pixel can be computed by using Eqs. (2.13) and (2.15). Figure 2.11 shows a digitized image $f_i(x,y)$, the average image $f(x,y)$ with $M = 16$, and the difference image between $f_i(x,y)$ and $f(x,y)$. The difference image shows a faint image of the chest, demonstrating that the noise in the imaging system is not random.

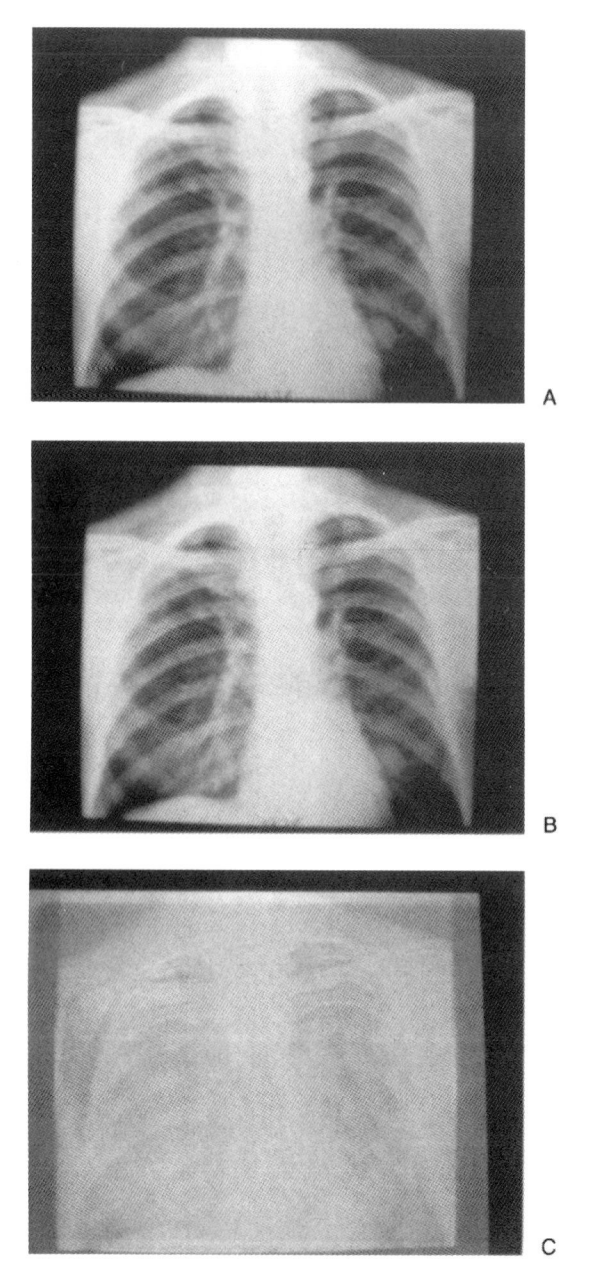

Figure 2.11 The difference between a digitized X-ray chest image before and after it has been averaged. (A) Chest X-ray film digitized with a video camera. (B) Digital image of the same chest X-ray film digitized 16 times and then averaged. (C) Image B subtracted from image A.

CHAPTER 3
Projection Radiography

3.1 PRINCIPLES OF CONVENTIONAL PROJECTION RADIOGRAPHY

Conventional projection radiography accounts for 70% of the total number of diagnostic imaging procedures. Therefore, to transform radiology from a film-based to a digital-based operation, we must understand conventional projection radiographic procedures and methods of digitizing radiographic films. This chapter discusses these two topics.

3.1.1 Some Standard Procedures Used in Conventional Projection Radiography

Conventional X-ray imaging procedures are used in all subspecialties of a radiology department, including neuroimaging, emergency, pediatric, breast imaging, chest, genitourinary, gastrointestinal, cardiovascular, and musculoskeletal. Although the detailed procedures differ within each subspecialty, the basic procedures can be summarized as follows:

0. Transfer patient-related information from the hospital information system (HIS), and radiology information system (RIS) to the X-ray procedure room before the arrival of the patient.
1. Check patient X-ray requisition for anatomical area of interest for imaging.
2. Place patient in position, standing up or on tabletop, for X-ray examination, and adjust the X-ray collimator for the size of the exposed area, or the field size.
3. Select a proper film screen cassette.
4. Place cassette in the holder located behind or on the table (under the patient).
5. Determine X-ray exposure factors for obtaining the best quality image with minimum exposure.
6. Turn on the X-rays to obtain a latent image of the patient on the film/screen cassette.
7. Process the exposed film through a film processor.
8. Retrieve the developed film from the film processor.
9. Inspect the radiograph through a light box for proper exposure or other errors (e.g., patient positioning, or movement).

10. Repeat steps 3–9 if the image on the film is unacceptable for diagnosis. Always keep in mind that the patient should not be subjected to unnecessary additional exposure.
11. Submit the film to a radiologist for approval.
12. Remove the patient from the table after the radiologist has determined that the quality of the radiograph is acceptable for diagnosis.
13. Release the patient.

Figure 3.1 shows a standard setup of a conventional radiographic procedure room and a diagnostic area. The numbers in the figure correspond to the preceding steps for a tabletop examination.

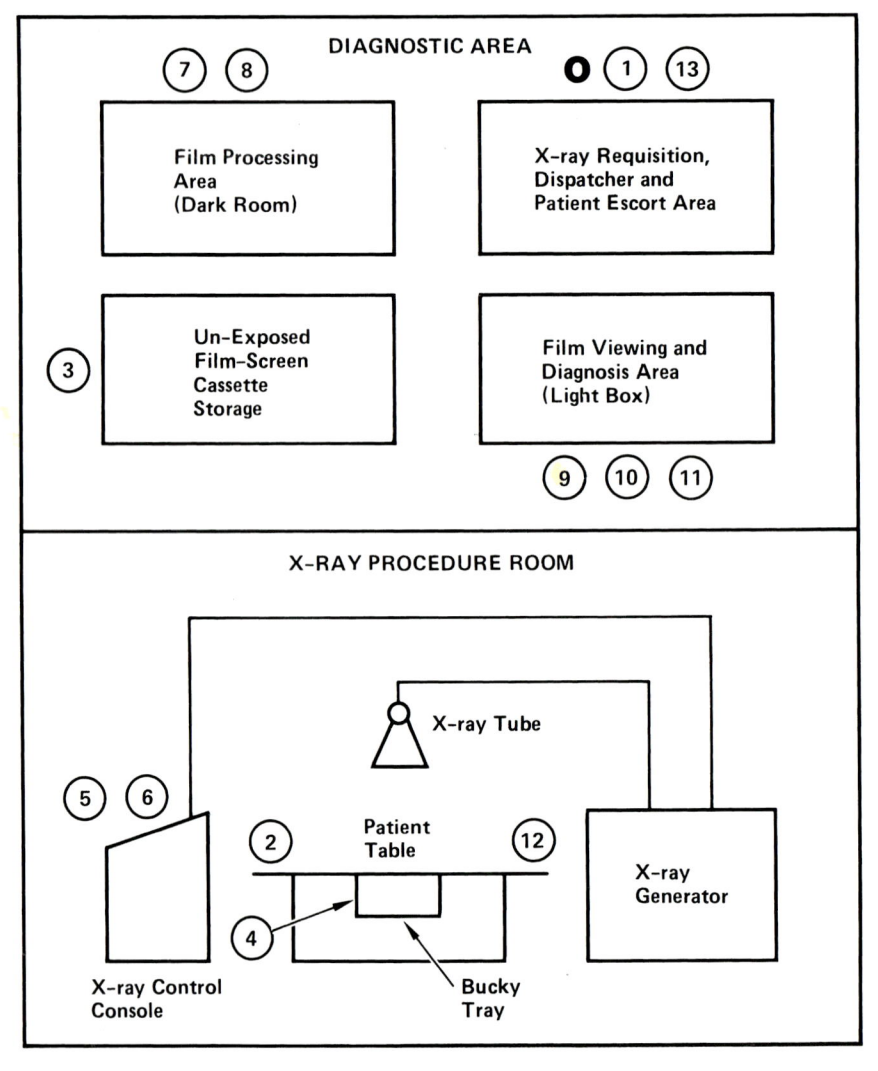

Figure 3.1 Standard setup of a radiographic procedure and diagnostic area.

3.1.1.1 The Effect of kVp, mA, and mAs Settings on the Appearance of a Radiograph

The radiographic image consists of structural patterns of various shades of gray. The degree of difference in shades of gray between selected areas on the images is referred to as the image contrast. Image contrast is a function of the following parameters:

- subject contrast
- film contrast
- X-ray scatter
- film fog level

Subject contrast is defined as the relative difference in X-ray intensity after transmission through anatomical structures and objects. It is affected by the inherent physical properties of the object under consideration: for example, effective atomic number, density, and object thickness. Subject contrast is also affected by extrinsic conditions—kVp, mA, and mAs of the X-ray settings—controllable during the examination procedure.

This section discusses these extrinsic conditions and their effect on the appearance of a radiographic image. The properties of film contrast and fog level, the characteristic curve of an X-ray film, and the effects of X-ray scatter are discussed in subsequent sections.

Before we consider the X-ray transmitted through an object, let us review the effects of kVp, mA, and mAs on the X-ray fluence (number of photons/unit area) incident on the surface of the object. X-ray fluence can be broken down into two components: the quantity (intensity of number) of X-ray photons and the quality (energy spectrum) of the X-ray photons. The quantity of the X-ray fluence incident on the subject is approximately proportional to:

- the square of the X-ray tube kilovolt potential difference $(kVp)^2$
- the X-ray tube current, in milliamperes
- the corresponding X-ray exposure time, in seconds

Subject contrast results when the fraction of photons absorbed in one area of the object is different from that absorbed in adjacent areas. The fraction of photons absorbed is called the absorption coefficient A and is a function of two variables, the property of the material with which the photons interact and the energies of the interacting photons. Thus we write

$$A = (Z, E) \tag{3.1}$$

where Z is the atomic number of the material and E is the X-ray photon energy.

For example, the absorption coefficients of bone and soft tissue plotted as a function of energy diverge at lower X-ray energies and then converge at higher energies. This pattern implies that a radiograph at a lower kVp will have a greater contrast between the bone and soft tissue than a radiograph of the same area acquired at a higher kVp. In general, a low kVp technique will produce a higher contrast image and a high kVp technique will produce a lower contrast image. However, most photons from an exposure taken at a low energy setting (low kVp) will be absorbed by the patient, hence will not penetrate through the patient. As a result, they cannot contribute to the formation of the image.

The tube current (mA), the time of exposure (s), or the product of the two, milliampere-seconds (mAs) contribute to the number of photons entering and leaving the patient. Therefore these are the factors determining the degree of darkness on the film. A low mAs setting may not have enough X-ray photons to form a good image (underexposed), and a high mAs setting may overexpose the film. If we increase the mAs in a procedure, an increased number of X-ray photons will reach the film screen. This will result in an increase in the exposure to this film, causing a darker appearance of the image. Thus, the darkening of the film is affected by both the kVp and the mAs.

3.1.1.2 Methods of Reducing X-Ray Scatter

So far the discussion of radiographic image contrast has been oversimplified because scattered radiation has not been considered. When X-ray photons travel through the patient, they are scattered, and the result is a radiograph with relatively low image contrast. Scattered X-ray photons tend to blur an image, since the actual location of the photon is misrepresented. For example, in chest radiography, the contribution to the film exposure from scattered X-ray photons can be equal to or greater than from the primary photons.

Scattered radiation is a primary cause of poor image quality in radiology. Methods of removing scattered X-rays generally result in increased patient exposure. Factors affecting the amount of scatter include kVp setting, patient thickness, and X-ray field size, which can be defined as follows:

1. *kVp setting:* the amount of scattered photons contributing to the image is a function of kVp because: (a) higher kVp results in greater percentage of Compton scatter interaction versus photoelectric interaction, the latter contributes to the formation of an image; and (b) higher energy photons undergoing Compton scatter tend to scatter more in the forward direction (onto the image receptor or film/screen), blurring the image.
2. *Patient thickness:* an increase in patient thickness increases the probability of Compton interaction before the photon can exit the patient.
3. *Field size:* the larger the X-ray field size (collimation), the greater the amount of scatter will be (plateau reached at approximately 30 cm × 30 cm field). The X-ray field size is an important factor for controlling scatter radiation. Smaller field sizes have the advantage of reducing patient dose.

There are several methods of minimizing the scattered photon contribution to the image; among these are the use of an air gap between the patient and the X-ray detector, and an external device called the radiographic grid, invented by Gustave Bucky in 1913. The radiographic grid is still the most effective way to minimize scatter. The physical device consists of lead foil strips separated by X-ray transparent spacers. The lead absorbs the scattered X-ray photons, thus improving the image quality.

Several parameters are used to characterize a radiographic grid: the grid ratio, the focal range, the number of lines per millimeter, and the mass of lead per unit area. The grid ratio is defined as the ratio of the height of the lead strips to the distance between them. An increase in this ratio decreases the amount of scattered photons reaching the film/screen cassette, hence increases the image contrast.

The focal range is the range of distances between the X-ray focal spot and the grid, at which point the divergence of the X-ray beam matches the lead strip divergence. Using the grid outside the recommended focal range results in fewer primary photons reaching the film/screen cassette. A higher value on lines/per millimeter and/or mass of lead/per area in the grid reduces the amount of scatter, but at the same time, the procedure will require a higher exposure. The radiographic grid reduces X-ray scatter and improves the image quality; on the other hand, it creates some potential problems during digitization because of the grid lines on the image. We will discuss this situation later in this chapter.

3.1.2 Image Receptor

3.1.2.1 Screen/Film Combination

The X-ray photons exiting the patient carry with them the information needed to form an image; the problem is that they cannot be visualized by human eyes. Rather, this information must be converted into a latent image, which in turn can be transformed into a visual image.

The common image receptor or detector used in diagnostic radiology is the film/screen combination consisting of a double-emulsion, radiation-sensitive film between two intensifying screens housed inside a lighttight cassette (Fig. 3.2) The X-ray film incorporates silver halide crystals suspended in a gelatin medium; its transparent (polyethylene terephthalate) plastic substrate, called the base, is coated on both sides by this emulsion. A slight blue tint is commonly incorporated in the base to give the radiograph a pleasing appearance. A photographic emulsion can be exposed to X-rays directly, but it is more sensitive to light photons of much less energy (~ 2.5–5 eV).

The intensifying screen, which is made of a thin phosphor layer (e.g., crystalline calcium tungstate), is more sensitive to the diagnostic X-ray energy (20–90 keV). The X-ray photons exiting the patient impinge onto such an intensifying screen, causing it to emit visible light photons that can be collected to form a visible image. X-ray photons that are not absorbed by the front screen in the cassette can be absorbed by the back screen. The light emitted from this second screen then exposes the emulsion on the back side of the film. The use of double-emulsion film thus can effectively reduce the patient exposure by half. With the film/screen as the image detector, the patient receives much lower exposure than is the case when film alone is used. Image blur due to patient motion can also be minimized when exposure times are shorter.

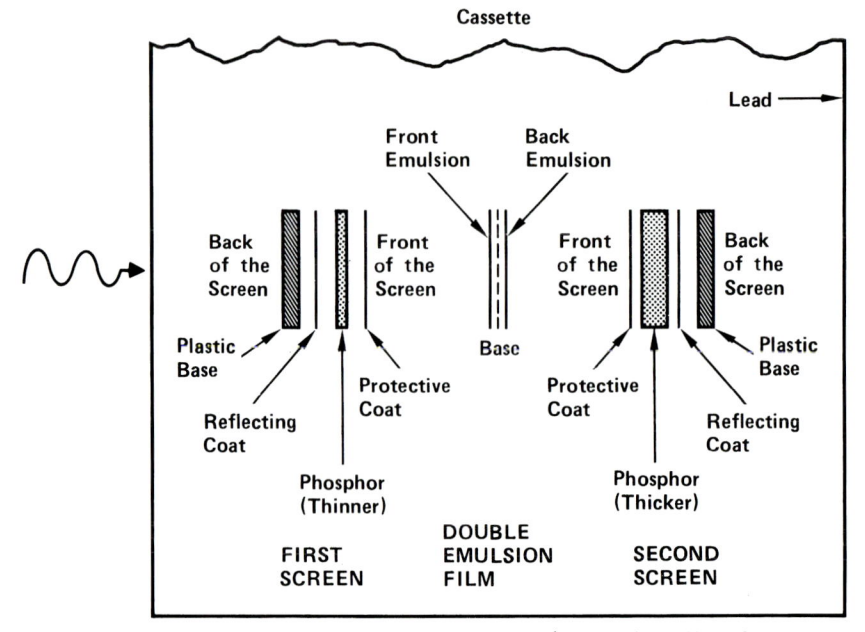

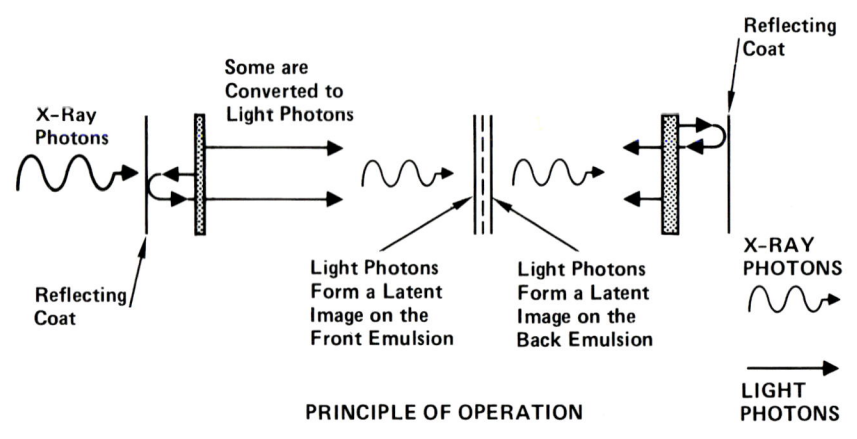

Figure 3.2 Schematic of a film/screen cassette and the formation of a latent image on the film. (Distances between screen, film, base material, and screen are used for illustrative purposes; the components are actually in contact with each other.)

Calcium tungstate phosphor was used in most screens until about 1971. New technology with rare earth phosphors has resulted in a more sensitive screen. Figure 3.2 presents a sectional view of the film/screen detector as well as its interaction with X-ray photons.

Formation of Latent Image The formation of the latent image on the film, called the *photographic effect,* is not well understood even now. The Gurney–Mott theory, summarized here, is an accepted, though incomplete, explanation of the latent image formation, which remains a topic of research.

The visible light photon output from the intensifying screen is absorbed by the photographic emulsion primarily by the photoelectric interaction of light photons with atoms of the silver halide crystals. These crystals consist of silver (Ag^+), bromine (Br)$^-$, and iodine (I)$^-$ ions, with about 90–99% silver bromide and 10–1% silver iodide suspended in the emulsion. Each crystal (grain) is about 1–2 μm in size. When X-ray film is exposed to light photons, electrons from the bromide ion are given enough energy to escape the ion. The free electrons move through the crystal and are trapped in one of the crystal defects, which are called *sensitivity specks.* The crystal has other defects, called *point defects,* which are responsible for photographic sensitivity. Point defects consist of silver ions that migrate through the crystal. When one silver ion mates with an electron in a sensitivity speck, the ion becomes a neutralized metallic silver atom.

$$Ag^+ + e^- \rightarrow Ag \qquad (3.2)$$

This process can be repeated in another crystal, in the same crystal within the same sensitivity speck, or in a different speck. More than one silver atom can exist within a sensitivity speck. A sensitivity speck is called a *latent image center* if it contains at least two silver atoms. Any crystal in the emulsion can have more than one latent image center, and this process of latent image formation can occur in any crystal in the emulsion. Once the latent image has formed on the exposed film, we need to develop the film to form a visible image.

Development of X-Ray Film   The development process of an exposed X-ray film consists of the following steps.

Developer. The basic reaction of the developer is to change into silver atoms the remaining silver ions in a single crystal (grain). Developers act as a supply of electrons, which become entrapped inside a sensitivity speck in the emulsion. Once within a sensitivity speck, the migrating silver ions can attach and reduce to a silver atom, as described in Eq. (3.2). This is the same physical phenomenon that occurs in crystals during exposure to light or X-ray photons. The speed of this reaction depends on the number of silver atoms within a latent image center and the number of latent image centers formed during exposure to light or X-ray photons. Therefore, time is a fundamental factor in the development process. Development should be discontinued when the ratio between the number of exposed, developed crystals to the number of unexposed, undeveloped crystals reaches a maximum.

Fixing. The fixing step removes remaining undeveloped silver halide crystals. If film is not fixed properly, it will appear cloudy because the remaining silver halide crystals act to disperse light.

Washing. Washing removes developing and fixing agents from the emulsion.

Drying. Drying removes water from the emulsion.

Film Optical Density The number of developed crystals per unit volume in the developed film will determine the fraction of light that can be transmitted through the unit volume. This transmission of light is referred to as the optical density of the film in that unit volume. Technically, the optical density (OD) is defined as the logarithm base 10 of 1 reciprocal transmittance of a unit intensity of light:

$$OD = \log_{10} (1/\text{transmittance}) \qquad (3.3)$$
$$= \log_{10} (I_0/I_t)$$

where I_0 = light intensity before transmission through the film
I_t = light intensity after transmission through the film

The film optical density is used to represent the degree of film darkening due to X-ray exposure.

Characteristic Curve of X-Ray Film The relationship between X-ray exposure and film optical density is called the *characteristic curve* or the *H and D curve* (after F. Hurter and V. C. Driffield, who first published such a curve in England in 1890). The logarithm of relative exposure is plotted instead of the exposure itself, partly because it compresses a large linear to a manageable logarithm scale, which makes analysis of the curve easier. Figure 3.3 shows an idealized curve with three segments: the toe, the linear segment, and the shoulder.

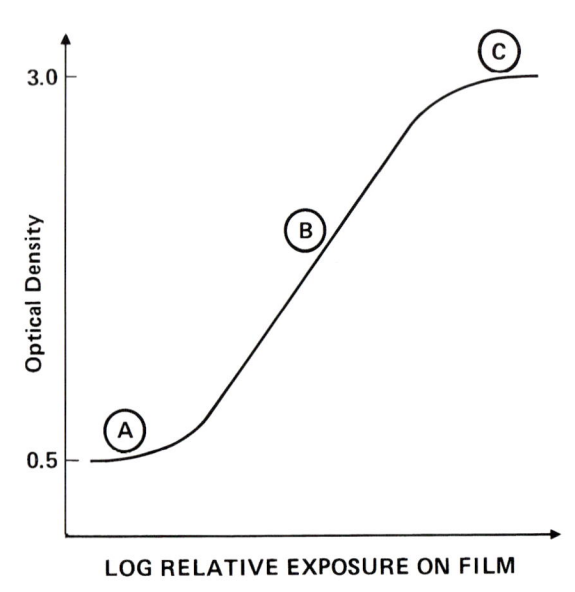

Figure 3.3 The relationship between the logarithm of relative X-ray exposure and the film optical density plotted as a curve, the characteristic curve or the H and D curve; see text for discussion of points A–C.

The toe is the base density or the base-plus-fog level (usually OD = 0.12–0.20). For very low exposures, the film optical density remains at the fog level and is independent of exposure level. Next is a linear segment over which the optical density and the logarithm of relative exposure are linearly related (usually between OD 0.3 and 2.2). The shoulder corresponds to high exposures or overexposures, where most of the silver halides are converted to metallic silver (usually OD 3.2). The film becomes saturated, and the optical density is no longer a function of exposure level.

The characteristic curve is usually described by one of the following parameters: film gamma, average gradient, film latitude, or film speed.

The film gamma (γ) is the maximum slope of the characteristic curve, and is described by the formula:

$$\text{gamma} = \frac{D_2 - D_1}{\log_{10} E_2 - \log_{10} E_1} \quad (3.4)$$

where D_2 = highest OD value within the steepest portion of the curve (B in Fig. 3.3) of curve
D_1 = lowest OD value within the steepest portion of curve
E_2 = exposure responsible for D_2
E_1 = exposure responsible for D_1

The average gradient of the characteristic curve is the slope of the characteristic curve calculated between optical density 0.25 and 2.00 above base plus fog level for the radiographic film under consideration. The optical density range between 0.25 to 2.00 is considered acceptable for diagnostic radiology application. For example, assuming a base and fog level of 0.15, the range of acceptable optical density is therefore 0.40–2.15. The average gradient can be represented by the following formula:

$$\text{average gradient} = \frac{D_2 - D_1}{\log_{10} E_2 - \log_{10} E_1} \quad (3.5)$$

where D_2 = 2.00 + base and fog level
D_1 = 0.25 + base and fog level
E_2 = exposure responsible for D_2
E_1 = exposure responsible for D_1

The film latitude describes the range of exposures used in the average gradient calculation. Thus, as described in Eq. (3.5), the film latitude is equal to $\log_{10} E_2 - \log_{10} E_1$.

The film speed, in units of reciprocal roentgens, can be defined as follows:

$$\text{speed} = \frac{1}{E} \quad (3.6)$$

where E is the exposure (in roentgens) required to produce a film optical density of 1.0 above base and fog. Generally speaking:

1. The latitude of a film varies inversely with film contrast, film speed, film gamma, and average gradient.
2. Film gamma and average gradient of a film vary directly with film contrast.
3. Film fog level varies inversely with film contrast.
4. Faster films require less exposure to achieve a specific density than slower films.

Large Latitude Film A film may have a latitude value that does not cover the range of exposures required in some imaging applications. Therefore, films with a larger latitude may be required. Large-latitude film can be helpful in imaging of the thorax area because X-ray photons passing through the mediastinum are attenuated to a much greater extent than those passing through the lungs.

If the range of exposures within an area to be imaged is too wide for the entire linear portion of the film response, some pertinent image information may fall into the toe and the shoulder of the characteristic curve. The result is an inaccurate portrayal, since the information in the toe and shoulder regions is low in contrast resolution. The solution is to use a film that has a linear region that covers a much wider range of exposures. Such a medium is referred to as large- or wide-latitude film.

Since film manufacturers have done much research on maximizing the performance of X-ray films to display latent images, they provide specific information on the type of film, with its specific characteristic curve, that should be used for a given radiologic examination. Therefore if the similar latent image is displayed with a video monitor, we need to consider how to utilize the monitor's display characteristic to best visualize the pertinent information in the image.

3.1.2.2 Image Intensifier Tube

Another image receptor used very often in projectional radiography is the image intensifier tube. The image intensifier tube is particularly useful for fluorographic and digital subtraction angiography procedures, which allow imaging of moving structures, like blood flow in the body, and dynamic processes in real time. Although X-ray films exposed rapidly in time can provide some information about these structures and processes, the use of an image intensifier can maximize the information available from the study and minimize the X-ray exposure to the patient. An image intensifier tube is shown schematically in Figure 3.4.

The X-rays exiting the patient enter the image intensifier tube through the glass envelope and are absorbed in the input phosphor intensifying screen. The input screen converts X-ray photons to light photons. The light emitted from the screen next strikes the light-sensitive photocathode, causing the emission of photoelectrons. These electrons are then accelerated across the tube (by approximately 25,000 V) and strike the output screen. In this way, the variance of the X-ray pattern that is due to attenuation

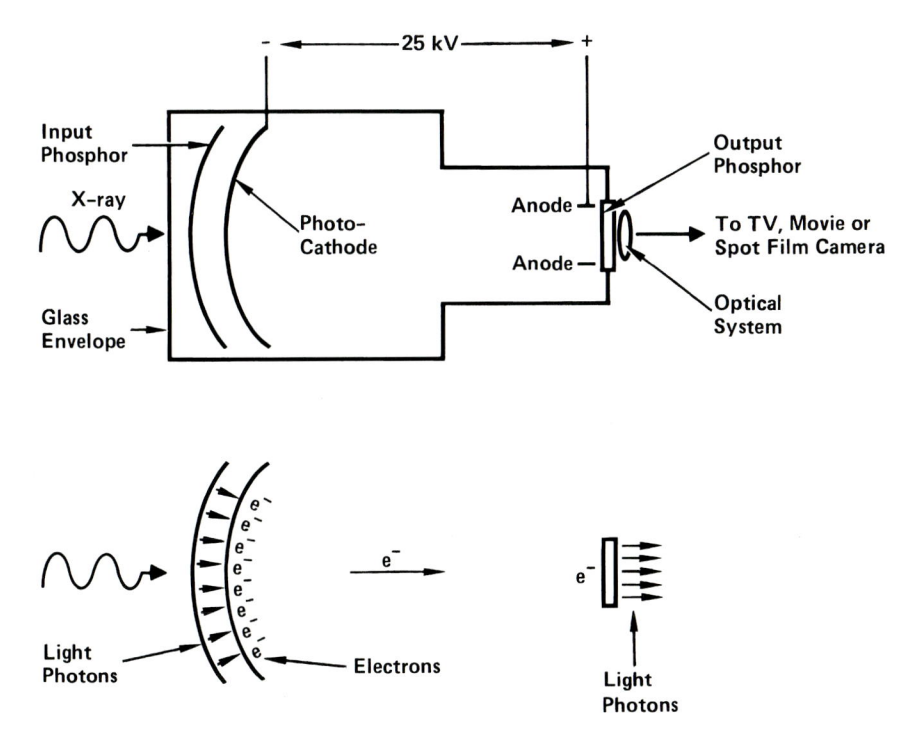

PRINCIPLES OF CONVENTIONAL PROJECTION RADIOGRAPHY 49

Figure 3.4 Schematic of the image intensifier tube and the formation of an image on the output screen.

upon passage through the body of the patient is converted into a variance of electron density. This stream of electrons is focused and converges on an output phosphor screen. At the time the electrons are absorbed by the output phosphor, the image information carried by the electron stream is once again converted to light of greater brightness than the light output from the input phosphor, hence the term image intensifier. The brightness gain in an image intensifier is the product two gains:

- *Minification gain:* the light intensity increases by a factor equal to the ratio of the areas between the input and output phosphors. Thus, the minification gain of an image intensifier with a 10-inch diameter input phosphor and a 1-inch diameter output phosphor is 100.
- *Flux gain:* each light photon emitted by the input phosphor will result in the generation of many light photons exiting the output phosphor. On average, this gain of light photons is about 50.

Therefore the brightness gain for this image intensifier is approximately $100 \times 50 = 5000$.

Image intensifiers are generally listed by the diameter of the input phosphor, ranging from 4.5 to 14 inches. The light from the output phosphor is then coupled to an optical system for recording using a movie camera (angiography), a TV camera (fluorography), or a spot film camera.

3.2 X-RAY FILM SCANNER

Since 70% of all radiographic procedures still use film as an output medium, it is necessary to investigate methods for converting images from films into digital format. This section discusses two types of film scanner: the video camera and the laser scanner.

As described in Chapter 2, when a radiographic film is digitized, the shades of gray in the film are quantized into a two-dimensional array of nonnegative integers called pixels or samples. The gray levels values of these pixels must represent the radiographic image favorably, to allow the reconstruction of the original image. Two factors have to be considered: the quality of the scanner and aliasing artifact. A low quality scanner with large pixel size and insufficient bits per pixel will yield a bad digitized image (see example in Fig. 2.1). On the other hand a good quality scanner may sometimes produce aliasing artifact in the digitized image owing to some special inherent patterns, such as grid lines, in the original film. The aliasing artifact can best be explained with the concept of data sampling. The well-known sampling theorem states that:

> If the Fourier transform of the image $f(x,y)$ vanishes for all u,v where $|u| \geq 2f_N$, $|v| \geq 2f_N$, then $f(x,y)$ can be exactly reconstructed from samples of its nonzero values taken $0.5f_N$ apart or closer. The frequency $2f_N$ is called the Nyquist frequency.

The theorem implies that if the pixel samples are taken more than $0.5f_N$ apart, complete reconstruction of the images from these samples will not be possible. The difference between the original image and the image reconstructed from these samples is due to aliasing error. The aliasing artifact creates new frequency components in the reconstructed image called moiré patterns. Examples of moiré patterns created by the laser scanning of radiographic images are given in later sections. These images all have certain fine patterns that cannot be resolved by the scanner.

3.2.1 Video Scanning System

The video scanner system is a low cost X-ray digitizer that produces either a 512 or 1K digitized image with 8 bits/pixel. The system consists of three major components: a scanning device with a video or a CCD (charge-coupled device) camera that scans the X-ray film, an analog/digital converter that converts the video signals from the camera to gray level values, and an image memory to store the digital signals from the A/D converter.

The image stored in the image memory is the digital representation of the X-ray film obtained by using the video camera. If the image memory is connected to a

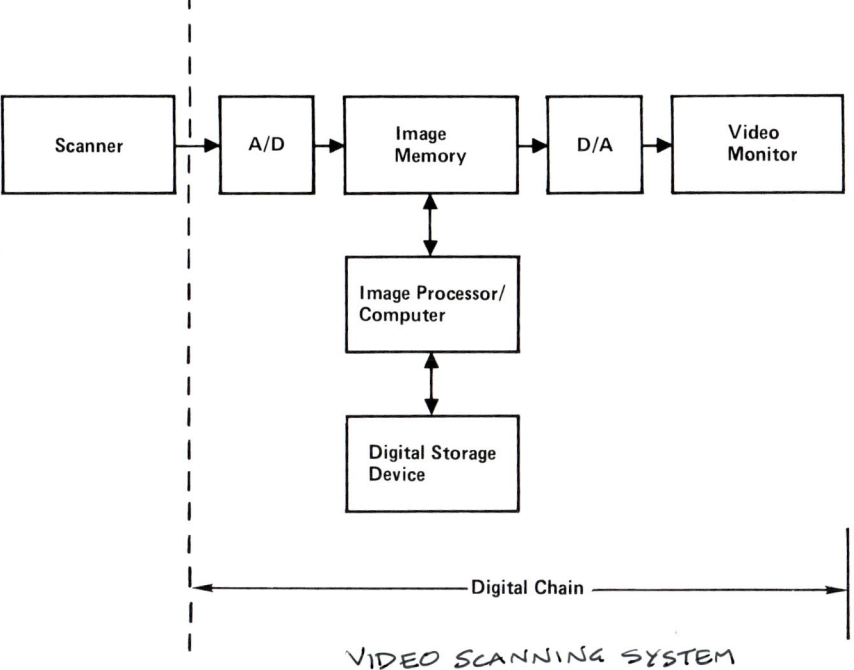

Figure 3.5 Block diagram of a film scanner showing the digital chain.

(VIDEO SCANNING SYSTEM)

digital-to-analog conversion circuitry and to a TV monitor, this digitized image can be displayed on the monitor (which is the video image) or a soft copy of the X-ray film. The memory can be connected to a peripheral storage device for long-term image archiving purposes, and to a computer or a processor for image manipulation. Figure 3.5 is a block diagram of a film video scanner; the digital chain shown is standard components of all other types of film scanner.

3.2.2 Laser Scanner

The laser scanner is the gold standard in film digitization. It normally converts a 14 in. $\times$ 17 in. X-ray film to a 2K $\times$ 2.5K $\times$ 12-bit image. The principle of laser scanning is shown in Figure 3.6. A rotating polygon mirror system is used to guide a collimated low power (5mW) laser beam (usually helium–neon) to scan across a line of the radiograph in a lighttight environment. The radiograph is advanced and the scan is repeated for the second lines and so forth. The optical density of the film is measured from the transmission of the laser through each small area (e.g., 175 μm $\times$ 175 μm) of the radiograph using a photomultiplier tube and a logarithmic amplifier. This electric signal is sent to a digital chain, where it is digitized to 8 to 12 bits from the A/D converter. The data are then sent to a computer, where a storage device is provided for the image. The scan process can be described as a repetition of the following sequential steps:

52 PROJECTION RADIOGRAPHY

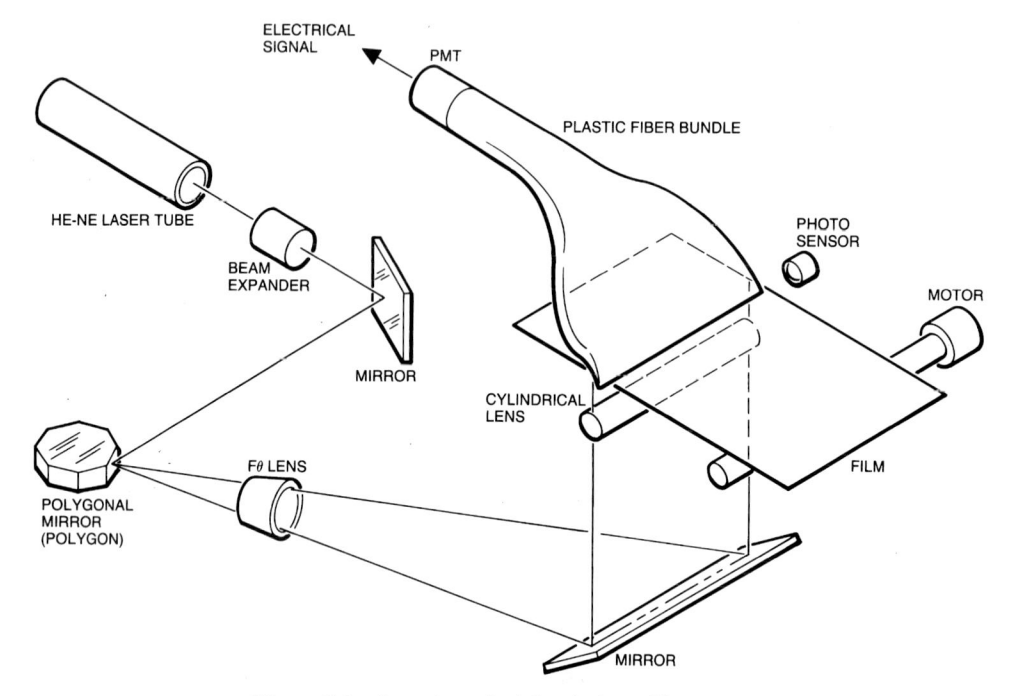

Figure 3.6 Scanning principle of a laser film scanner.

1. Laser beam scans one line of the radiograph.
2. Photomultiplier detects light transmission one pixel at a time.
3. Amplifier and signal conditioners perform analog signal processing.
4. Analog-to-digital converter digitizes signal to 8 to 12 bits.
5. Data controller mediates data transmission to computer.
6. Mechanical transport system moves the film to the next scan line.

Figure 3.7 shows the schematic block diagram of a laser scanner system.

3.3 DIGITIZATION

3.3.1 Parameters Affecting the Quality of Digitization

Before the film scanner is ready for clinical use, it is important to evaluate its specifications and to verify the quality of the digitized image. This section describes some standard tests used routinely to evaluate the quality of a film scanner. The laser scanner described in Table 3.1 is used as an example.

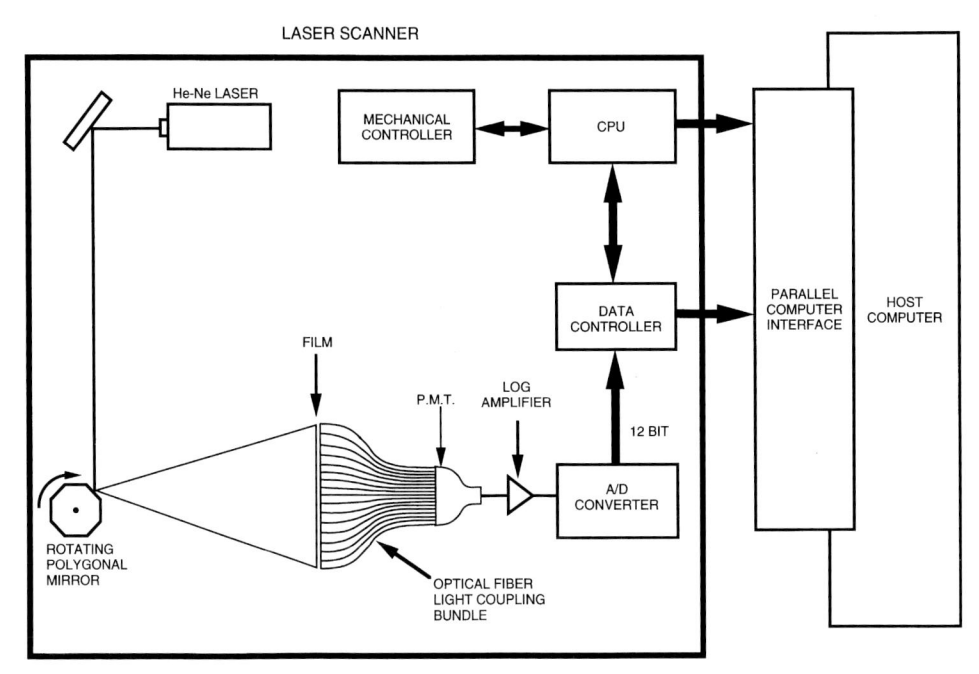

Figure 3.7 Block diagram of a laser film scanner interfacing to a host computer.

3.3.1.1 Optical Density Versus Gray Level Value

The mapping of optical densities of the film to gray levels from the laser scanner can be measured by scanning a calibrated Kodak 310-ST-252 photographic step wedge (composed of silver halide particles suspended in a gelatin) and recording the optical density of each step and the resulting digital output value. The quoted accuracy of the step wedge is 2% of the optical density value. The table consists of 21 optical densi-

TABLE 3.1 Specifications of a Laser Scanner

Film size supported, in. × in.	14 × 17, 14 × 14, 12 × 14, 10 × 12, 8 × 10
Pixel size, μm	50–200
Sampling distance, μm	50, 75, 100, 125, 150, 175, 200
Optical density range	0–2, 0–4
Bits/pixel	12
Hardware interface	SCSI*
Laser power	5 mW
Scanning speed	200 lines/s
Data format	DICOM

*SCSI: small computer systems interface.

54 PROJECTION RADIOGRAPHY

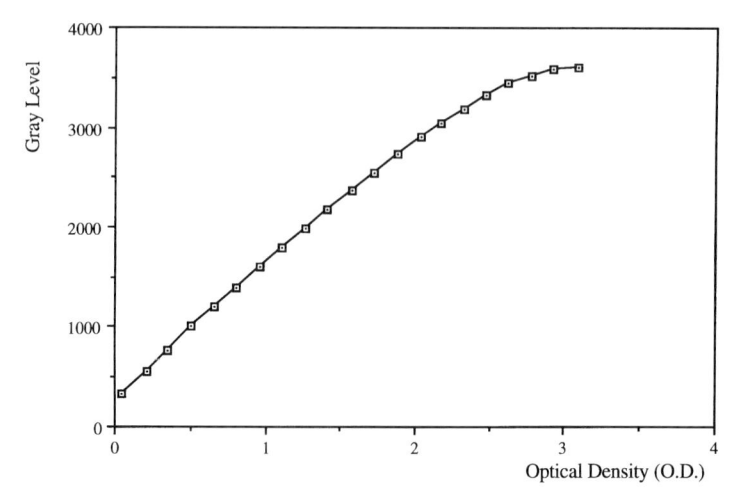

Figure 3.8 Relationship between the input film optical density and gray level values of a laser scanner: it is Linear up to OD = 2.5.

ty steps ranging from 0.06 OD to 3.09 OD. A rectangular region consisting of 2000 pixels used for averaging the digital output value for each step should be sufficient.

Figure 3.8, the optical density to gray level transfer curve of the scanner, shows that the digitization of optical density is highly linear over the step wedge range (0.06–2.50 OD). It has a range from 500 to 3500 gray levels over this optical density range. Linearity in this range covers essentially most of the diagnostic films produced in today's radiology departments.

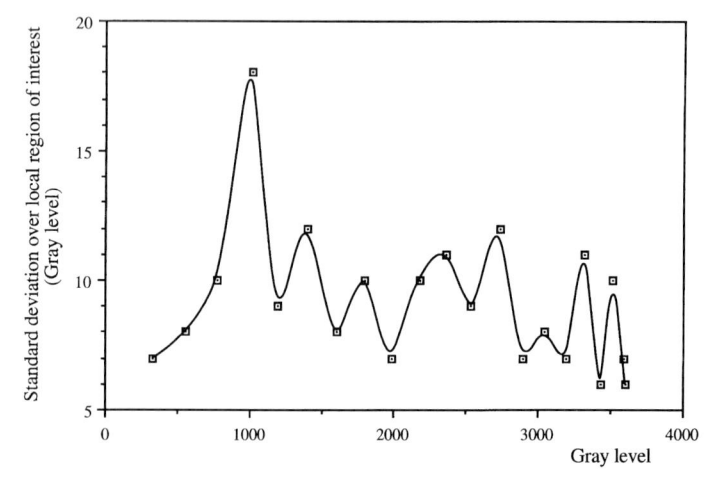

Figure 3.9 Flat field response: plot showing the change in the standard deviation of optical density over the density range of a laser scanner. Data are accumulated over the entire imaging field (global variations). In general, the standard deviation is less than 1%.

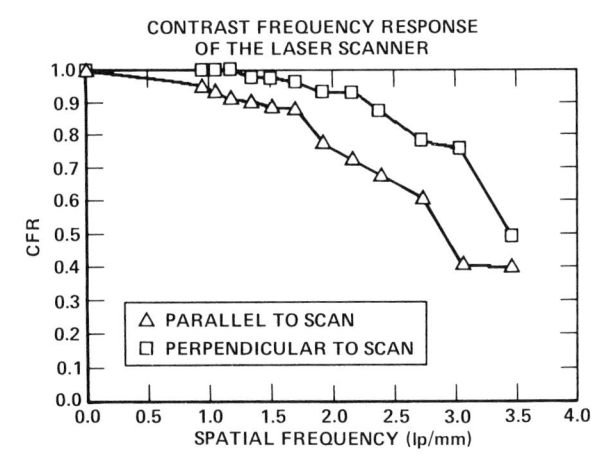

Figure 3.10 Contrast frequency response (CFR) of a laser scanner in both the parallel and perpendicular scan directions.

3.3.1.2 Accuracy of the Laser Scanner Digitization

It is difficult to measure the accuracy of the digital representation of an optical density value because there is no film that is perfectly uniform in optical density and free of noise. To measure the nonuniformity (overall constancy) and noise (local constancy), we can use 10×10 pixel area blocks of the Kodak step wedge. The 10×10 areas should be large enough for statistical accuracy and small enough to avoid any nonuniformities presented on the step wedge.

Field uniformity can be measured by scanning the calibrated step wedge at five

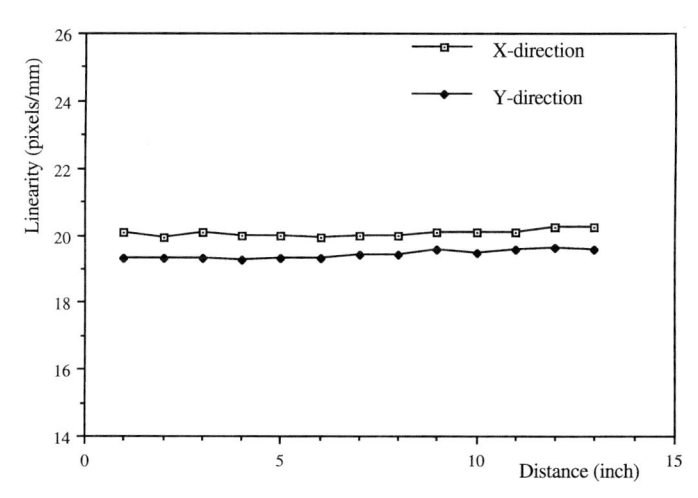

Figure 3.11 Linearity of the scanner. The number of pixels per millimeter is counted from the left of the film to the right, and from the top to the bottom.

different locations along the scan direction. These locations correspond to various degrees of offset from the center of the scanning field. The scanning line should cover a distance of 14 inches. The 500 pixels from each step (100 pixels from each location) can then be used to calculate the root mean square (rms) fluctuation from a constant input to the system. Figure 3.9 summarizes the overall conversion accuracy of the scanner.

Field nonuniformities parallel to the scan direction arise mainly from fluctuations in the laser output intensity, nonuniformities in the fiber-optic light coupling, and quantum noise in the light detection system. Nonuniformities perpendicular to the scan direction arise from longer term drift of the laser intensity and from lower frequency noise and drift in the detection electronics. The overall flat field response of the system is the combined responses in the parallel and perpendicular directions.

Noise values can be determined by scanning 10×10 square pixel area blocks and calculating the standard deviation of the resultant gray level values. The standard deviation from the five different locations along the scan direction can be averaged.

3.3.1.3 Contrast Frequency Response of the Scanner

The laser scanner's frequency response can be tested by scanning a high precision microlithographed line pair (lp) pattern consisting of alternating and equally spaced dark and light stripes at different spatial frequencies. One such pattern (USAF, 1951) was developed by the U.S. Air Force. The dark and light areas correspond to optical densities 0.05 and 3.40, respectively. The average gray level for the dark and light stripes can be obtained from the digitized image, and the contrast frequency response (CFR) can be calculated for each frequency. The CFR parallel to the scan direction can be determined from line pair patterns oriented perpendicular to the beam traversal direction and the perpendicular CFR from line pair patterns oriented parallel to the scanning laser beam. These values indicate the degree to which contrast depends on spatial frequency and are given by:

$$\text{CFR}(f) = \frac{D_{\max}(f) - D_{\min}(f)}{D_{\max}(f)} \quad (3.7)$$

where $D_{\max}(f)$ = digital value of dark stripe
$D_{\min}(f)$ = digital value of light stripe
f = spatial frequency of the stripes

The laser scanner with the specification shown in Table 3.1 has "full width at half-maximum" spot sizes of 50 μm in the scanning direction and 50 μm perpendicular to the scan direction. The sampling distance in both directions is 50 μm. The contrast frequency response curves for this laser scanner in directions parallel and perpendicular to the scan direction are given in Figure 3.10. The response drops to 0.5 at a frequency of 2.9 cycles/mm in the direction parallel to scan direction and 3.5 cycle/mm in the direction perpendicular to the scan. To measure the linearity of the scanner, we count the number of pixels in one millimeter from the left of the film to the right and from the top to the bottom. Figure 3.11 shows the results.

3.3.2 Aliasing Artifacts

3.3.2.1 Practical Consideration

Aliasing artifacts are low spatial frequency components introduced to the digitized image as a result of undersampling during digitization. They appear most often when a high resolution digitization device like a laser scanner is used on X-ray films with patterns of certain types, like grid patterns.

Films produced by today's radiology departments can be categorized into four classes, depending on how the film was obtained:

1. Conventional X-ray films obtained without a grid.
2. Digital images (CT, MRI) printed by a laser film printer.
3. Films produced by a video multiformat camera.
4. Conventional X-ray films obtained with a grid.

Normally, digitized images obtained from films with a low resolution scanner (e.g., a video camera) do not contain any noticeable aliasing artifacts. This is because the low modulation transfer function (MTF) of the scanner filters out much of the high frequency content of the image, with the result that frequencies above the Nyquist frequency are negligible. Category 1 X-ray films obtained without a grid and category 2 films produced by a laser film printer, when digitized with a high resolution laser scanner, may or may not contain aliasing artifacts, depending on the frequency contents of the image. In almost all cases, the artifacts will be weak and not visually prominent.

Care must be exercised, however, in the digitization of category 3 X-ray films with a grid and category 4 films produced by a multiformat camera. Close examination of these two categories reveals a structured background of periodic line patterns superimposed on the image. For films produced with a grid, the background pattern consists of the septa of the grid used, while for films obtained with a multiformat camera, they are the raster video scan lines. Table 3.2 shows some typical line pattern frequencies produced by grids and multiformat cameras on film obtained from various imaging modalities.

To examine the effect of these high spatial frequency background line patterns on the digitized image, let us assume that these films are digitized with the laser scanner with a spot size of 100 μm and a sampling distance of 175 μm. The sampling theory states that these background periodic lines will produce moiré patterns because of aliasing, unless the following condition is satisfied:

$$\Delta x = 175 < \frac{1}{2f} \qquad (3.8)$$

TABLE 3.2 Some Moiré Patterns Observed in Digitized Images of X-Ray Films Obtained Using the Grid and Films Produced with Multiformat

X-Ray Film with Grid (lead strips/mm)		Multiformat Camera (scan line pair/mm)		
80 lines/in.	100 lines/in.	DSA	CT	MRI
3.1*	4.0*	2.7	3.4	5.7

*Without a magnification factor. With a magnification factor, the value should be lower.

where Δx is the sampling interval and f is the frequency of the background line pattern.

The highest allowable frequency to avoid moiré patterns for the case of the laser scanner is 2.86 cycles/mm. Examination of the frequency values in Table 3.2 reveals that digitized images from films containing background line patterns with frequencies above 2.8 cycles/mm (CT and MRI images produced by the multiformat camera and the X-ray image obtained using a grid) will contain moiré patterns, since Eq. (3.8) is violated.

Figure 3.12 shows some examples. The four digitized images in the left-hand column come from films with background line patterns obtained from four different modalities (see also Table 3.2). The display contrast and the brightness of each digitized image were adjusted to highlight the moiré patterns, which depend on the frequency and contrast of the line patterns, the orientation of the line patterns with respect to the scanning direction, and the MTF of the scanner.

To minimize the occurrence of distracting moiré patterns in the resultant image, the film should be scanned with the background line patterns oriented perpendicular to the direction in which the resolution of the scanner is worst. This is because more of the high frequency components due to the periodic line patterns will be filtered out, and therefore the spectral content above the Nyquist frequency of the scanner will be diminished. In this case, the resolution is worse in the direction parallel to the scan direction. This is a trade-off between higher resolution and the avoidance of aliasing artifacts.

The right-hand column in Figure 3.12 shows the corresponding images digitized with the scanning beam traversing perpendicular to the background line patterns, that →

Figure 3.12 Some examples of moiré patterns on images digitized with a laser scanner. These films all have background periodic line patterns. 1, Arteriogram: moiré pattern (slanted vertical lines) appears on both left and right images; 2, MRI: moiré pattern (woven horizontal lines) on left-hand image only; 3, CT: moiré pattern (horizontal lines) on left-hand image only. The level and window settings on the left-hand image are adjusted to highlight the moiré pattern in the background. 4, DSA: (no moiré pattern seen). left-hand image: line patterns oriented parallel to scan direction (scanner resolved lines well), moiré patterns are more severe; right-hand image: lines patterns oriented perpendicular to scan direction (scanner does not resolve lines as well), moiré patterns are less severe.

59

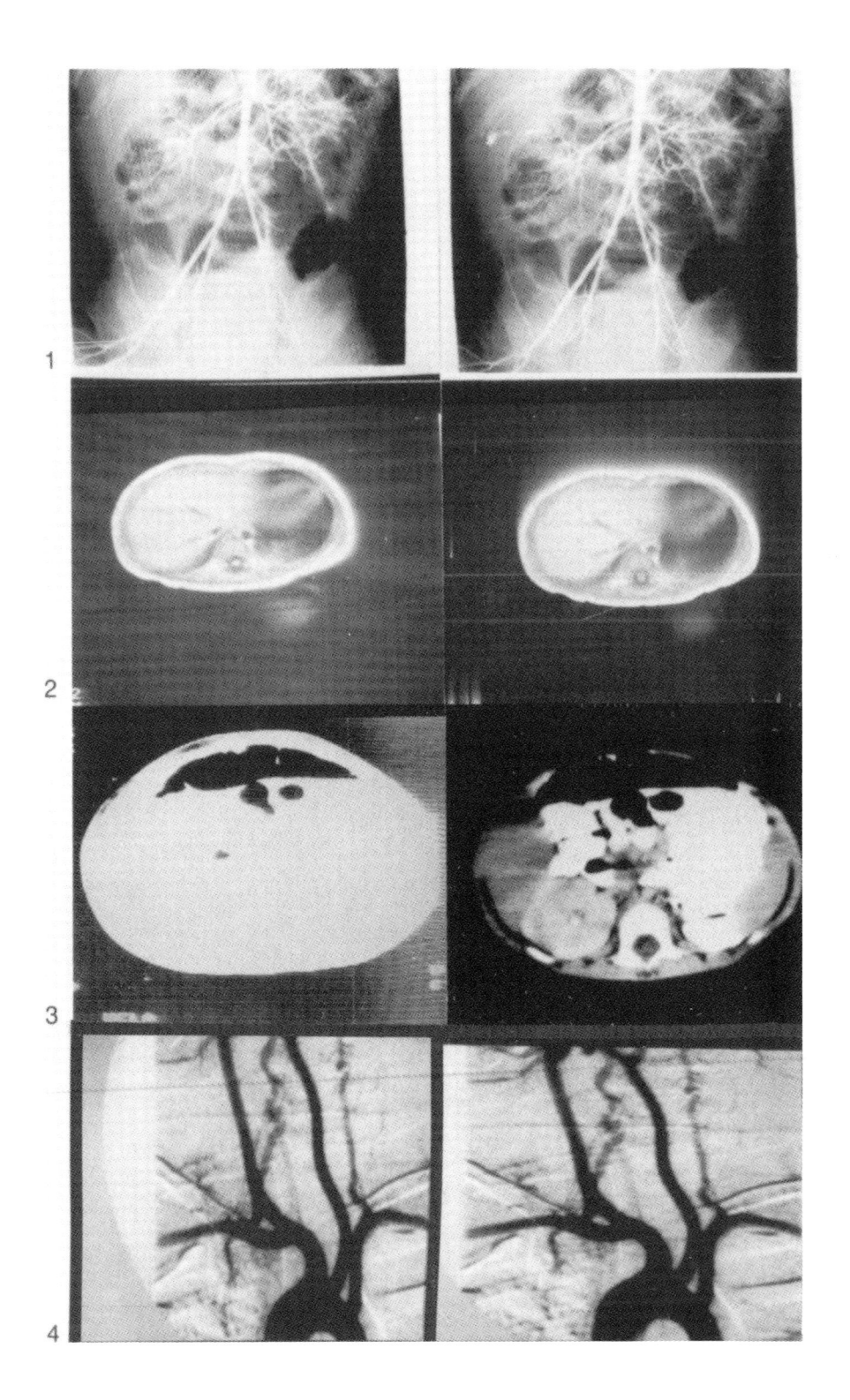

is, in the direction perpendicular to the direction in which the scanner's MTF is lowest. It can be seen that the presence of moiré patterns due to aliasing has been minimized.

The appearance of moiré patterns due to inadequate sampling of images with high frequency components has been documented for many digitizing systems. Figure 3.12 shows some interesting cases from diagnostic radiology.

3.3.2.2 Sampling Artifacts Arising from Grid Patterns

During the past several years the multiformat camera has been eliminated for filming CT/MR images, and therefore we only have to worry about older CT/MR films. On the other hand, scatter grid is still used in most X-ray examinations to minimize scattering. For this reason we have to be careful during digitization of conventional X-ray films.

Two phenomena can be puzzling. First, why the aliasing artifacts appear to be more prominent under certain digitization conditions? Second, why does the orientation of the moiré pattern change abruptly when there is only a slightly change in the digitization condition? To explain these apparent anomalies, Wang (1996) developed a three-parameter model to explain sampling artifacts arising from an antiscatter grid: the laser spot size of the digitizer, the sampling distance, and the angle between the grid lines, and the direction perpendicular to the laser beam scanning direction. The first two parameters are adjustable with the scanner, and the third parameter can be manipulated by angling the film during digitization. After the digitization, whether the aliasing artifacts on the digitized image is visible depends on three factors: the amplitude of the aliasing frequency, the frequency response of the display, and the visual sensitivity of the human interpreting the image. The amplitude of the aliasing artifacts is independent of the sampling frequency, but may depend on the orientation of the grid line pattern. Generally speaking, the smaller the amplitude, the less dominant the aliasing artifacts. The human visual response, which varies with grid frequency, has been reported to be at its highest response around 1–2 cycle/mm, and decreasing on both sides.

Figure 3.13 shows that the orientation of the moiré pattern depends on the specif-

Figure 3.13 (a) Chest phantom film with a scarcely visible grid line pattern. The square is the digitization region. (b) Digitized images with a 105 μm focal spot size laser scanner at different sampling distances and angles. Images in rows 1–3 from top to bottom were digitized with the film tilted 0°, 5°, and 10°, respectively. Images in columns 1–4 from left to right were digitized with sampling distances 200, 254, 293, and 352 μm, respectively. The aliasing artifacts are most prominent at 254 and 293 μm. Some aliasing artifacts are seen at 200 μm with 0° and 5°. Observe the abrupt change of the moiré pattern orientation in column 2. (c) Digitized image with a 210 μm focal spot size at different sampling distances and angles. Images in rows 1–3 from top to bottom were digitized with the film tilted 0°, 5°, and 10° respectively. Images in columns 1–4 from left to right were digitized with sampling distances 200, 254, 293, and 352 μm, respectively. For this large focal spot size, no appreciable aliasing artifacts are seen regardless of sampling distance and tilted angle.

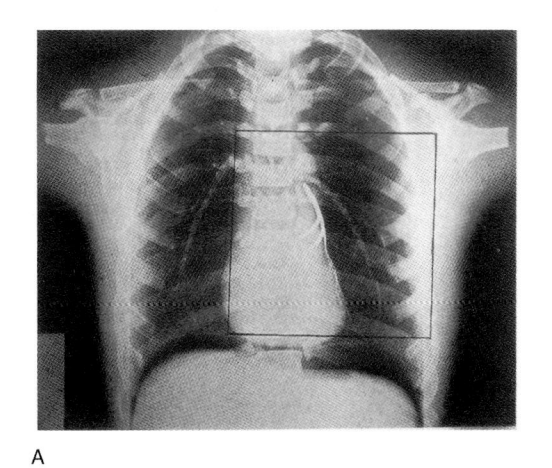

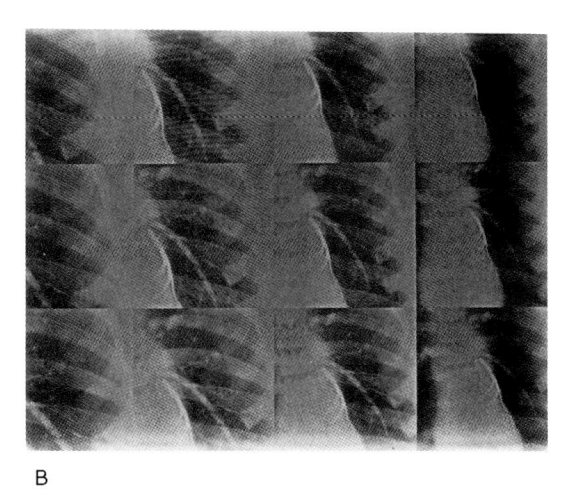

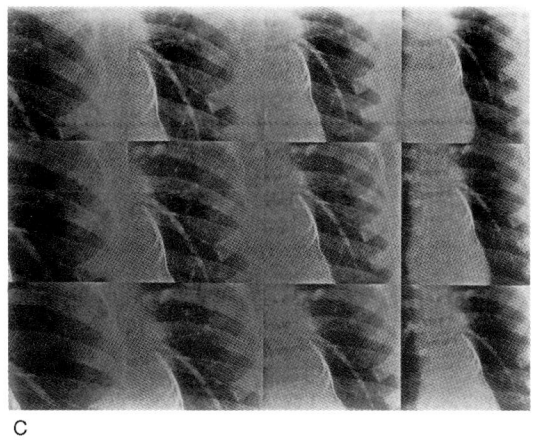

A

B

C

61

ic set of digitizing parameters: these images are in the anatomical position, and each is rotated 90° clockwise with respect to the digitizing position. For example, the images in the first row in Figure 3.13b have aliasing patterns almost parallel to the x direction. The images in the second row were digitized with the film tilted 5°, and the angles of aliasing patterns vary from $-70°$ to 35°. The images in the third row were digitized with the film tilted 10°, and the angles of the aliasing patterns vary from $-80°$ to 55°.

Digitization using a laser film digitizer cannot totally eliminate the aliasing artifacts without losing imaging resolution. But with a proper choice of digitization parameters, we can minimize the visibility of the aliasing artifacts. During digitization, the film should be positioned such that the grid lines are perpendicular to the scanning direction. This way we may be able to take advantage of the high frequency attenuation characteristic of the photomultiplier–amplifier component in the scanner to reduce the amplitude of the gird lines. The amplitude of the aliasing artifacts is independent of the sampling frequency. We cannot reduce the aliasing amplitude by varying the sampling frequency. If the Nyquist frequency condition cannot be satisfied, we can select a sampling frequency from which the scanner will give a higher aliasing frequency. The reason for this is that the display system functions as a low pass filter. The aliasing artifacts will be less prominent owing to the high frequency attenuation characteristic of the display system. Besides, a digital image can be postprocessed. The high frequency aliasing artifacts are more easily to be removed than the low frequency components because the original image is dominated by low frequency components. Once the sampling distance has been selected, the laser spot size should be selected to be the same as the sampling distance.

Since it is difficult to remove the grid line aliasing artifacts in the digitizing process, it is more desirable to remove them from the digitized image. One method is to transform the image to the frequency domain, search for sharp high frequency peaks corresponding to the grid lines, and remove them.

CHAPTER 4
Digital Radiography

As mentioned earlier, 70% of radiographic procedures are conventional projection radiographic examinations. For the radiology department to move from a film-based to digital-based operation, it is essential to derive new imaging acquisition systems that can directly convert this 70% of radiographic examinations to digital format.

This chapter discusses two approaches. The first is to utilize existing equipment in the radiographic procedure room and change only the image receptor component. This approach is represented by two technologies, both based on the use of phosphors: computed radiography (CR), using the photostimulable phosphor imaging plate technology, and digital fluorography. The method does not require any modification in the procedure room and is therefore more easily adopted for daily clinical practice. The second approach is to redesign the conventional radiographic procedure equipment, including the geometry of the X-ray beams and the image receptor. This method is therefore more expensive to adopt, but it offers special features like low X-ray scatter, which would not otherwise be available in the conventional procedure.

Imaging plate technology was introduced in the late 1970s and early 1980s. Work done by researchers at Xerox Medical Systems (xeroradiography, electronic scanning of selenium plate), Image Systems Division/3M (electroradiography), M.D. Anderson Hospital, in Texas (laser scanning of selenium plate), Fuji Photo Film Company, Ltd. (laser-stimulated luminescence phosphor plate), and Philips Medical Systems (electrophoretic devices) have stimulated growth in this field.

An imaging plate (IP) system consists of two components: an imaging plate to store the latent image and the scanning mechanism to extract the latent image from the plate to form a digital image. In the past, the development of plate technology was hindered by the low spatial resolution and signal-to-noise ratio of the IP compared to the X-ray film, and the difficulty of displaying and storing IP images. At the present time, most of these technical problems have been resolved. More and more hospitals are installing imaging plate systems to replace the conventional screen/film receptor, in particular, in intensive care, portable, and emergency medicine applications.

4.1 IMAGING PLATE TECHNOLOGY

Use of the laser scanner to digitize X-ray films was discussed in detail in Chapter 3. Reading a laser-stimulated luminescence phosphor imaging plate uses scanning principles similar to those familiar from the laser scanner. The only difference is that instead of scanning an X-ray film, the laser scans an image receptor called a *laser-stimulated luminescence phosphor plate* (or imaging plate, IP). An imaging plate system, commonly called computed radiography, consists of two components: the imaging plate and the scanning mechanism. This section describes the principle of the imaging plate, the system specifications and operation, and some clinical considerations.

4.1.1 Principle of the Laser-Stimulated Luminescence Phosphor Plate

The physical size of the imaging plate is similar to that of a conventional radiographic screen; it consists of a support coated with a photostimulable phosphorus layer made of BaFX:Eu^{2+}(X = Cl, Br, I), europium-activated barium fluorohalide compounds. After the X-ray exposure, the photostimulable phosphor crystal is able to store a part of the absorbed X-ray energy in a quasi-stable state. Stimulation of the plate by a helium–neon laser beam having a wavelength of 633 nm leads to emission of luminescence radiation, the amount of which is a function of the absorbed X-ray energy.

The luminescence radiation stimulated by the laser scanning is collected through a focusing lens and a light guide into a photomultiplier tube, which converts it into electrical signals. Figure 4.1 shows the physical principle of the laser-stimulated luminescence phosphor imaging plate. The size of the imaging plate can be 8 × 10, 10 × 12, 14 × 14, or 14 × 17 square inches.

4.1.2 A Computed Radiography System Block Diagram and Its Principle of Operation

The imaging plate is housed inside a light-tight cassette just like a screen–film system. Exposure of the IP to X-ray radiation results in the formation of a latent image on the plate (similar to the latent image formed in a screen/film receptor). The exposed plate is then processed through a computed radiographic (CR) system for extracting the latent image—analogous to the exposure of film that is developed by a film developer.

There are four major components in the computed radiographic system: the image reader, the image processor, the image storage devices, and the image recorder. The output of this system can be a printed film or a digital image; the latter can be stored in a digital storage device and be displayed on a video monitor. The first commercial computed radiographic system (FCR-101) was introduced in 1987 by the Fuji Medical Systems of Japan. A recent model, the FCR-9000 system, is shown in Figure 4.2. Figure 4.3 shows the principle of CR operation.

The CR system also has an automatic patient recording component that transmits

Figure 4.1 Physical principle of laser-stimulated luminescence phosphor imaging plate. (A) From the X-ray photons exposing the imaging plate to the formation of the light image. (B) The scanning laser beam (b) and the emitted light (a) from the imaging plate have two distinguished wavelengths to avoid cross talk. (Courtesy of J. Miyahara, Fuji Photo Film Co., Ltd.)

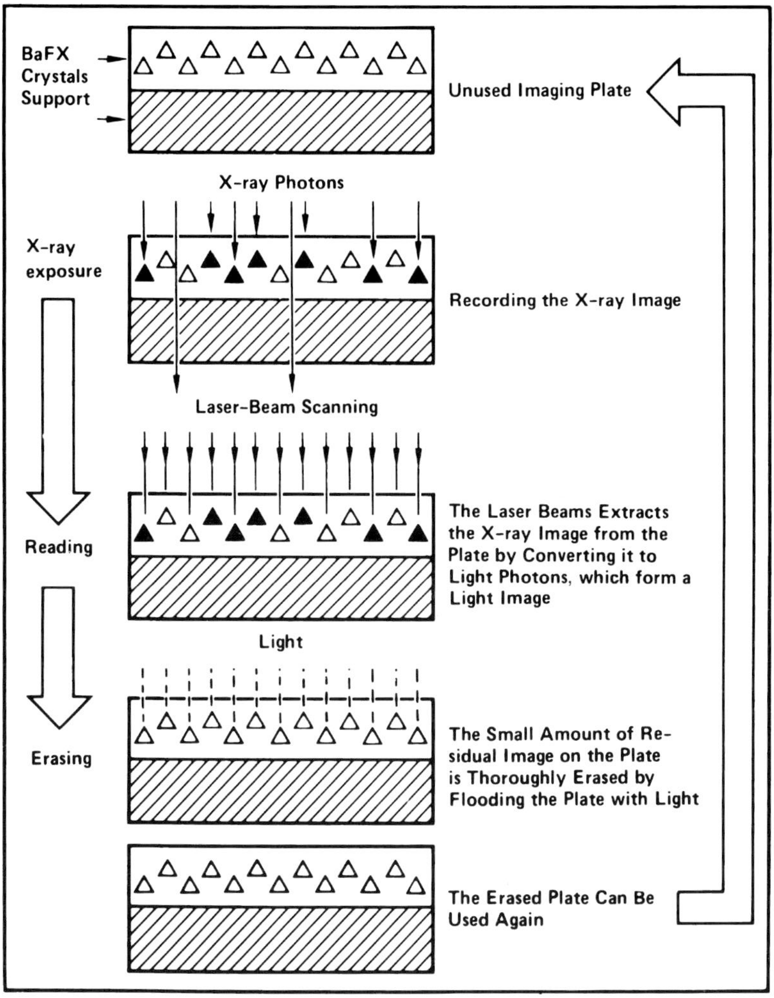
BaFX
Crystals
Support
Unused Imaging Plate
X-ray Photons
X-ray
exposure
Recording the X-ray Image
Laser-Beam Scanning
Reading
The Laser Beams Extracts the X-ray Image from the Plate by Converting it to Light Photons, which form a Light Image
Light
Erasing
The Small Amount of Residual Image on the Plate is Thoroughly Erased by Flooding the Plate with Light
The Erased Plate Can Be Used Again

A

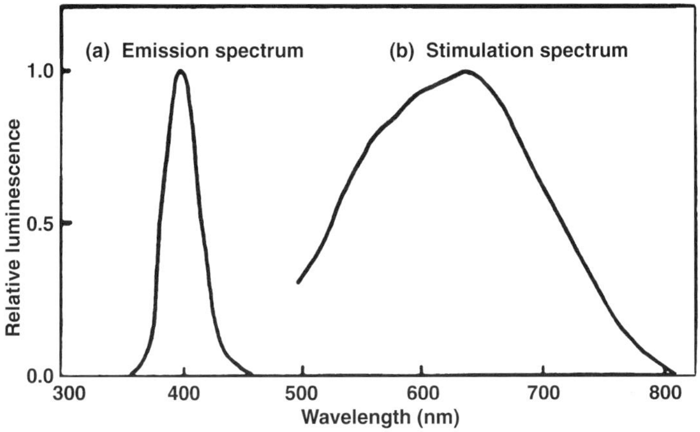
(a) Emission spectrum
(b) Stimulation spectrum
Relative luminescence
1.0
0.5
0.0
300
400
500
600
700
800
Wavelength (nm)

B

66 DIGITAL RADIOGRAPHY

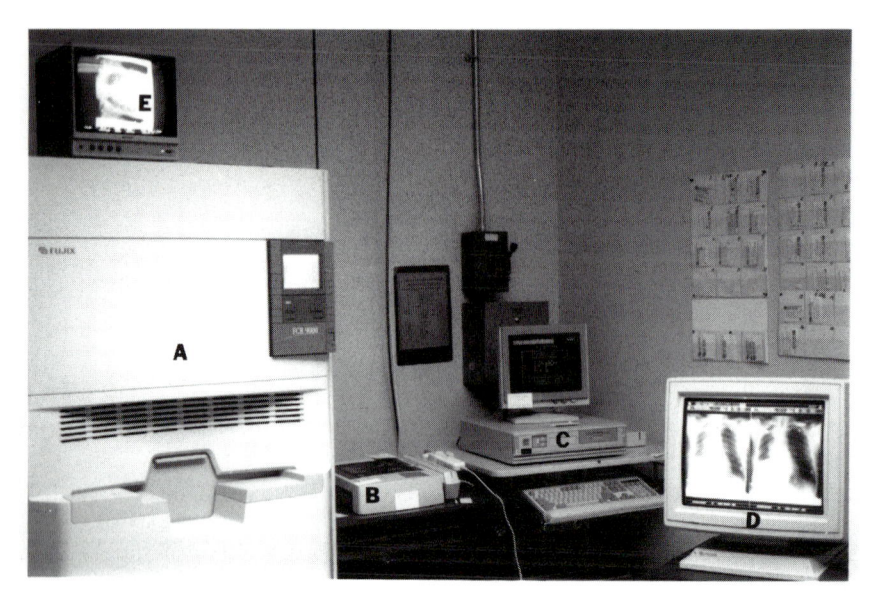

Figure 4.2 Photograph of the FCR 9000 system: A, imaging plate reader; B, patient ID card reader; C, ID terminal; D, image processing workstation, and E, quality assurance monitor.

the patient information from an ID card, the size of a conventional credit card, through an ID terminal to the system database. Selected information in this ID card is merged with the image and is printed on top of the film or displayed with the image on the video monitor for identification purposes.

We have described the removable-IP plate CR system. Another type of CR is the nonremovable IP system. There are several plates circulating inside this CR system, but no cassette. Two configurations are possible: the standing type (patient is in an upright position) and the recumbent type (patient lies on an examination table). Dur-

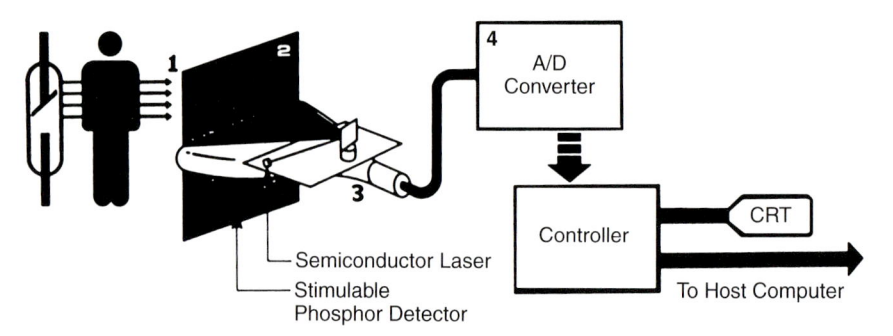

Figure 4.3 Schematic showing formation of the latent image on the CR imaging plate (1), the plate being scanned by the laser beam (2), light photons being converted to electrical signal (3), and electrical signals being converted to digital signals, which form a CR image (4). (Courtesy of Konica Corporation.)

ing the exposure, the conveyor transports an IP to the proper position aligned with the region of interest of the patient. After the exposure, the conveyor transports the exposed IP to the IP reader for scanning and an unexposed plate to the proper position for a possible second exposure. Nonremovable IP systems are good for special-procedure rooms, (e.g., chest examination rooms), because less time is needed to load and unload the cassette. These systems also minimize the mechanical handling of the IP associated with loading and unloading, which tend to break the IP more easily. The disadvantage of the nonremovable IP system is that it requires modifying the procedure room.

4.1.3 Operating Characteristics of the CR System

A major advantage of the CR system compared to the conventional screen/film system is that the imaging plate is linear and has a large dynamic range between the X-ray exposure and the relative intensity of the stimulated phosphors. Hence, under similar X-ray exposure conditions, the image reader is capable of producing images with density resolution comparable or superior to those from conventional screen/film systems. Since the image reader automatically adjusts the amount of exposure received by the plate, over- or underexposure within a certain limit will not affect the appearance of the image. This useful feature can best be explained by the two examples given in Figure 4.4.

In quadrant A of Figure 4.4, example I represents the plate exposed to a higher relative exposure level but a narrower exposure range (10^3–10^4). The linear response of the plate after laser scanning yields a high level but narrow light intensity (photostimulable luminescence, PSL) range from 10^3 to 10^4. These light photons are converted into electric output signals representing the latent image stored in the image plate. The image processor senses a narrow range of electric signal and selects a special lookup table (the linear line in Fig. 4.4B), which converts the narrow dynamic range 10^3–10^4 to a large light relative exposure of 1 to 50 (Fig. 4.4 B). If a large latitude film is used that covers the dynamic range of the light exposure from 1 to 50, as shown in quadrant C (see discussion on large-latitude film in Section 3.1.2.1), these output signals will register the entire optical density range from OD 0.2 to OD 2.8 on the film. The total system response, including the imaging plate, the lookup table, and the film subject to this exposure range, is depicted as curve I in quadrant D. The system–response curve, relating the relative exposure on the plate and the OD of the output film, shows a high gamma value and is quite linear. This example demonstrates how the system accommodates a high exposure level but a narrow exposure range.

Returning now to quadrant A in Figure 4.4, consider example II, in which the plate receives a lower exposure level but wider exposure range. The CR system automatically selects a different lookup table in the image processor to accommodate this range of exposure so that the output signals again span the entire light exposure range from 1 to 50. The system–response curve is shown as curve II in quadrant D. The key to selecting the correct lookup table is the range of the exposure: it must span the total light exposure of the film, namely from 1 to 50. It is noted that in both examples, the entire useful optical density range for diagnostic radiology is utilized.

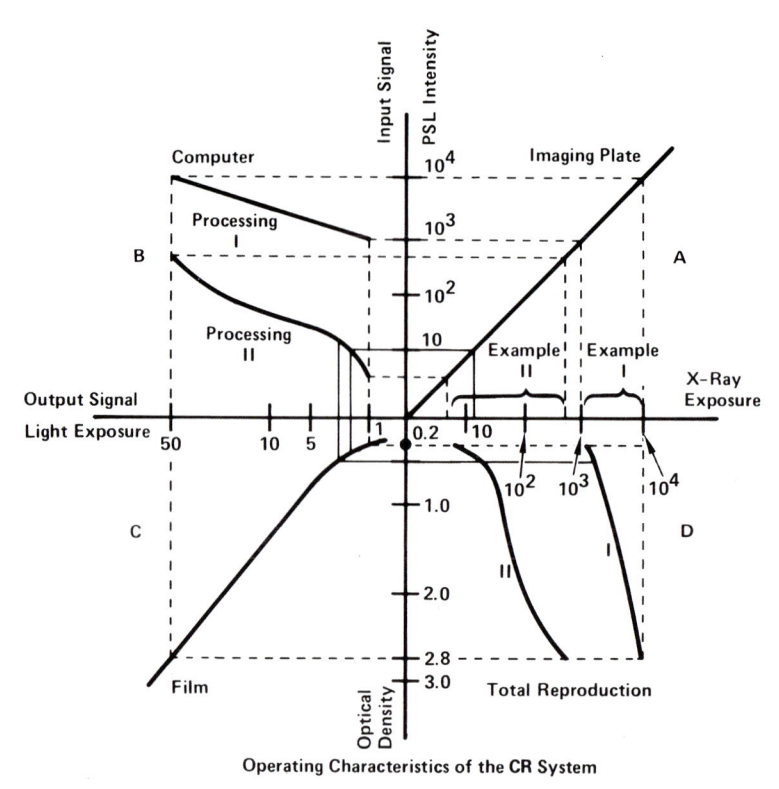

Figure 4.4 Two examples illustrating the operating characteristics of the CR system.

If a conventional screen/film combination system was used, exposure on example I in Figure 4.4 would utilize only the higher optical density region of the film, whereas in example II the lower region would be used. Neither case would utilize the full dynamic range of the optical density in the film. From these two examples it is seen that the CR system allows the utilization of the full optical density dynamic range, regardless of whether the plate is overexposed or underexposed. The same effect will be achieved if the image recorder is not used to produce a hard copy of the digital image formed from the output signal. That is, the digital image produced from the image reader and the image processor will also utilize the full dynamic range of the 10-bit digital number. The principle of the laser scanner system discussed in Chapter 3 can be applied to the rationalization of these phenomena, as well.

4.1.4 Imaging Plate Reader and Recorder

To extract the latent image from the imaging plate after it has been exposed to X-rays, an imaging plate reader is needed. The principle of the imaging plate reader in the CR system is similar to that of the laser scanner, discussed in Chapter 3. The only difference is that the laser scanner scans an X-ray film, whereas the imaging plate reader

TABLE 4.1 General Specifications of the Imaging Plate Reader and Recorder in a Computed Radiographic System

	Reader	Recorder
Image format, cm^2	43.2 × 35.6	21.4 × 17.6
	35.6 × 35.6	17.6 × 17.6
	30.5 × 25.4	20.1 × 16.7
	20.3 × 25.4	20.0 × 25.1
Sampling raster, pixels/mm	5–10	10
Laser spot size, μm	100	120
Gray levels	10 bits (A/D)	10 bits (D/A)
Speed, s	90 (for 43.2 cm × 35.6 cm)	90 (for 21.4 cm × 17.6 cm)
Laser power, mW	15	0.1

scans the plate. After the scanning, a light image is formed that can be either recorded on film or displayed on a video monitor. In the case of recording on film, a laser recorder is used which operates almost identically to a conventional laser printer for other imaging modalities; the digital image is written onto a single emulsion film. For direct display on a video monitor, soft copy display technology is needed. The details of both types of display are discussed in Chapter 12.

Table 4.1 shows the specifications of the image reader and the recorder. In general, the size of the digital image generated by the imaging plate reader is 2000 × 2000 × 10 bits or higher, depending on the size of the film and the sampling raster. Note that due to various sizes of IP, the dimensions of a CR image are also variable. For convenience, we generally say that a CR image is 2K. Upon comparison of Tables 3.1, 4.1, and 12.5, the similarities between the characteristics of the laser scanner and the image reader, and the laser printer and the image recorder, are quite evident.

4.1.5 Some Clinical Applications

The CR system is an excellent method of converting conventional projectional radiographic images into digital format. It does not require recording the image on film first and later digitizing it through a scanner. Instead, the image is stored as a latent image in the imaging plate, whereupon the laser reader reads the latent image from the plate and converts it into digital form directly. The imaging plate can be erased and reused. Other value-added clinical applications of this system include the following:

1. Since the CR system can automatically adjust for under- or overexposure, acceptable diagnostic images can be produced at exposures that would have provided unacceptable, or at least marginal, radiographs if used with conventional screen/film techniques. This characteristic is important for intensive care units and emergency room applications, since it is often difficult to obtain radiographs of proper exposure in these clinical environments.

2. The large latitude in the digital image allows excellent visualization of both soft tissue and bone detail.
3. Because of the wide dynamic range of the system, it is possible to reduce X-ray dose to patients based on the information required. For example, in a screening procedure (e.g., scoliosis assessment and follow-up of fracture alignment), 5–10% of the conventional dose will produce acceptable images—a substantial benefit to the patient.
4. It is possible to virtually eliminate the need for repeat examinations due to exposure errors, especially for the portable radiographic units. Figure 4.5 shows a series of skull films taken with different exposures comparing the conventional screen/film technique and the CR technique.

4.1.6 CR Background Removal

4.1.6.1 What Is Background Removal?

Under normal operating conditions, images obtained by projection radiography contain unexposed areas due to X-ray collimation: for example, areas outside the circle of the imaging field in digital fluorography (DF), and areas outside the collimator of CR for skeletal and pediatric radiology. In digital images, unexposed areas appearing white on a display monitor will be called background in this context. Figure 4.6 is a pediatric CR image with white background as seen on a monitor. Background removal in this context means that the brightness of the background is converted from white to black.

Three major advantages are gained by performing background removal in digital projection radiography. First, background removal immediately provides lossless data compression, an important cost-effective parameter in digital radiography when one is dealing with large images. Second, a background-removed image has better image visual quality for the following reason: diagnosis from radiography is the result of information processing based on observation with the eye. Since the contrast sensitivity of the eye is proportional to the Weber ratio $\Delta B/B$, where B is brightness of the background and ΔB is the difference in brightness between the region of interest in the image and the background, removing or decreasing the unwanted background in projection radiography images makes these images more easily readable and greatly improves their diagnostic effects. Once the background in a digital projectional radiograph has been removed (e.g., in CR), the radiologist can assign to the image a more representative lookup table (see Section 12.3.2.2), pertinent to only the range of gray scales in the image, not the background. Thus, it can improve the visual quality of the images. Third, in portable CR, it is often difficult to examine injured or weakened patients in an anatomical position aligned with the standard image orientation for reading. As a result, the orientation of the image during reading may need to be adjusted. In film interpretation, it is easy to rotate or flip the film. But in soft copy display, sophisticated software programs are needed to automatically recognize that such adjustments are necessary, and to correct the orientation of the digital image. These software algorithms often fail if the background of the image is not re-

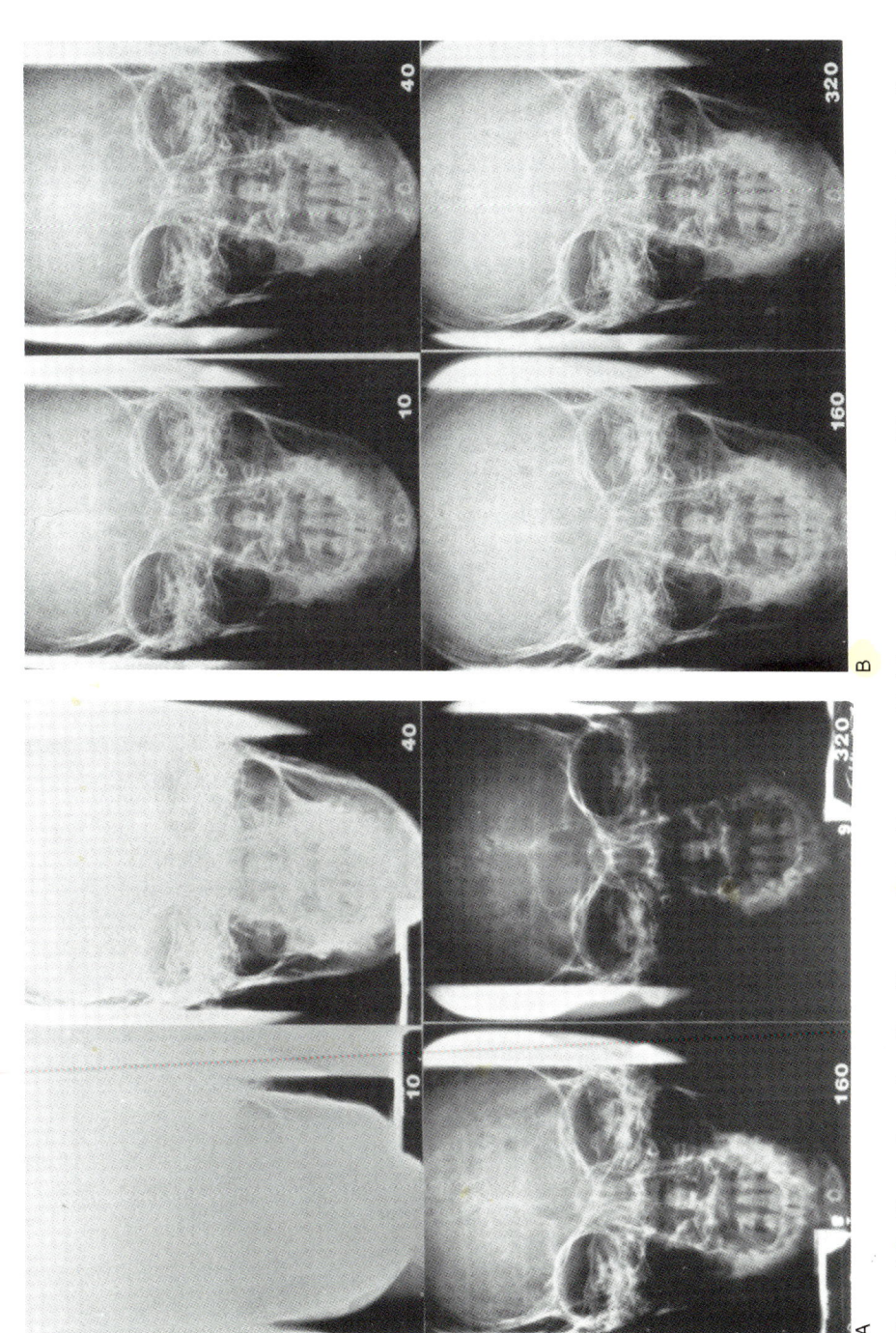

Figure 4.5 Comparison of quality of images obtained by means of (A) the conventional screen/film method and (B) CR techniques. Exposures were 70 kVp and 10, 40, 160, and 320 mAs on a skull phantom. In this example, the CR technique is almost dose independent. (Courtesy of Dr. S. Balter.)

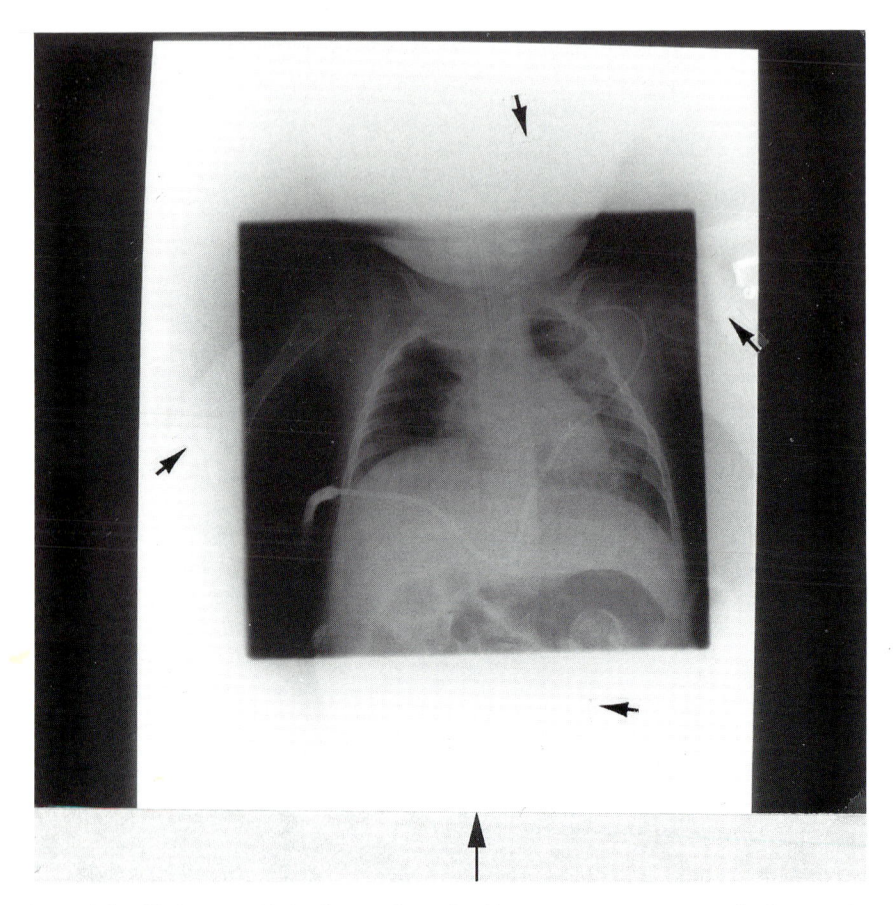

Figure 4.6 CR image with background, marked by arrows as seen on a display monitor. Three regions are visible: the image, the background, and the black screen, which is the result of a small image on a large display surface.

moved. A background-removed image will improve the successful rate of automatic image orientation. Thus background removal is a crucial preprocessing step in computer-aided detection, and diagnosis (CAD). A background-removed image can improve the diagnostic accuracy of CAD algorithms, since the cost functions in the algorithms can be assigned to the image only rather than to the image and its background combined.

In the cases of digital fluorography and the film digitizer, the background removal procedure is straightforward. In the former, since the size of the image field is a predetermined parameter, the background can be removed by converting every pixel outside the diameter of the image field to black. In the latter, since the digital image is obtained in a two-step procedure (first a film is obtained, then it is digitized), the boundaries between the background and the exposed area can be determined interactively by the user, and the corner points may be input during the digitizing step.

```
┌─────────────────────────────────────────────┐
│ Analysis of intensity distribution of CR image │
│                 background                  │
└─────────────────────────────────────────────┘
                      ↓
┌─────────────────────────────────────────────┐
│ Statistical description of CR image background signals │
└─────────────────────────────────────────────┘
                      ↓
┌─────────────────────────────────────────────┐
│ Sampling, filtering, and lock-in angle of background │
│                edge signals                 │
└─────────────────────────────────────────────┘
                      ↓
┌─────────────────────────────────────────────┐
│ Adaptive adjustment of threshold parameters based on │
│   statistical description of CR image background    │
└─────────────────────────────────────────────┘
                      ↓
┌─────────────────────────────────────────────┐
│ Reliable estimation of CR image background removal │
└─────────────────────────────────────────────┘
```

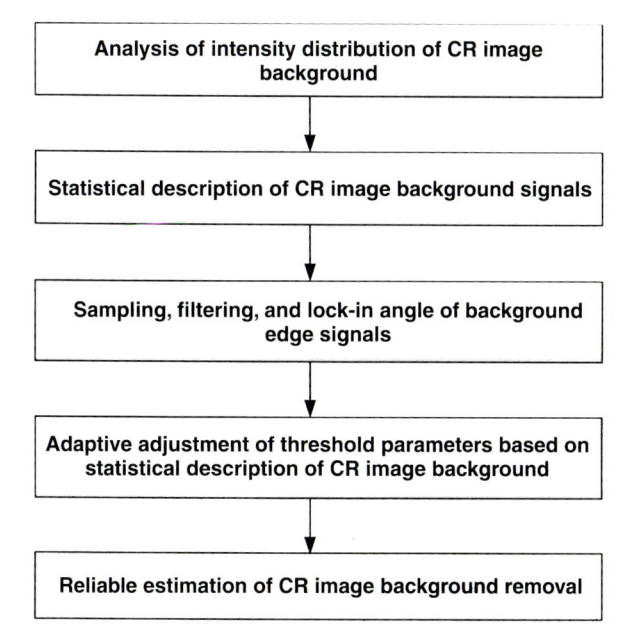

Figure 4.7 Block diagram of the background recognition and removal procedure developed by Zhang.

Background removal is a more complex procedure in the case of CR, since it has to be done automatically during image acquisition or preprocessing time. Automatic removal of CR background is difficult because the algorithm has to recognize different body part contours as well as various collimator sizes and shapes. Since the background distribution in CR images is complex and removal is irreversible, it is difficult to achieve a high ratio of full background removal and yet ensure that no valid information is removed from the image. Earlier methods to remove the background of CR images can achieve only 42% background removal. One of the better methods, developed by J. Zhang (1997b), is based on a statistical description of the intensity distribution of the CR background, signal processing, and consistent and reliable estimations of background removal operations. Figure 4.7 is a block diagram of the background recognition and removal procedures. With this method implemented in the CR preprocessing unit, very high ratios of full background removal without deleting valid information from the image is possible.

4.1.6.2 *Examples of CR Images After Background Removal*

Figures 4.8 to 4.11 show examples of CR images before and after the application of Zhang's automatic background removal method. The characteristic of Figure 4.8 is that there are more than two edges on the right side of the original image; Figure 4.9 shows that the odd-shaped abdominal collimator is on the bottom side; Figure 4.10 shows that there are anatomical structures on both sides of the background of an elon-

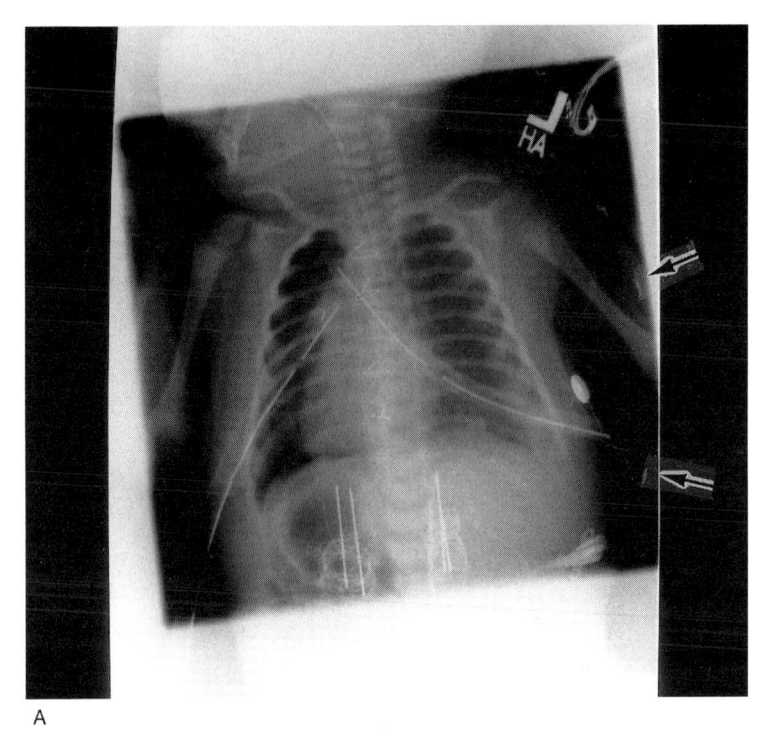

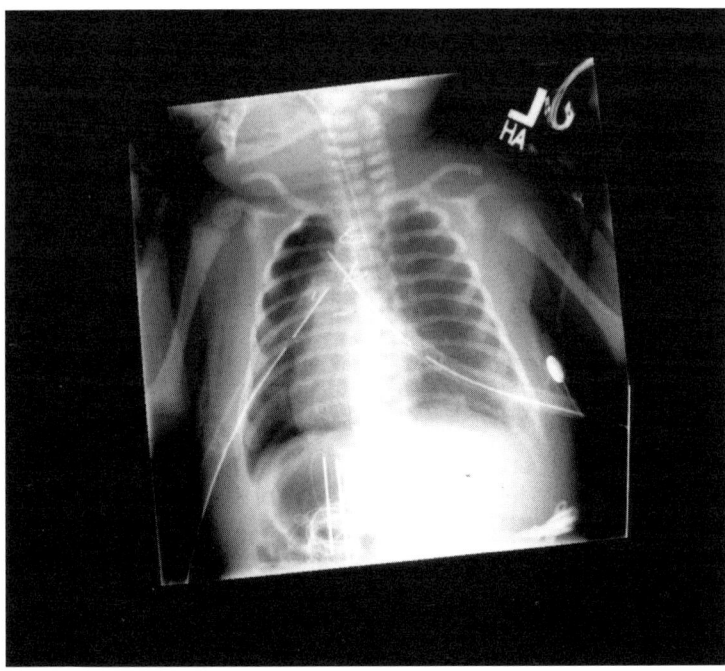

Figure 4.8 (A) Original image and (B) background-removed image. Characteristics: more than two edges on the right side, marked by arrows.

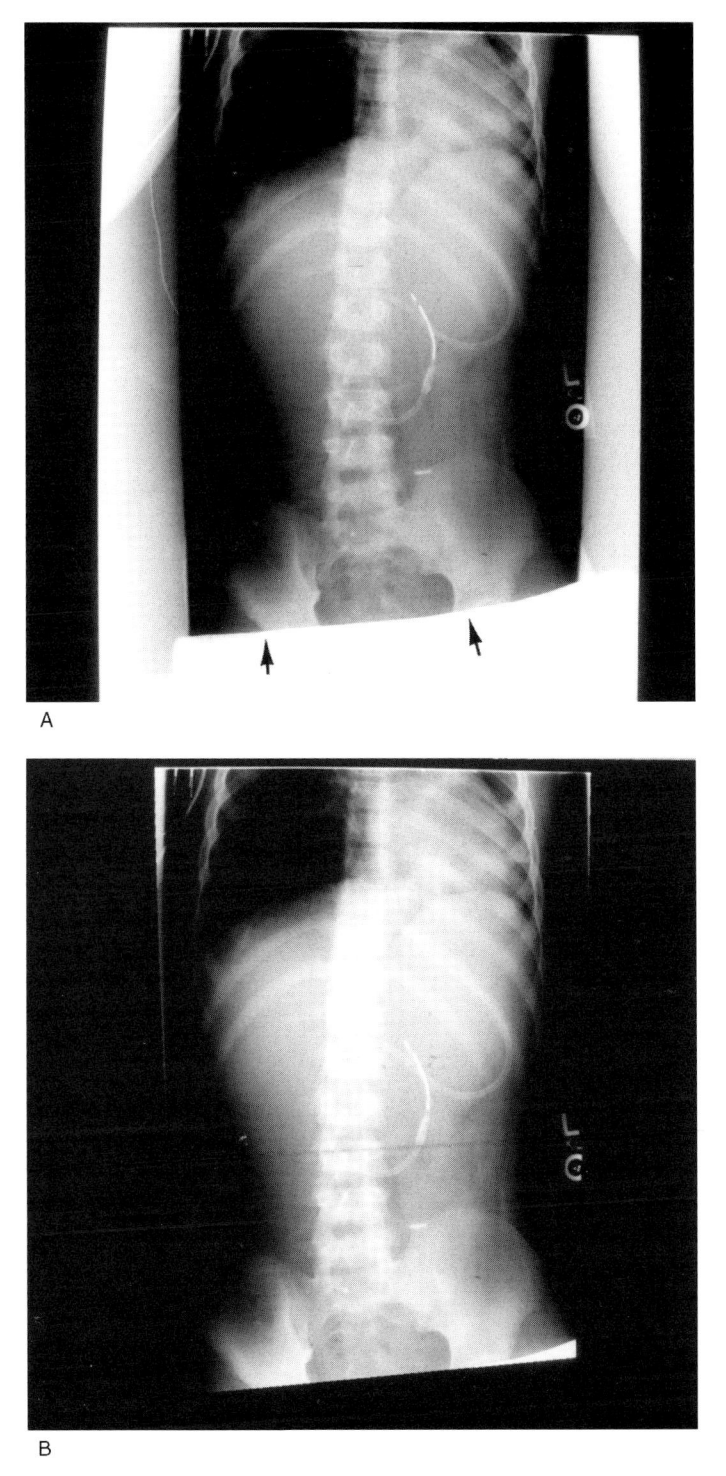

Figure 4.9 (A) Original image and (B) background-removed image. Characteristics: an odd-shaped abdominal collimator, marked by arrows.

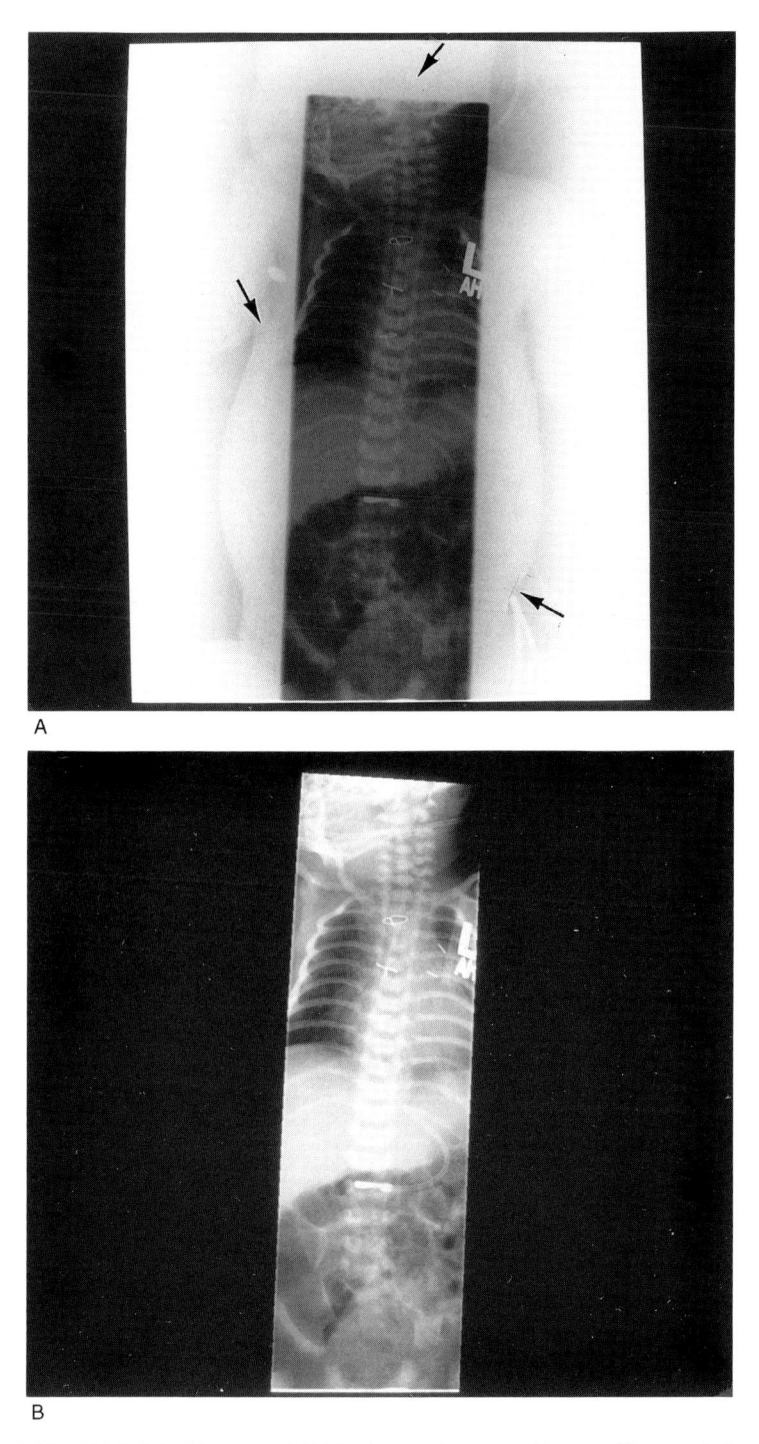

Figure 4.10 (A) Original image and (B) background-removed image. Characteristics: a longitudinal collimator. Background shows anatomical structures, marked by arrows.

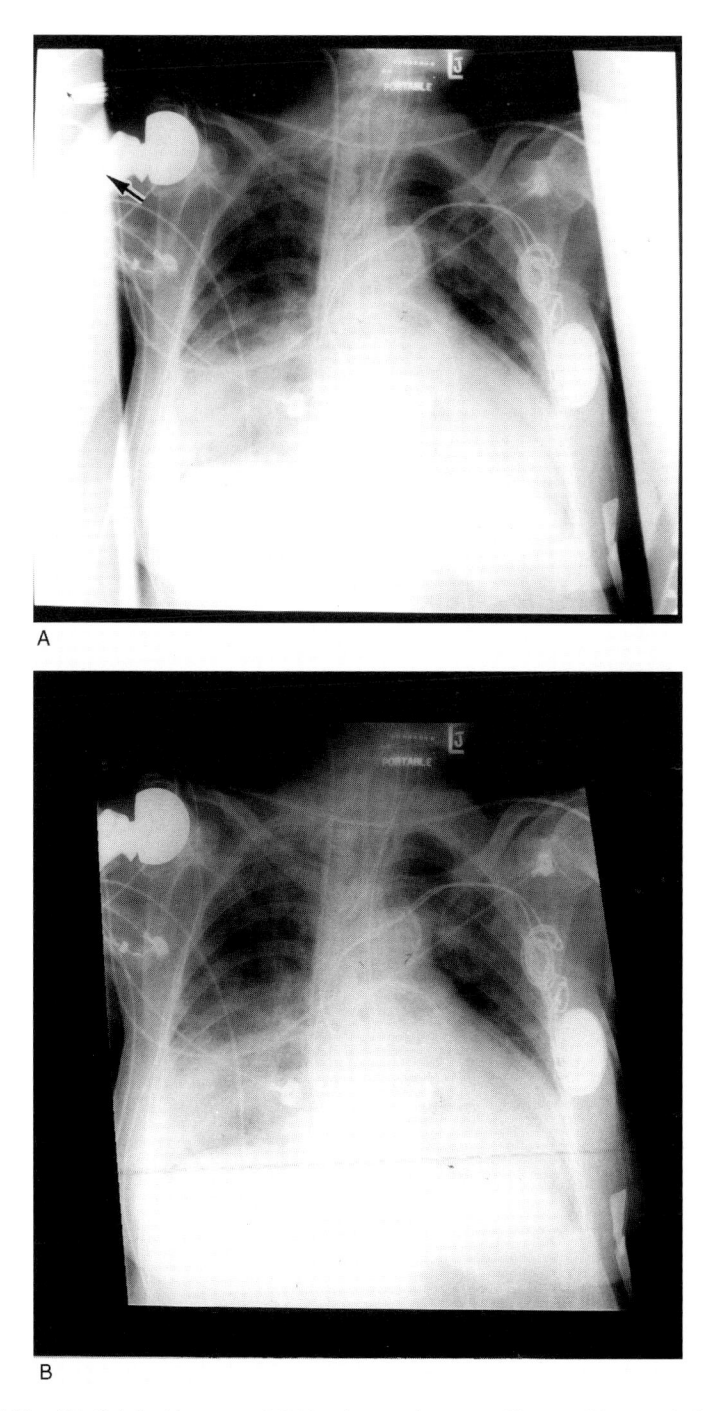

Figure 4.11 (A) Original image and (B) background-removed image. Characteristics: a prosthetic device at the left side of the image, marked by arrow.

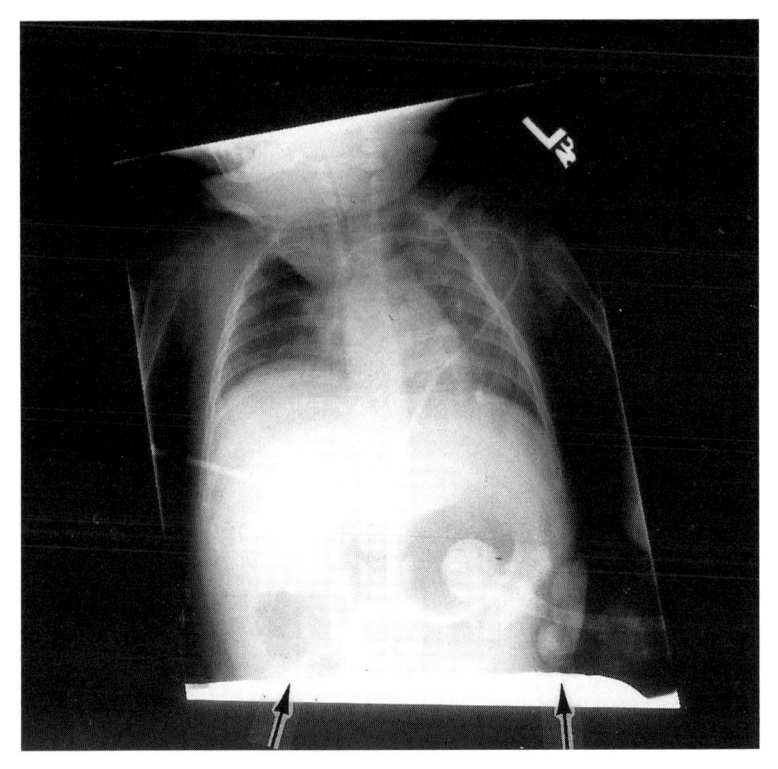

Figure 4.12 CR image with an odd-shaped abdominal collimator, marked by arrows; only partial background was removed from the image.

gated pediatric spine CR image; and Figure 4.11 shows a prosthetic device at the left. These images reveal that the visual contrast of the background-removed images (Fig. 4.11b) is much better than that of the original images (Fig. 4.11a) because a higher portion of each histogram is shifted after background removal, which renders a better lookup table determination. Also, image sizes are reduced without loss of image information.

As a test of its accuracy, the method was implemented in a clinical PACS at the University of California, San Francisco. Three hundred thirty consecutive intensive care unit CR images were used as the sample over a period of 5 days, of which 246 had background and 84 did not. The evaluation of this method using this sample was based on the following measures: (1) correct recognition of background; (2) full background removal (see Figs. 4.8–4.11); (3) partial background removal (see Fig. 4.12, bottom); (4) little or no background removal (see Fig. 4.13); and (5) removal of valid image data.

Table 4.2 summarizes the evaluation of Zhang's background removal method as applied to these images: background recognition was 99% correct. In this sample set, the algorithm achieves 91, 8.8, and 0.2% full, partial and no background removal, respectively. Most importantly, no valid data were removed from any of these images.

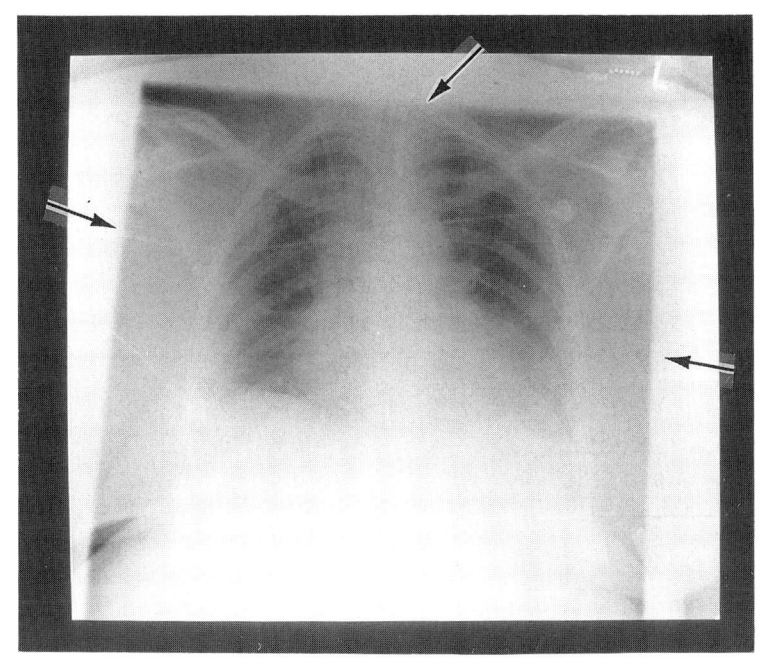

Figure 4.13 CR image with no background removal due to nondistinct separation between the image and background pixels; background remains marked by arrows.

The table also shows that the percentage of full background removal is less than that of correct recognition. This means that even though the recognition is correct, several built-in checking mechanisms prevent the removal of background with certain degrees of uncertainty. These mechanisms safeguard the irreversible process of deleting valid image data, and provide a trade-off between sensitivity and specificity.

Automatic removal from CR images of background due to X-ray collimation during projection radiographic examinations is a very important step in effectively displaying CR images with soft copy. A good method must correctly recognize background signals in CR images, provide a very high ratio of full background removal, and guarantee that no valid image information will be removed from the operation

TABLE 4.2 Measure of Success of the Automatic Background (BKGD) Recognition and Removal Algorithm*

Evaluative Measure			Cases (%)
Recognition of BKGD	243 (BKGD)	87 (no BKGD)	99.0%
Full removal	223		91.0%
Partial removal	21		8.8%
No Removal	2		0.2%
Removal of valid information	0		0.0%

*Total images = 330; with BKGD = 246, no BKGD = 84.

even with asymmetrical and complex background signals. There are at least four immediate benefits to CR images after they have been processed with automatic background removal: (1) the visual quality perceived by the eye in reading these processed images can be improved greatly; (2) the background-removed images offer immediate lossless data compression; (3) automatic orientation algorithms will perform better on images with background removed; and (4) the processed images facilitate some computer-aided diagnosis methods applied to digital projection radiography. Automatic background removal is an important step toward the implementation of a successful soft copy display of CR in PACS. In addition, background removal can be used in digital radiography as described in Sections 4.4 and 4.5.

4.2 DIGITAL FLUOROGRAPHY

Digital fluorography (DF) is another method that can produce a digital X-ray image without substantial changes in the radiographic procedure room. This technique requires an add-on unit in the conventional fluorographic system.

Recall that fluorography is the procedure of displaying fluoroscopic images on a video monitor by means of an image intensifier coupling with a video camera (see Section 3.2.1). This technique is used to visualize motion inside body compartments (e.g., blood flow, heart beat), and the movement of a catheter during an intervention procedure, as well as to pinpoint a body region for making a film image for subsequent detailed diagnosis. Each exposure required in a fluorographic procedure is very minimal compared with a conventional X-ray procedure.

Digital fluorography is considered to be an add-on system because a digital chain is added to an existing fluorographic unit. This method utilizes the established X-ray tube assembly, image intensifier, video scanning, and digital technologies. The output from a digital fluorographic system is a sequence of digital images displayed on a video monitor.

Digital fluorography has an advantage over conventional fluorography in that it gives a larger dynamic range image and can remove uninteresting structures in the images by performing digital subtraction.

When image processing is introduced to the digital fluorographic system, dependent on the application, other names are used: digital subtraction angiography (DSA), digital subtraction arteriography (DSA), digital video angiography (DVA), intravenous video arteriography (IVA), computerized fluoroscopy (CF), and digital video subtraction angiography (DVSA) are examples.

4.2.1 Description of System Components

A complete digital fluorographic system consists of four major components; the numbered items in the list that follows correspond to numbered areas in Figure 4.14.

1. *X-ray source.* The X-ray tube itself and a grid to minimize the scattering were described in Section 3.1.1. The X-ray source also includes a collimator.

DIGITAL FLUOROGRAPHY   81

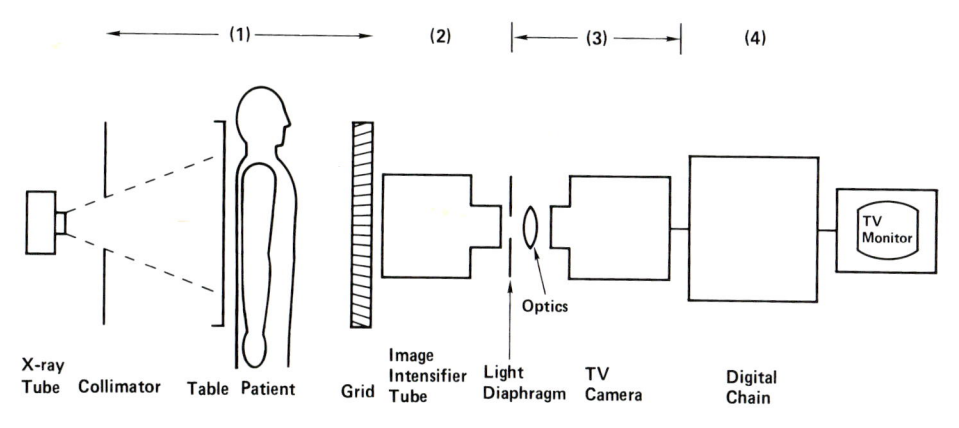

Figure 4.14 Schematic of a digital fluorographic system; see text for key to numbers.

2. *Image receptor.* The image receptor used in a digital fluorographic system is an image intensifier tube; its functions was described in Section 3.1.2.2.
3. *Video camera plus optical system.* The light from the image intensifier goes through an optical system, which allows the video camera to be adjusted for focusing. The amount of light going into the camera is controlled by means of a

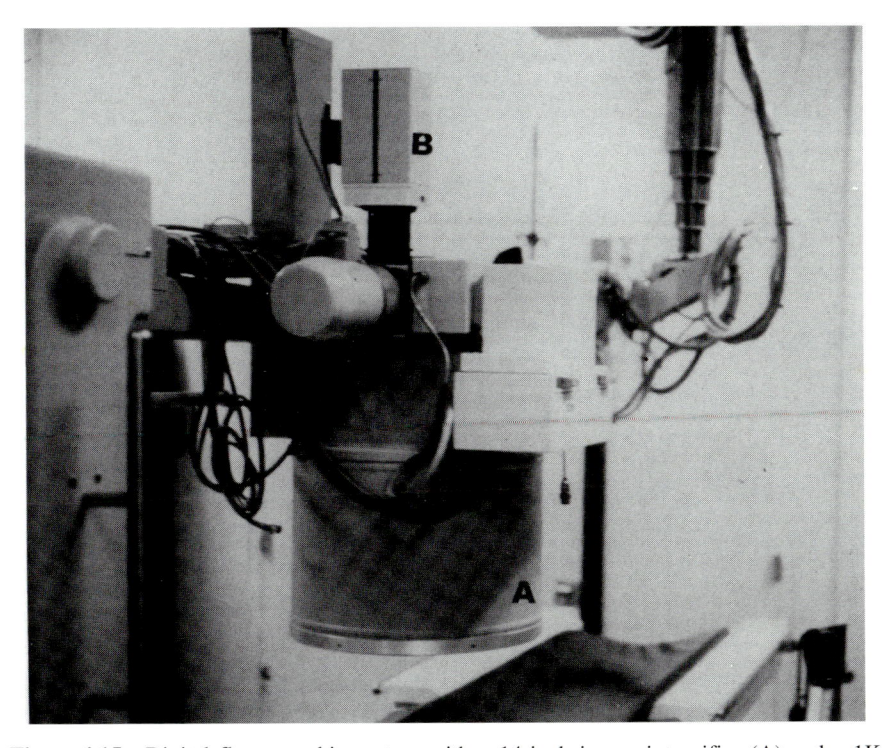

Figure 4.15 Digital fluorographic system with a 14-inch image intensifier (A) and a 1K plumbicon camera attached to a digital chain (B).

TABLE 4.3 Spatial Resolution of a Digital Fluorographic System Without Geometric Magnification

Image Intensifier Mode (in.)	Image Intensifier Resolution (lp/mm)	Nyquist Resolution Limitation for DSA (lp/mm)		Measured Resolution (lp/mm)	
		512 System	1024 System	512 System	1024 System
14				0.85	0.90
9	3	1.1	2.2		
6	4	1.5	3.0	1.5	1.75
4.5	5	2.1	4.2		

light diaphragm. The operating procedure of the TV camera was described in Section 3.2.1. The type of camera used in digital fluorography is usually a plumbicon or a CCD. The scanning mechanism can either be interlaced or progressive, and the camera matrix size can be from 512 to 1024 pixels per line.

4. *Digital chain.* The add-on unit is the digital chain, which consists of an A/D converter, image memories, image processor, digital storage, and video display. The A/D converter, the image memory, and the digital storage can handle 512 × 512 × 8 bit images at 30 frames per second, or 1024 × 1024 × 8 bit images at 7.5 frames per second. Sometime the redundant array of inexpensive disks (RAID) configuration is used to handle such a high speed data transfer. Figure 4.15 illustrates a digital fluorographic system showing a 14-inch image intensifier and a plumbicon camera. Table 4.3 gives the spatial resolution limitations and some typical parameters of a DF unit. As this table indicates, the spatial resolution of the DF is limited by the size of the digital image, not by the image intensifier tube.

4.2.2 Operational Procedure

A digital fluorography imaging session proceeds as follows.

1. The patient is positioned according to conventional fluorographic procedure.
2. Mask images without contrast material injection are taken.
3. An intravenous or intra-arterial bolus injection of a contrast medium is administered, either manually or through a power injector.
4. The X-ray source is turned on and sequential digital images are obtained with the proper imaging mode.
5. Selected sequential images in a bolus injection cycle are stored in the digital disk for future review and process.
6. Another bolus injection is administered if necessary, and the cycle is repeated.
7. The result is a sequence (or sequences) of digital images showing the contrast medium flowing through a region of interest.

8. Any such sequence of images can be enhanced with the mask images through digital subtraction.

4.3 LOW-SCATTERING DIGITAL RADIOGRAPHIC SYSTEM

Both imaging plate technology and a digital fluorographic system can be run without changing the X-ray source, after only minimal modifications to the image detector system. The low-scattering digital radiographic systems discussed in this section—the line scan and flying-spot scanning technique—require substantial modifications in both the configurations of the X-ray source and the detector system.

4.3.1 Line Scan Technique

In the line scan technique, the X-ray source is first collimated with a lead slit. The linear X-ray beam is transmitted through the patient and detected by a linear detector array (see Fig. 4.16). The collimated X-ray source and the detector array form a functional unit that defines a vertical beam. An image is obtained by moving the unit transversely across the region of interest of the patient. In the direction parallel to the detector array, the sampling distance is defined by the detector-to-detector spacing; while in the direction perpendicular to the detector array, it is determined by the distance between two sets of detector readings. If multiple detector arrays are used in a line providing multiple readings during a transverse scan, then it is called a "slot scan." An example of the line scan technique is the digital mammography system described in Section 4.4.

4.3.2 Flying-Spot Scan Technique

In the flying-spot scan technique (see Fig. 4.17), the X-ray source (a) is first collimated with a slit (b), the slit is further collimated into a pencil beam (d) by a rotating disk with radial slits (c) perpendicular to the beam. The pencil beam scans horizontally from left to right across the patient while the disk rotates, and the attenuation is measured by a system of solid state scintillators and photomultiplier tubes (e). The crystals are large enough to intercept a whole plane of X-rays formed by (b) independent of the rotational position of the disk.

Therefore, regardless of the position of the disk, the detector can measure the X-ray transmission through the slit. The continuous rotation of the disk allows measurements of adjacent points along the same transverse plane. The disk rotates at about 1800 rpm; an independent optical system determines this rotational position as a function of time. The output of the detector as a function of time can then be correlated with the disk's rotational position to give the X-ray transmission as a function position within the X-ray plane. This generates a one-dimensional transverse line through the subject. To generate the second dimension, the X-ray tube, collimator, rotating disk, and detector functioning as a unit translates through to the patient (two arrows in Fig. 4.17). The detector output is then sent to a digital chain to form a digital image.

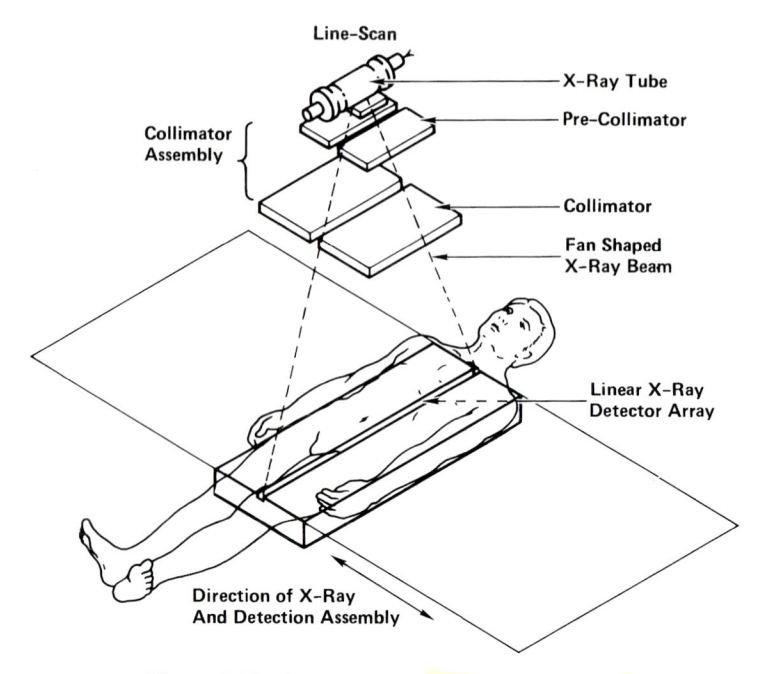

Figure 4.16 Schematic of a line scanning system.

The advantage of flying-spot scanning is the low dosage to the patient (because of the minimal amount of scattering as the X-ray source is collimated to a pencil beam). There are two principal disadvantages. First, the utilization of the X-ray energy is low, since most X-ray photons are blocked by the collimators and, as a result, the X-ray source tends to have a short life. Second, a low signal-to-noise ratio, which is due to the low photon counts per pixel, in turn yields a noisier image.

4.4 FULL-FIELD DIGITAL MAMMOGRAPHY

4.4.1 Screen/Film and Digital Mammography

Breast cancer is the fourth most common cause of death among women in the United States. There is no known means of preventing the disease, and available therapy has been unsuccessful in reducing the national mortality rate over the past 60 years. Current attempts at controlling breast cancer concentrate on early detection by means of mass screening, using periodic mammography and physical examinations, because ample evidence indicates that such screening indeed can be effective in lowering the death rate.

Conventional screen/film mammography has certain technical limitations which reduce its effectiveness: the film gradient must be balanced against the need for wide latitude and detection of microcalcifications. In addition, portrayal of the clarity of

FLYING-SPOT SCAN

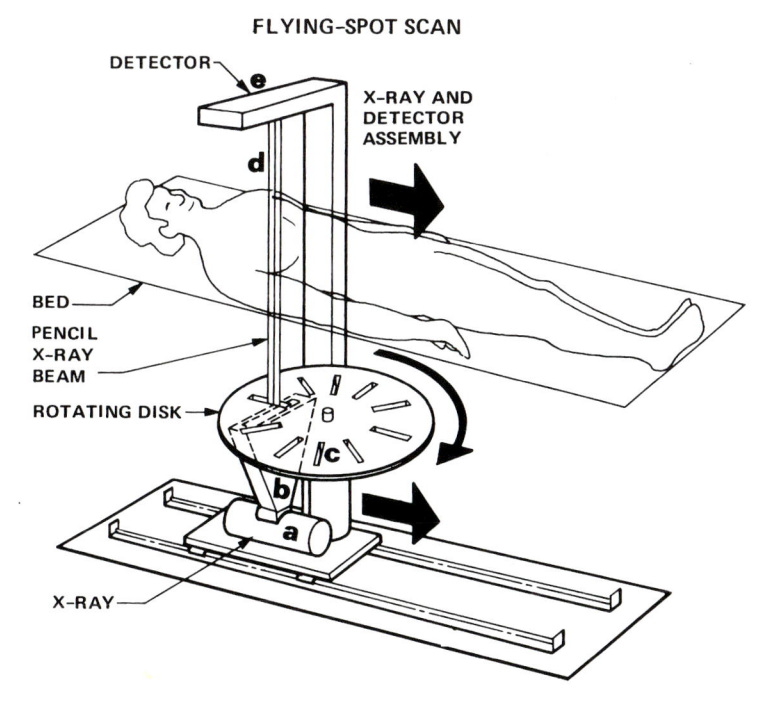

Figure 4.17 Schematic of a flying-spot scanning system.

the margins of breast masses is reduced because of the presence of film noise in the image, film processing artifacts can degrade the mammographic image, and the day-to-day variability inherent in automated film processors can produce suboptimal image quality. Digital mammography is a method of alleviating some of these limitations.

Early digital mammography applications acquired data by digitizing conventional mammography films according to the procedure described in Section 3.2.2. This approach severely limited the potential of digital mammography, since the resultant images contained no more radiographic information than the standard films from which they were produced. Indeed, currently most digitized images are slightly inferior in quality to their corresponding parent films, accounting in no small part for the general lack of clinical acceptance of digital mammography applications.

Digital mammography can overcome most of these problems, at the same time providing additional features not available with standard mammographic imaging such as contrast enhancement, digital archiving, and computer-aided diagnosis. In addition, applications of real-time telemammography add to these advantages the utilization of expert mammographers (rather than general radiologists) to interpret mammography examinations. During the past several years, as a result of concentrated efforts by the National Cancer Institute and the U.S. Army Medical Research and Material Command, some prototype digital mammography systems were developed in joint efforts by academic institutions and private industry. Some of these systems are ready for clinical evaluation. In the next section we describe the principle of digital mammography, a very critical component in a totally digital imaging system.

4.4.2 Full-Field Digital Mammography (FFDM)

Currently, four major manufacturers are developing full-field digital mammography systems: Trex (formerly Bennett and Lorad, Danbury, CT), General Electric Medical Systems (Milwaukee, WI), Fischer Imaging Company (Denver, CO), and Planmed (Finland). The Senoscan, developed by Fischer Imaging Company, is used for the discussion here not because of its superiority over the others, but because of our experience with the system.

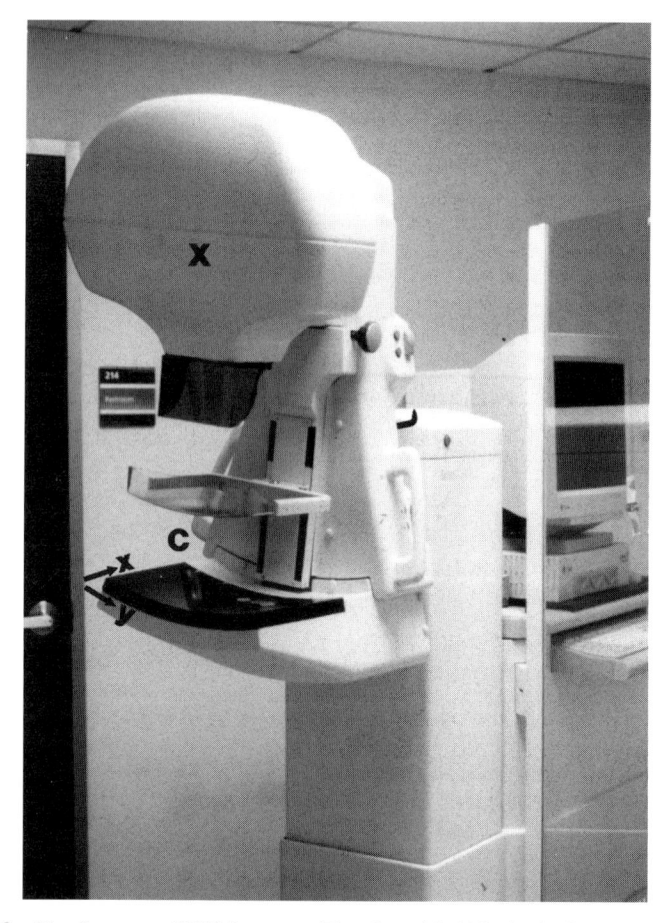

Figure 4.18 The Senoscan FFDM system. The slot with 300 pixel width covers the x axis (4400 pixels); the X-ray beam sweeps (arrow) in the y direction, producing over 5500 pixels. X, X-ray and collimator housing; C, compressor.

4.4.2.1 Slot-Scanning FFDM Technology

The imaging principle of the Senoscan FFDM system is similar to conventional mammography systems. They all utilize X-rays to expose a patient's breast, employ a Bucky device to support the breast, and all incorporate a detector system into the Bucky to record the mammogram. However, they differ mainly in two aspects: the scanning mechanism and the detector system. In a conventional system, a patient's entire breast is exposed to X-rays concurrently and the latent image is detected by a screen/film cassette, which is contained in the Bucky. Unlike conventional mammography systems, the Senoscan uses a slot-scanning technology in which a breast is scanned by an X-ray fan beam and the image is recorded by a charged-couple device camera encompassed in the Bucky. Figure 4.18 shows a picture of the Senoscan FFDM system. The scanning mechanism is very similar to that shown in Figure 4.16.

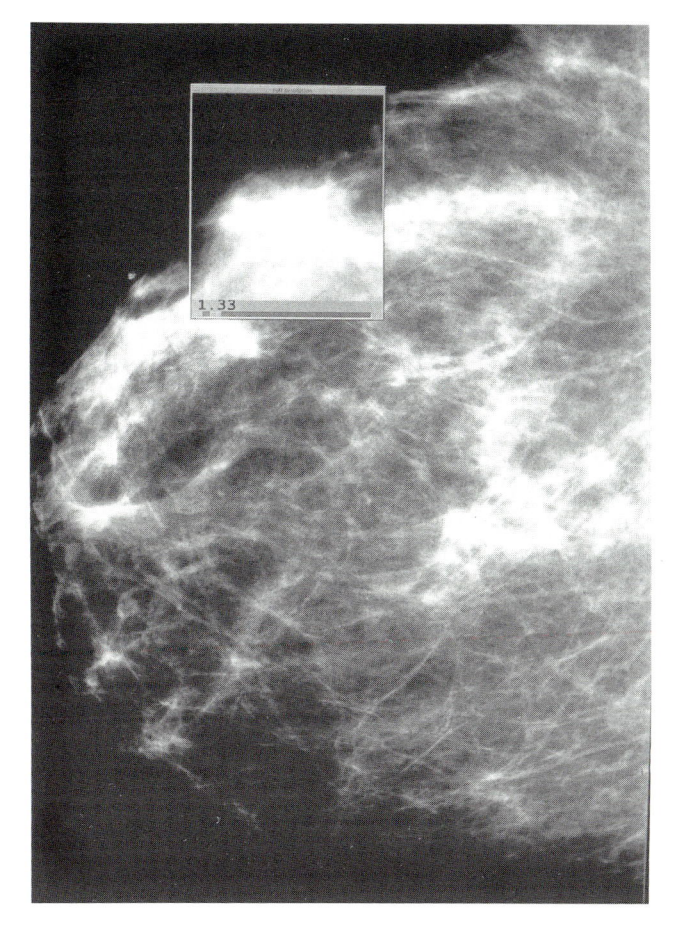

Figure 4.19 Digital mammogram (4K × 5K × 12 bit) obtained with the Senoscan FFDDM shown on a 2K × 2.5K monitor . The window at the upper part of the image is the magnified glass showing a true 4K × 5K region. (Courtesy of Drs. E. Sickles and S.L. Lou.)

The X-ray photons emitted from the X-ray tube are shaped by a collimator to become a fan beam. The width of the fan beam covers one dimension of the image area (e.g., x axis), and the fan beam sweeps in the other direction (y axis). The movement of the detector system is synchronous with the scan of the fan beam.

The detector system of the FFDM is composed of a thin phosphor screen coupled with four CCD detector arrays via a tapered fiber-optic bundle. Each CCD array is composed of four 1100 × 300 CCD cells. The gap between any two adjacent CCD arrays is only one pixel wide, a design feature that simplifies the task of butting the gap. The phosphor screen converts the penetrated X-ray photons (i.e., the latent image) to light photons. The light photons pass through the fiber-optic bundle, reach the CCD cells, and then are transformed to electrical signals. The more light photons received by each CCD cell, the larger the signal transformed. The electrical signals are quantized by an analog-to-digital converter to create a digital image. Finally, the image pixels travel through a data channel into the system memory of the FFDM acquisition computer. Figure 4.19 shows a 4K × 5K × 12 bit digital mammogram obtained with the Senoscan system.

4.4.2.2 FFDM Imaging Characteristics

Conventional mammography utilizes an adjustable scatter-reduced Bucky device, whereas the FFDM uses a fixed-size Bucky. The size of the Bucky device in a conventional mammography system can be from 18×24 cm^2 to 24×30 cm^2, adjustable depending on the patient's breast size. However, the Bucky size of the Senoscan FFDM system is fixed with an image area of 24×30 cm^2, to accommodate large breast sizes. For a pixel size of 54×54 μm^2 at the phosphor screen, the FFDM system generates an image matrix of 4096×5625 square pixels. This spatial resolution is equivalent to approximately 9 line pairs per millimeter. For each pixel, the gray level ranges from 0 to 4095 (i.e., 12-bit), where gray level 0 is black and 4095 is white.

Table 4.4 summarizes the imaging specifications of the Senoscan FFDM system.

TABLE 4.4 Specifications of the Senoscan FFDM System

Image area	240×300 mm^2
Detector	Charge-coupled devices
Image scan time	Slot scan, 4.5 seconds (nominal)
kV Range	25–50 kVp
Tube current	200 mA at 45 kVp
Focal spot size	0.30 mm (nominal)
Pixel Size	Nominal mode: 54×54 μm^2; high resolution: 27×27 μm^2
Image matrix	$4,096 \times 5,625$ pixels (nominal), 12 bits/pixel
Spatial Resolution	9 lp/mm (nominal), 18 lp/mm (high resolution)
Detective quantum efficiency	$\leq 50\%$ at $f(0)$
Scatter-to-primary ratio	$\leq 0.15\%$

The digital mammography system generates an image of 40 MByte, and an examination normally requires four images totaling 160 MBytes (see Table 2.1). To handle such a large image file requires innovative technologies for image display, communication, and storage. These topics are discussed in later chapters.

4.5 RECENT ADVANCES IN DIGITAL RADIOGRAPHY

Since 70% of radiological procedures still rely on projection radiography, new methods of digital image capture are needed to achieve a digital-based operation in the medical center. These systems should produce digital images of high quality and deliver low dosages to patients; they should be easily operated, compact in size, and able to offer competitive cost savings to conventional screen/film system. During the past several years, major X-ray equipment companies have devoted efforts to develop new digital radiography systems, in particular, in flat panel detectors.

Let us first revisit the three methods of obtaining a digital radiograph, the areal, the line (or slot) scan, and the flying-spot mode. Computed radiography and digital fluorography, two prevailing methods of obtaining digital images without using a film digitizer, use the areal mode. The digital mammography system, using a slot scanning mode described in Section 4.4, is a prototype system being clinically evaluated. All these systems have one commonality: they use the indirect image capture method. In this technology, attenuated X-ray photons are first converted to light photons by the phosphor or scintillator, and the light photons are converted to electrical signals from which the image is formed.

There is another method, called direct image capture, which can generate a digital image without going through the light photon conversion process. Figure 4.20 shows the difference between the direct and the indirect digital capture methods. The advantage of the former is that it eliminates the intermediate step of light photon conversion. The engineering involved in direct digital capture is tremendous, however, and it is difficult to use the detector for dynamic image capture because the detector has to be recharged after each readout.

In the areal scan method, the current technology being pursued relies on flat-panel sensors, either amorphous silicon (scintillator or phosphor) panels, or selenium-based semiconductor detectors. The flat panel can be one large or several smaller panels butted together. The amorphous silicon panel uses the indirect capture method, whereas the amorphous selenium panel uses direct capture. Examples of the amorphous silicon panels are the systems being developed by Trixell (a consortium among Siemens, Philips, and Thomson) for chest radiography and fluoroscopy; and the GE detector system for mammography, radiography, and fluoroscopy applications. Examples of semiconductor detectors using amorphous selenium are Sterling's system for direct digital radiography and the modified Trex Medical system for real-time fluoroscopy. It appears that the direct capture method, which eliminates an intermediate step of light photon conversion, has the advantage over the indirect capture method. However, because of engineering difficulties, it may be several years before com-

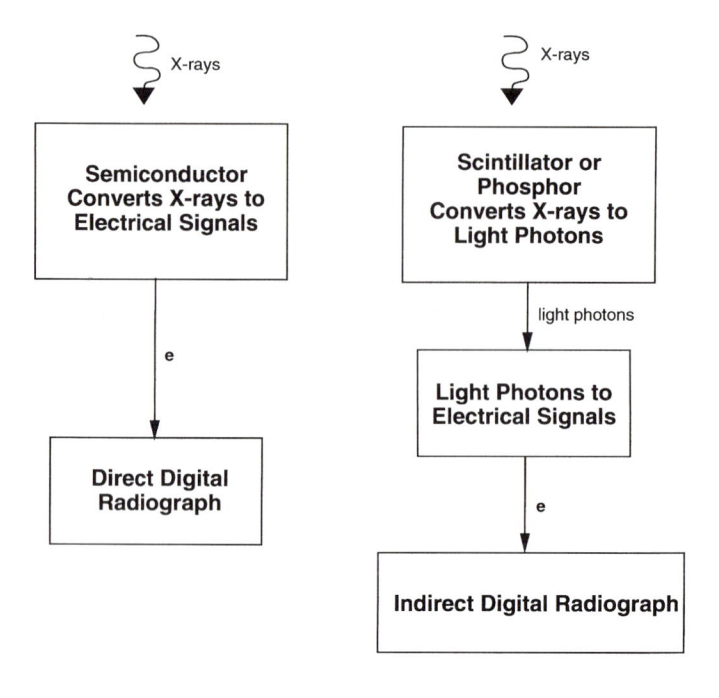

DIGITAL RADIOGRAPHY

```
         X-rays                                X-rays
           │                                     │
           ▼                                     ▼
  ┌──────────────────┐               ┌──────────────────┐
  │  Semiconductor   │               │  Scintillator or │
  │ Converts X-rays to│              │     Phosphor     │
  │ Electrical Signals│              │ Converts X-rays to│
  └──────────────────┘               │   Light Photons  │
           │                         └──────────────────┘
           │ e                                 │ light photons
           │                                   ▼
           │                         ┌──────────────────┐
           │                         │  Light Photons to│
           │                         │ Electrical Signals│
           │                         └──────────────────┘
           ▼                                   │ e
  ┌──────────────────┐                         ▼
  │  Direct Digital  │               ┌──────────────────┐
  │    Radiograph    │               │Indirect Digital Radiograph│
  └──────────────────┘               └──────────────────┘

  A. Direct Digital Radiography    B. Indirect Digital Radiography
```

Figure 4.20 Direct and indirect image capture methods.

mercial products based on direct capture will be available for clinical use. The areal scan method has the advantage of being fast in image capture, but it also has two disadvantages: the high X-ray scatter, as described earlier, and the difficulty of manufacturing the flat panels. The supply base for radiologic flat panels is limited to several companies, which can create a slow production cycle.

CHAPTER 5

Computed Tomography, Magnetic Resonance, Ultrasound, Nuclear Medicine, and Microscopic Imaging

This chapter considers medical images acquired and presented in digital format: X-ray computed tomography (CT), magnetic resonance imaging (MRI), ultrasound (US) imaging, single photon and positron emission computed tomography (ECT and PET), and digital microscopic imaging. Computed tomography and magnetic resonance imaging, introduced in the early 1970s and 1980s, respectively, are now standard diagnostic imaging techniques. The ultrasound scanner was originally an analog imaging device, but digital technology has become an integral part of the instrumentation, and US images are now rendered in digital format. ECT and PET use tomographic techniques similar to those required for XCT, but the energy sources used are different. Digital microscopy, a prerequisite for telepathology and telemedicine applications, provides quantitative data from microscopic slides.

5.1 IMAGE RECONSTRUCTION FROM PROJECTIONS

Most sectional images, like MR and CT, are generated based on image reconstruction from projections. For this reason, we will summarize the Fourier projection theorem, the algebraic reconstruction, and the filtered back-projection method before discussing imaging modalities.

5.1.1 The Fourier Projection Theorem

Let $f(x,y)$ be a two-dimensional cross-sectional image of a three-dimensional object. The image reconstruction theorem states that $f(x,y)$ can be reconstructed from the cross-sectional one-dimensional projections. In general, 180 different projections in one-degree increments are necessary to produce a satisfactory image, and using more projections always results in a better reconstructed image.

Mathematically, the image reconstruction theorem can be described with the help of the Fourier transform (FT) discussed in Section 2.4. Let $f(x,y)$ represent the two-dimensional image to be reconstructed and let $p(x)$ be the one-dimensional projection of $f(x,y)$ onto the horizontal axis, which can be measured experimentally (see Fig. 5.1,

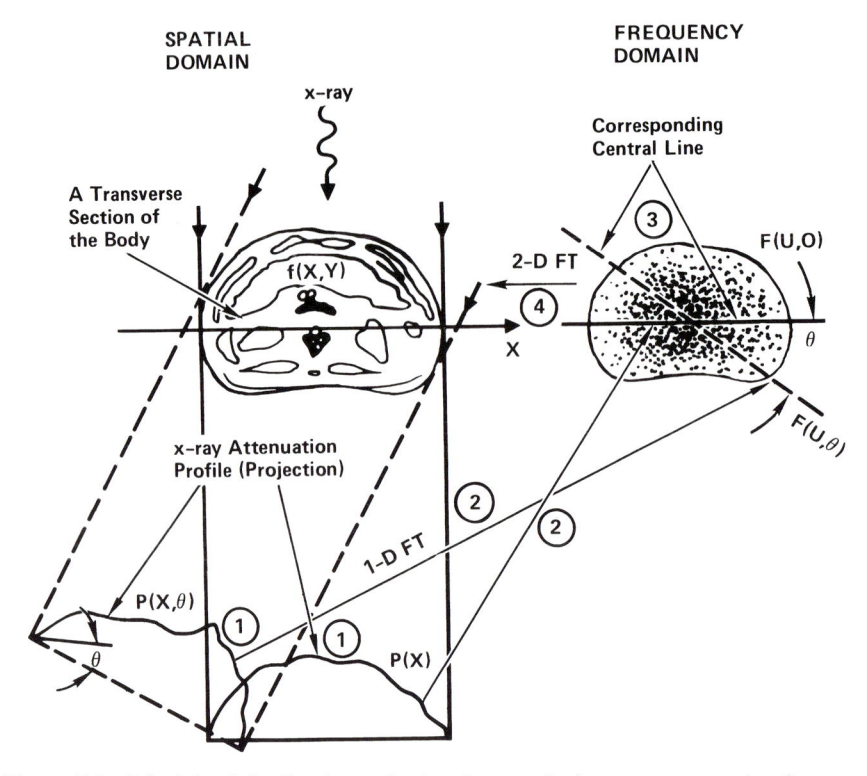

Figure 5.1 Principle of the Fourier projection theorem for image reconstruction from projections. The numerals represent the steps described in the text.

the zero-degree projection). In the case of X-ray CT, we can consider $p(x)$ to be the total linear attenuation of tissues transverses by a collimated X-ray beam at location x. Then

$$p(x,0) = \int_{-\infty}^{+\infty} f(x,y)dy \tag{5.1}$$

The 1-D Fourier transform of $p(x)$ has the form

$$P(u) = \int_{-\infty}^{+\infty} \left(\int_{-\infty}^{+\infty} f(x,y)dy \right) \exp(-i2\pi ux)\,dx \tag{5.2}$$

Equations (5.1) and (5.2) imply that the 1-D Fourier transform of a one-dimensional projection of a two-dimensional image is identical to the corresponding central section of the two-dimensional Fourier transform of the object. For example, the two-dimensional image can be a transverse (cross-) sectional X-ray image of the body, and the one-dimensional projections can be the X-ray attenuation profiles (projection) of

IMAGE RECONSTRUCTION FROM PROJECTIONS   93

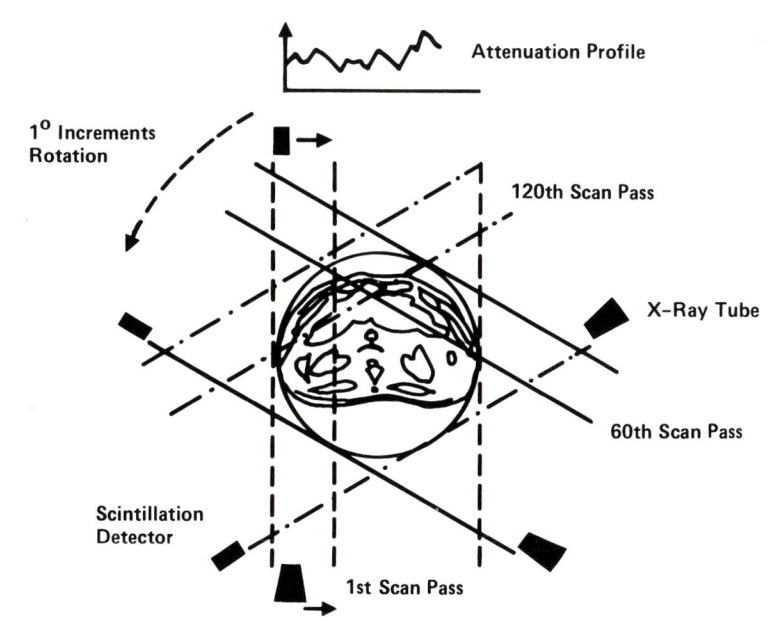

Figure 5.2 Schematic of the translation and rotation scanning mode using a pencil-thin collimated X-ray beam. During each scan pass, an X-ray attenuation profile is generated. It takes 180 of these profiles at one-degree increments to compile enough data for the computer to reconstruct the cross-sectional image.

the same section obtained from a linear X-ray scan at certain angles. If 180 projections at one-degree increments are accumulated and their 1-D FTs performed, each of these 180 1-D Fourier transform projections in one direction will represent a corresponding central line of the two-dimensional Fourier transform of the X-ray cross-sectional image. The collection of all these transformed projections is the 2-D Fourier transform of $f(x,y)$

The steps of a 2-D image reconstruction from its 1-D projections are as follows (see also Fig. 5.1):

1. Obtain 180 1-D projections of $f(x,y)$, $p(x,\theta)$.
2. Perform the FT on each 1-D projection.
3. Arrange all these 1-D FTs according to their corresponding angles in the frequency domain: the result is the 2-D FT of $f(x,y)$.
4. Perform the inverse 2-D FT, which gives $f(x,y)$.

The Fourier projection theorem forms the basis of tomographic image reconstruction. Other methods that also can be used to reconstruct a 2-D image from its projections are discussed later in this chapter. It is emphasized that the reconstructed image from projections is not always exact; it is only an approximation of the original image. A different reconstruction method will give a slightly different version of the original image. Since all these methods require extensive computation, a computer or special hardware is needed to implement the procedure. The term "computerized (computed) tomography" is often used to indicate that the image is obtained from its projections by means of a reconstruction method. If the 1-D projections are obtained from X-ray transmission (attenuation) profiles, the procedure is called XCT; the method of obtaining projects from γ-ray emission profiles is called ECT.

5.1.2 The Algebraic Reconstruction Method

The algebraic reconstruction method is often used for the reconstruction of images from an incomplete number of projections (i.e., < 180°). We use a numerical example to illustrate the method.

Let $f(x,y)$ be a 2 × 2 image with the following pixel value:

$$f(x,y) = \begin{array}{|c|c|} \hline 1 & 2 \\ \hline 3 & 4 \\ \hline \end{array}$$

The four projections of this image are as follows:

0°	projection	4,6
45°	projection	5(1 and 4 are ignored for simplicity)
90°	projection	3,7
135°	projection	5((3 and 2 are ignored for simplicity)

Combining this information, one obtains:

the 0° projection: 4 6
↓ ↓   ╱5 the 45° projection

1	2	←3
3	4	←7

} the 90° projection

╲5 the 135° projection

The problem is to reconstruct the 2 × 2 image $f(x,y)$, which is unknown, from these four known projections, which may be obtained from direct measurements. The algebraic reconstruction of the 2 × 2 image from these four known projections proceeds stepwise as follows:

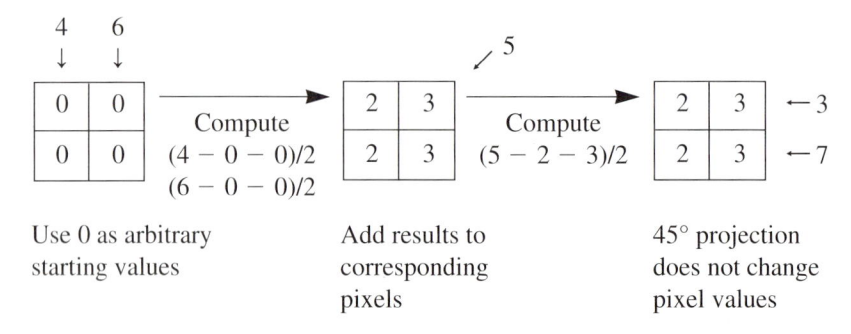

4 6
↓ ↓

0	0
0	0

Compute
(4 − 0 − 0)/2
(6 − 0 − 0)/2

→

╱5

2	3
2	3

Compute
(5 − 2 − 3)/2

→

2	3	←3
2	3	←7

Use 0 as arbitrary starting values

Add results to corresponding pixels

45° projection does not change pixel values

Compute
(3 − 2 − 3)/2
(7 − 2 − 3)/2

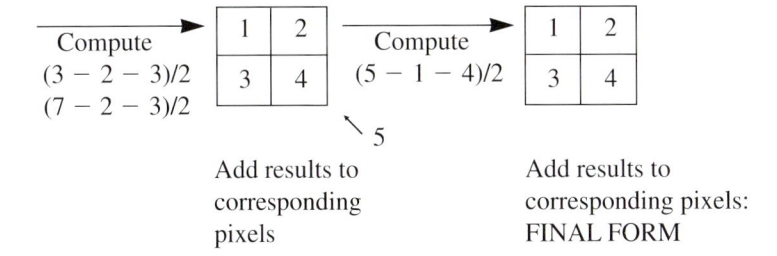

1	2
3	4

Compute
(5 − 1 − 4)/2

1	2
3	4

5

Add results to
corresponding
pixels

Add results to
corresponding pixels:
FINAL FORM

From the last step, it is seen that the result is an exact reconstruction (a pure chance) of the original 2 × 2 image $f(x,y)$ It requires only four projections because $f(x,y)$ is a 2 × 2 image. A 512 × 512 image would require 180 projections, each with sufficient data points, to render a good quality image.

5.1.3 The Filtered (Convolution) Back-Projection Method

The selection of the proper filter is the key to obtaining a good reconstruction from filtered (convolution) back-projection. This is the method of choice for almost all XCT scanners.

5.1.3.1 A Numerical Example

Consider the example introduced in Section 5.1.2. We now wish to reconstruct the 2 × 2 matrix $f(x,y)$ from its four known projections using the filtered back-projection method. The procedure is to first convolve each projection with a preselected filter function and then back-project the convolution result to form an image.

For this example, the filter function $(-1/2, 1, -1/2)$ will be used. This means that when each projection is convolving with this filter function, the point on the projection under consideration will be multiplied by "1" and both points one pixel away from this point will be multiplied by "$-1/2$." Thus, when the projection [4,6] is convolved with $(-1/2, 1, -1/2)$, the result is $(-2, 1, 4, -3)$, since

$$
\begin{array}{rrrrr}
  & -2 & 4 & -2 & \\
+ &   & -3 & 6 & -3 \\
\hline
  & -2 & 1 & 4 & -3 \\
\end{array}
$$

Back-projecting this result to the picture, we have:

−2	1	4	−3
−2	1	4	−3

The data points −2, −3 outside the 2 × 2 reconstructed picture domain are truncated. The result of the following step-by-step illustration of this method, which uses the numerical example described in Section 5.1.2, is an exact reconstruction (again, by pure chance) of the original $f(x,y)$:

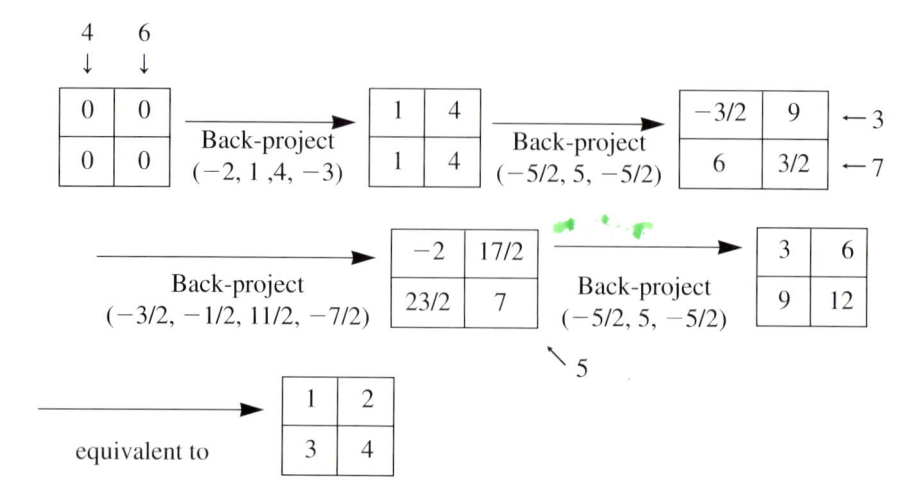

```
 4   6
 ↓   ↓
┌───┬───┐                    ┌───┬───┐                       ┌─────┬───┐
│ 0 │ 0 │                    │ 1 │ 4 │                       │-3/2 │ 9 │ ← 3
├───┼───┤  Back-project      ├───┼───┤   Back-project        ├─────┼───┤
│ 0 │ 0 │  (−2, 1, 4, −3)    │ 1 │ 4 │   (−5/2, 5, −5/2)     │  6  │3/2│ ← 7
└───┴───┘                    └───┴───┘                       └─────┴───┘
```

```
                              ┌─────┬─────┐                    ┌───┬────┐
                              │ −2  │17/2 │                    │ 3 │ 6  │
       Back-project           ├─────┼─────┤   Back-project     ├───┼────┤
   (−3/2, −1/2, 11/2, −7/2)   │23/2 │  7  │   (−5/2, 5, −5/2)  │ 9 │ 12 │
                              └─────┴─────┘                    └───┴────┘
                                       ↘
                                        5
```

```
                    ┌───┬───┐
                    │ 1 │ 2 │
   equivalent to    ├───┼───┤
                    │ 3 │ 4 │
                    └───┴───┘
```

5.1.3.2 Mathematical Formulation

In a CT scanner, the image $f(x,y)$ can been reconstructed by using Eq. (5.3):

$$f(x,y) = \int_0^\pi h(t) * m(t,\phi)\, d\phi \qquad (5.3)$$

where $m(t,\phi)$ is the "t" sampling point at "ϕ" angle projection, $h(t)$ is the filtered function, and the asterisk is the convolution operator.

5.2 TRANSMISSION X-RAY COMPUTED TOMOGRAPHY (XCT)

5.2.1 Conventional XCT

A CT scanner consists of a scanning gantry housing an X-ray tube and a detector unit, and a movable bed that can align a specific cross section of the patient with the gantry. The gantry provides a fixed relative position between the X-ray tube and the detector unit. A scanning mode is the procedure of collecting X-ray attenuation profiles (projections) from a transverse (cross) section of the body. From these projections, the CT scanner's computer program reconstructs the corresponding cross-sectional image of the body.

When the CT scanner was first introduced, it utilized a single, pencil-thin X-ray beam as the energy source and took approximately 4.5 minutes to collect the necessary data to perform the picture reconstruction. Figure 5.2 shows the schematic of a first generation CT scanner. Comparing Figure 5.1 with Figure 5.2 shows the similarity between the Fourier projection theorem and the actual hardware apparatus.

During this long 4.5-minute interval, many factors work against the system, in-

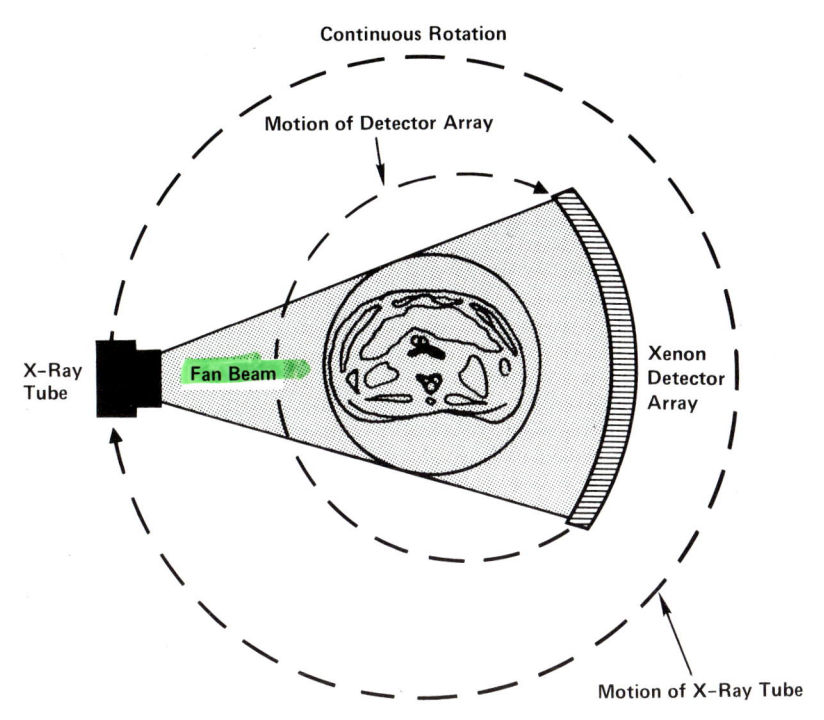

Figure 5.3 Schematic of the rotation scanning mode using a fan-beam X-ray. The detector array (usually pressurized xenon ionization chambers, for compactness) rotates with the X-ray tube as a unit.

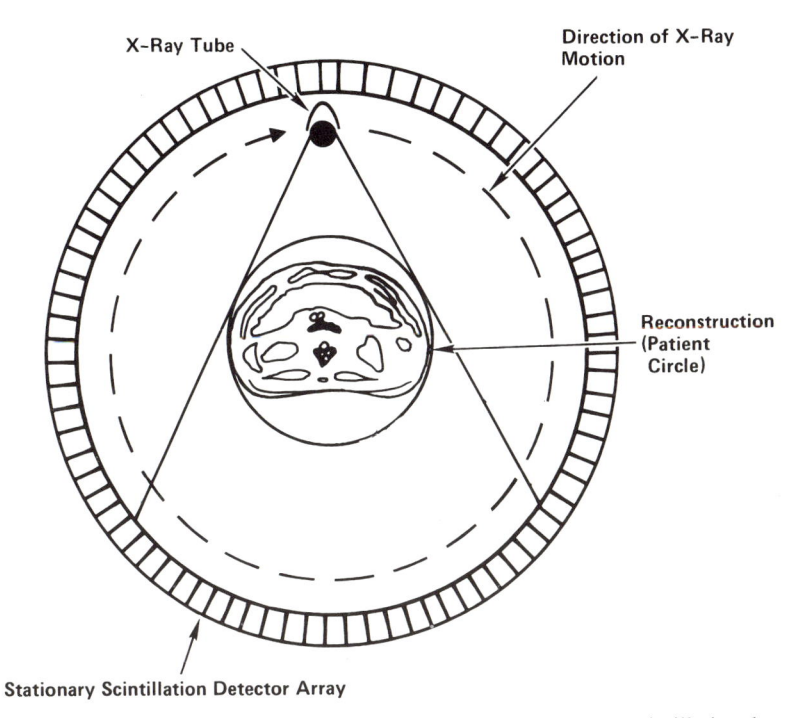

Figure 5.4 Schematic of the rotation scanning mode with a stationary scintillation detector array.

cluding motion from the patient. Patient motion can be categorized into two types: actual physical movement and physiological movement (e.g., heartbeat, respiratory motion, peristalsis). Because of these motions, the reconstructed image will have certain motion artifacts characterized by lines radiating from the center of the movement which can degrade the quality of the image. To overcome this problem, it is necessary to speed up the scanning speed by modifying the scanning gantry. Figures 5.3 and 5.4 show the schematic of the third and the fourth generation state-of-the-art XCT scanners, respectively.

5.2.2 Spiral (Helical) XCT

Two other configurations can further improve the scanning speed: the helical (spiral), discussed here, and the cine (see Section 5.2.3). The helical CT is based on the design of the third- and fourth-generation scanners, whereas the cine CT uses a scanning electron beam X-ray tube.

The CT configurations described earlier have one common characteristic: the patient's bed remains stationary during the scanning; after a complete scan, the patient's bed advances a certain distance and the second scan begins. The start-and-stop motions retard the scanning operation, however. If the patient's bed could assume a forward motion at constant speed while the scanning gantry rotated continuously, the total scanning time of a multiple section examination could be reduced. Such a configuration is not possible, however, because of the high voltage cables connected to the gantry and the transformer, which is external to the gantry. To prevent the cables from becoming tangled, the rotation must be oscillatory. Thus, in the spiral or helical CT configuration, the rotation of the gantry and the linear movement of the patient's bed occur simultaneously during the projectional data acquisition.

Figure 5.5 illustrates the principle of spiral CT. There are two possible scanning modes: single helical and cluster helical. In the single helical mode, the bed continuously advances while the gantry rotates for a longer period of time, say 30 seconds. In the cluster helical mode, the simultaneous rotation and translation lasts only 15 seconds, whereupon both motions stop for 7 seconds before resuming again. The single helical mode is used for patients who can hold their breath for a longer period of time, while the cluster helical mode is for patients who need to take a breath after 15 seconds.

The design of the helical XCT, introduced in the late 1980s, is based on three technological advances: the slip-ring gantry, improved detector efficiency, and greater X-ray tube cooling capability. The slip-ring gantry contains a set of rings and electrical components that rotate, slide, and make contact to generate both high energy (to supply the X-ray tube and generator) and standard energy (to supply power to other electrical and computer components). For this reason, no electrical cables are necessary to connect the gantry and its components. During the helical scanning, the term "pitch" is used to define the relationship between the X-ray beam collimation and the velocity of the bed movement. Thus, a pitch of 1:1 means that the collimation is 1.0 cm and the bed is moving at 1.0 cm/s. A complete 360° rotation is complete as the bed advances 1.0 cm in one second. During this time, raw data are collected covering 360 degrees and 1.0 cm. For the single helical scan mode, raw data are taken

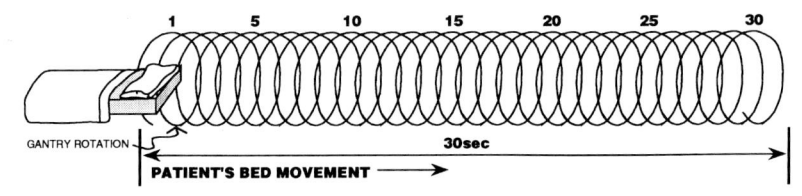

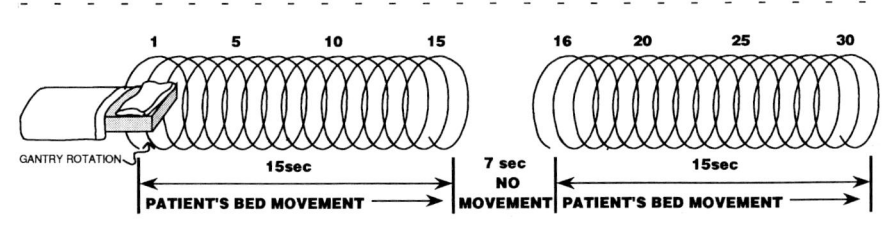

Figure 5.5 Helical (spiral) CT scanning modes.

continuously for 30 seconds while the bed moves 30 cm. After the data collection phase, the raw data are interpolated and/or extrapolated to projections. These projections thus organized are used to reconstruct sectional images. Reconstruction slice thickness can be from 2 mm to 1 cm, depending on the interpolation and extrapolation used.

The advantages of the spiral CT scans are speed of scanning (allowing the user to select slices from continuous data to reconstruct slices with peak contrast medium), retrospective creation of overlapping or thin slices, and volumetric data collection. The disadvantages are the helical reconstruction artifacts and potential object boundary unsharpness.

5.2.3 Cine XCT

Cine XCT, introduced in 1982, uses a completely different X-ray technology, namely, an electron beam X-ray tube: this scanner is fast enough to capture the motion of the heart. The detector array of the system is based on the fourth-generation stationary detector array (scintillator and photodiode). As shown schematically in Figure 5.6, an electron beam (1) is accelerated through the X-ray tube and bent by the deflection coil (2) toward one of the four target rings (3). Collimators at the exit of the tube restrict the X-ray beam to a 30° fan beam, which forms the energy source of scanning. Since there are four tungsten target rings, each of which has a fairly large area (210° tungsten, 90 cm radius) for heat dissipation, the X-ray fan beam can sustain the energy level required for scanning continuously for various scanning modes. In addition, the detector and data collection technologies used in this system allow very rapid data acquisition. Two detector rings (indicated by 4 in Fig. 5.6) allow data acquisi-

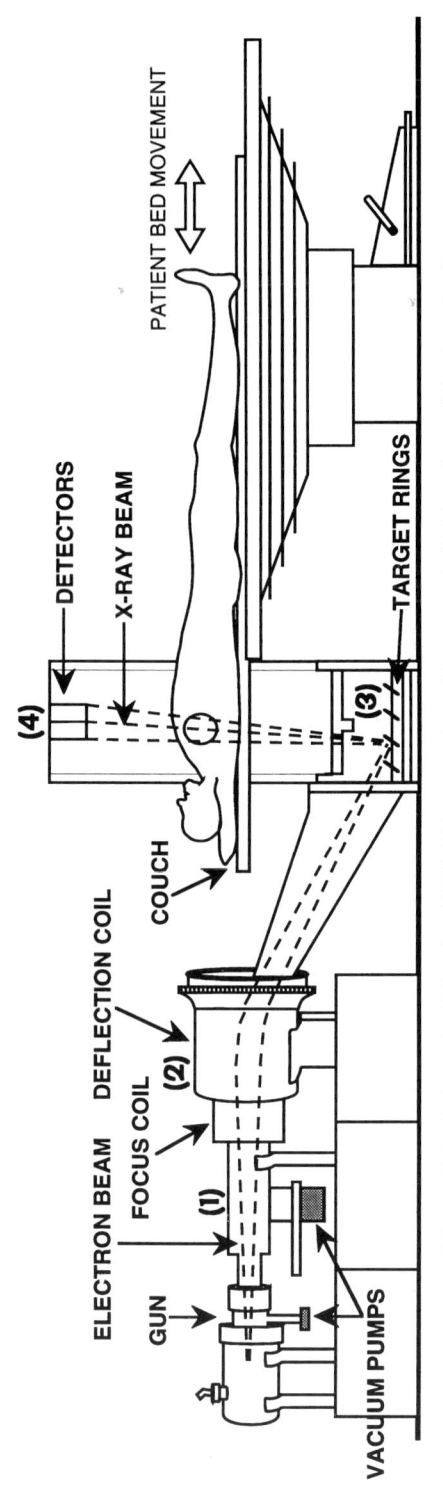

Figure 5.6 Schematic of the cine XCT. (Diagram adapted from a technical brochure of Imatron, Inc.)

tion for two consecutive sections simultaneously. For example, in the slow acquisition mode with a 100 ms scanning time, and an 8 ms interscan delay, cine XCT can provide 9 scans/s, or in the fast acquisition mode with a 20 ms scanning time, 34 scans/s.

The scanning can be done continuously on the same body section (to collect dynamic motion data of the section) or along the axis of the patient (to observe the vascular motion). Because of its fast scanning speed, cine XCT is used for cardiac motion and vascular studies and emergency room scans.

5.2.4 Operation Principle of an XCT Scanner

Figure 5.7 shows the components of a fourth-generation X-ray CT scanner and their interconnections. Included are a gantry housing the X-ray tube, the detectors, and signal processing/conditioning circuits, a front-end preprocessor unit for data corrections and data reformatting, an image data buffer memory, a controlling computer, a high speed computational processor, a hardware back-projector unit, and a video controller for displaying CT images. The following terms are among those commonly used in CT.

1. *Detector circle radius:* the distance from the center of the gantry to the placement of the detectors.
2. *Source circle radius:* the distance from the center of the gantry to the focal spot of the X-ray source.
3. *Scan circle radius:* the distance from the center of the gantry to the edge of the object of interest.
4. *Detector specifications:* the number of detectors used (typically 600–1400) and the detector material composition (e.g., BGO, CaF, Cd_2WO_4).
5. *Scan speed:* the length of time the X-ray tube is turned on during scanning— a factor contributing to the dose received by the patient.
6. *Source fan:* a data file that consists of readings from all detectors for a given source position.
7. *Detector fan:* a data file that consists of all readings from a single detector, with the X-ray source rotating to all necessary angle positions.
8. *Convolution:* a mathematical operation used in image reconstruction to minimize artifacts.
9. *Back-projector:* a hardware processor that can quickly perform the back-projection (see Eq. 5.3) reconstruction algorithm commonly used in CT.
10. *Slice thickness:* the amount of X-ray collimation with respect to the patient's body axis. This collimation defines the slice thickness, the third dimension of a picture element or pixel. The term "voxel" is sometimes used instead of "pixel."
11. *CT or Hounsfield number:* a number assigned to a voxel which represents the relative X-ray attenuation coefficient, defined as follows:

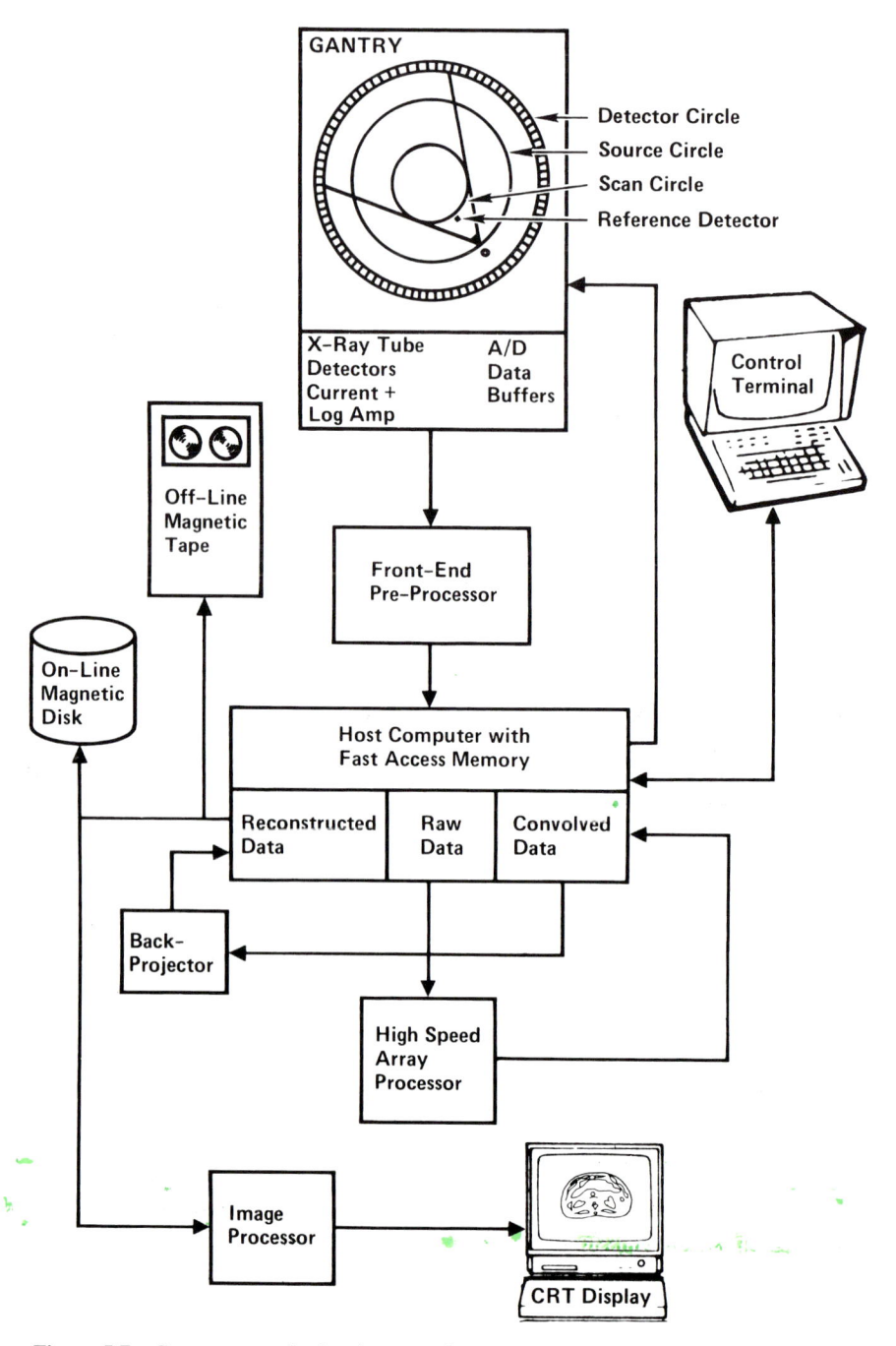

Figure 5.7 Components of a fourth-generation XCT scanner and their interconnections.

$$\frac{K(\mu - \mu_W)}{\mu_W}$$

where μ is the attenuation coefficient of the material under consideration, μ_W is the attenuation coefficient of water, and K is a constant set by the manufacturer.

12. *Reconstruction matrix size:* the number of voxels in the resulting reconstructed image, typically, 512×512 with 12 bits/voxel.
13. *Reconstruction times:* average time required to perform the image reconstruction for a given matrix size.
14. *System storage disk size:* the capacity of magnetic disks available in the system to store images. Images stored in these disks can be quickly accessed and displayed. For long-term storage, images are archived onto magnetic tapes or optical disks.

5.3 EMISSION COMPUTED TOMOGRAPHY

Emission computed tomography (ECT) has many characteristics in common with transmission X-ray CT. The main difference between these two techniques is the source of radiation used. In ECT the radionuclide, which is administered to a patients in the form of radiopharmaceuticals either by injection or by inhalation, is used as a source instead of an external X-ray energy. The basic principle of ECT is based on nuclear medicine scanning, which is discussed in Section 5.4.

It is important to select a dose-efficient detector system for an ECT system for two reasons. First, the quantity to be measured in ECT is the distribution of the radionuclide in the body, which changes with time as a result of flow and biochemical kinetics in the body. Thus, all the necessary measurements must be made in a short period of time. Second, the amount of isotope administered is limited because of the usual dose considerations. Therefore, detector efficiency plays a crucial role in selecting a scintillator for ECT systems.

The basic principle of image reconstruction is the same in ECT as in transmission CT except that the signal in ECT is the attenuation of γ-rays during their flight from the emitting nuclei to the detectors. To minimize the contribution from scattered radiation, the ECT uses the characteristics of monoenergetic energy in setting up a counting window to discriminate the lower energy scattered radiation from the high energy primary radiation. There are two major categories in ECT: single photon emission CT and positron emission CT.

5.3.1 Single Photon Emission CT (SPECT)

There are many different designs for the SPECT, but only rotating gamma camera systems (see Section 5.4) are commercially available. In a rotating camera system, the gamma camera is rotated around the object, and images in a two-dimensional se-

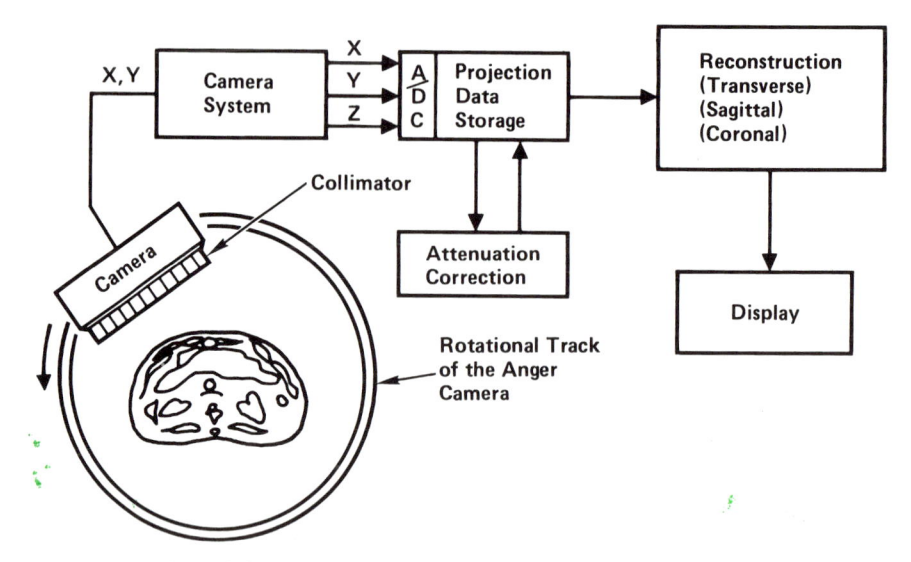

Figure 5.8 Schematic of a single photon emission CT (SPECT).

ries are reconstructed and stored for processing. The camera is composed of a large scintillation crystal with a diameter of 30–50 cm and a number of photomultiplier tubes (PMTs) attached to the opposite surface of the crystal. When a γ-ray photon interacts with the crystal, the light generated from the photoelectric effect is uniformly distributed among the neighboring PMTs. By measuring the relative signal of each PMT, the camera can locate the interaction position for each event. The drawback of this system is the difficulty of maintaining uniform speed of rotation of a rather heavy camera. Figure 5.8 shows the schematic of a SPECT.

Since a typical tomographic study takes 15–20 minutes to complete, it is important to have adequate patient immobilization. To provide the best sensitivity and resolution, it is desirable to have the camera as close to the patient as possible. Since the dimension of the body width is greater than its thickness, an elliptical orbit of rotation of the camera tends to produce a higher resolution image. Different collimators are used for different applications. In general, the reconstruction algorithm must be modified and the attenuation values corrected for each type of collimator. For example, a single-plane converging collimator will need a fan beam reconstruction algorithm, and a parallel collimator will need a parallel beam algorithm.

Three methods of correcting attenuation values based on the assumption of a constant attenuation value are summarized as follows.

1. *Geometric mean modification.* Each data point in a projection is corrected by the geometric mean of the projection data, which is obtained by taking the square root of the product of two opposite projection data points.
2. *Iterative modification.* This method is similar to the iteration reconstruction method for XCT described earlier. A reconstruction without corrections is first

performed, and each pixel in the reconstructed image is compensated by a correction factor that is the inverse of the average measured attenuation from that point to the boundary pixels. The projections of this modified image are obtained, and the differences between each of the corrected projections and the original measured projections are computed. These difference projections are reconstructed to obtain an error image. The error image is then added back to the modified image to form the corrected image.

3. *Convolution method.* Each data point in the projection is modified by a factor that depends on the distance from a centerline to the edge of the object. The modified projection data points are filtered with a proper filter function and then back-projected with an exponential weighting factor to obtain the image (see Section 5.1.3).

Currently, SPECT is mostly used for studies of the brain, including brain blood volume (^{99m}Tc-labeled blood cells), regional cerebral blood flow (^{123}I-labeled iodoantipyrine or inhaled ^{133}Xe), and physiological condition measurements.

5.3.2 Positron Emission CT (PET)

In PET, a positron instead of single photon is used as a radionuclide source. The positron emitted from a radionuclide is rapidly slowed down, and is annihilated by a combination yielding two 511 keV γ-rays oriented about 180° to each other. The PET system utilizes this unique property of positrons by employing a detector system that requires simultaneous detection of both photons from annihilation, and thus avoids the need for collimators. With a pair of detectors, placed on the two opposite sides of the patient, only events that are detected in coincidence are recorded. Simultaneous detection of two annihilation photons by the detector system thus signals the decay of a positron anywhere along a line connecting the two points of detection (Fig. 5.9). Because of this multiple coincidence logic, PET systems have higher sensitivity than SPECT.

The correction of attenuation is easier in PET than in SPECT because the probability that annihilated photons will reach both detectors simultaneously is a function of the thickness of the body between the two opposite detectors. The correction factor can be obtained by means of a preliminary scan of the body with an external γ-ray source, or a correction table based on a simple geometric shape resembling the attenuation medium to be used. Patient movements, oversimplified geometric shape, and nonuniform medium will cause errors in attenuation correction.

Thallium-drifted sodium iodide NaI(Tl), bismuth germanate (BGO), and cesium fluoride (CsF) are being used as detector materials. Because of the high energy of the annihilation photon, detector efficiency plays a crucial role in selecting a scintillator for a PET system. Bismuth germanate is considered to be the most prominent candidate for PET detector material because of its high detection efficiency, which is due to its high physical density (7.13 g/cm^3) and large atomic number (83), as well as its nonhygroscopicity (which makes for easy packing) and its lack of afterglow.

A typical whole-body PET scanner consists of 512 BGO detectors placed in 16 circular array banks with 32 detectors in each bank. During scanning, the system is capa-

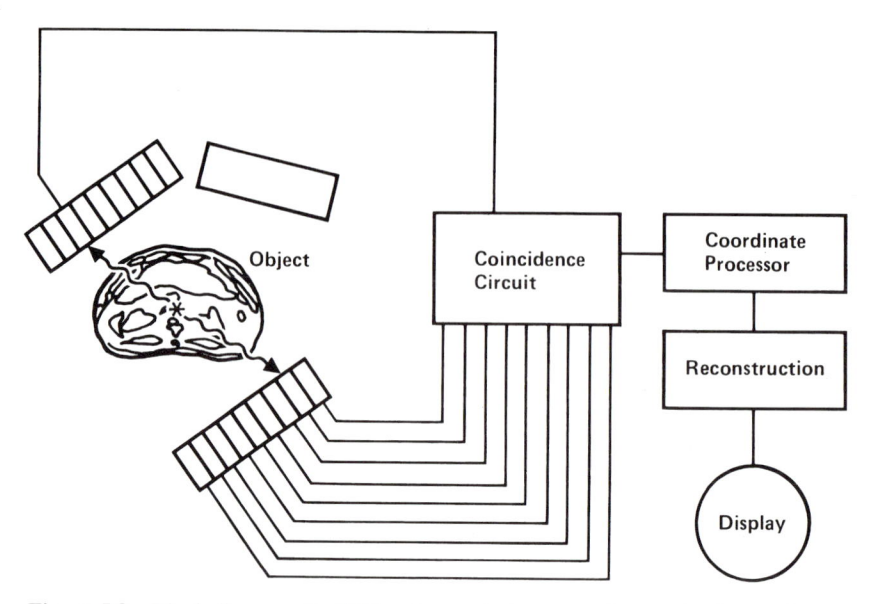

Figure 5.9 Block diagram of a PET system; only two array detector banks are shown.

ble of wobbling to achieve higher resolution via finer sampling. The image spatial resolution for the stationary and wobbled modes are 5–6 and 4.5–5 mm, respectively.

A recent PET engineering development is the *whole-body imaging technique*, which produces tomographic images of the entire body with equal spatial resolution in orthogonal image planes. Since the body longitudinal axis is, in general, longer than the other two axes, the patient bed is required to advance during the scanning process to permit the entire body length to be scanned. A complicated data acquisition system in synchrony with the bed motion is necessary to monitor the data collection process. Figure 5.10 illustrates images of the transaxial, coronal, and sagittal orthogonal planes, as well as the anterior–posterior projection image of the whole-body PET image with a fluoride ion isotope ($^{18}F^-$).

5.4 NUCLEAR MEDICINE

5.4.1 Principles of Nuclear Medicine Scanning

Although ECT is sectional imaging, nuclear medicine scanning is projectional. The principle of nuclear medicine is needed to explain the concept of ECT. The formation of an image in nuclear medicine relies on administering a radiopharmaceutical agent that can be used to differentiate between a normal and an abnormal physiological process. A radiopharmaceutical agent consists of a tracer substance and a radionuclide for highlighting the tracer's position. The tracer typically consists of a molecule that resembles a constituent of the tissue of interest, a colloidal substance that is attacked by reticuloendothelial cells, for example, or a capillary blocking agent. A gam-

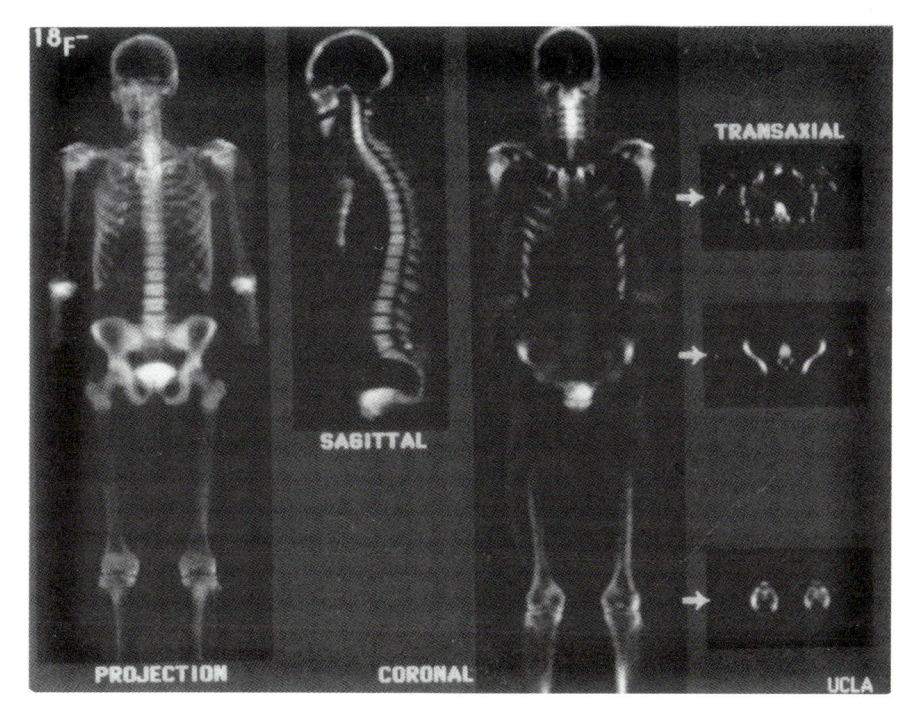

Figure 5.10 From right to left, images of transaxial, coronal, and sagittal orthogonal planes, as well as the anterior–posterior projection image of the whole-body PET image with fluoride ion ($^{18}F^-$). (Courtesy of R.A. Hawkins.)

ma camera (Section 5.4.2) is then used to obtain an image of the distribution of the radioactivity in an organ.

The radionuclide is chosen on the basis of its specific activity, half-life, energy spectrum, and ability to bond with the desired tracer molecule. Its activity is important because, in general, one would like to perform scans in the shortest possible time while nevertheless accumulating sufficient nuclear counting decay statistics. As always, the half-life must be reasonably short to minimize the radiation dose to the patient. The energy spectrum of the isotope is important because if the energy emitted is too low, the radiation will be severely attenuated when it passes through the body; hence nuclear statistics will be poor or scan times unacceptable. If the energy is too high, there may not be enough photoelectric interaction, and absorption in the detector crystal will be low. Typical isotopes used in nuclear medicine have γ-ray emission energies of 100–400 keV.

5.4.2 The Gamma Camera and Associated Imaging System

As with most imaging systems, nuclear medicine imagers (e.g., gamma cameras) contain subsystems for data acquisition, data processing, data display, and data archival. A computer is used to control the flow of data and coordinate these subsystems into

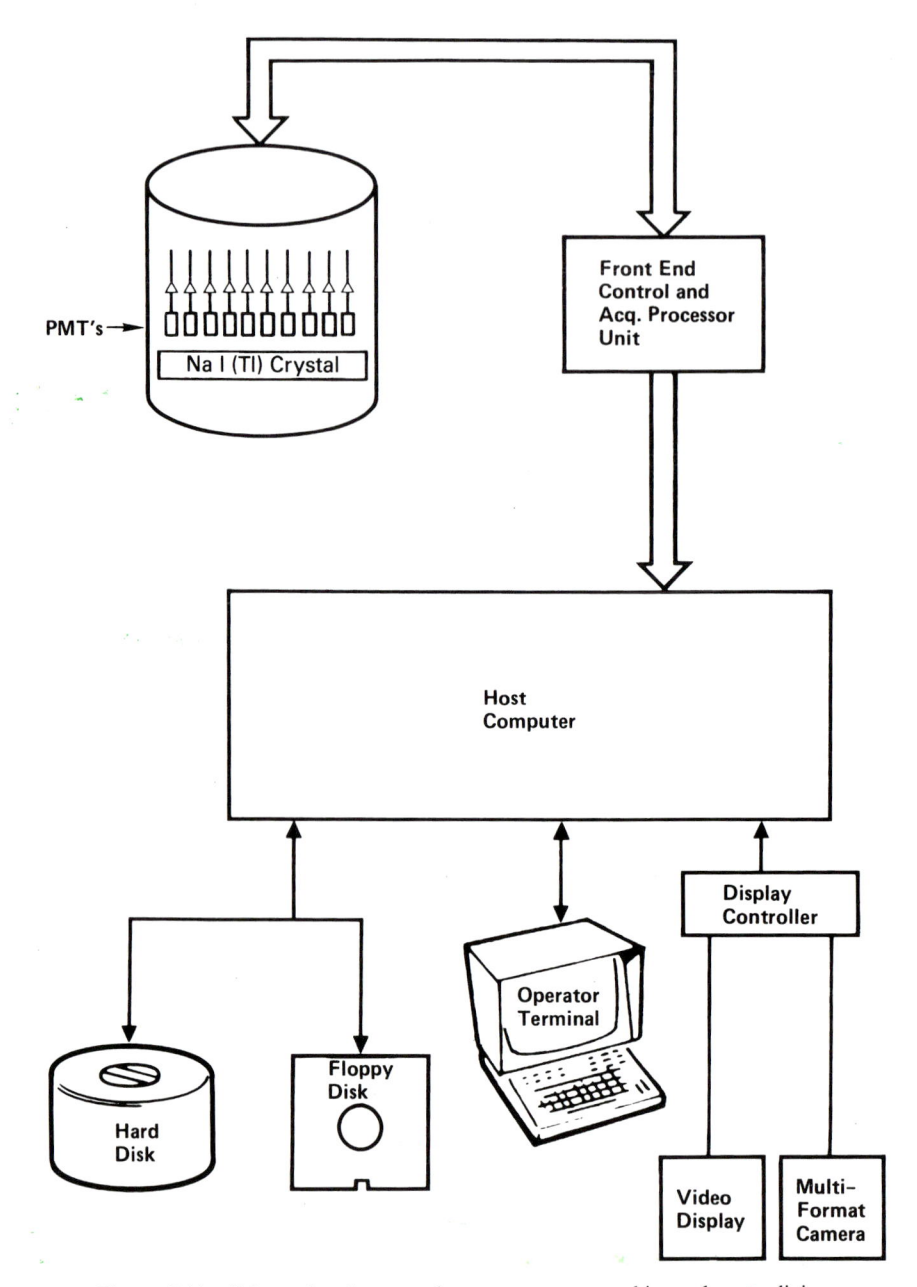

Figure 5.11 Schematic of a general gamma camera used in nuclear medicine.

a functional unit. The operator interactively communicates with the computer via commands from a computer terminal or predefined push buttons on the system's control terminal. Figure 5.11 shows a schematic of a typical digital nuclear medicine gamma camera. Typical matrix sizes of nuclear medicine image are 64×64 or 128×128 by 16 bits, with a maximum of 30 frames per cardiac cycle. In gated mode, useful parameter values such as ejection fraction and stroke volume may be calculated. In addition, the frames of a cardiac cycle may be displayed consecutively and rapidly in cine fashion to evaluate heart wall motion.

5.5 ULTRASOUND IMAGING

Ultrasound imaging has gained widespread application in many areas of medicine including obstetrics, gynecology, pediatrics, ophthalmology, mammography, abdominal imaging, and cardiology, as well as in the imaging of small organs such as the thyroid, prostate, and testicles, and recently in endoscopy. Its wide acceptance is partially due to its noninvasiveness, its use of nonionizing radiation, and its low procedural costs. An ultrasound examination is a widely used as first step in attempting to diagnose a presented ailment.

5.5.1 Principles of B-Mode Ultrasound Scanning

B-mode ultrasound imaging attempts to reconstruct a cross-sectional view of the patient by way of detecting the amplitudes of acoustical reflections (echoes) that occur at the interface of tissues having different acoustical properties.

Ultrasonic waves are introduced into the body by pressing against the skin with a transducer that generates pulses of high frequency sound waves, which are directed toward the structures of interest. A coupling gel is used to provide efficient transfer of acoustical energy into the body. The acoustical wave propagates through the body tissue, and its radiation pattern will demonstrate high directivity in the near field or Fresnel zone close to the body surface (see Fig. 5.12); it will begin to diverge in the far field or Fraunhofer zone. The range of the near and far fields is determined mainly by the wavelength λ of the sonic waves used and the diameter of the transducer. In general, it is preferable to image objects that are in the Fresnel zone, where lateral resolving power is better.

The fate of the acoustical wave is highly dependent on the acoustical properties of the medium in which the wave is propagating. The speed of the wave in media depends on the elasticity and density of the material and affects the degree of refraction (deviation from a straight path) that occurs at a boundary between tissues. The characteristic impedance of the material, which determines the degree of reflection that occurs when a wave is incident at a boundary, depends on the material's density and the speed of sound in the material. The larger the difference between the acoustic impedances of two materials forming a boundary, the greater will be the strength of the reflected wave.

5.5.2 System Block Diagram and Operational Procedure

Figure 5.13 shows a general block diagram of a typical B-mode ultrasound scanner. It is composed of a transducer, a high voltage pulse generator, a transmitter circuit, a receiver circuit with time gain compensation (TGC), a mechanical scanning arm with position encoders, a digital scan converter (DSC), and a video display monitor.

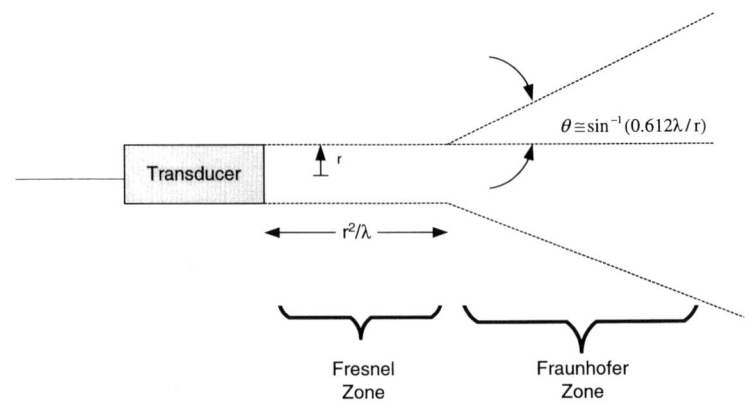

Figure 5.12 Principle of the ultrasound wave produced by a transducer made of piezoelectric material: λ wavelength of the sound wave used.

$\theta \cong \sin^{-1}(0.612\lambda/r)$

λ: Wavelength of the Sound Wave Used

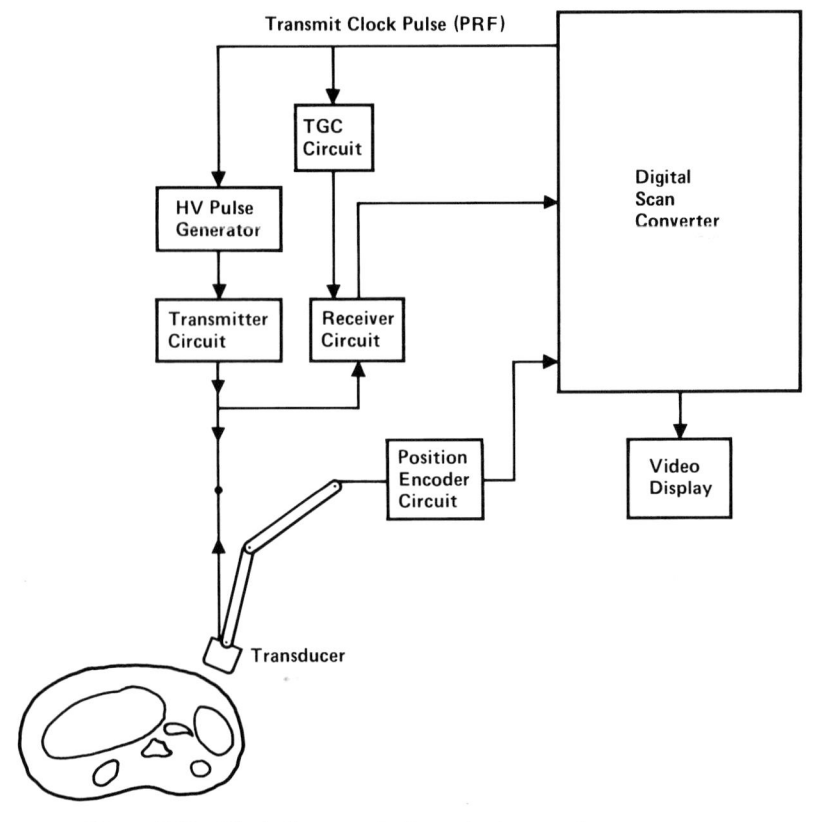

Figure 5.13 Block diagram of a B-mode ultrasound scanner system.

The acoustical waves are generated by applying a high voltage pulse to a piezoelectric crystal, resulting in the creation of a longitudinal pressure sonic wave. The rate at which pulses are supplied by the transmitter circuit to the transducer, as determined by a transmit clock, is called the pulse repetition frequency (PRF). Typical PRF values range from 0.5 to 2.5 kHz. The frequency of the acoustic wave, which is determined by the thickness of the piezoelectric crystal, may range from 1 to 15 MHz. The transducer can serve as acoustical transmitter as well as receiver, since mechanical pressure waves interacting with the crystal will result in the creation of an electrical signal.

Received echo amplitude pulses, which eventually form an ultrasound image, are transferred into electrical signals by the transducer. A radio frequency receiver circuit then amplifies and demodulates the signal. The receiver circuit, a crucial element in an ultrasound scanner, must have a huge dynamic range (30–40 dB) to be able to detect the wide range of reflected signals, which are typically 1–2 V at interfaces near the surface and microvolts at deeper structures. In addition, the receiver must introduce little noise and must have a wide amplification bandwidth.

The time gain compensator circuit allows the operator to amplify the echoed signal according to its depth of origin. This feature helps compensate for the higher attenuation of the signal seen from echoes originating from deeper interfaces and results in a more uniform image (i.e., interfaces are not darker closer to the body surface on the image display solely because they are closer to the transducer). The operator is able to obtain the best possible image by controlling the amount of gain at a particular depth.

The output of the receiver is fed into the digital scan converter and used to determine the depth (Z *dimension*) at which the echo occurred. The depth at which the echo originated is calculated by determining the time the echo takes to return to the transducer. The depth of the reflector can be obtained because time and depth are related, and the depth is half the time interval from the transmission of the signal pulse to signal return times the velocity of sound in the traversal medium.

The encoding of the x and y positions of the face of the transducer and the angular orientation of the transducer with respect to the normal of the scanning surface is accomplished by the scanning arm position encoder circuit. The scanning arm is restricted to moving in one linear direction at a time. The arm contains four potentiometers whose resistance will correspond to the x and y positions and cosine and sine directions (with angle with respect to the normal of the body surface) of the transducer.

For example, if the transducer is moved in the y direction while x and the angle of rotation are kept fixed, then only the Y potentiometer will change its resistance. Position encoders on the arm will generate signals proportional to the position of the transducer and the direction of the ultrasound beam. The x, y, and z data are fed into the digital scan converter to generate addresses that will permit the echo strength signals to be stored in the appropriate memory locations.

The digital scan converter (DSC) performs A/D conversions of data, data preprocessing, pixel generation, image storage, data postprocessing, and image display. The analog echo signals from the receiver circuit are digitized by an analog-to-digital converter in the DSC, typically to 8 bits (256 gray levels). Fast A/D converters are normally used because most ultrasound echo signals have a wide bandwidth, and the sampling frequency should be at least twice the highest frequency of interest in the image. Typical A/D sampling rates range from 10 to 20 MHz. The DSC image memory is a random access memory that is normally $512 \times 512 \times 8$ bits for each memory plane.

The data may be preprocessed to enhance the visual display of the data and to match the dynamic range of the subsequent hardware components. Echo signals are typically rescaled, and often nonlinear (e.g., logarithmic) circuits are used to emphasize and de-emphasize certain echo amplitudes.

5.5.3 Sampling Modes and Image Display

Three different sampling modes are available on most ultrasound units: the *survey mode,* in which the data stored in memory are continually updated and displayed, *the static mode,* in which only maximum values during a scanning session are stored and displayed, and an *averaging mode,* in which the average of all scans for a particular scan location are stored and displayed.

Once stored in memory, the digital data are subjected to postprocessing operations of several types. These can be categorized according to changes in the gray level display of the stored image, temporal smoothing of the data, or spatial operations. Gray scale mean and windowing, and nonlinear gray scale transformations are common.

Image display is performed by a video processor and controller unit that can quickly access the image memory and modulate an electron beam to show the image on a video monitor. The digital scan converter allows for echo data to be read continuously from the fast access image memory. This helps to avoid flicker on the display video monitor in real-time imaging. Hard copies of the image are normally obtained using a laser camera.

5.5.4 Color Doppler Ultrasound Imaging

Ultrasound scanning using the Doppler principle can detect the movement of blood inside vessels. In particular, it can detect whether the blood is moving away from or toward the scanning plane. When several blood vessels are in the scanning plane, it is advantageous to use different colors to represent the blood flow direction and speed with respect to the stationary anatomical structures. Thus, colors coupling with the gray scale ultrasound image results in a duplex Doppler ultrasound image. This coupling permits simultaneously imaging of anatomical structures as well as characterization of circulatory physiology from known reference planes within the body. The resulting image is called color Doppler or color-flow imaging. For a $512 \times 512 \times 8$ bit ultrasound gray scale image, a color Doppler image will need $512 \times 512 \times 24$ bits, a threefold increase in storage requirement. Figure 5.14 shows a color Doppler US image of a liver scan.

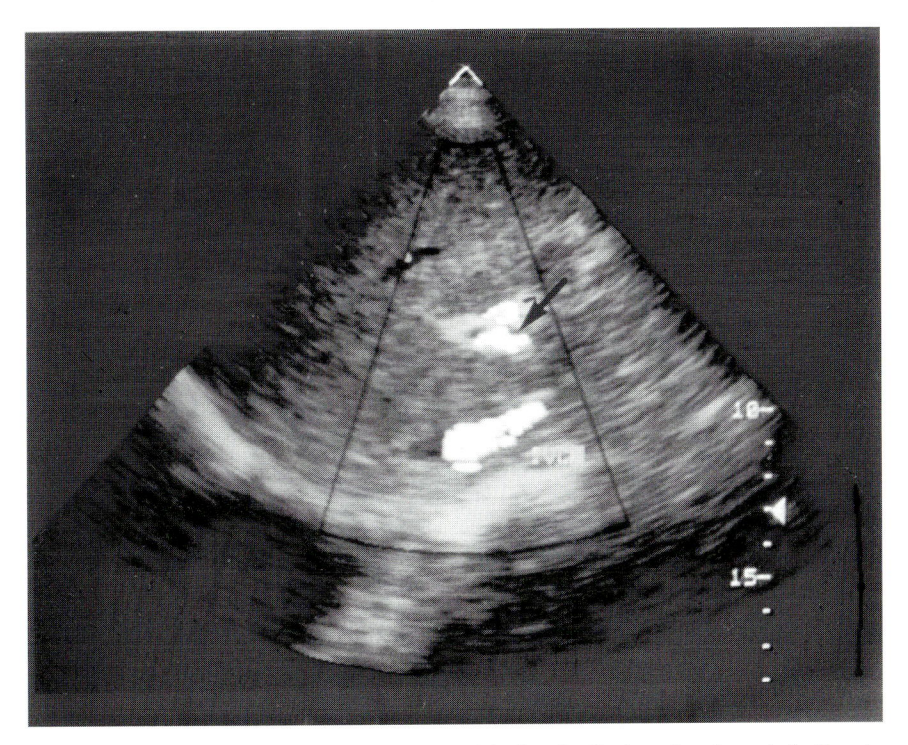

Figure 5.14 Color Doppler ultrasound image of the longitudinal section through the liver indicates that the flow in the inferior vena cava (IVC) is reversed: blood flow (in red) is directed toward the US scanning plane. Flow in the portal vein (arrow) is hepatopetal. (See color plate.) (Courtesy of E. Grant.)

5.5.5 Cine Loop Ultrasound Imaging

One advantage of ultrasound imaging over other imaging modalities is its noninvasive nature, which permits the accumulation of ultrasound images continuously through time without adverse effects on the patient. Such images can be played back in a cine loop, which can reveal the dynamic motion of a body organ—for example, the heart beat (see also Section 5.2.3: Cine XCT). Several seconds of cine loop ultrasound images can produce a very large image file. For example, a 10-second series of color Doppler cine loop ultrasound images will yield $(10 \times 30) \times 0.75 \times 10^6$ bytes ($= 225$ Mbyte) of image information, a very large file to be handled digitally. We will consider how to manage such large data files for storage and for communication in later chapters.

5.6 MAGNETIC RESONANCE IMAGING

5.6.1 MR Imaging Basics

Magnetic resonance imaging (MRI) devices form images of objects through probing the magnetic moments of nuclei, at present usually protons, employing radio frequency (RF) radiation and strong magnetic fields. Information concerning the spatial distribution of nuclear magnetization in the sample is determined from RF signal emission by these stimulated nuclei. The received signal intensity is dependent on five parameters: hydrogen density (ρ_H), spin–lattice relaxation time (T_1), spin–spin relaxation time (T_2), flow velocity (e.g., arterial blood), and chemical shift.

The purpose of MR imaging is to ascertain spatial (anatomical) information from the returned RF signals through filtered back-projection reconstruction or Fourier analysis, ultimately displaying a two-dimensional section or a three-dimensional volume of the object for diagnostic evaluation.

There exists distinct advantages for utilizing MRI over other modalities (e.g., XCT) in certain types of examination. The interaction between the static magnetic field, RF radiation, and atomic nuclei is free of ionizing radiation; therefore, the imaging procedure is apparently safe. Since, in addition, the scanning mechanism is completely electronic, requiring no moving parts to perform a scan, it is possible to obtain two-dimensional slices of the coronal, sagittal, and transaxial planes, and any oblique section, as well as a three-dimensional volume. However, the major disadvantage at present is lower spatial resolution compared with XCT.

5.6.2 Magnetic Resonance Image Production

A simplified block diagram of a typical MR imaging device (Fig. 5.15) illustrates the components necessary for the production, detection, and display of the MRI signal. The system includes the following:

1. The magnet to produce the static magnetic H_0 field.
2. RF equipment to (a) produce the magnitude of the RF magnetic H_1 field (transmitter, amplifier, and coil for transmitting mode), and (b) detect the free induction decay (FID), which is the response of the net magnetization to an RF pulse (coil for receiving mode, preamplifier, receiver, and signal demodulator).
3. $x, y,$ and z gradient power supplies and coils providing the magnetic field gradients needed for encoding spatial position.
4. The electronics and computer facility to orchestrate the whole imaging process (control interface with computer), digitize the MR image data (A/D converter), reconstruct the image (computer algorithms), and display it (computer, disk storage, image processor, and display system).

5.6.3 Steps in Producing an MR Image

An MR image is obtained by using a selected pulse sequence that perturbs the external magnetic field H_0. For this reason, a set of MR images is named based on the selected pulse sequence. Some useful pulse sequences in radiology applications are spin echo, inversion recovery, gradient echo, and echo planar. Each of these pulse sequence highlights certain chemical compositions in the tissues under consideration. For example, a spin–echo MR image is produced in the following manner. First, the object is placed inside an RF coil situated in the homogeneous portion of the main

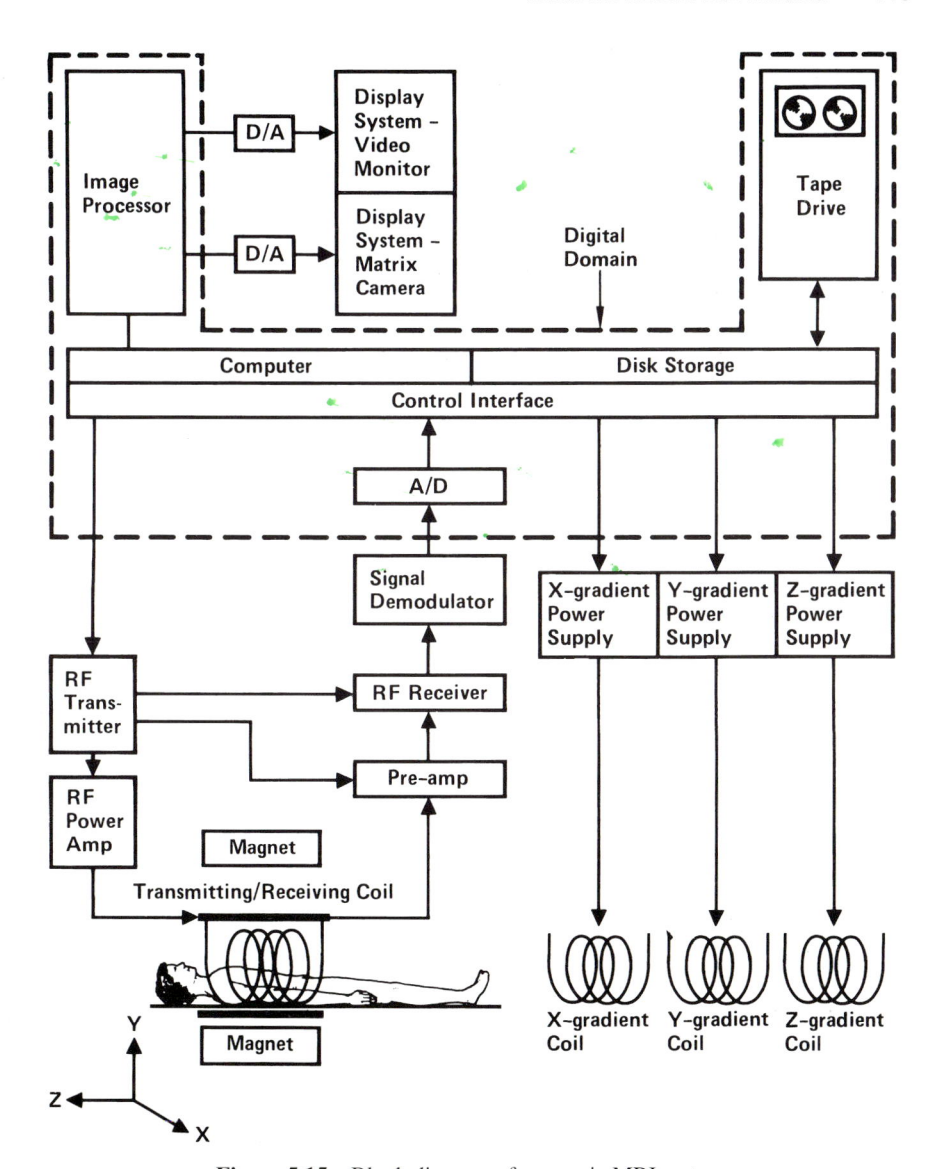

Figure 5.15 Block diagram of a generic MRI system.

magnetic field, H_0. Next, a pulsing sequence with two RF pulses is applied to the imaging volume (hence spin–echo). At the same time a magnetic gradient is applied to the field H_0 to identify the relative position of the spin–echo (FID) signals. The FID signal is demodulated from the RF signal, sampled with an analog-to-digital converter, and stored in a digital data array for processing. This set of data is analogous to one set of projection data in XCT. After the repetition time has elapsed, the pulsing sequence is applied and the FID is sampled repeatedly with alternate gradient magnitudes until the desired number of projections have been acquired.

During and after data collection, computed tomographic reconstruction algorithms as described in Section 5.1 are performed on the acquired projections (digital data) using filtered back-projection or inverse two-dimensional fast Fourier transform (FFT). This yields the final result, a digital image (digital data file) of localized magnetization in the spatial domain whose magnitude follows the spin-echo dependence on hydrogen density, relaxation times, flow, and chemical shift. The inverse Fourier transform (IFT) produces an image in the spatial domain. This procedure can be represented as follows:

$$\text{frequency spectrum} \xrightarrow{FT} \text{FID} \xrightarrow{IFT} \text{spatial distribution (image)}$$

This digital image can then be archived on disk storage. Figure 5.16 demonstrates the image information flow.

5.6.4 Image Format, Resolution, and Contrast

5.6.4.1 *Image Format*

The basic image format of an MR scanner is different from that of other modalities (e.g., XCT). Although both display two-dimensional tomographic slices, MRI, in addition to the transaxial cross sections characteristic of XCT, can acquire sagittal, coronal, and oblique planes (Fig. 5.17), as well as three-dimensional images.

Not only is MRI different from XCT in image plane orientation flexibility, but the observable in the MRI scan (the FID) contains information involving many parameters (e.g., T_1 and T_2). In XCT, however, the only observable is the X-ray linear attenuation coefficient. The challenge of MRI is attempting to decipher the wealth of information bound up in the FID (ρ_H, T_1, T_2,), flow velocity, and chemical shift, and determining how to display all this information adequately. Usually, only the magnetization magnitude is displayed, which is a function of all the above-mentioned parameters, though one may predominate to yield a so-called weighted image. Much work has been performed to obtain true T_1 and T_2 maps for MRI tissue characterization.

5.6.4.2 *Image Quality*

Discussions of image quality entail considerations of three parameters: spatial resolution, density (contrast) resolution, and signal-to-noise ratio. The density resolution of MRI at the present time is about 8 bits deep, although the A/D converters used to sample the demodulated FID usually sample 2 bytes deep (Fig. 5.18). The spatial resolution of MRI typically varies between 0.3 and 2.0 mm, depending on the gradient strength and on the coils used to send/receive the RF signal. Because there exists only a 6.8 ppm/T (parts per million/tesla) excess of magnetic moments in the lower energy state, the magnetization vector is very small; thus the MR phenomena is inherently noisy, with low signal-to-noise ratio. This is why the image data are only really about 8 bits deep.

Even though the S/N ratio is lower in MRI than in XCT, MR images rival or excel XCT images in some regions of the body, especially in the brain, the spinal col-

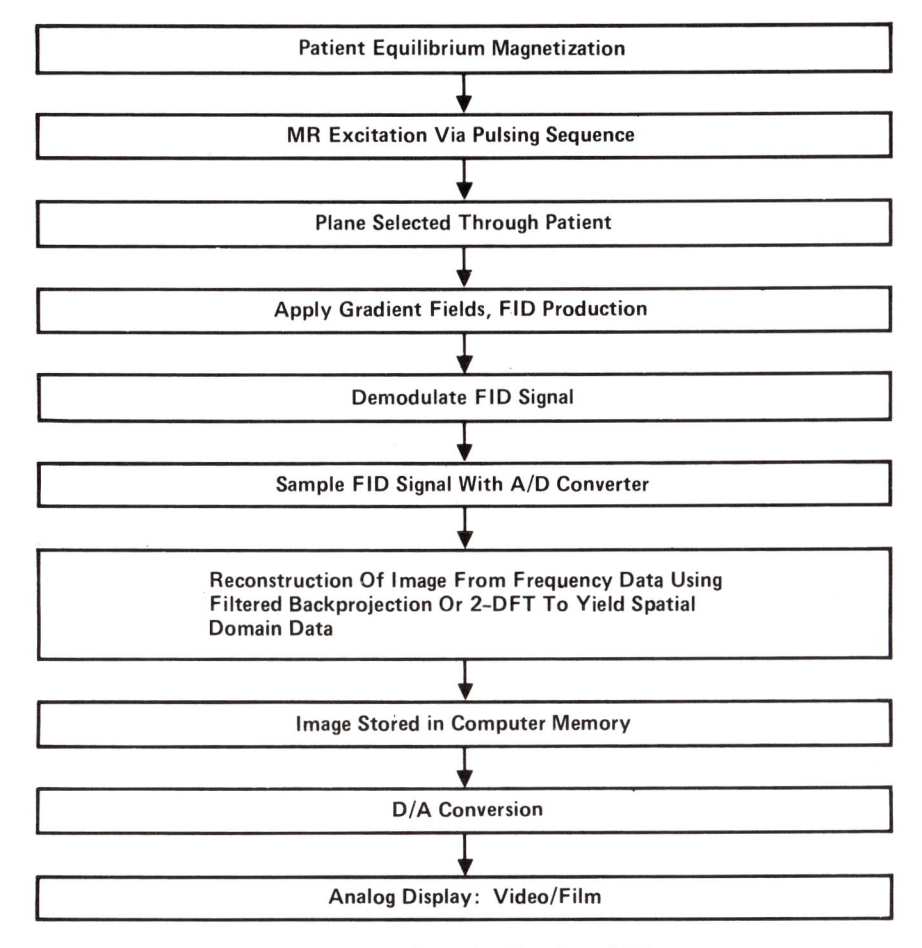

```
┌─────────────────────────────────────────┐
│    Patient Equilibrium Magnetization    │
└─────────────────────────────────────────┘
                    ↓
┌─────────────────────────────────────────┐
│     MR Excitation Via Pulsing Sequence  │
└─────────────────────────────────────────┘
                    ↓
┌─────────────────────────────────────────┐
│       Plane Selected Through Patient    │
└─────────────────────────────────────────┘
                    ↓
┌─────────────────────────────────────────┐
│     Apply Gradient Fields, FID Production│
└─────────────────────────────────────────┘
                    ↓
┌─────────────────────────────────────────┐
│           Demodulate FID Signal         │
└─────────────────────────────────────────┘
                    ↓
┌─────────────────────────────────────────┐
│    Sample FID Signal With A/D Converter │
└─────────────────────────────────────────┘
                    ↓
┌─────────────────────────────────────────┐
│ Reconstruction Of Image From Frequency  │
│ Data Using Filtered Backprojection Or   │
│ 2-DFT To Yield Spatial Domain Data      │
└─────────────────────────────────────────┘
                    ↓
┌─────────────────────────────────────────┐
│       Image Stored in Computer Memory   │
└─────────────────────────────────────────┘
                    ↓
┌─────────────────────────────────────────┐
│              D/A Conversion             │
└─────────────────────────────────────────┘
                    ↓
┌─────────────────────────────────────────┐
│       Analog Display: Video/Film        │
└─────────────────────────────────────────┘
```

Figure 5.16 Image information flow in an MRI scanner.

umn, and skeletal joints, because of the significantly better tissue contrast realized in MRI. Tissue contrast may be manipulated through choice of pulsing sequence and sequence parameters (e.g., repetition time T_R, echo time T_E). The major drawback to MRI is the inherently poor signal-to-noise ratio. In fact, the three parameters—spatial resolution, contrast resolution, and S/N are inextricably related, one being augmented only at the expense of one or both of the other two.

5.7 MICROSCOPIC IMAGING

5.7.1 Instrumentation

Digital microscopy is used to extract sectional quantitative information from biomedical microscopic slides. A digital microscopic imaging system consists of the following six components:

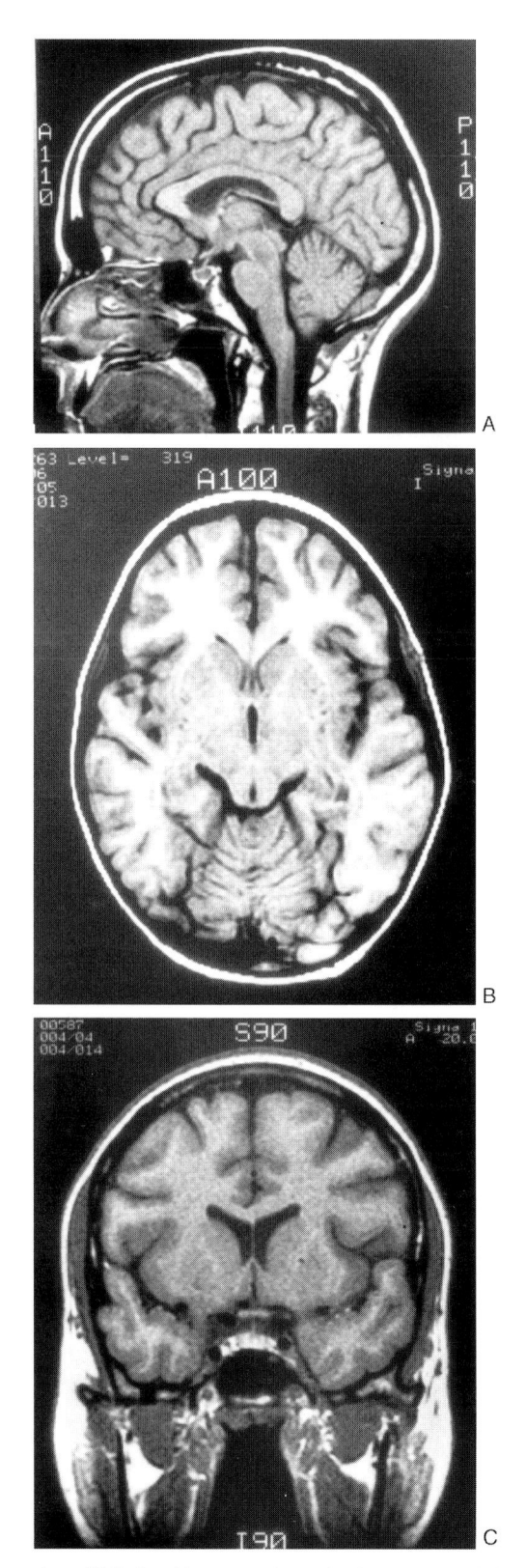

Figure 5.17 Examples of MR head images: (A) sagittal, (B) transaxial, and (C) coronal.

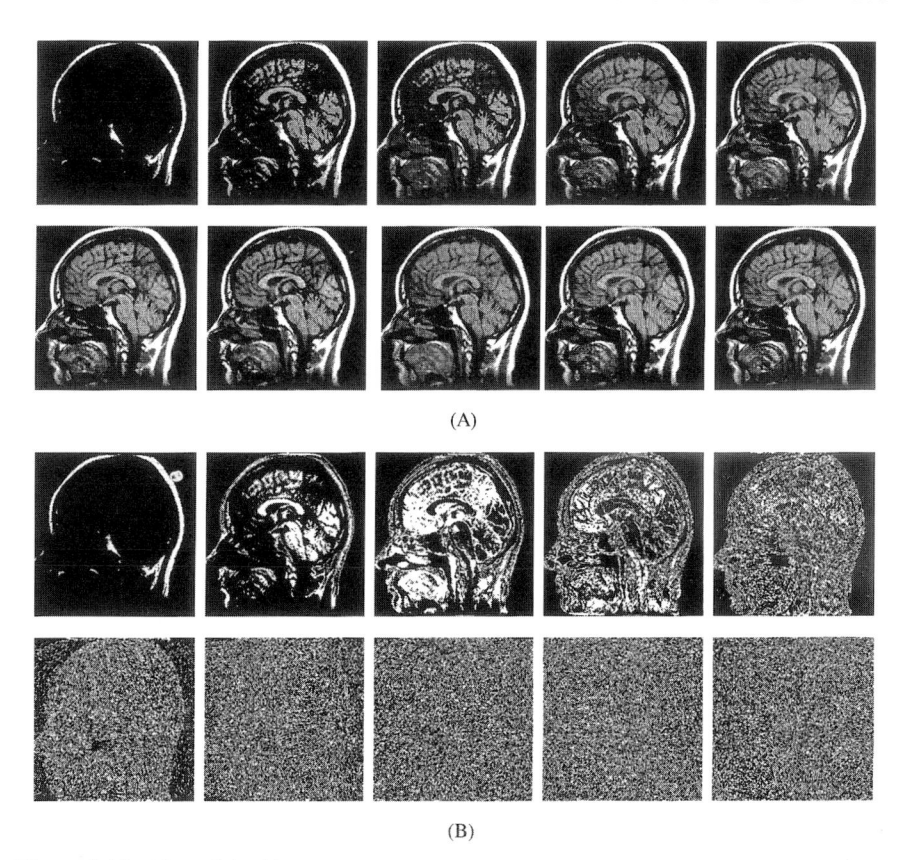

Figure 5.18 The original image (second row, last image) was obtained digitally from a GE Signa 5X MR scanner with 12 bits/pixel. These pictures explore the depth information of the MR image using bit planes. (A) The accumulative bit planes; the top left image displays the most significant bit (1). Moving from left to right, and top to bottom, the next highest bit is added to the previous one: 1 + 2, 1 + 2 + 3, 1 + 2 + 3 + 4, 1 + 2 + 3 + 4 + 5, ... The last image in the second row is the original. No visual differences between the original and rest of the images in the second row are observed. Furthermore, individual bit planes may be observed to determine whether image information is presented at each bit. (B) The individual bit planes. The left-most image in the top row displays the most significant bit (1). Moving from left to right, and top to bottom, the next highest bit is displayed: 2, 3, 4, 5, 6, 7, 8, 9, 10. The bit plane images contain noticeable structural information up to the seventh bit plane. The eighth, ninth, and tenth bit planes offer little, if any structural information.

- a compound microscope with proper illumination for specimen input
- a vidicon (or CCD) camera for scanning microscopic images
- TV monitors for displaying the image
- an analog-to-digital (A/D) converter
- an image memory
- a computer (or image processor) to process the digital image

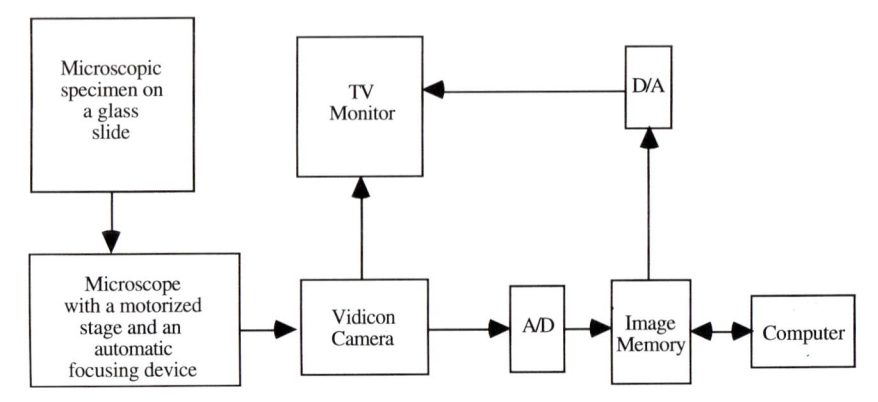

Figure 5.19 Block diagram showing the instrumentation for digital microscopy.

Figure 5.19 shows the block diagram and the physical setup of the instrumentation.

To do effective quantitative analysis with the microscope, two additional attachments to the microscope are necessary: a motorized stage assembly and an automatic focusing device.

5.7.1.1 Motorized Stage Assembly

A motorized stage assembly promotes rapid screening and locating exact position of objects of interest for subsequent detailed analysis. The motorized stage assembly consists of a high precision x-y stage with a specially designed holder for the slide to minimize the vibration due to transmission when the stage is moving. Two stepping motors are used for driving the stage in the x and the y directions. A typical motor step is about 2.5 μm, with an accuracy and repeatability to within ± 1.25 μm. The motors can move the stage in either direction with a maximum speed of 650 steps, or 0.165 cm, per second. The two stepping motors can be controlled manually, or they can be under automatic control by the computer.

5.7.1.2 Automatic Focusing Device

The automatic focusing device ensures that the microscope is focusing all the time when the stepping motors are moving the stage from one field to another. It is essential to have the microscope in focus before the vidicon/CCD camera starts to scan.

Two common methods for automatic focusing are using a third stepping motor in the z direction, and using an air pump. To achieve automatic focusing by means of a third motor, this z-direction motor moves the stage up and down with respect to the objective lens. The z movements are nested in large $+z$ and $-z$ values initially and then gradually to smaller $+z$ and $-z$ values. After each movement, a video scan of the specimen is made through the microscope and some optical parameters are derived from the scan. A focused image is defined as the scan with these optical parameters above certain threshold values. Since nested upward and downward movements of the stage in the z direction are necessary, although the method is automatic, computer processing time to perform the automatic focusing is needed each time the stage moves.

The use of an air pump for automatic focusing is based on the assumption that to have automatic focusing, the specimen lying on the upper surface of a glass slide must be on a perfect horizontal plane with respect to the objective lens at all times. The glass slide is not of uniform thickness, however, and when it rests on the horizontal stage, the lower surface of the slide will form a horizontal plane with respect to the objective, but the upper surface will not, contributing to the imperfect focus of the slide. If an air pump is used to create a vacuum from above, such that the upper surface of the slide is suctioned from above to form a perfect horizontal plane with respective to the objective, then the slide will be focused all the time. Using an air pump for automatic focusing does not require additional time during operation, but it does require precision machinery. Figure 5.20 shows a digital microscopic system.

5.7.2 Resolution

The resolution is defined as the minimum distance between two objects in the specimen which can be resolved by the microscope. The following three factors control the resolution of a microscope.

1. The angle subtended by the object of interest in the specimen and the objective lens: the larger the angle, the higher the resolution.
2. The medium between the objective lens and the coverslip of the glass slide: the higher the refractive index of the medium, the higher the resolution.
3. The wavelength of light employed: the shorter the wavelength, the higher the resolution.

These three factors can be combined into a single equation (Ernst Abbe, 1840–1905)

$$s = \frac{\lambda}{2(\text{NA})} = \frac{\lambda}{2n \sin i} \tag{5.4}$$

where s is the distance between two objects in the specimen that can be resolved (the smaller the s, the greater the resolution), λ is the wavelength of the light employed, n is the refractive index of the medium, i is the half-angle subtended by the object at the objective lens, and NA is the numerical aperture commonly used for defining the resolution (the larger the NA, the higher the resolution).

Therefore, to obtain a higher resolution for a microscopic image, an oil immersion objective lens (large n) with a large angular aperture and select a shorter wavelength of light source for illumination.

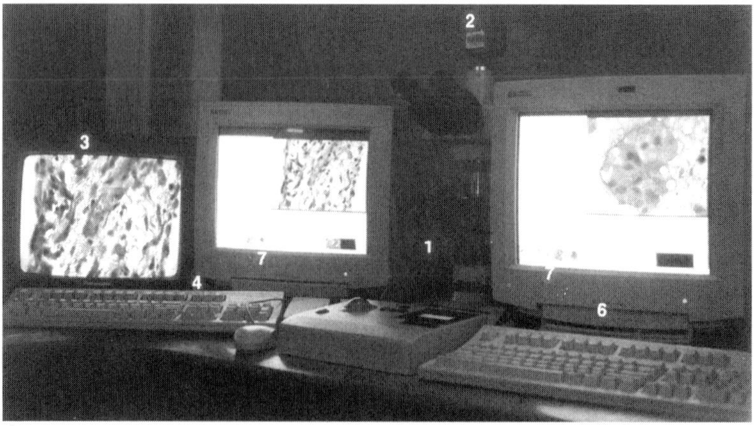
2
3
7
1
4
7
6

A

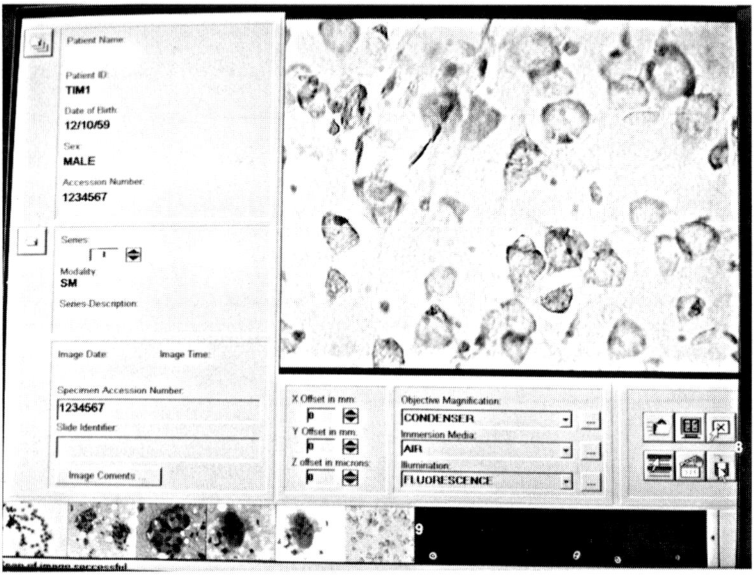
Patient Name
Patient ID
TIM1
Date of Birth
12/10/59
Sex
MALE
Accession Number
1234567
Series
Modality
SM
Series Description
Image Date
Image Time
Specimen Accession Number
1234567
Slide Identifier
Image Coments
X Offset in mm
Y Offset in mm
Z offset in microns
Objective Magnification
CONDENSER
Immersion Media
AIR
Illumination
FLUORESCENCE
8
9

B

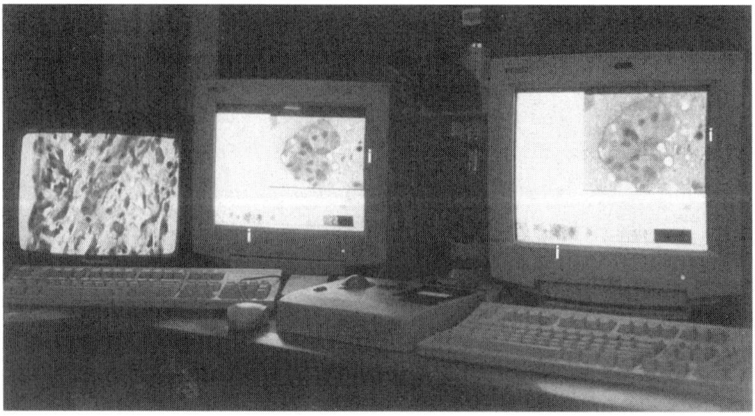

C

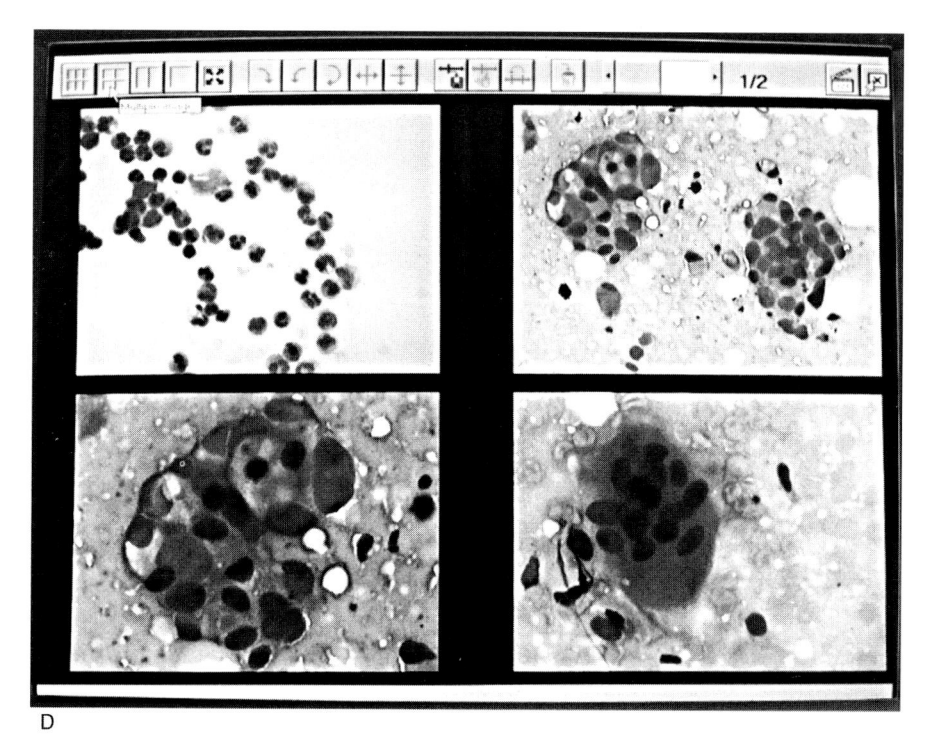

Figure 5.20 A digital telemicroscopic system. (A) *Left:* Image acquisition workstation, automatic microscope (1); CCD camera (2); video monitor (3); computer with an A/D converter attached to the CCD, an image memory, a database to manage the patient image file (4); the video monitor (3) showing a real-time image from the microscope, which is being digitized and shown on the workstation monitor (5). *Right:* Remote diagnostic workstation (6). Thumbnail images at bottom of both workstations are images have been captured and sent to the diagnostic workstation from the acquisition workstation (7). (B) Close-up of the acquisition workstation. Pertinent data related to the exam are shown in various windows. Icons on the bottom right (8) are six simple click-and-play functions: transmit, display, exit, patient information, video capture, digitize, and store. The last captured image (9) is shown on the workstation monitor. (C) Both the acquisition and the diagnostic workstations are displaying the same image for teleconsultation (i). (D) Four-on-one display format showing the first four thumbnail images (see b, bottom row) on one screen of the workstation. The top-row icons are simple image display, manipulation, and transmission functions. (E) Sample patient directory page. The top-row icons are basic user interface functions. [Prototype telemicroscopic imaging system at the Laboratory for Radiological Informatic Lab, UCSF. Courtesy of Drs. S. Atwater, T. Hamill, and H. Sanchez (images); and Nikon Research Corp. and Mitra Imaging, Inc. (equipment).] (See color plate.)

5.7.3 Contrast

Contrast is the ability to differentiate various components in the specimen with different intensity levels. Black-and-white contrast is equivalent to the range of the gray scale (the larger the range, the better the contrast). Color contrast is an important parameter in microscopic image processing; to bring out the color contrast from the image, various color filters must be used with the adjusted illumination.

It is clear that the spatial and density resolutions of a digital image are limited by the resolution and contrast of a microscope, respectively.

5.7.4 Vidicon/CCD Camera and Scanning

When the specimen is focused under the microscope, a vidicon or a charge-coupled device (CCD) camera (see Section 3.2.1) can be attached to the microscope tube to detect the light emitted from the specimen within the microscopic field of view. The camera scans the specimen pixel by pixel from left to right, top to bottom, and forms a light image of the specimen on the photosensitive face of the camera. The brightness $B(x,y)$ of each pixel is converted into an electrical voltage (video signal), which is transmitted to the display monitor. This voltage is used to control the brightness of a corresponding spot on the fluorescent screen of the monitor. These spots reconstruct a video image of the specimen on the TV screen. If the camera is to perform satisfactorily for microscopic imaging, the following specifications should be met:

Gamma (γ) of the camera	0.65 or less
Dynamic range	200:1
Resolution	The MTF (modulation transfer function derived by plotting the video amplitude versus the number of line per unit length) should be comparable to that of an ideal Gaussian spot with diameter 1/500 of the image width.
Linearity	$\pm$ 0.5% of the pixel value for all pixels

5.7.5 A/D Conversion

There are two methods for digitizing the microscopic image from the vidicon camera. The first is real-time digitizing with a fast A/D converter, usually in the 10 MHz range. It converts the video signal $B(x,y)$ into a digital number $f(x,y)$ and sends it to the (x,y) location of the image memory. A complete TV frame (512×512 pixels with 8 bits/pixel) can be digitized in 1/30 second. Because of the high speed A/D conversion, the signal-to-noise ratio of the real-time digitized image tends to be low. To improve the SNR, it is common to digitize the same frame many times and take the average value for each pixel (Section 2.5.2).

The second method, featuring a high resolution digitizer, uses a slower but better signal-to-noise ratio A/D converter, and the digital image thus obtained is of better quality. Since the A/D conversion rate is much slower than the TV scanning rate, the same microscopic field must be scanned many times to produce a complete digital image.

5.7.6 Image Memory

The image memory stores and displays the digitized microscopic image. Once digitized and stored in the memory, the image is continuously refreshed in synchrony with the video scan.

The image memory is not a component of the main computer and should be considered as a very fast peripheral storage device; the stored image can be accessed by the computer for image processing. The image memory is generally organized into memory planes, each plane has the storage capacity to refresh a 512×512 one-bit gray level image. The most commonly used refresh memory for imaging has 8 or 12 memory planes, which give 256 to 4096 gray levels. In addition, there should be one extra memory plane for graphic overlay on top of the image memory for interactive image processing.

If a real color microscopic image is needed, the color specimen is generally digitized in three separate steps, with a red, a blue, and a green filter. The three color-filtered images are then stored in the corresponding three image memories, the red, blue, and green, each of which with eight planes. Thus, a true color image has 24 bits/pixel. The computer will treat the contents of the three image memories as individual microscopic images and process them separately. The real color digital microscopic image can be displayed back on a color monitor from these three memories through a color composite video control. Figure 5.21 shows the block diagram of a true color

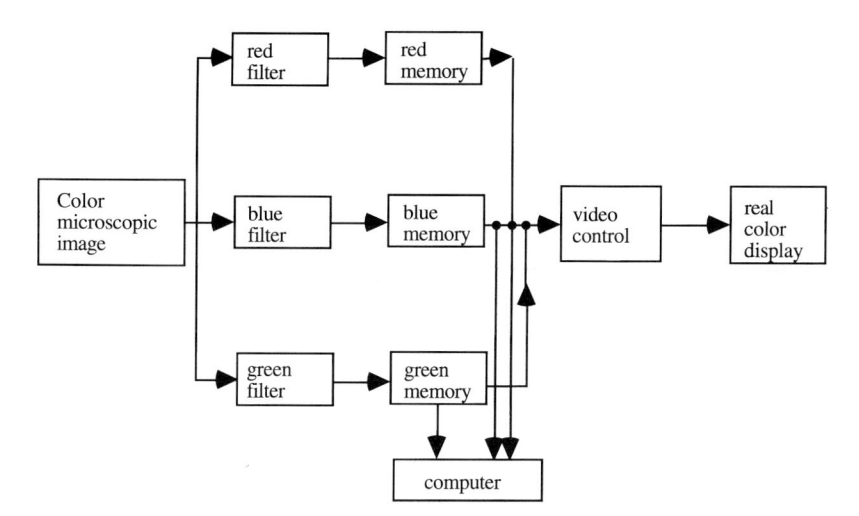

Figure 5.21 Color image processing block diagram. Red, blue, and green filters are used to filter the image before digitization. The three digitized, filtered images are stored in the red, blue, and green memories, respectively. The real color image can be displayed back on the color monitor from these three memories through the composite video control.

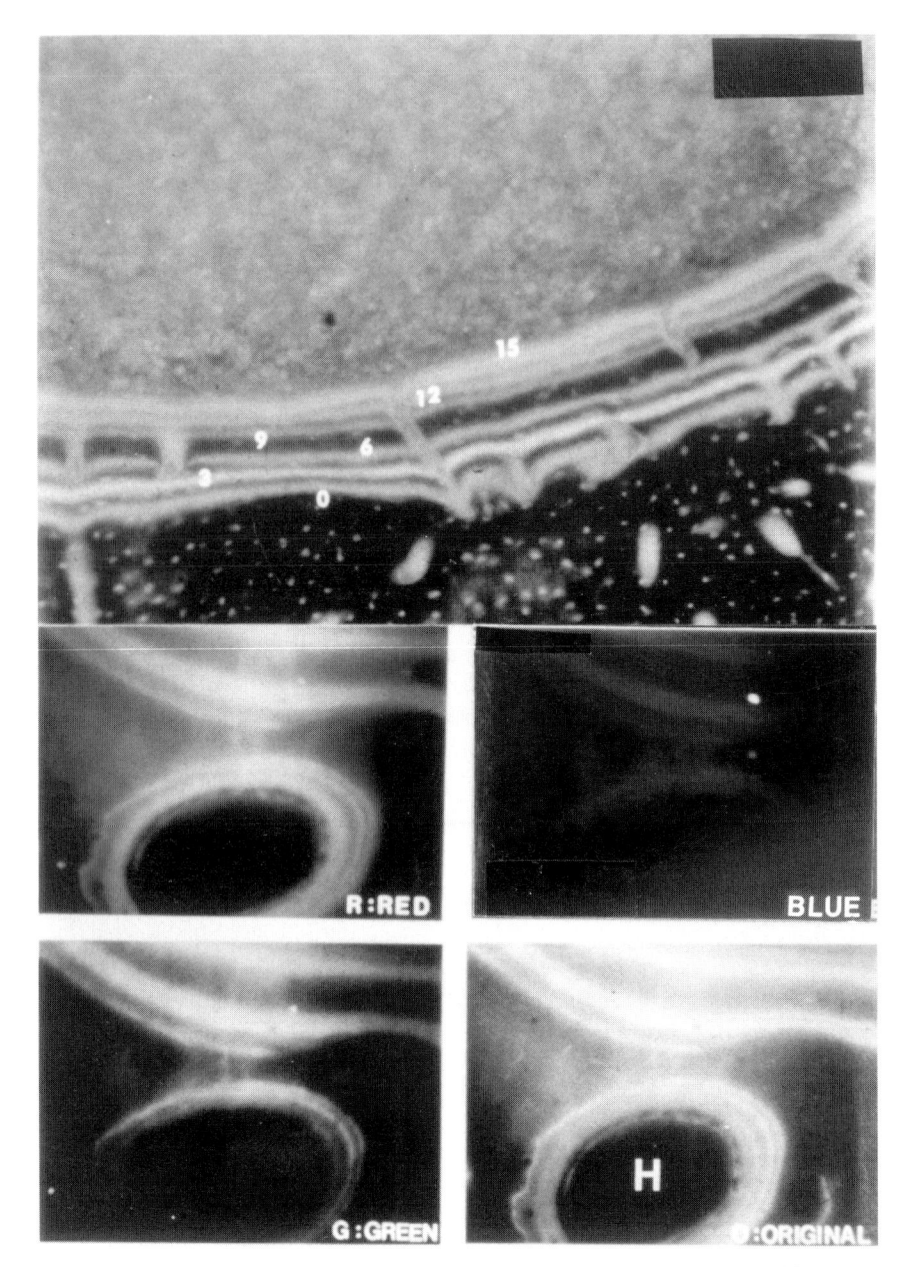

Figure 5.22 *Top:* Fluorochromic image of a bone cell from the tibia of a rat bone biopsy sample with tetracycline labels shown in orange-red. Each label has its own color characteristics: day 0, oxytetracycline label; day 3, DCAF; day 6, xylenol orange, 90 mg/kg; day 9, hematoporphyrin, 300 mg/kg (did not stain); day 12, doxycycline; day 15, alizarin red 5. The dose is 20 mg/kg. *Lower series:* Partial osteonal unit depicting the osteoid and the Haversian canal (H); one tetracycline label is shown in orange-red, the inside ring immediately adjacent to H. The three color images red, blue, and green are also shown. (See color plate.)

microscopic imaging system. In the fluorochromic image of a bone cell with tetracycline labels of Figure 5.22, a partial osteonal unit is shown in the red, blue, green, and the composite color images.

5.7.7 Computer

The computer, usually a personal computer with necessary peripherals, serves as a control as well as performing image analysis in the system. The following are the major control functions:

movement of the x-y stepping motors
control of the automatic focusing
control of the color filtering
control of the digitization of the microscopic image
image processing

For examples of digitized images of a cell, refer again to Figure 2.2, the lymphocyte shown in various spatial and density resolutions.

CHAPTER 6

Image Compression

Compressing a radiologic image can save image storage space and transmission time. This chapter describes some compression techniques that are applicable to radiologic images.

6.1 TERMINOLOGY

The half-dozen definitions that follow are essential to an understanding of image compression/reconstruction.

Original image. The original image is a digital radiologic image $f(x,y)$, where f is a nonnegative integer function, and x and y can be from 0 to 255, 0 to 511, 0 to 1023, and 0 to 2047. In the three-dimensional (3-D) case, $f(x,y,z)$ is a 3-D data block. The original image is a two-dimensional rectangular array or a 3-D data block to be compressed into a one-dimensional data file.

Transformed image. The transformed image $F(u,v)$ of the original image $f(x,y)$ is the two-dimensional array after a mathematical transformation. If the transformation is the forward discrete cosine transform, then u, v are nonnegative integers representing the frequencies. In the case of 3-D, the transformed data block is also a 3-D data block.

Compressed image file. The compressed image file is a one-dimensional array of encoded information derived from the original or the transformed image by an image compression technique.

Reconstructed image from a compressed image file. The reconstructed image from a compressed image file is a two-dimensional rectangular array $f_c(x,y)$, or a 3-D data block $f_c(x,y,z)$. The technique used for the reconstruction (or decoding) depends on the method of compression. In the case of error-free compression, the reconstructed image is identical to the original image, whereas in irreversible image compression, some information will be lost between the original and the reconstructed image. The term "reconstructed image from a compressed image file" should not be confused with the image reconstruction accomplished by means of projections used in computed tomography as described in Chapter 5.

Difference image. The difference image is defined as the subtracted image or a 3-D data block between the original and the reconstructed image, $f(x,y) - f_c(x,y)$, or $f(x,y,z) - f_c(x,y,z)$. In the case of error-free compression, the difference image is the zero image. In the case of irreversible compression, the difference image is the difference between the original image and the reconstructed image. The amount of the difference depends on the compression technique used as well as the compression ratio.

Compression ratio. The compression ratio between the original image and the compressed image file is the ratio between computer storage required to save the original image and that of the compressed data. Thus, a 4:1 compression on a 512 × 512 × 8 = 2,097,152-bit image requires only 524,288-bit storage, 25% of the original image storage required.

6.2 BACKGROUND

Picture archiving and communication systems (PACS) require image compression for obvious reasons: to speed up image transmission rate and to save on storage requirements. The number of digital radiologic images captured per year in the United States alone is of the order of petabytes (i.e., 10^{15} bytes) and is increasing rapidly every year. Image compression provides an impetus for storage and communication of this voluminous supply of digital image data. First, it reduces the bit size required to store and represent images, while maintaining relevant diagnostic information. Second, it enables fast transmission of large medical image files over a network for display at workstations, where diagnostic, review, and teaching purposes can be served.

Technically, all image data compression schemes can be broadly categorized into two types. One is *reversible* or "lossless" *compression*, shown in Figure 6.1. A reversible scheme achieves modest compression ratios of the order of 2 to 3, but will allow exact recovery of the original image from the compressed version. An *irreversible scheme* will not allow exact recovery after compression but can achieve much higher compression ratios (e.g., ranging from 10 to 50 or more). Generally speaking, more compression is obtained at the expense of more image degradation; that is, image quality declines as the compression ratio increases. Another type of compression used in medical imaging is *clinical image compression*, which stores a few medically relevant images, as determined by the physicians, out of a series of real-time images or a multiple sequence examination, thus reducing the total number of images in an examination file. The stored images may or may not be further compressed by the reversible or irreversible scheme. In an ultrasound examination, for example, the radiologist may collect data for several seconds, at 30 images per second of data collection, but keep only 4 to 8 frames for recording, discarding the rest. In an MR head study, a multiple sequence examination can accumulate up to 200 images, of which only several may be of importance for the diagnosis.

Image degradation from irreversible compression may or may not be visually apparent. The term "visually lossless" has been used to characterize lossy schemes that result in no visible loss under normal radiologic viewing conditions. An image reconstructed from a compression algorithm that is visually lossless under certain viewing conditions (e.g., a 19-in. video monitor with 1024 × 1024 pixels at a viewing dis-

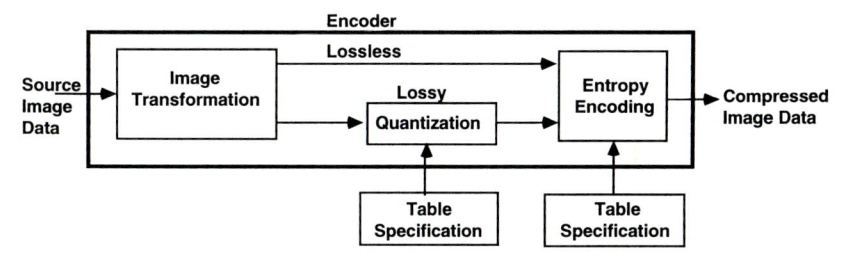

Figure 6.1 The general framework for image data compression. Image transformation can be as simple as a shift of a row and a subtraction, or a more complicated mathematical transformation can result. The decoder is the reverse of the encoder. The quantization determines whether the compression is lossless or lossy.

tance of 4 ft) could result in visible degradations under more stringent conditions (e.g., printed on a 14 in. × 17 in. film).

A related term used by the American College of Radiology and National Electrical Manufacturing Association (ACR-NEMA), or Digital Imaging and Communication in Medicine (DICOM) is *information preserving*. The ACR-NEMA standard report defines a compression scheme as "information preserving" if the resulting image retains all the significant information of the original image. Both "visually lossless" and "information preserving" are subjective terms, and extreme caution must be taken in their interpretation.

Currently, lossy algorithms are not being used by radiologists in primary diagnoses because physicians and radiologists are concerned with the legal consequences of an incorrect diagnosis based on a lossy compressed image. Indeed, lossy compression has raised new legal questions for manufacturers and users alike, and the U.S. Food and Drug Administration (FDA) has instituted new regulatory policies. However, large-scale clinical tests are under way by several research laboratories to develop reasonable policies and acceptable standards for the use of lossy processing on medical images. This topic is discussed in Section 6.8.

6.3 ERROR-FREE COMPRESSION

This section presents three error-free image compression techniques. The first technique is based on some inherent properties of the image under consideration; the second and third are standard data compression methods.

6.3.1 Background Removal

Compression, by means of background removal is applied to two different categories of images: cross-sectional images obtained from picture reconstructions from projections like MR, CT, PET, and SPECT; and digital projectional images like CR and digital mammography. A cross-sectional image is first compressed through a clipping

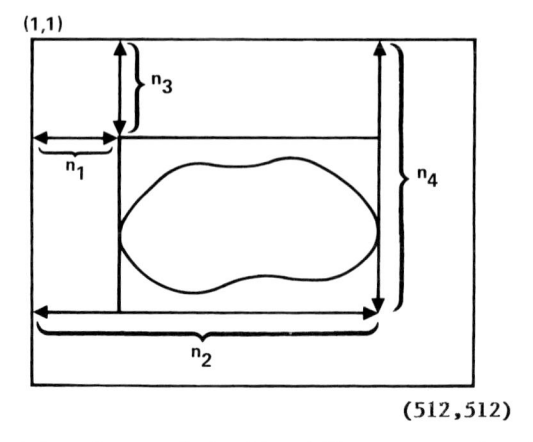

Figure 6.2 A simple boundary search algorithm yields n_1, n_2, n_3, and n_4, the four parameters required to compress a 512 × 512 CT image to a smaller rectangular area with dimensions of $(n_2 - n_1) \times (n_4 - n_3)$. These parameters also give the relative location of the rectangle with respect to the original image. Each pixel in this rectangle area can be compressed further by means of a lossless procedure.

procedure as shown in Figure 6.2. In this case, only the information within the rectangle, including the outer boundary of the cross section, is retained. The size and relative location of the rectangle with respect to the original image are saved in the image header for image reconstruction. In the case of CR and digital mammography, the background outside of anatomical boundary can be discarded through a background removal technique as described in Section 4.1.6: Figures 4.8 to 4.12 showed some background-removed CR images. Figure 6.3 shows a digital mammogram from which the background was removed automatically. In these cases, background-removed images have been compressed by discarding background information that has no diagnostic value. The value of each pixel within the rectangle, or anatomical boundary, can be further compressed through a lossless compression, described in Section 6.3.2.

6.3.2 Run-Length Coding

Run-length coding, which is based on the repeatability of adjacent pixel values, can be used to compress an image rowwise or columnwise. A run-length code consists of three sequential numbers: the mark, the length, and the gray level. The compression procedure starts with obtaining a histogram of the image. The histogram of an image is a plot of the frequency of occurrence versus the pixel value of the entire image. The mark is chosen as the gray level in the image that has the least frequency of occurrence. If more than one gray level has the same least frequency of occurrence, the higher gray level will be chosen as the mark. The image is then searched line by line, and sets of three sequential numbers are encoded.

For example, assume that the lowest frequency of occurrence gray level in a 512

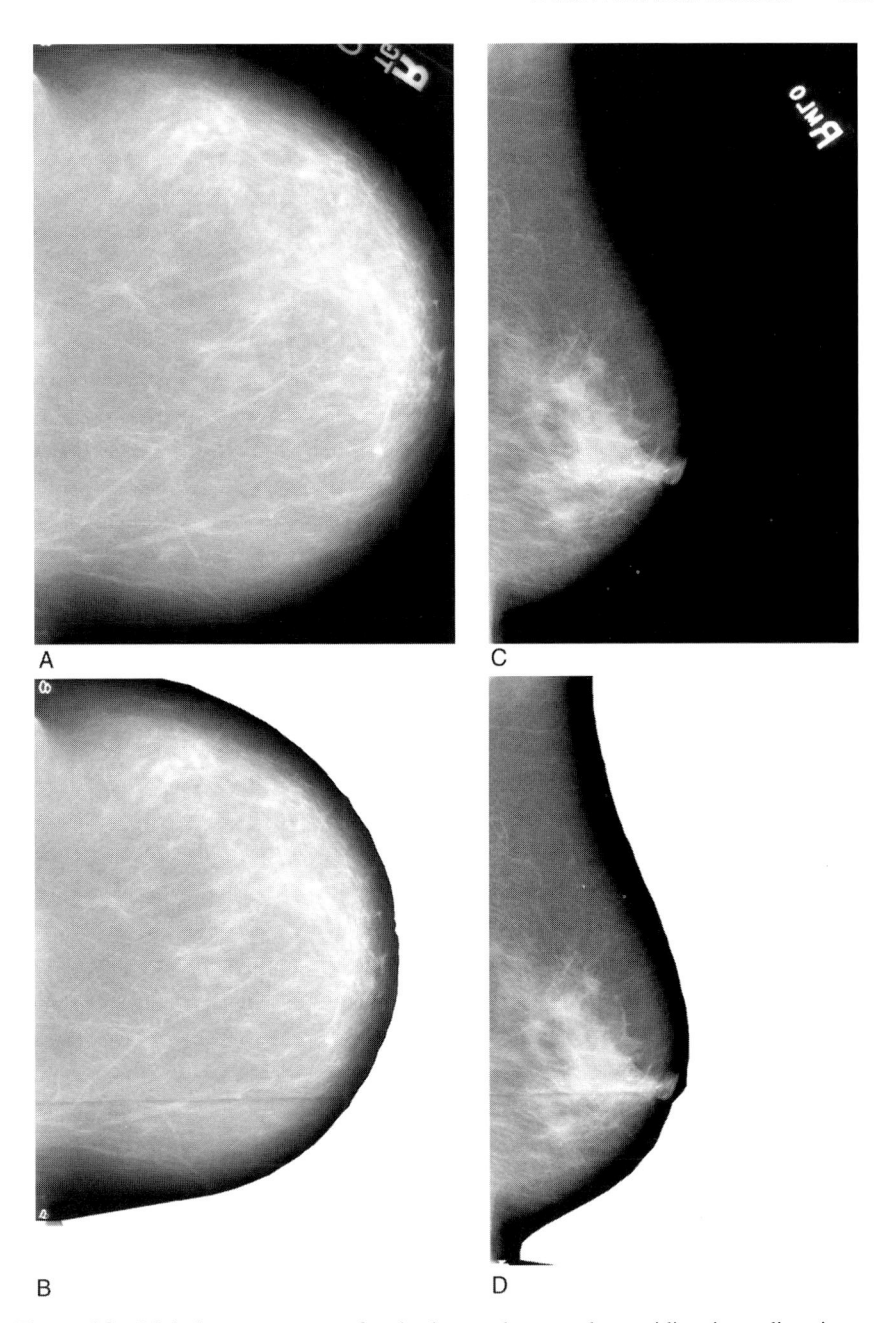

Figure 6.3 Digital mammogram after background removal, providing immediate image compression. (A) A large breast occupies most of the image. (B) Background-removed image, compression ratio 3.1:1. (C) A small breast occupies a small portion of the image. (D) Background-removed image, compression ratio 6.3:1. (Courtesy of Jun Wang, 1996.)

× 512 × 8 image is 128. During the search, suppose the search program encounters 25 pixels, all of which have a value of 10. The run-length code for these numbers would then be:

128	25	10
MARK	LENGTH	GRAY LEVEL

When the length is the same as the mark, the three-number set should be split into two sets. For example, the set 128 128 34 should be split into two sets: 128 4 34 and 128 124 34; the lengths 4 and 124 are arbitrary but should be predetermined before the encoding.

There are two special cases in the run-length code:

1. Since each run-length code set requires three numbers, there is no advantage in compressing adjacent pixels with value repeating fewer than four times. In this case each of these pixel values are used as the code.
2. The code can consist of two sequential numbers only:

    128 128: next pixel value is 128
    128 0: end of the coding

To decode the run-length coding, the procedure checks the coded data sequentially. If a mark is found, the following two codes must be the length and the gray level, except for the two special cases. In the first case, if a mark is not found, the code itself is the gray level. In the second case, a 128 following a 128 means that the next pixel value is 128, and a 0 following a 128 means the end of the coding.

Figure 6.4 provides an example: the run-length codes of two horizontal lines from a CT head scan (Fig. 6.4C, E) yield compression ratios for these lines of about 9.1:1 and 1.5:1, respectively.

A modified run-length coding called run-zero coding is sometimes more practical to use. In this case, the original image is first shifted one pixel to the right and a shifted image is formed. A subtracted image between the original and the shifted image is obtained, which is to be coded. A run-length code on the subtracted image requires only the mark and the length because the third code is not necessary: either it is zero or it is not, given the two special cases described earlier. The run-zero coding requires that the pixel values of the left-most column of the original image be saved for the decoding procedure.

6.3.3 Huffman Coding

Huffman coding, which is based on the probability (or the frequency) of occurrence of gray levels in the image, can be used to compress the original image. The encoding procedure is best described with an example.

1. *The original image.* Consider the 10 × 10 image with eight gray levels (C, F, G, B, E, D, H, A) shown in Figure 6.5A.

ERROR-FREE COMPRESSION **135**

(A) Selective run-length coding for CT image application

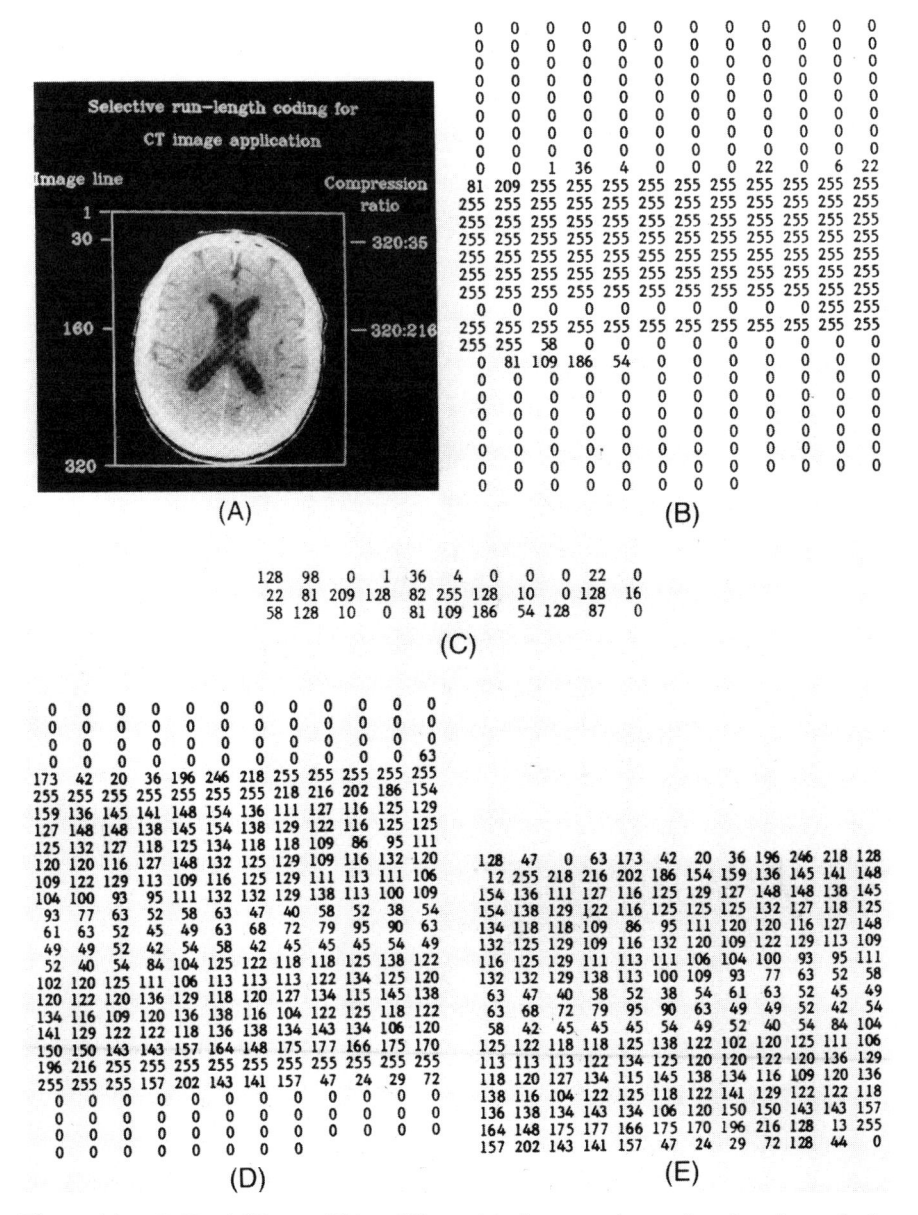

(B)
```
  0   0   0   0   0   0   0   0   0   0   0   0
  0   0   0   0   0   0   0   0   0   0   0   0
  0   0   0   0   0   0   0   0   0   0   0   0
  0   0   0   0   0   0   0   0   0   0   0   0
  0   0   0   0   0   0   0   0   0   0   0   0
  0   0   0   0   0   0   0   0   0   0   0   0
  0   0   0   0   0   0   0   0   0   0   0   0
  0   0   1  36   4   0   0   0  22   0   6  22
 81 209 255 255 255 255 255 255 255 255 255 255
255 255 255 255 255 255 255 255 255 255 255 255
255 255 255 255 255 255 255 255 255 255 255 255
255 255 255 255 255 255 255 255 255 255 255 255
255 255 255 255 255 255 255 255 255 255 255 255
255 255 255 255 255 255 255 255 255 255 255 255
255 255 255 255 255 255 255 255 255 255 255 255
  0   0   0   0   0   0   0   0   0   0 255 255
255 255 255 255 255 255 255 255 255 255 255 255
255 255  58   0   0   0   0   0   0   0   0   0
  0  81 109 186  54   0   0   0   0   0   0   0
  0   0   0   0   0   0   0   0   0   0   0   0
  0   0   0   0   0   0   0   0   0   0   0   0
  0   0   0   0   0   0   0   0   0   0   0   0
  0   0   0   0   0   0   0   0   0   0   0   0
  0   0   0   0   0   0   0   0   0   0   0   0
  0   0   0   0   0   0   0   0   0   0   0   0
  0   0   0   0   0   0   0
```

(C)
```
128  98   0   1  36   4   0   0  22   0
 22  81 209 128  82 255 128  10   0 128  16
 58 128  10   0  81 109 186  54 128  87   0
```

(D)
```
  0   0   0   0   0   0   0   0   0   0   0
  0   0   0   0   0   0   0   0   0   0   0
  0   0   0   0   0   0   0   0   0   0   0
  0   0   0   0   0   0   0   0   0   0  63
173  42  20  36 196 246 218 255 255 255 255 255
255 255 255 255 255 255 255 218 216 202 186 154
159 136 145 141 148 154 136 111 127 116 125 129
127 148 148 138 145 154 138 129 122 116 125 125
125 132 127 118 125 134 118 118 109  86  95 111
120 120 116 127 148 132 125 129 109 116 132 120
109 122 129 113 109 116 125 129 111 113 111 106
104 100  93  95 111 132 132 138 113 100 109
 93  77  63  52  58  63  47  40  58  52  38  54
 61  63  52  45  49  63  68  72  79  95  90  63
 49  49  52  42  54  58  42  45  45  54  54  49
 52  40  54  84 104 125 122 118 118 125 138 122
102 120 125 111 106 113 113 122 134 125 120
120 122 120 136 129 118 120 127 134 115 145 138
134 116 109 120 136 138 116 104 122 125 118 122
141 129 122 122 118 136 138 134 143 134 106 120
150 150 143 143 157 164 148 175 177 166 175 170
196 216 255 255 255 255 255 255 255 255 255 255
255 255 255 157 202 143 141 157  47  24  29  72
  0   0   0   0   0   0   0   0   0   0   0
  0   0   0   0   0   0   0   0   0   0   0
  0   0   0   0   0   0   0   0   0   0   0
  0   0   0   0   0   0   0
```

(E)
```
128  47   0  63 173  42  20  36 196 246 218 128
 12 255 218 216 202 186 154 159 136 145 141 148
154 136 111 127 116 125 129 127 148 148 138 145
154 138 129 122 116 125 125 125 132 127 118 125
134 118 118 109  86  95 111 120 120 116 127 148
132 125 129 109 116 132 120 109 122 129 113 109
116 125 129 111 113 111 106 104 100  93  95 111
132 132 129 138 113 100 109  93  77  63  52  58
 63  47  40  58  52  38  54  61  63  52  45  49
 63  68  72  79  95  90  63  49  49  52  42  54
 58  42  45  45  54  49  52  40  54  84 104
125 122 118 118 125 138 122 102 120 125 111 106
113 113 113 122 134 125 120 120 122 120 136 129
118 120 127 134 115 145 138 134 116 109 120 136
138 116 104 122 125 118 122 141 129 122 118
136 138 134 143 134 106 120 150 150 143 143 157
164 148 175 177 166 175 170 196 216 128  13 255
157 202 143 141 157  47  24  29  72 128  44   0
```

Figure 6.4 (A) Head CT scan (320 × 320 matrix); for convenience of explanation, only the 8 most significant bits per pixel (0 to 255) are used during the compression. (B) Pixel values in horizontal line 30 of the head CT scan: total bytes, 320. (C) Run-length coding for line 30: code mark, 128; total bytes required, 35; compression ratio, 320/35, (9.1:1). (D) Pixel values in horizontal line 160 of the head CT scan, total bytes, 320. (E) Run-length coding for line 160: code mark, 128; total bytes required, 216; compression ratio, 320/216, (1.5:1). The compression ratios in C and E are quite different because of the backgrounds outside the CT image.

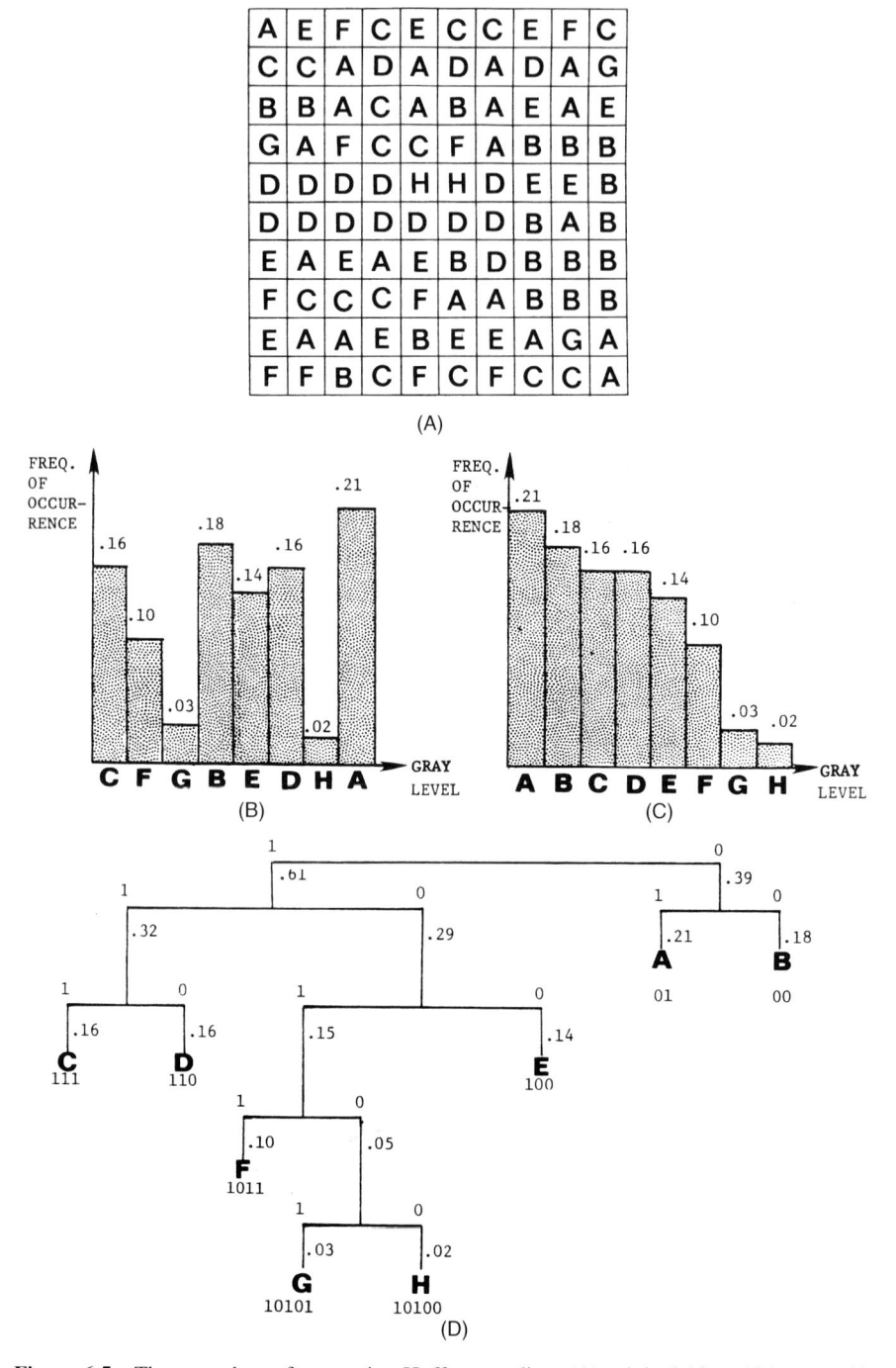

Figure 6.5 The procedure of generating Huffman coding: (A) original 10 × 10 image with eight gray levels (C, F, G, B, E, D, H, A), (B) histogram of the original image, (C) the rearranged histogram, and (D) the Huffman tree and its corresponding codes.

2. *The histogram.* Obtain the histogram of the original image (Fig. 6.5B).

3. *Rearrangement of the histogram.* Rearrange the histogram according to the probability (or frequency) of occurrence of the gray levels and form a new histogram (Fig. 6.5C).

4. *The Huffman tree.* A Huffman tree with two nodes at each level is built as follows (Fig. 6.5D). To start, take the two gray levels with the lowest probability of occurrence, in this case G and H, to form the first level; always put the gray level with a higher probability value to the left. Add the total probabilities of these two nodes (.03 + .02 = .05). Take the next gray level in the rearranged histogram (F) and form a higher level branch with G and H; put F at the left because of its higher probability value (0.1). Continue until the branch has reached a probability of 0.29. At this point no gray levels in the rearranged histogram have a higher probability value than 0.29. Take the next two available gray levels in the rearranged histogram (C and D) and form a new branch. Always place the higher probability gray level on the left. Join this new branch with the previously established branches, which gives a probability of 0.61. Return to the rearranged histogram and repeat the procedure until all the gray levels have been used. This completes the first step of forming a Huffman tree.

Next, designate a "1" to the left and a "0" to the right node throughout all branches of the tree, starting from the highest probability branches. The last step is to assign bits to each gray level according to its location in the tree. For example, gray level H would be assigned "10100" because it is at the fifth level, with the trace of the probabilities as follows:

```
1————0————1————0————0————"H"
  .61     .29    .15    .05    .02
```

The complete Huffman tree is shown in Figure 6.5D.

5. *The Huffman code.* The Huffman code for these eight gray levels are:

A:01   2 bits
B:00   2 bits
C:111   3 bits
D:110   3 bits
E:100   3 bits
F:1011   4 bits
G:10101 5 bits
H:10100 5 bits

Therefore, the first row of the original image (Fig. 6.5A) can be encoded as:

```
  01    100   1011   111   100   ...
   A     E     F      C     E    ...
```

138 IMAGE COMPRESSION

6. *Compression ratio.* To compute the compression ratio, assume that each pixel in the original image requires 3 bits to preserve the information ($2^3 = 8$ gray levels). The average number of bits required to compress this image using this Huffman code can be computed by:

$$\text{average number of bits} = \sum_{i=1}^{8} P_i[\text{bit is required for gray level ``}i\text{''}]$$
$$= 0.21 \times 2 + 0.18 \times 2 + 0.16 \times 3 + 0.16 \times 3 + 0.14 \times 3 + 0.1 \times 4 + 0.03 \times 5 + 0.02 \times 5$$
$$= 2.81$$

where i is any of A, B, ..., H and P_i is the probability of occurrence of gray level "i."

The compression ratio, in this case, 3:2.81 = 1.1:1, is not a very good result. In general, Huffman coding will give low compression ratios for flat histogram images and higher compression ratios for sharp histograms.

In practice, Huffman coding should also be applied to the subtracted image obtained from the original and the shifted image as described in Section 6.3.2. To reconstruct the image, the compressed image file is searched sequentially, bit by bit, to match the Huffman code, and then decoded accordingly.

Figure 6.6 presents an example of an error-free image compression using the Huffman coding on a shifted-then-subtracted digitized chest X-ray image ($512 \times 512 \times 8$).

To obtain higher error-free compression ratios, the run-length method can be used first, followed by the Huffman coding.

6.4 TWO-DIMENSIONAL IRREVERSIBLE IMAGE COMPRESSION

6.4.1 Introduction

Irreversible compression is most often done in the transform domain and is called transform coding. The procedure of transform coding is to first transform the original image into the transform domain with a two-dimensional transformation—for example, Fourier, Hadamard, cosine, Karhunen–Loeve, or wavelet. The transform coefficients are then quantized and encoded (see Fig. 6.1). The result is a highly compressed data file.

The image can be compressed in blocks or in its entirety. In block compression, before the image transformation, the entire image can be subdivided into equal sized blocks (e.g., 8×8), whereupon the transformation is applied to each block. A statistical quantitation method is then used to encode the 8×8 transform coefficients of each block. In the block compression technique, all blocks can be compressed in parallel, and it is easier to perform the computation for a small block transformation than for an entire image. However a blocky artifact, which is not desirable for radiologic applications, may appear in the reconstructed image when the compression ratios are

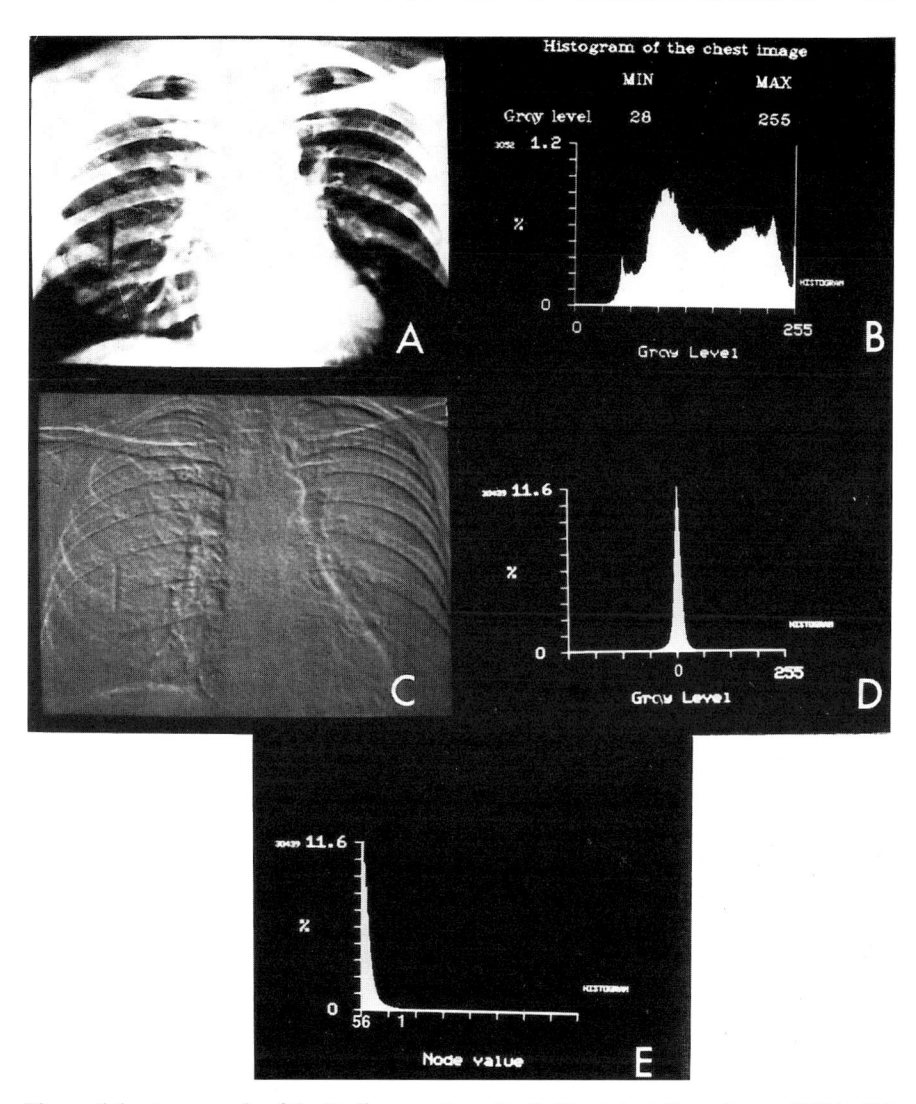

Figure 6.6 An example of the Huffman coding of a digitized chest X-ray image (512 × 512 × 8): (A) the original digitized chest image, (B) histogram of the original image, (C) the subtracted image, (D) histogram of the subtracted image, and (E) the rearranged histogram. The compression ratio of the subtracted image is about 2.1:1. Shifting the image one pixel down and one pixel to the right produces a subtracted image between the original and the shifted image. Huffman coding of the subtracted image yields a higher compression ratio than that of the original image. The first row and the left-most column of the original image are needed during the decoding process.

high. Further image processing on the reconstructed image is sometimes necessary to smooth out such an artifact.

The full-frame compression technique, on the other hand, transforms the entire image into the transform domain. Quantitation is applied to *all* the transform coefficients of the entire transformed image. The full-frame technique is computationally tedious, expensive, and time-consuming. Since, however, it does not produce a blocky artifact, it is more suitable for radiologic application in principle.

6.4.2 Block Compression Technique

The most popular block compression technique using forward two-dimensional discrete cosine transform is the JPEG (Joint Photographic Experts Group) standard. Sections 6.4.2.1 to 6.4.2.4 summarize this method, which consists of four steps: two-dimensional forward discrete cosine transform (DCT), bit allocation table and quantitation, DCT coding, and entropy coding.

6.4.2.1 Two-Dimensional Discrete Cosine Transform

Discrete cosine transform, a special case of discrete Fourier transform discussed in Section 2.4.3, has been proven to be an effective method for image compression because the energy in the transform domain is concentrated in a small region. As a result, the DCT method can yield larger compression ratios and maintain the image quality compared with other methods. The forward discrete cosine transform of the original image $f(j, k)$ is given by

$$F(u,v) = \left(\frac{2}{N}\right)^2 C(u)C(v) \left(\sum_{k=0}^{N-1} \sum_{j=0}^{N-1} f(j,k) \cos\frac{u(j+0.5)}{N} \cos\frac{v(k+0.5)}{N} \right) \quad (6.1)$$

The inverse discrete cosine transform of $F(u,v)$ is the original image $f(j,k)$:

$$f(j,k) = \sum_{v=0}^{N-1} \sum_{u=0}^{N-1} F(u,v) C(u) C(v) \cos\frac{u(j+0.5)}{N} \cos\frac{v(k+0.5)}{N} \quad (6.2)$$

where $C(O) = (1/2)^{[1/2]}$ for $u, v \neq 0$
$\qquad\qquad = 1$ for $u, v = 0$
and $N \times N$ is the size of the image.

Thus, for the block transform, $N \times N = 8 \times 8$, whereas for the full-frame compression of a 2048 × 2,048 image, $N = 2048$.

6.4.2.2 Bit Allocation Table and Quantization

The 2-D DCT of an 8 × 8 block yields 64 DCT coefficients. The energy of these coefficients is concentrated among the lower frequency components. To achieve a higher compression ratio, these coefficients are quantized with no greater precision than is necessary to achieve the desired image quality. Since, however, quantization compromises the original values of the coefficients, some information lost. Quantization of the DCT coefficient $F(u,v)$ can be obtained by

$$F_q(u,v) = \text{NINT}\frac{F(u,v)}{Q(u,v)} \qquad (6.3)$$

where $Q(u,v)$ is the quantizer step size, and NINT is the nearest integer function.

One method of determining the quantizer step size is by manipulating a bit allocation table $B(u,v)$ which is defined by

$$\begin{aligned}B(u,v) &= \log_2\big[|F(u,v)|\big] + K & \text{if } |F(u,v)| \geq 1 \\ &= K & \text{otherwise}\end{aligned} \qquad (6.4)$$

where $|F(u,v)|$ is the absolute value of the cosine transform coefficient, and K is a real number that determines the compression ratio. Notice that each pixel in the transformed image $F(u,v)$ corresponds to one value of the table $B(u,v)$. Each value in this table represents the number of computer memory bits for saving the corresponding pixel value in the transformed image. The value in the bit allocation table can be adjusted to increase or decrease the amount of compression by assigning a certain value to K. Thus, for example, if a pixel located at (p,q) and $F(p,q) = 3822$, then $B(p,q) = 11.905 + K$. If one selects $K = +0.095$, then $B(p,q) = 12$ (i.e., 12 bits are allocated to save the value 3822). On the other hand, if one selects $K = -0.905$, then $B(p,q) = 11$ [i.e., $F(p,q)$ is compressed to 11 bits].

Based on Eq. (6.4), we can rewrite Eq. (6.3) as follows:

$$F_q(u,v) = \text{NINT}\left[(2^{|B(m,n)-1|} - 1)\frac{F(u,v)}{|F(m,n)|}\right] \qquad (6.5)$$

where $F(u,v)$ is the coefficient of the transformed image, $F_q(u,v)$ is the corresponding quantized value, (m,n) is the location of the maximum value of $|F(u,v)|$ for $0 < u,v < N - 1$, and $B(m,n)$ is the corresponding number of bits in the bit allocation table assigned to save $|F(m,n)|$. It is seen in Eq. (6.5) that $F(u,v)$ has been normalized with respect to $(2^{|B(m,n)-1|} - 1)/|F(m,n)|$

The quantized value $F_q(u,v)$ is an approximate value of $F(u,v)$ because of the value K described in Eq. (6.4). This quantized procedure introduces an approximation to the compressed image file.

6.4.2.3 DCT Coding and Entropy Coding

For block quantization with an 8 × 8 matrix, the $F(0,0)$ is the DC coefficient and is normally the maximum value of $|F(u,v)|$. Starting from $F(0,0)$, the rest of the 63 coefficients can be coded in a zigzag sequence shown in Figure 6.7. This zigzag se-

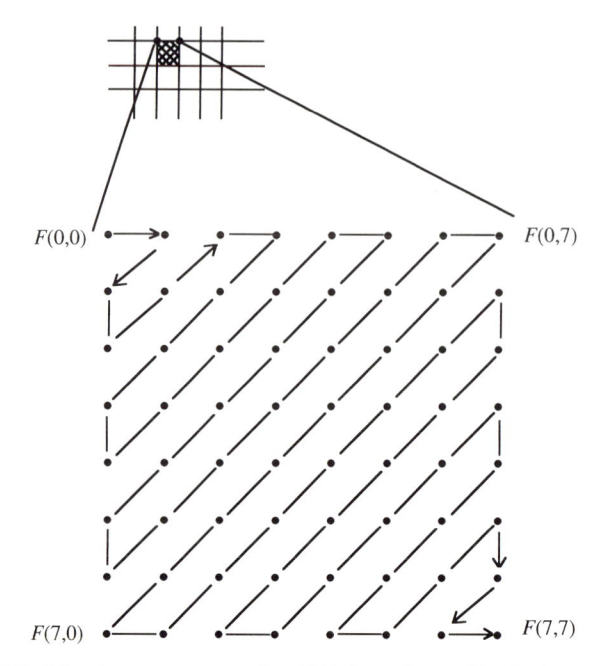

Figure 6.7 The zigzag sequence of an 8 × 8 matrix used in block quantization.

quence will facilitate entropy coding by placing low frequency components, which normally have larger coefficients, before high frequency components.

The last step in block compression is the entropy coding, which provides additional lossless compression by using a reversible technique—for example, run-length coding or Huffman coding, as described in Sections 6.3.2 and 6.3.3.

6.4.2.4 Decoding and Inverse Transform

The block-compressed image file is a sequential file containing the following information: entropy coding, zigzag sequence, bit allocation table, and the quantization. This information can be used in reverse order to reconstruct the compressed image. The compressed image file is decoded by using the bit allocation table as a guide to form a two-dimensional array $F_A(u,v)$, which is the approximate transformed image. The value of $F_A(u,v)$ is computed by

$$F_A(u,v) = \frac{|F(m,n)| \cdot F_q(u,v)}{2^{|B(m,n)-1|} - 1} \tag{6.6}$$

Equation (6.6) is almost the inverse of Eq. (6.5), and $F_A(u,v)$ is the approximation of $F(u,v)$. Inverse cosine transform Eq. (6.2) is then applied on $F_A(u,v)$, which gives $f_A(x,y)$, the reconstructed image. Since $F_A(u,v)$ is an approximation of $F(u,v)$, some differences exist between the original image $f(x,y)$ and the reconstructed image

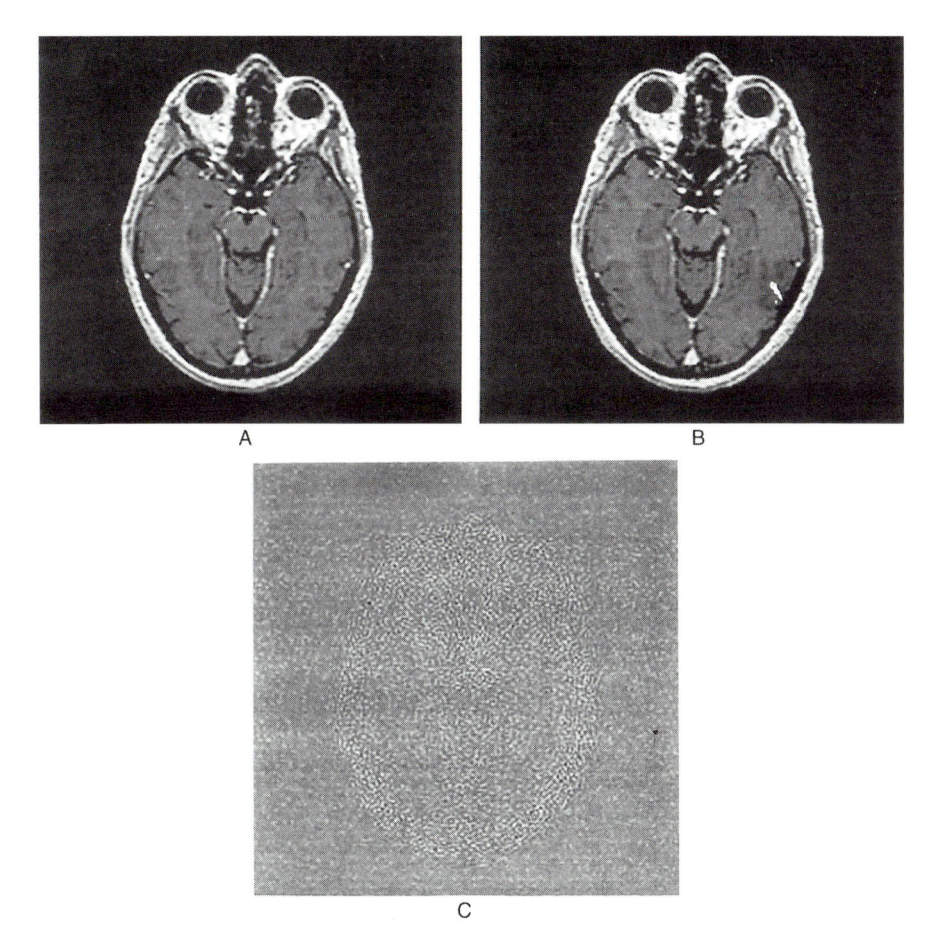

Figure 6.8 MR image compressed at a compression ratio of 20:1, in accordance with the JPEG standard: (a) the original image, (b) the reconstructed image, and (c) the difference image. Compared this result with that by the wavelet transform method discussed in section 6.6.3 (Fig. 6.30).

$f_A(x,y)$. The compression ratio is dependent on the amount of quantization and the efficiency of the entropy coding. Figure 6.8 shows some block compression results with a compression ratio of 20:1 obtained by means of the JPEG standard.

6.4.3 Full-Frame Compression

6.4.3.1 The Full-Frame Bit Allocation Algorithm

The full-frame bit allocation (FFBA) compression technique in the cosine transform domain is developed primarily for radiologic images. It is different from the JPEG block method in that the transform is done on the entire image. Image compression using blocks of the image gives blocky artifacts that might affect diagnostic accuracy.

Figure 6.9 Data flow of the full-frame bit allocation technique.

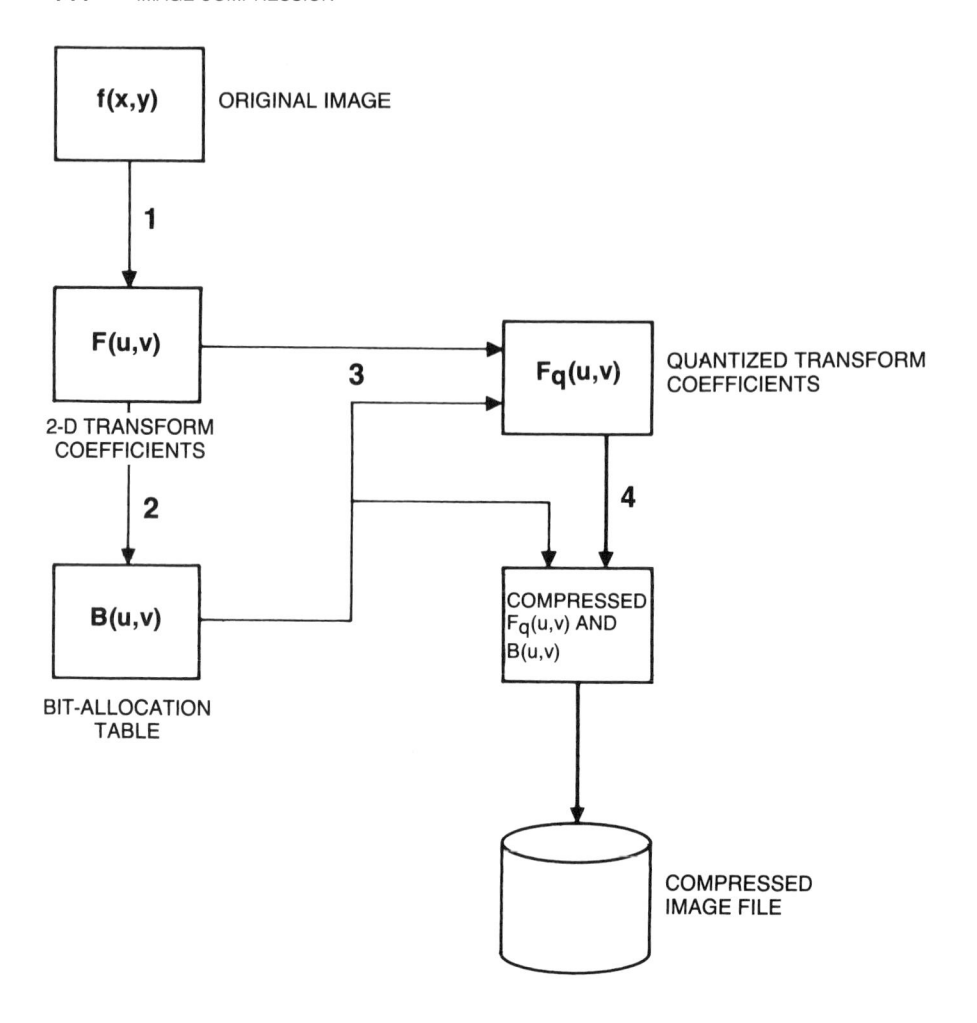

OPERATIONS:
1. FORWARD DISCRETE COSINE TRANSFORM
2. BIT-ALLOCATION PROCESS
3. QUANTIZATION
4. BIT-ALLOCATION ENCODING

Basically, the FFBA is similar to the block compression technique, as indicated by the following steps. The transformed image of the entire image is first obtained by using the cosine transformation (Eq. 6.1). A bit allocation table (Eq. 6.4) designating the number of bits for each pixel in this transformed image is then generated, the value of each pixel is quantized based on a predetermined rule (Eq. 6.5), and the bit

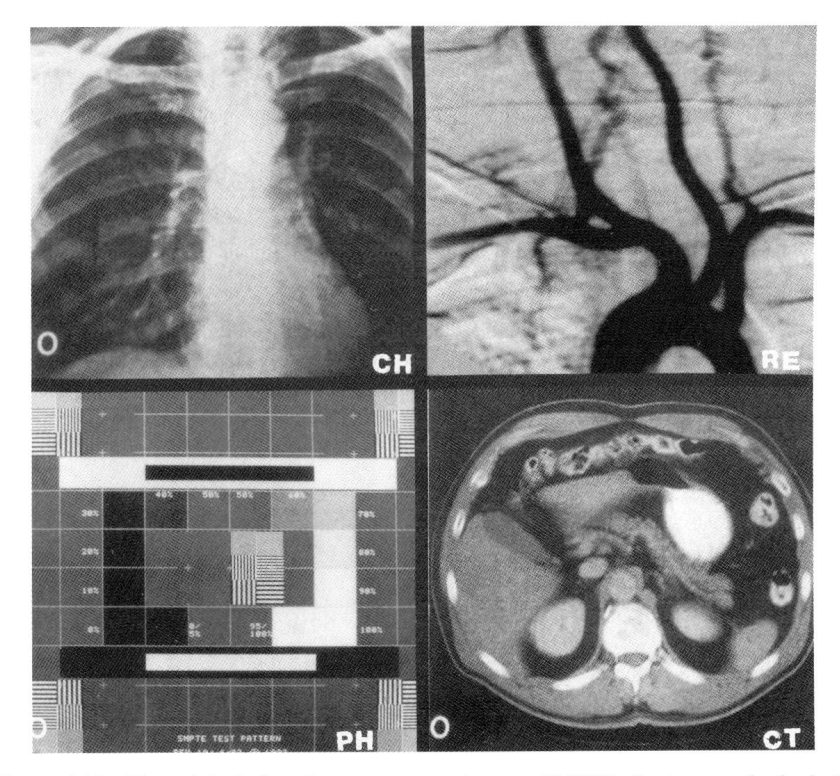

Figure 6.10 The original chest image, renoarteriogram, SMPTE phantom, and a body CT image.

allocation table is used to encode the quantized image, forming a one-dimensional sequentially compressed image file. The one-dimensional image file is further compressed by means of lossless entropy coding. The compression ratio between the original image and the compressed image file depends on the information in the bit allocation table, the amount of quantization on the transformed image, and the entropy coding. The compressed image file and the bit allocation table are saved and used to reconstruct the image. Figure 6.9 shows the data flow of the full-frame bit allocation technique. The bit allocation table is of the same size of the original image, but it can be compressed substantially by means of the property of radial symmetry in the transform domain or a predetermined zone map.

During image reconstruction, the bit allocation table is used to decode the one-dimensional compressed image file back to a two-dimensional array. An inverse cosine transform is performed on the two-dimensional array to form the reconstructed image. The reconstructed image does not exactly equal the original image because approximation is introduced in the bit allocation table generation and in the quantization procedure.

Despite this similarity, however, the implementation of the FFBA is quite different from the block compression method for several reasons. First, it is computationally tedious and time-consuming to carry out the 2-D DCT when the image size is

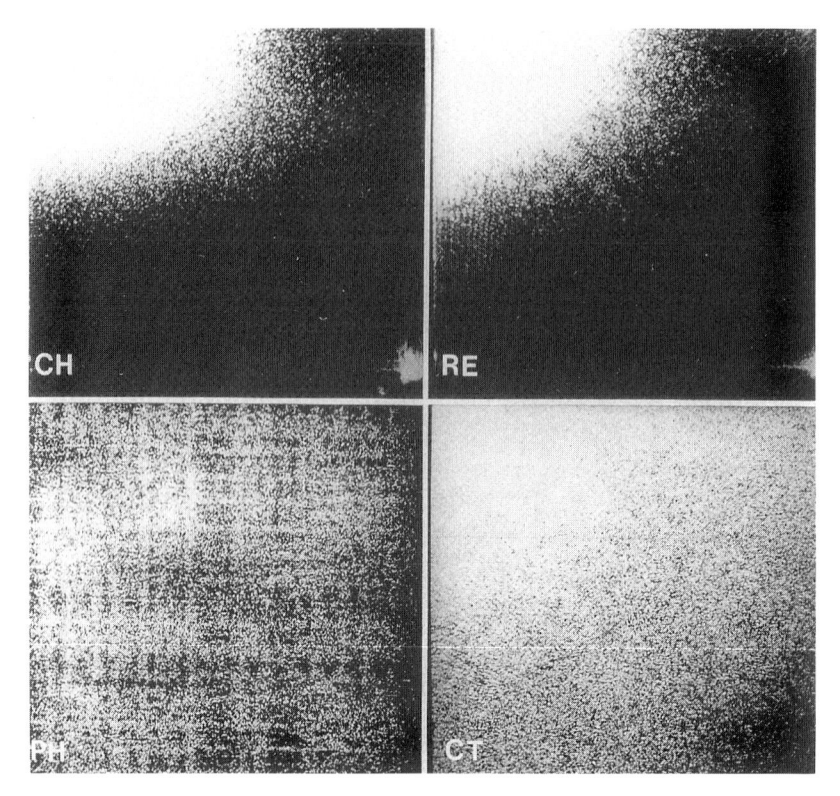

Figure 6.11 The cosine transforms of the entire chest radiograph (CH), the renoarteriogram (RE), the SMPTE phantom (PH), and the CT scan (CT) shown in Figure 6.10. The origin is located at the upper left-hand corner of each image. It is seen that the frequency distribution of the cosine transforms of the chest radiograph, and the renoarteriogram are quite similar: they concentrate in the upper left corner, representing the lower frequency components. The frequency distribution of the cosine transform of the CT is spread more toward the higher frequency region, whereas in the case of the SMPTE phantom, the frequency distribution of the cosine transform is all over the transform domain.

large. Second, the bit allocation table given in Eq. (6.4) is large when the image size is large, and therefore it becomes an overhead in the compressed file. In the case of block compression, one 8×8 bit allocation table is sufficient for all blocks. Third, zigzag sequencing provides an efficient arrangement for the entropy coding in a small block of data. In the FFBA, zigzag sequencing is not a good method for rearranging DCT coefficients because of the large matrix size. The implementation of the FFBA is best accomplished by using a fast DCT method and a compact full-frame bit allocation table, along with consideration of computational precision; a specially designed hardware module is essential. For details of these topics, refer to the references at the back of the book. Figure 6.10 shows a chest radiograph (CH), a renoarteriogram (RE), the SMPTE phantom (PH), and a body CT (CT) image; and Figure 6.11 gives the corresponding cosine transforms of these images.

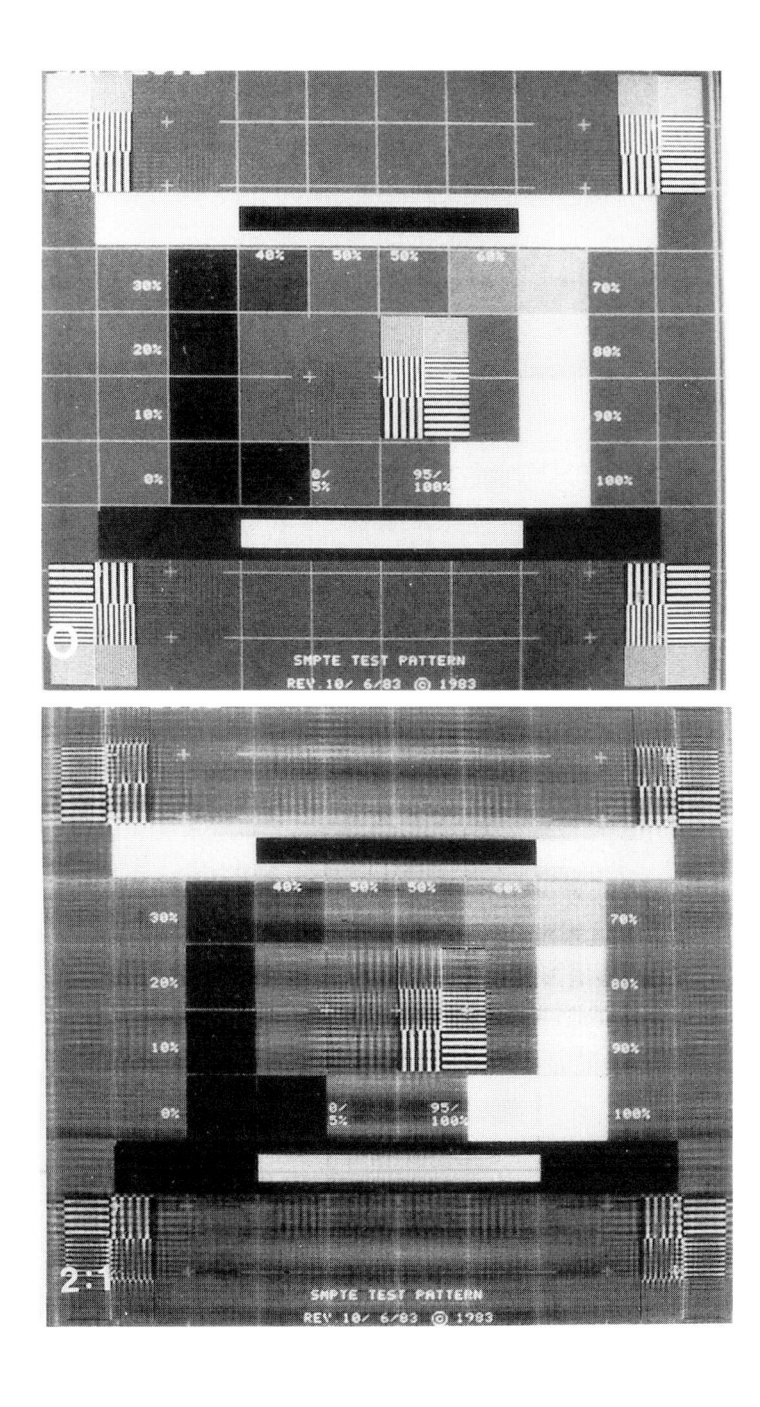

Figure 6.12 The digital SMPTE phantom and the reconstructed image, with compression ratio of 2:1. Observe the vertical and horizontal edge artifacts in the reconstructed image.

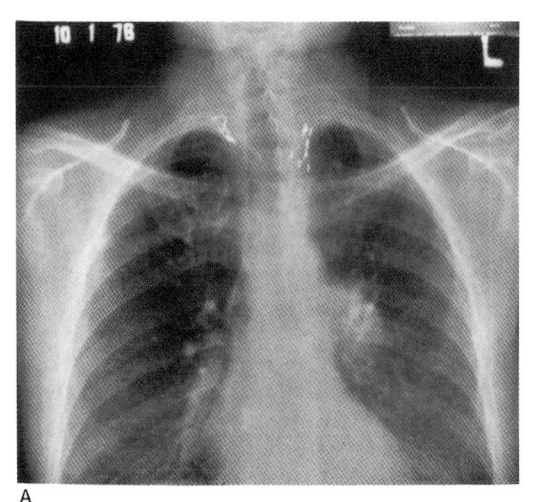

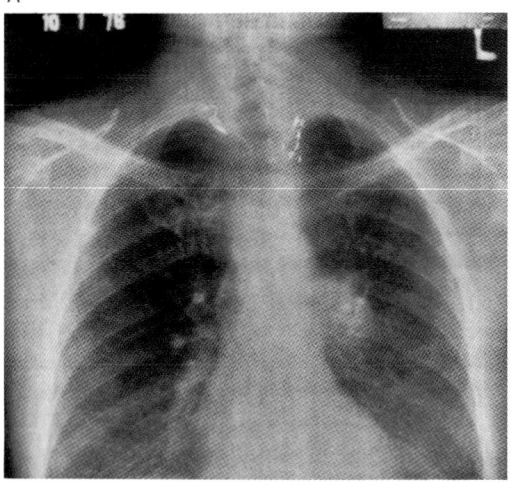

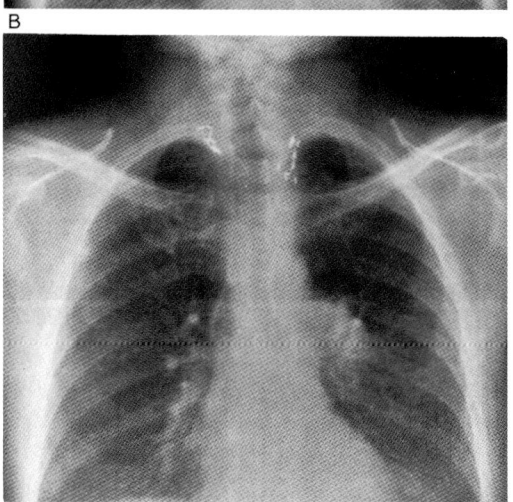

A

B

C

148

6.4.3.2 Variations of the Full-Frame Compression Technique

The full-frame compression technique is very sensitive to anatomical or artificial sharp edges, especially when the bit allocation table is condensed on the basis of radial symmetry. Under these conditions, the high frequency components of the transform are compromised, resulting in edge artifacts. Figures 6.12, 6.13, and 6.14 show three examples. Figure 6.12 is a digital SMPTE phantom and the reconstructed image with a compression ratio of 2:1. Figure 6.13A is a digitized chest radiograph with the patient's identification label; the reconstructed image (Fig. 6.13B) has a compression ratio 9:1. Figure 6.14A is a CT head image; its reconstructed image (Fig. 6.14B) has a compression ratio 12:1. The first two cases show vertical and horizontal edge artifacts adjacent to the edges, and artificially induced identification label, respectively, whereas the third case shows the ringing artifacts due to the anatomical feature in the edge of the skull. Artifacts from many edges in an SMPTE phantom are difficult to remove; other artifacts can be minimized with a composite compression, however. If we consider the CT head scan as an example, the composite compression consists of the following steps, as shown in Figure 6.15:

1. The original image is first subdivided into two regions, the brain and the skull. This can be done by means of a standard automatic segmentation image processing technique.
2. A brain tissue image is formed by filling the region outside the brain tissue with the average CT value of the brain tissue.
3. The FFBA method is applied to the brain tissue image and forms a compressed data file.
4. A skull image is formed by filling in zeros inside and outside the skull.
5. The skull image is compressed with a conventional error-free method (e.g., run-length coding), and a second compressed data file is formed.

The skull image and the brain tissue image are reconstructed separately from their corresponding compressed data files by using the proper decoding method. A single substitution algorithm can be used to assemble the two reconstructed images into one reconstructed CT image. Figures 6.13C and 6.14C show the reconstructed chest radiograph and the CT head image using the composite compression technique with compression ratios identical to those of Figures 6.13B and 6.14B. Both the horizontal and vertical line artifacts and the ringing artifacts disappear.

←

Figure 6.13 (A) Digitized 512 × 512 chest radiograph with the patient's identification label (top right). (B) The reconstructed image from A with compression ratio 9:1. Observe the vertical and horizontal edge artifacts near the label. (C) The reconstructed image from A with composite compression, after removal of the patient's identification label; compression ratio is also 9:1.

150 IMAGE COMPRESSION

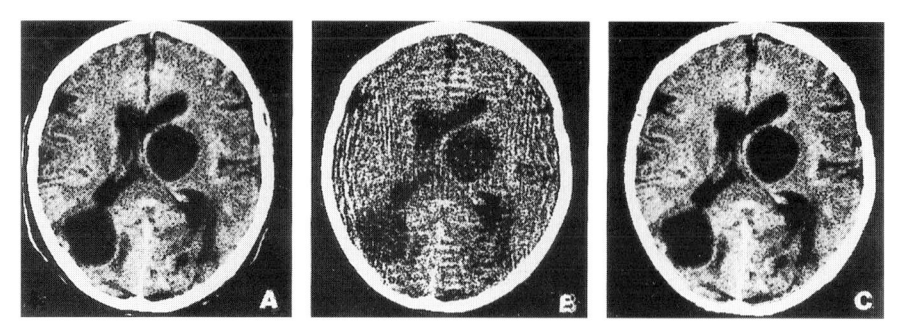

Figure 6.14 Application of the FFBA technique to a CT image of the head. (A) Original image. (B) Reconstructed image from a 12:1 compression ratio obtained without the use of the composite compression. Observe the ringing artifacts in the brain. (C) Reconstructed image from a 12:1 compressed ratio with the use of the composite compression.

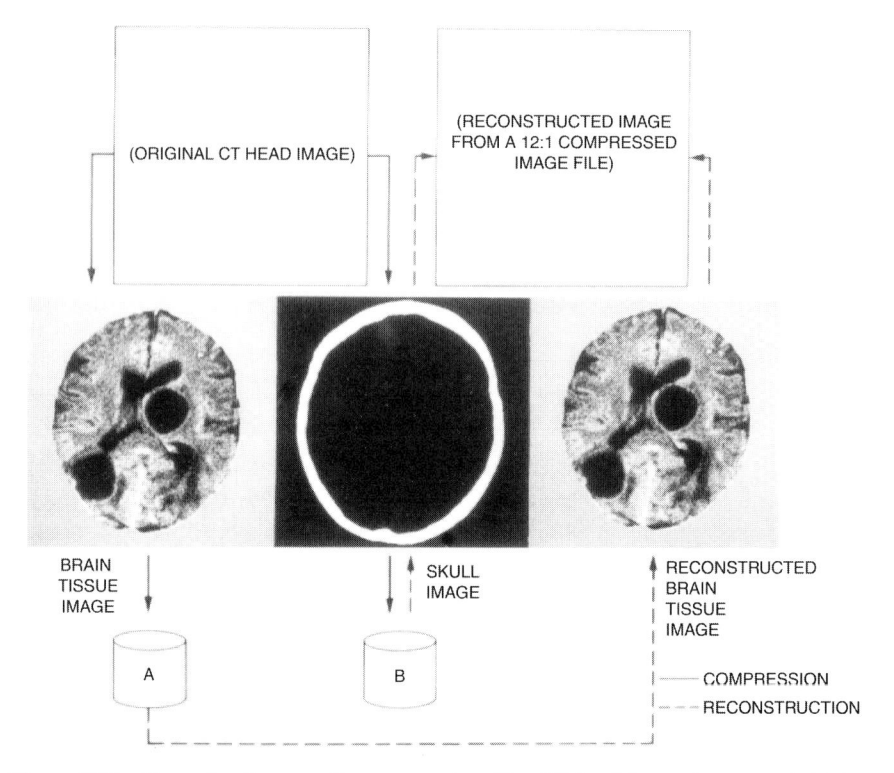

Figure 6.15 Example of composite compression. The CT head image is segmented into a brain and a skull image. The FFBA is used to compress the brain image, and run-length coding is used for the skull image. The composite reconstructed image is obtained by assembling the brain and the skull reconstructed images.

6.5 MEASUREMENT OF THE DIFFERENCE BETWEEN THE ORIGINAL AND THE RECONSTRUCTED IMAGE

It is natural to raise the question of how much an image can be compressed and still preserve sufficient information for a given clinical application. This section discusses some parameters and methods used to measure the trade-off between image quality and compression ratio.

6.5.1 Quantitative Parameters

6.5.1.1 Normalized Mean-Square Error

The normalized mean-square error (NMSE) between the original $f(x,y)$ and the reconstructed $f_A(x,y)$ image can be used as a quantitative measure on the closeness between the reconstructed image to the original image. The formula for the normalized mean-square error is given by

$$\text{NMSE} = \frac{\sum_{x=0}^{N-1}\sum_{y=0}^{N-1}[f(x,y) - f_A(x,y)]^2}{\sum_{x=0}^{N-1}\sum_{y=0}^{N-1}f(x,y)^2} \quad (6.7)$$

or

$$\text{NMSE} = \frac{\sum_{u=0}^{N-1}\sum_{v=0}^{N-1}[F(u,v) - F_A(u,v)]^2}{\sum_{u=0}^{N-1}\sum_{v=0}^{N-1}F(u,v)^2} \quad (6.8)$$

because cosine transform is a unitary transformation.

NMSE is a global measurement on the quality of the reconstructed image; it does not provide information on the local measurement. It is obvious that the NMSE is a function of the compression ratio. A high compression ratio will yield a high NMSE value.

6.5.1.2 Peak Signal-to-Noise Ratio

Another quantitative measure is the peak signal-to-noise ratio (PSNR), based on the root-mean-square error of the reconstructed image, which is very similar to the NMSE:

$$\text{PSNR} = \frac{20\log(f(x,y)_{\max})}{\left(\sum_{x=0}^{N-1}\sum_{y=0}^{N-1}(f(x,y) - f_A(x,y))^2\right)^{1/2} / (N \times N)} \quad (6.9)$$

where $f(x,y)_{max}$ is the maximum value of the entire image, $N \times N$ is the total number of pixels in the image, and the denominator is the root-mean-square error of the reconstructed image.

6.5.2 Qualitative Measurement: Difference Image and Its Histogram

The difference image between the original and the reconstructed image gives a qualitative measurement that compares the quality of the reconstructed image with that of the original image. The corresponding histogram of the difference image provides a global qualitative measurement of the difference between the original and the reconstructed images. A very narrow histogram means a small difference, whereas a broad histogram means a very large difference.

6.5.3 Acceptable Compression Ratio

Consider the following experiment. Compress a $512 \times 512 \times 8$ bit digitized chest X-ray film using the FFBA with compression ratios 4:1, 7:1, 12:1, 19:1, and 32:1. The original digitized image and the five reconstructed images are shown in Figure 6.16. All these six images are displayed simultaneously in random order on a multiviewing workstation with six identical video monitors. Observers are to evaluate these images qualitatively. Only the original image is identified, and the observers are requested to write down the comparative order of the five reconstructed images based on the quality of each image.

Table 6.1 shows one of the tabulated results, which demonstrates that most observers can order only three of the images correctly. To understand the reason for this,

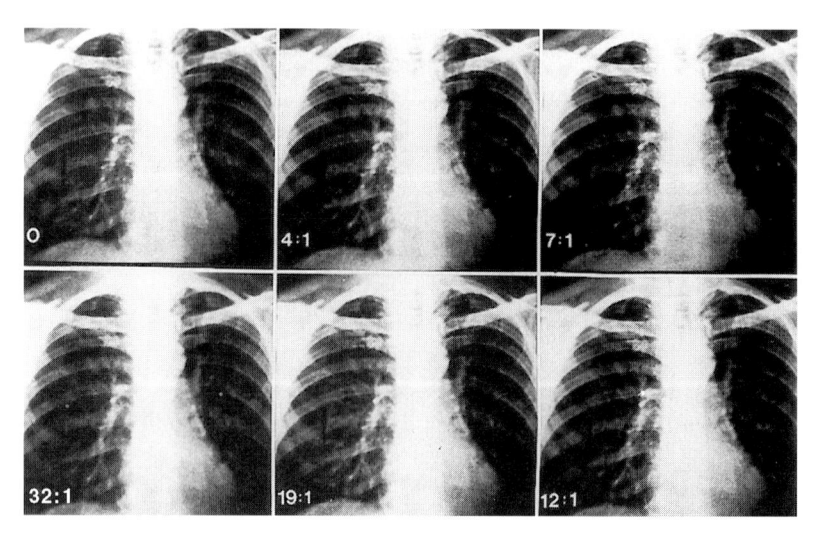

Figure 6.16 Reconstructed images: upper left, a chest radiograph digitized to $512 \times 512 \times 8$; clockwise, five reconstructed images with compression ratios of 4:1, 7:1, 12:1, 19:1, and 32:1. (The FFBA method was used.)

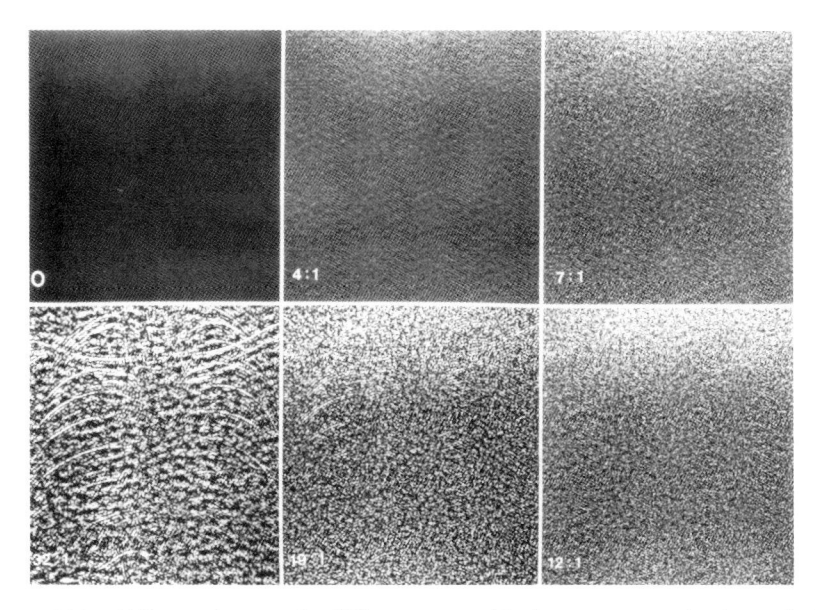

Figure 6.17 Difference images: the difference created by image compression is evenly distributed throughout the whole image; the higher the compression ratio, the larger the difference. To afford better visualization of the difference images, each pixel value in the difference image has been magnified by a factor of 10 and added to a constant 127 before the display. Clockwise from upper left, difference images between the original (Fig. 6.16, O) and the O, 4:1, 7:1, 12:1, 19:1, and 32:1 reconstructed images.

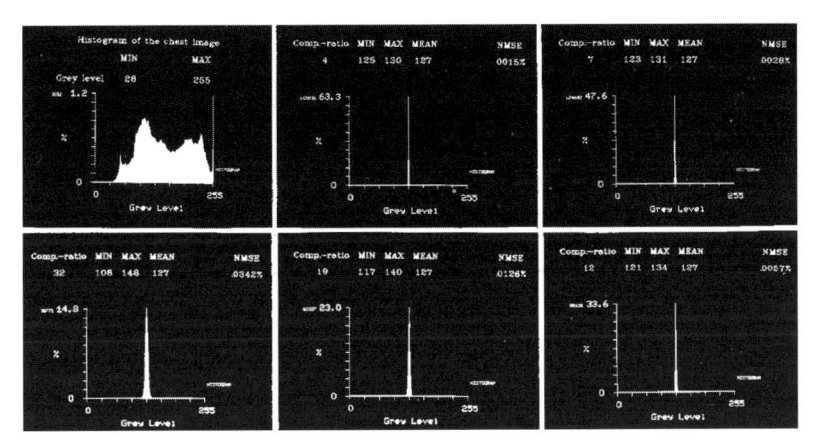

Figure 6.18 Histograms of the original image and the difference images, showing minimum, maximum, mean, and standard deviation of each histogram on the top. The normalized mean-square error (NMSE) between the original and the reconstructed image is also depicted Clockwise from upper left: histograms of the original image (Fig. 6.16, O), and the corresponding 4:1, 7:1, 12:1, 19:1, and 32:1 difference images (Fig. 6.17). It is seen that the range of the 4:1 compression ratio histogram is very narrow; and as the compression ratio becomes higher, the range of the corresponding histogram becomes broader.

TABLE 6.1 Evaluation of Quality of Reconstruction Images with Compression Ratios 4:1, 7:1, 12:1, 16:1, and 32:1 on a Chest Radiograph (see Figs. 6.16–6.18)

Non-Radiologist with Some Image Processing Background: 25 Total Samples		
Score*	Number of Observers	Correct Evaluations (%)
5	1	4
4	0	0
3	1	4
2	4	16
1	7	28
0	12	48
Identify 4:1 correctly	2	8
Identify 32:1 correctly	9	36
Radiologists: 12 Total Samples		
Score*	Number of Observers	Correct Evaluations (%)
5	0	0
4	0	0
3	5	41.0
2	5	41.7
1	2	16.7
0	0	0
Identify 4:1 correctly	2	16.7
32:1 correctly	11	91.7

*A score of 5 means that the observer identified the order of all five reconstructed images correctly based on the quality of the displayed images. A score of 3 means that the observer identified the order of any three of the five reconstructed images.

consider Figure 6.17, which shows the difference images between the original and the reconstructed images. It is difficult to detect any residual anatomical structures from these images for compression ratios lower than 12:1; hence the observers have difficulty putting the 4:1, 7:1, and 12:1 images in a proper order.

Figure 6.18 shows the histograms of the original and all the difference images. The range of the 4:1 compression ratio histogram is very narrow, and as the compression ratio becomes higher, the range of corresponding histogram becomes broader. Figure 6.18 also displays the normalized mean-square errors between the original image and the reconstructed images (upper right-hand corner, under NMSE): for compression ratios 4:1, 7:1, 12:1, 19:1, and 32:1, they are 0.0015, 0.0028, 0.0057, 0.0126, and 0.0342, respectively. Clearly, the NMSEs of all these difference images are very small.

The body CT image shown in Figure 6.19 offers another example. Reconstructed images with compression ratios less than and equal to 8:1 do not exhibit visible deterioration in image quality. The experiment described illustrates that for this particular image, reconstructed images from compression ratios less than 10:1 are visually

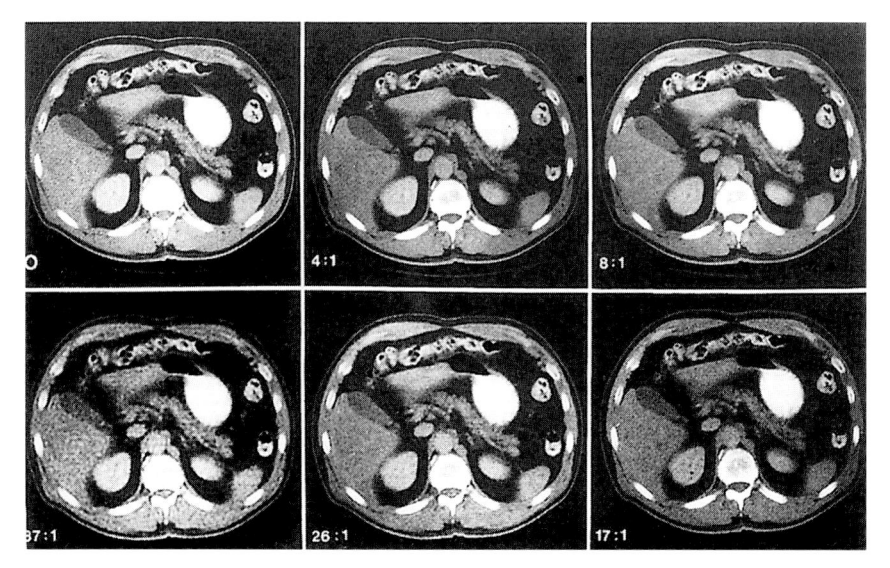

Figure 6.19 Body CT scan (upper left), followed clockwise by reconstructed images with compression ratios of 4:1, 8:1, 17:1, 26:1, and 37:1. (The FFBA method was used.)

indistinguishable from the original image; that is, there are no residual anatomical structures appearing in the difference image. In other words, compression ratio 10:1 or less is acceptable for this image. It is obvious that compression ratio is a function of many variables, such as type and quality of the image to be compressed, the digitizer used, the size of the digitized image, and the display method; there is no universally acceptable ratio.

6.5.4 Quality of the Reconstructed Image

Radiologic image compression has been studied extensively during the past 10 years. Based on these studies, we can summarize certain observations, as follows.

1. A digitized X-ray film with a larger matrix always yields a higher acceptable compression ratio. This is true for all categories projectional radiography. One explanation is that when a projectional radiograph is digitized into a larger matrix, the correlation between pixels is higher. A higher correlation image gives a higher acceptable compression ratio.
2. An image with many edges (e.g., pulmonary arteriograms) and/or with high contrast regions (e.g., barium inside the stomach and the gastrointestinal tract) always gives a lower acceptable compression ratio compared to that of a similar radiograph without the contrast medium.
3. The acceptable compression ratio of all anterior–posterior (AP) chest X-rays is quite predictable. This is probably the result of three factors:
   (a) A chest X-ray has relatively few sharp edges.
   (b) The background area outside the chest wall for an adult is small.

156 IMAGE COMPRESSION

  (c) The image is relatively symmetrical with respect to the medial line of the image.
4. The acceptable compression ratio for lateral chest X-rays is comparatively lower than that of the AP chest image. This effect is probably attributable to three characteristics of the lateral view:
   (a) The background outside the chest wall in the image is relatively larger than that in the AP view.
   (b) The boundary between the image and the background is relatively sharp compared to the AP view.
   (c) The image has a relatively larger area in the neck region, the optical density of which contrasts quite markedly to the adjacent background area.
5. In the case of barium contrast studies in the gastrointestinal region, a high contrast image and/or image with large contrast regions always gives a lower acceptable compression ratio.
6. In digital subtraction angiography, the area outside the circular field of the image intensifier and the area inside the four edges of the X-ray field in conventional radiography do not create problems in image compression. However, the background area between the skull and the circular field of the image intensifier in a neuroangiogram, which shows up as an overexposed (black) area, will lower the acceptable image compression ratio. The reason is similar to that given in item 5 with respect to a high contrast area inside the image.
7. The patient identification label in each radiograph will also lower the acceptable image compression ratio. This label, which is quite large and has four sharp edges, will give horizontal and vertical edge artifacts on the reconstructed images even at a very low compression ratio. It is advantageous to perform some image preprocessing before the image is compressed. Preprocessing includes deleting labels, and filling up the area with pixel values similar to the background in the digital image (see Fig. 6.13).
8. For body CT images, scans in the lower abdominal region always give a lower acceptable compression ratio than scans in the chest and the upper abdominal region. This is because the small intestine, in the lower abdominal region, contains air, which results in high contrast compared to the organs.
9. CT head images can be preprocessed and separated into a skull image and a brain tissue image (see Fig. 6.15). Error-free compression can be used to compress the skull image, and the full-frame bit allocation technique can be applied for the brain tissue image.

Table 6.2 summarizes the relationship between image compression ratio, matrix size, number bits per pixel, and digitizer quality.

6.5.5 Receiver Operating Characteristic Analysis

Another method of measuring the difference between the quality of original and reconstructed images is receiver operating characteristic (ROC) analysis, based on the

TABLE 6.2 Relationship Between Image Compression Ratio, Matrix Size, Number of Bits per Pixel, and Quality of the Digitizer

Case 1:	Use the same digitizer on the same film. Adjust to the same normalized mean-square error.
To digitize the film to a larger matrix size (same bits/pixel) gives ↓ a higher compression ratio	To digitize the film to more bits per pixel (same matrix size) gives ↓ a lower compression ratio
Case 2:	Use different digitizers on the same film. Adjust to the same normalized mean-square error with the same image size.
Film digitized with a lower quality digitizer gives ↓ a higher compression ratio	Film digitized with a higher quality digitizer gives ↓ a lower compression ratio

work of Swets and Pickett, and Metz. This method was developed for comparing the quality of images produced by two modalities. To begin, a set of good quality images of a certain category (e.g., AP chest radiographs) is selected by a panel of experts. The selection process includes considerations of types of disease, method of determination of the "truth" of the disease, number of images, distribution between normal and abnormal images, and the subtlety of the disease appearing on images. The images in the set are then compressed to a predetermined compression ratio and reconstructed. The result is two sets of images: the original and the reconstructed.

Observers with expertise in diagnosing the subject diseases participate as observers to review all the images. For each image, an individual observer is asked to give an ROC confidence rating on a scale of 1 to 5 representing his or her impression of the likelihood of the presence of the disease. A confidence value of 1 indicates that the disease is definitely not present, and a confidence value of 5 indicates that the disease is present. Confidence values 2 and 4 indicate that the disease process is probably not present or probably present, respectively. A confidence value of 3 indicates that the presence of the disease process is equivocal or indeterminate. Every image is read by every observer. The ratings of all images by a single observer is graded based on the "truth." The two plots that result show true positive (TP) versus false positive (FP). The first plot is an ROC curve representing the observer's performance of diagnosing the selected disease from the original images; the curve in the second plot indicates performance on the reconstructed images. The area A_z under the ROC curve is an index of quantitative measure of the observer's performance on this image. Thus, if the A_z (original) and the A_z (reconstructed) of the two ROC curves are very close to each other, we can say that diagnoses of this disease based on the reconstructed image with the predetermined compression ratio will be as good as those made (by this observer) from the original image. In other words, this compression ratio is acceptable for this image type with the given disease.

In doing the ROC analysis, the statistical "power" of the study is important: the higher the power, the more confidence can be placed in the result. The statistical power is determined by the number of images used and the number of observers. A meaningful ROC analysis often requires many images (100 or more) and five to six observers to determine one type of image with several diseases. Although performing an ROC analysis is tedious, time-consuming, and expensive, this method for determination of the quality of the reconstructed image is accepted by the radiology community .

Sections 6.5.5.1 and 6.5.5.2 show examples of two ROC analyses: thoracic images of various types of intrathoracic pathology and hand radiographs revealing subperiosteal resorption. The compression method used was the FFBA with zone bit allocation table implemented in a hardware module described in Section 6.4.3.

6.5.5.1 Thoracic Imaging with Lung Nodules and Interstitial Lung Disease

In a study based on work by Aberle et al. (1993), 122 posteroanterior chest radiographs were obtained on patients in an ambulatory patient setting: 30 cases of interstitial lung disease, 45 images containing combinations of lung nodules ($N = 37$) or mediastinal masses ($N = 39$), and 47 normal images containing none of these pathologies. The images were digitized (nominal 2K × 2K × 12 bit resolution), printed on a hard copy format (14 in. × 14 in.), and compressed at an approximate compression ratio of 20:1. Figure 6.20 shows three images: original, reconstructed, and subtracted. Observer performance tests were conducted in which five radiologists used ROC analysis on digitized uncompressed and compressed hard copy images. Tables 6.3 and 6.4 show the ROC area (A_z) for interstitial disease and lung nodules, respectively: there are no significant differences between the two display conditions for the detectability of either thoracic abnormality. Thus, irreversible image compression at ratios of 20:1 may be acceptable for use in digital thoracic imaging.

6.5.5.2 Hand Radiographs with Subperiosteal Resorption

A study based on work by Sayre et al. (1992) entailed the analysis of 71 hand radiographs, of which 45 were normal and 26 had subperiosteal resorption. The images were digitized to 2K × 2K × 12 bit resolution and printed on film (14 in. × 17 in.). The digitized images were compressed to 20:1 using the FFBA method and printed on film of the same size. Figure 6.21 shows original, reconstructed, and subtracted

Figure 6.20 Example of using the full-frame image compression hardware in thoracic imaging. (A) Digitized 2048 × 2048 × 12 bit AP chest image printed back on a film. (B) Reconstructed image with a compression ratio of 20:1. (C) The difference image between the original and the reconstructed image. (From Aberle et al., 1993.)

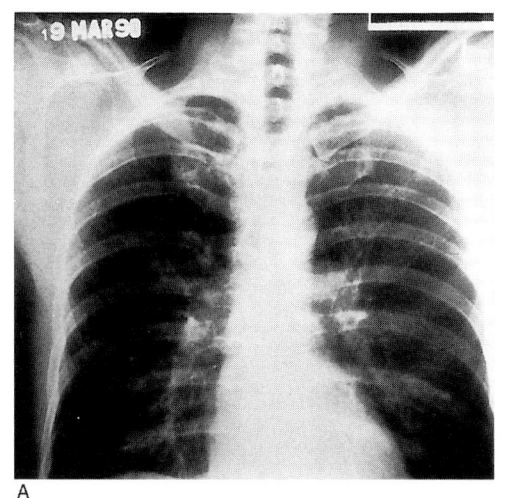

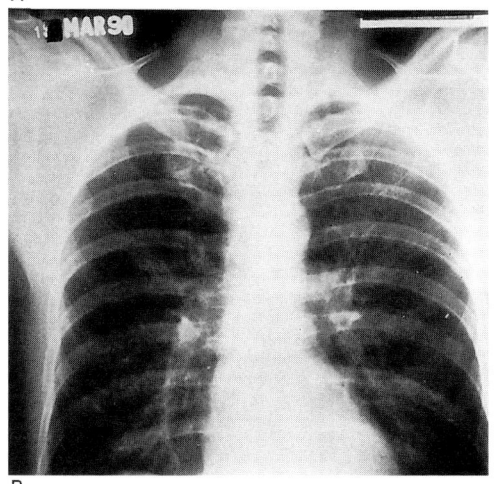

A

B

C

TABLE 6.3 Reader-Specific Areas Under the ROC Curves (A_z) for Interstitial Disease*

Observer	A_z ($\pm$SD) Digitized Image	A_z ($\pm$SD) Compressed Image	P Value	95% Confidence Intervals for Area Differences
A	.967 ($\pm$ .024)	.988 ($\pm$ .011)	.16	$-$.063, .021
B	.956 ($\pm$ .028)	.889 ($\pm$ .055)	.12	$-$.013, .147
C	.947 ($\pm$ .047)	.957 ($\pm$ .031)	.42	$-$.092, .072
D	.978 ($\pm$ .017)	.989 ($\pm$ .011)	.27	$-$.041, .019
E	.884 ($\pm$ .065)	.902 ($\pm$ .059)	.38	$-$.041, .019
Mean score	.946 ($\pm$ .036)	.945 ($\pm$ .033)	.43	$-$.151, .115

*All values refer to the A_z ($\pm$SD).
Source: Aberle et al.(1993).

TABLE 6.4 Reader-Specific Areas Under the ROC Curves (A_z) for Lung Nodules*

Observer	A_z ($\pm$SD) Digitized Image	A_z ($\pm$SD) Compressed Image	P Value	95% Confidence Intervals for Area Differences
A	.871 ($\pm$ .053)	.902 ($\pm$ .039)	.23	$-$.131, .069
B	.848 ($\pm$ .073)	.900 ($\pm$ .047)	.20	$-$.185, .081
C	.839 ($\pm$ .061)	.846 ($\pm$ .051)	.45	$-$.141, .128
D	.915 ($\pm$ .066)	.886 ($\pm$ .072)	.25	$-$.113, .172
E	.856 ($\pm$ .050)	.876 ($\pm$ .053)	.32	$-$.121, .081
Mean score	.866 ($\pm$ .061)	.882 ($\pm$ .052)	.30	$-$.148, .116

* All values refer to the A_z ($\pm$SD).
Source: Aberle et al. (1993).

images. An ROC analysis with five observers was performed. Figure 6.22 shows the ROC curves of the original and the reconstructed images from the five observers: statistics demonstrate that there is no significant difference between using the original or the reconstructed images with 20:1 compression ratio for the diagnosis of subperiosteal resorption from hand radiographs.

6.6 THREE-DIMENSIONAL IMAGE COMPRESSION

6.6.1 Background

So far, we have discussed only two-dimensional image compression. However, acquisition of three- and four-dimensional medical images are becoming more common in CT, MR, and digital subtraction angiography (DSA). The third dimension can be in the spatial domain (e.g., sectional images) or in the time domain (e.g., in an angiographic study). Such processes significantly increase the volume of data gathered per study. To compress 3-D data efficiently, one must consider decorrelation images. Some work done on 3-D compression reported by Sun and Goldberg (1988), Lee et al. (1993), and Koo et al. (1992) considered the correlation between adjacent sections. In 1989, Chan, Lou, and Huang reported a full-frame DCT method for DSA, CT, and MR. They found that when four to eight slices were grouped as a 3-D volume, compression was twice as efficient as it was with 2-D full-frame DCT for DSA. The 3-D method of compressing CT images was also more efficient than 2-D. However, 3-D compression did not achieve very high efficiency in the case of MR images. In Sections 6.6.2 and 6.6.3, we discuss the wavelet transform in 3-D image compression based on Wang's work (1996).

The wavelet transform has drawn significant attention since the publication of the papers by Daubechies (1988) and Mallat (1989). Wavelet theory and its applications have been developed substantially in the past few years. Wavelet transform data supply both spatial and frequency information, whereas conventionally in the Fourier transform there is only frequency information. Because of this characteristic, wavelet image compression has lately shown promising results.

6.6.2 Wavelet Theory and Multiresolution Analysis

6.6.2.1 Wavelet Theory

A transform operation maps a function from one domain to another. The basis is a set of functions that is used for the transformation. In the Fourier transform, the basis functions are a series of sine and cosine functions and the resulting domain is the frequency domain.

In a one-dimensional wavelet transform, there exists a mother wavelet function $\psi(x)$. The basis functions are formed by dilation and translation of the mother wavelet

$$\psi_{a,b}(x) = \frac{1}{\sqrt{a}} \psi\left(\frac{x-b}{a}\right) \qquad (6.10)$$

where a and b are the dilation and translation factors, respectively. The continuous wavelet transform of a function $f(x)$ can be expressed as follows:

$$F_w(a,b) = \frac{1}{\sqrt{a}} \int_{-\infty}^{\infty} f(x) \psi^*\left(\frac{x-b}{a}\right) dx \qquad (6.11)$$

where * is the complex conjugate operator.

The basis functions given in Eq. (6.10) are redundant when a and b are continuous. It is possible, however, to discretize a and b so as to form an orthonormal basis. One way of discretizing a and b is to let $a = 2^m$, $b = 2^m n$, so that Eq. (6.10) becomes

$$\psi_{m,n}(x) = 2^{-m/2} \psi(2^{-m} x - n) \qquad (6.12)$$

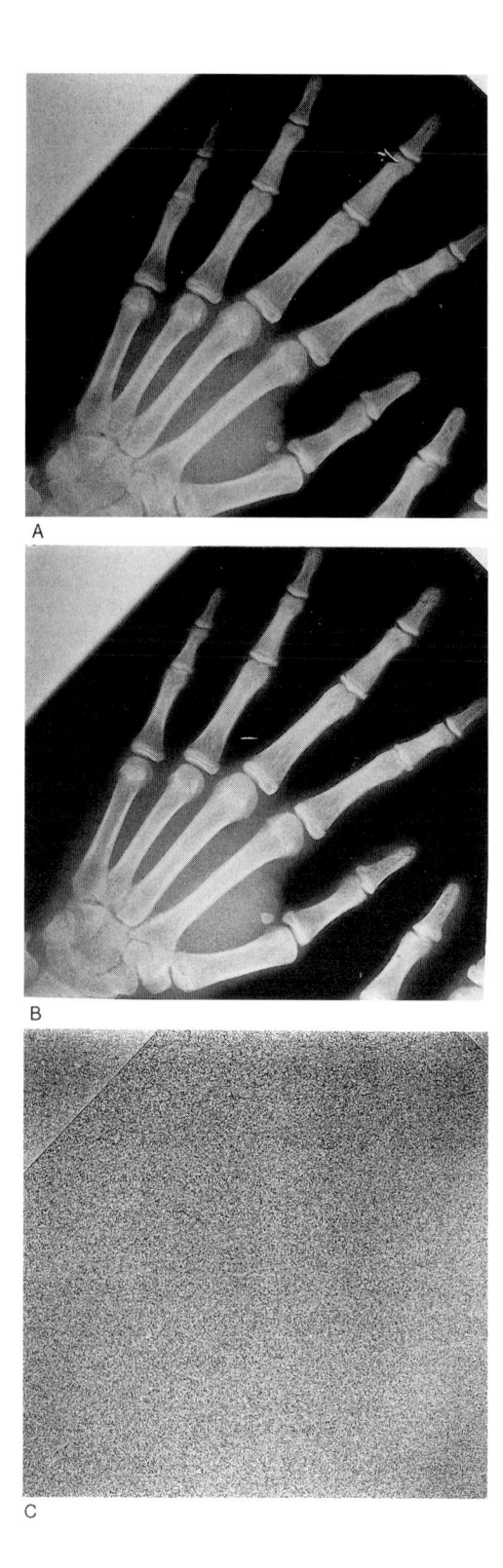

A

B

C

162

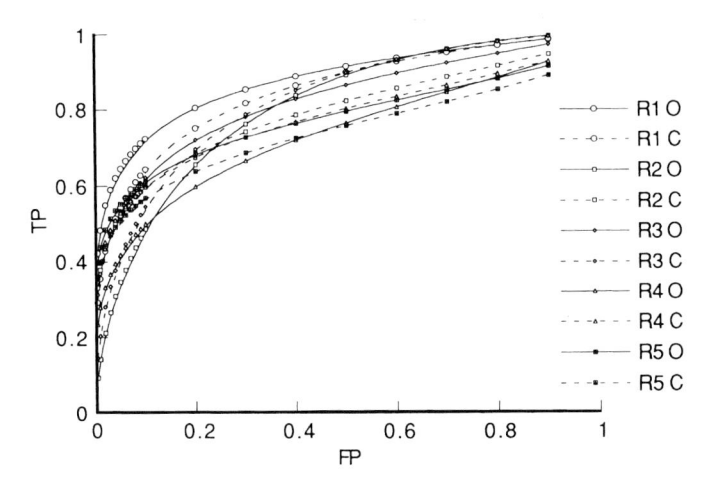

Figure 6.22 Comparison of five observer ROC curves obtained from a hand image compression study: *TP*, true-positive; *FP* false-positive; O, original; C, reconstructed image, R, radiologist.

where m and n are integers. The wavelet transform then becomes

$$F_w(m,n) = 2^{-m/2} \int_{-\infty}^{\infty} f(x)\psi(2^{-m}x - n)\,dx \qquad (6.13)$$

Since m and n are integers, Eq. (6.13) is called a wavelet series. It is seen from this representation that the transform contains both the spatial and frequency information.

6.6.2.2 Multiresolution Analysis

Multiresolution analysis decomposes a signal into a series of smooth signals and their associated detailed signals at different resolution levels. At each level, the smooth signal and its detailed signal can be used to reconstruct the smooth signal in the next higher resolution level. The multiresolution-decomposed signal lies between the spatial and frequency domains. The 3-D wavelet method discussed here is based on Mallat's definition of multiresolution theory using a pyramid algorithm.

We use a one-dimensional case to explain the concept of multiresolution analysis. Consider the discrete signal f_m at level m, which can be decomposed into the $m + 1$ level by convoluting it with h (low pass) and g (high pass) filters to form a smooth signal f_{m+1} and a detailed signal f'_{m+1} as shown in Figure 6.23. This can be implemented in the following equations using the pyramidal algorithm,

---

Figure 6.21 Example of using the full-frame image compression hardware in hand radiographs with evidence of subperiosteal resorption (arrows). (A) A digitized 2048 × 2048 × 12 bit hand image printed on a film. (B) Reconstructed image with a compression ratio of 20:1. (C) The subtracted image. (From Sayre et al., 1992.)

164   IMAGE COMPRESSION

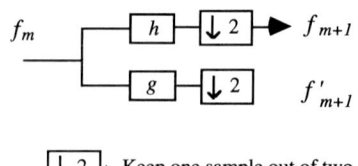

⎣ 2 ⎦ : Keep one sample out of two

Figure 6.23   Decomposition of a signal f_m into a smooth resolution f_{m+1} and a detailed signal f'_{m+1}.

$$f_{m+1}(n) = \sum_k h(2n-k) f_m(k)$$

$$f'_{m+1}(n) = \sum_k g(2n-k) f_m(k) \quad (6.14)$$

where f_{m+1} is the smooth signal and f'_{m+1} is the detailed signal at the resolution level $m+1$.

The total number of discrete points in f_m is equal to that of the sum of f_{m+1} and f'_{m+1}. The same process can be further applied to f_m+1, creating the detailed and smooth signal at the next lower resolution level, until the desired level is reached.

Figure 6.24 depicts the components resulting from three levels of decomposition of the signal f_1. The horizontal axis indicates the total number of discrete points of the original signal, and the vertical axis is the level of the decomposition. At the resolution level $m = 3$, the final signal is composed of the detailed signals of the other resolution levels $f'_1, f'_2,$ and f'_3 plus one smooth signal f_3. Signals at each level can be compressed by quantization and encoding methods described in earlier sections. Accumulation on all these compressed signals at different levels can be used to reconstruct the original signal.

In the case of 2-D, the first level will result in four components, the x-direction and the y-direction (see Figure 6.27). Figure 6.25 shows a digital mammogram with its wavelet transformation in two levels.

The primary advantage of the wavelet transform over the Fourier transform is that the wavelet transform is localized in both the spatial and frequency domains; therefore, the transformation of a given signal will contain both spatial and frequency information of that signal. On the other hand, the Fourier transform basis extends infinitely, with the result that any local space is spread out over the whole frequency domain.

6.6.3   Three-Dimensional Image Compression with Wavelet Transform

6.6.3.1   The Block Diagrams

Figure 6.26 shows the block diagrams of three-dimensional wavelet compression and decompression. In the compression process, a 3-D wavelet transform is first applied to the 3-D image data, resulting in a 3-D multiresolution representation of the image. Then the wavelet coefficients are quantized using scalar quantization. Finally, entropy coding is imposed on the quantized data by means of run-length and Huffman coding.

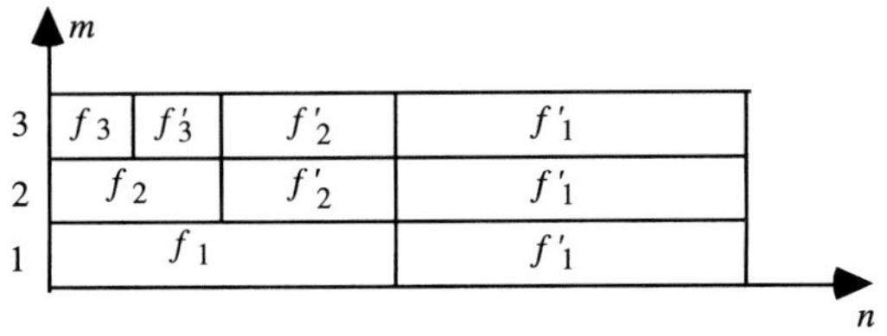

3	f_3	f'_3	f'_2	f'_1
2	f_2		f'_2	f'_1
1	f_1			f'_1

Figure 6.24 Three-level wavelet decomposition of a signal. Note that the total number of pixels in each level is the same.

The decompression process is the inverse of the compression process. The compressed data are first entropy-decoded. Second, a dequantization procedure is applied to the decoded data. Finally, an inverse 3-D wavelet transform is applied, resulting in the reconstructed 3-D image data.

6.6.3.2 Three-Dimensional Wavelet Transform

For the three-dimensional case, a wavelet ψ and a scaling function ϕ are chosen such that the three-dimensional scaling and wavelet functions are separable. That is, the scaling function has the form

$$\Phi(x,y,z) = \phi(x)\phi(y)\phi(z) \tag{6.15}$$

and the wavelet functions are given as follows:

$$\Psi^1(x,y,z) = \phi(x)\phi(y)\psi(z) \quad \Psi^2(x,y,z) = \phi(x)\psi(y)\phi(z) \quad \Psi^3(x,y,z) = \psi(x)\phi(y)\phi(z)$$
$$\Psi^4(x,y,z) = \phi(x)\psi(y)\psi(z) \quad \Psi^5(x,y,z) = \psi(x)\phi(y)\psi(z) \quad \Psi^6(x,y,z) = \psi(x)\psi(y)\phi(z)$$
$$\Psi^7(x,y,z) = \psi(x)\psi(y)\psi(z). \tag{6.16}$$

Three-dimensional wavelet transforms can be computed by extension of the one-dimensional pyramidal algorithm. One level of the decomposition process from f_m to

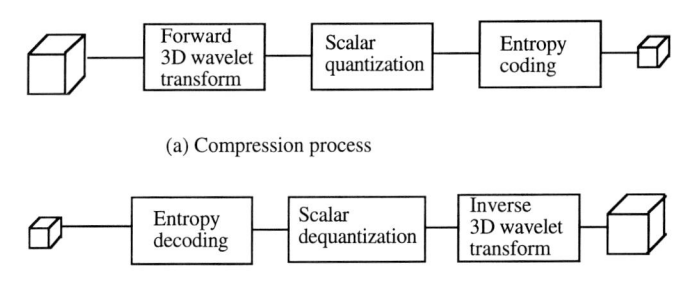

(a) Compression process

(b) Decompression process

Figure 6.26 Block diagrams of the compression and decompression using the 3-D wavelet transform.

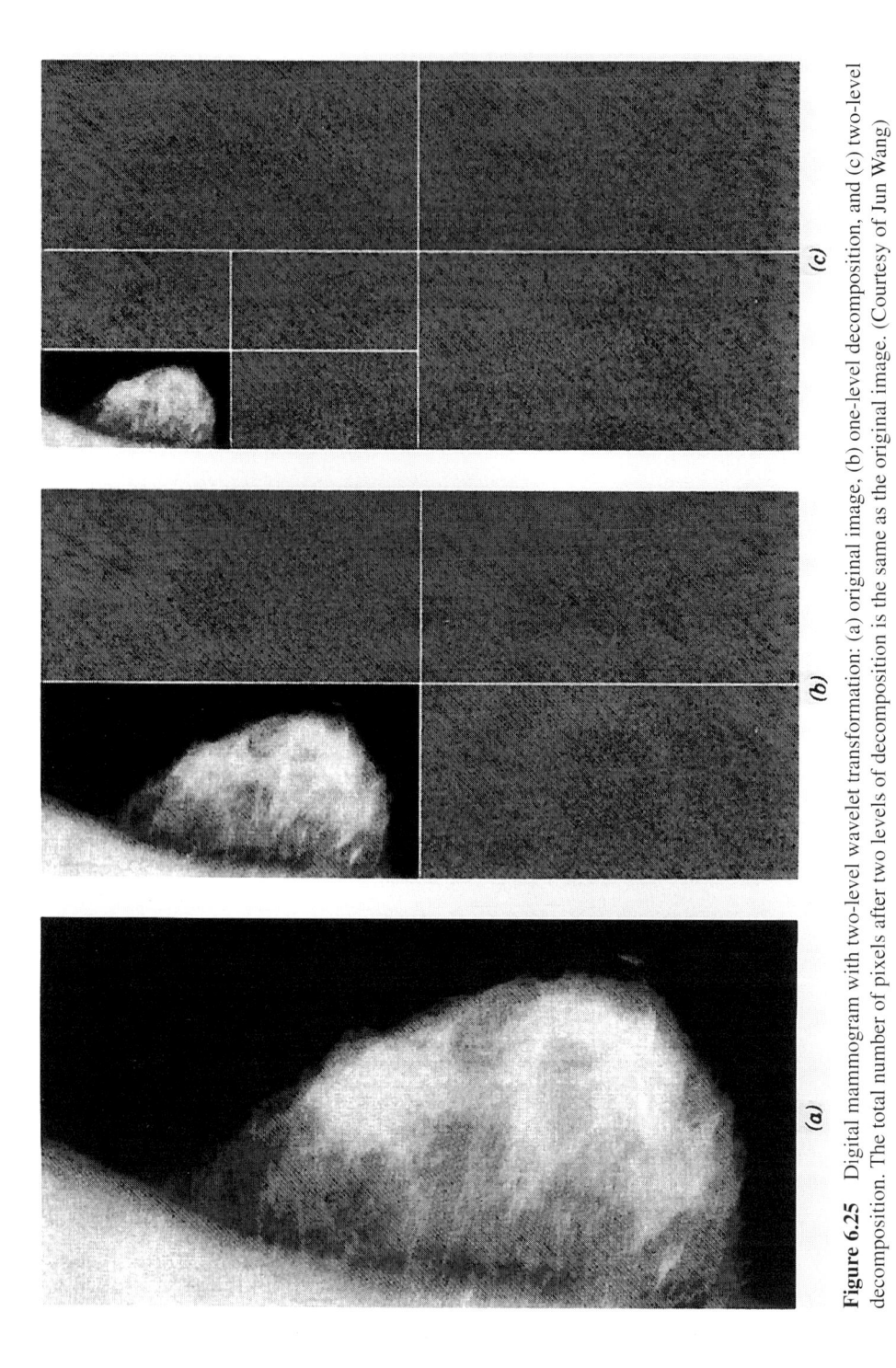

Figure 6.25 Digital mammogram with two-level wavelet transformation: (a) original image, (b) one-level decomposition, and (c) two-level decomposition. The total number of pixels after two levels of decomposition is the same as the original image. (Courtesy of Jun Wang)

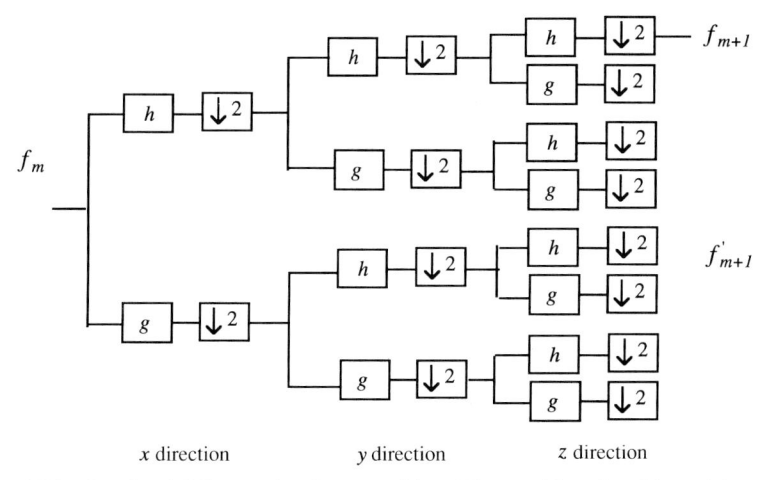

Figure 6.27 One-level 3-D wavelet decomposition. The resulting signal has eight components.

f_{m+1} is shown in Figure 6.27. We first convolute each line in the x direction with filters h and g, followed by subsampling every other pixel. The resulting signals are convoluted with h and g in the y direction, again followed with subsampling. Finally the same procedure is applied to the z direction.

The resulting signal has eight components. Since h is a low pass filter, only one component contains low frequency information, f_{m+1}. The rest of the components convolute at least once with the high pass filter g, and therefore contain the detailed signals f'_{m+1} in different directions. The same process is repeated for the low frequency signal, f_{m+1}, until the desired level is reached.

Figure 6.28 shows two levels of 3-D wavelet transform on a volume data set. The first level decomposes the data into eight components: f_1 is the low resolution portion of the image data, and the remaining blocks are high resolution components. As Figure 6.28 indicates, f_1 can be further decomposed into eight smaller volumes labeled f_2 and f'_2. The detailed images on level 1 contain higher frequency components than those of level 2 f'_2.

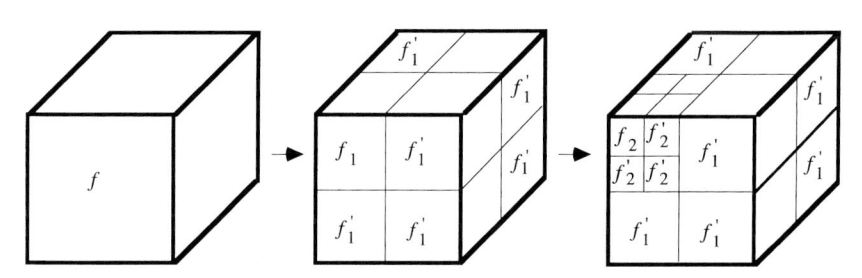

Figure 6.28 Representation of a 3-D wavelet transform on a volume data set after two-level decomposition.

With properly chosen wavelets, the low resolution component in the m level is $1/(2^3)^m$ of the original image size after the transformation, but contains about 90% of the total energy in the m level, where m is the level of the decomposition and the high resolution components are separated into different resolution levels. For these reasons, the wavelet transform yields a better presentation of the original image for compression purposes. Different levels of representation can be coded differently to achieve a desired compression ratio.

6.6.3.3 Quantization

The second step of compression is quantization. The purpose of quantization is to map a large number of input values into a smaller set of output values by reducing the precision of the data. This is the step in which information may be lost. Wavelet-transformed data are floating point values and consist of two types: low resolution image components, which contains most of the energy, and high resolution image components, which contain the information from sharp edges.

Since the low resolution components have most of the energy, we want to maintain the integrity of such data. To minimize data loss in this portion, we map each floating point value to its nearest integer neighbor (NINT). The high resolution components of the wavelet coefficients, contain many coefficients of small magnitude that correspond to the flat areas in the original image. These coefficients contain very little energy, and we can eliminate them without creating significant distortions in the reconstructed image. A threshold number T_m, is chosen, such that any coefficients less than T_m will be set to zero. Above the T_m, a range of floating point values are mapped into a single integer. If the quantization number is Q_m, quantized high frequency coefficients can be written as follows:

$$a_q(i,j,k) = \text{NINT}\left[\frac{a(i,j,k) - T_m}{Q_m}\right] \quad a(i,j,k) > T_m$$

$$a_q(i,j,k) = 0 \quad -T_m \leq a(i,j,k) \leq T_m$$

$$a_q(i,j,k) = \text{NINT}\left[\frac{a(i,j,k) + T_m}{Q_m}\right] \quad a(i,j,k) < -T_m \quad (6.17)$$

where $a(i,j,k)$ is the wavelet coefficient, $a_q(i,j,k)$ is the quantized wavelet coefficient, and m is the number of the level in the wavelet transform; T_m and Q_m are functions of the wavelet transform level. The function T_m can be set as a constant, and $Q_m = Q2^{m-1}$, where Q is a constant.

6.6.3.4 Entropy Coding

In the third step, the quantized data are subjected to run-length coding followed by the Huffman coding. Run-length coding is effective when there are pixels with the same gray level in a sequence. Since thresholding of the high resolution components

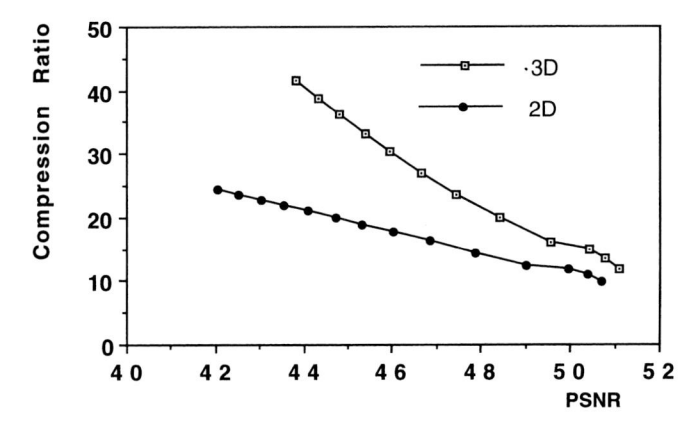

Figure 6.29 Comparison between 3-D and 2-D wavelet compression results on MR head images.

results a large number of zeros, run-length coding can be expected to significantly reduce the size of data. Applying Huffman coding after run-length coding can further improve the compression ratio.

6.6.3.5 Some Results

This section presents some compression results using a 3-D MR data set from a GE 5x Signa MR Scanner with 124 images and 256 × 256 × 12 bits per image. A 2-D wavelet compression is also applied to the same data set, and the results are compared with the 3-D compression results. The 2-D compression algorithm is similar to that of the 3-D compression algorithm except that a two-dimensional wavelet transform is applied to each slice.

Figure 6.29 compares the compression ratios for the 3-D and 2-D algorithms; the horizontal axis is the peak signal-to-noise ratio (PSNR) defined in Section 6.5.1.2, and the vertical axis represents the compression ratio.

At the same PSNR, compression ratios of the 3-D method are about 40–90% higher than that of the 2-D method. From Figure 6.30, a slice of MR volume image data compressed with 3-D wavelet method, we can see that the compression ratio of 20:1 the decompressed image quality is nearly the same as that of the original image.

6.7 COLOR IMAGE COMPRESSION

6.7.1 Examples of Color Image in Radiology

Color images are very important in microscopy but very seldom used in radiology because traditionally, radiology uses an X-ray source, which produces monochromatic images. Color, when used, is mostly for enhancement purposes. In this case, a certain gray level or a range of gray levels is converted to colors, to enhance visual appear-

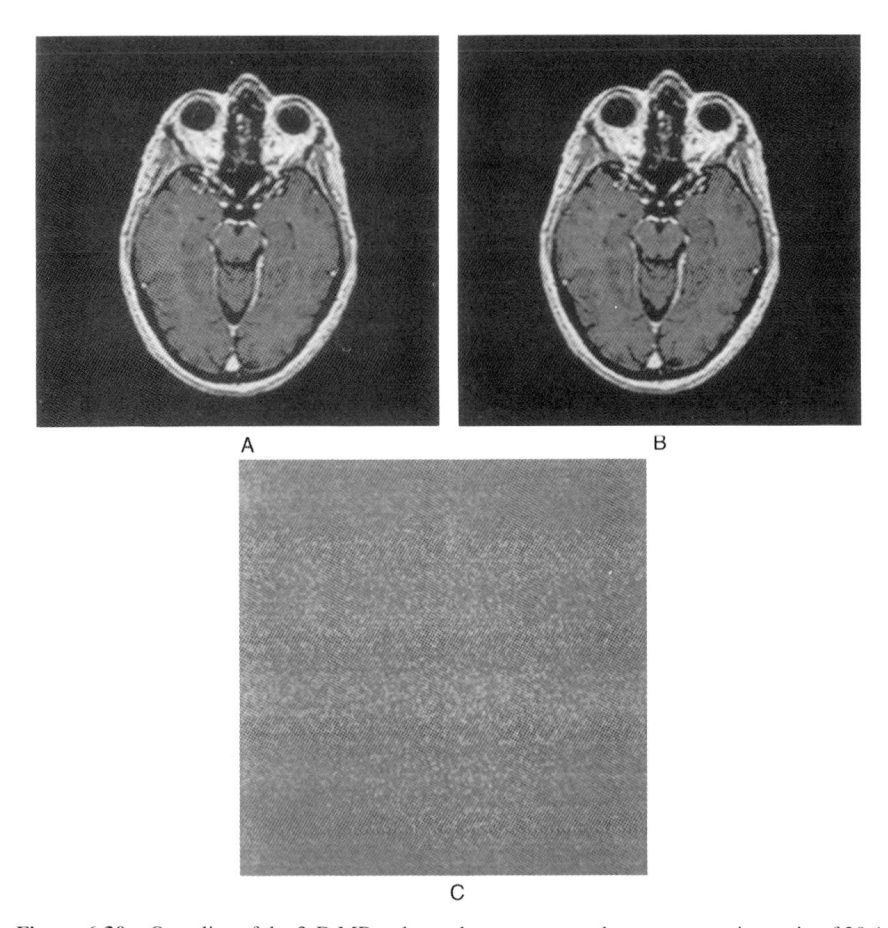

Figure 6.30 One slice of the 3-D MR volume data compressed at a compression ratio of 20:1 with the 3-D wavelet compression method: compared with Figure 6.8. (a) Original image. (b) Reconstructed image. (c) Difference image. (Courtesy of Jun Wang, 1995.)

ance. Examples are found in nuclear medicine, PET, and most recently, in Doppler ultrasound (US) (see Fig. 5.14). In Section 5.5.4, we noted that a 10-second Doppler US study can produce an image file as large as 225 Mbyte because of the pseudocolor images. We now discuss a method of compressing US color images.

6.7.2 The Color Spaces

Traditionally, a color $512 \times 512 \times 24$ bit image is decomposed into a red, a green, and a blue image in the RGB color space, each with $512 \times 512 \times 8$ bits (see Sections 5.5.4 and 5.7.6). Each image is treated independently as an individual image. For display, the display system combines the images on a color monitor through a color composite video control. This scheme is referred to as the color space, and the three-color decomposition is determined by drawing a triangle on a special color chart developed by the Commission Internationale de L'Eclairage (CIE) with each of the base colors as an end point. The CIE color chart is characterized by isolating the luminance (or brightness) from the chrominance (or hue). Based on this characteristic as a guideline, the National Television System Committee (NTSC) defined a new color space YIQ, representing the luminance, in-phase chrominance, and quadrature chrominance coordinates, respectively. In digital imaging, a color space called YCbCr is used, where Cr and Cb represent two chrominance components. The conversion between the standard RGB space to YCbCr is given by

$$\begin{bmatrix} Y \\ Cb \\ Cr \end{bmatrix} = \begin{bmatrix} 0.2990 & 0.587 & 0.114 \\ -0.1687 & -0.3313 & 0.5 \\ 0.5 & -0.4187 & -0.0813 \end{bmatrix} \begin{bmatrix} R \\ G \\ B \end{bmatrix} \quad (6.18)$$

where R, G, and B pixel values are between 0 and 255.

There are two advantages of using the YCbCr system. First, it distributes most of the image information into the luminance component (Y), with less going to chrominance (Cb and Cr). As a result, the YCbCr elements are less correlated and, therefore, can be compressed separately without loss in efficiency. Second, through field experience, the variations in the Cb and Cr planes are known to be less than that in the Y plane. Therefore, Cb and Cr can be subsampled in both the horizontal and the vertical direction without losing much of the chrominance. The immediate compression from converting the RGB to YCbCr is 2:1. This can be computed as follows:

Original color image size: $512 \times 512 \times 24$ bits
YCbCr image size: $512 \times 512 \times 8$ + 2 × ($0.25 \times 512 \times 512 \times 8$) bits
                      (Y)   (Cb and Cr)   subsampling

That is, after the conversion, each YCbCr pixel is represented by 12 bits: 8 bits for the luminance (Y), and eight bits for each of the chrominances (Cb and Cr) for every other pixel and every other line. The Y, Cb, and Cr image can be compressed further as three individual images by using error-free compression. JPEG, the Joint Photographic Experts Group, uses this technique for color image compression.

6.7.3 Compression of Color Ultrasound Images

Normal US Doppler studies generate an average of 13 ± 6 Mbyte per image file. There are cases that can go up to 80–100 Mbyte. To compress a color Doppler image (see Fig. 5.14), the color RGB image is first transformed to the YCbCr space by means of Eq. (6.18). But instead of a subsampling of the Cb and the Cr images as described earlier, all three images are subjected to a run-length coding independently. Two factors favor this approach. First, a US image possesses information within a sector. Outside the sector, the image contains only background information. Background information can yield a very high compression ratio. Second, the Cb and Cr images contain little information except at the flow regions, which are very small compared with the entire anatomical structures in the image. Thus, run-length coding of Cb and Cr can give very high compression ratio, eliminating the need for subsampling. On average, two-dimensional, error-free, run-length coding can give a compression ratio of 3.5:1, or as high as 6:1. Even higher compression ratios can result if the third dimension (time) of a temporal US study is considered.

6.8 LEGAL AND REGULATORY ISSUES

In this section, we discuss the legal and regulatory issues of radiologic image compression. Reversible or lossless compression does not cause any legal complications but does provide modest reduction in image size, with a compression ratio of 2:1. Therefore intense research effort has been focused on lossy compression schemes of low bit rate that discard image data of no diagnostic significance but retain medically relevant information in an examination. The results of many studies indicate that a digital chest image conceivably can be compressed to 10:1 or higher with acceptable diagnostic quality.

Image compression is influenced by the standards of two major organizations: ACR-NEMA (American College of Radiology–National Electrical Manufacturers Association) and DICOM (Digital Imaging and Communication in Medicine), and by the Center for Devices and Radiological Health (CDRH) of the U.S. Food and Drug Administration (FDA). For example, in the DICOM 3.0 Standards, Part 5 Annex A.4.1 is dedicated to the specifications of JPEG image compression. A summary of premarket notifications reviewed by the FDA in 1992 indicated that most PACS devices submitted for marketing clearance are all-new products or are significant modifications of existing products. Of the 19 products reviewed, 15 implement some form of compression and 6 incorporate lossy compression; some even have a compression ratio as high as 80:1.

The availability of lossy compression has raised new regulatory and legal questions for manufacturers, users, and the FDA. The regulatory policy, however, is concerned less about patents and copyright matters, as in commercial software systems, and more with the safety and the quality of medical devices that incorporate compression hardware and software, including the following considerations: indication for use and labeling, existence of a suitable measure of compression that properly characterizes the degree of information, and the effects of compression on image postprocessing. The legal questions frequently asked involved the possibility of legal standards for image compression and product liability guidelines. All these pertinent questions and issues raised are interrelated. To transfer lossy compression technology into the marketplace, the researchers, as well as the developers, must properly understand the technical implications and the challenges derived from these issues.

6.8.1 Use of Irreversible Compression

Should the lossy coding techniques be restricted to uses other than primary diagnosis? Lossy techniques are being used for teaching files, reviewing reports, long-term archiving of images with known diagnosis, and presenting research conclusions. Radiologists are concerned, however, that the use of lossy compression at the primary diagnosis might cause loss of fine details or subtle information of original images and result in incorrect diagnosis or interpretation, with the accompanying possibility of malpractice suits. Since primary diagnosis is an important activity that has a significant impact on the health care service, excluding the use of lossy coding from its practice hinders the move toward a digital radiology environment. Thus, another regulatory issue to be undertaken is the rendering of an informed decision as to whether lossy compression can be used for specific primary diagnoses that do not require high resolution. Also worthy of study is the issue of tailoring the degree of lossy compression for radiological applications of different kinds.

6.8.2 Measure of Image Compression

Although there exist many methods of evaluating image quality, such as subjective ratings, paired comparisons, free response ROC, sensitivity and specificity, and signal-to-noise ratio. Classical ROC analyses as described in Section 6.5.5 are still the radiologist's most credible and acceptable way of measuring image quality. A great deal of work has been done to determine ROC curves for different specific radiological tasks using images reconstructed under various degrees of lossy compression. It would be almost impossible, however, to attempt this work as the basis of regulation. This is because there is a wide variety of diagnostic radiological tasks, and the acceptable degree of compression is task-dependent.

The FDA has chosen to place such a decision in the hands of the user. The agency, however, has taken steps to ensure that the user has the information needed to make the decision by requiring that the lossy compression statement as well as the approximate compression ratio be attached to lossy images. The manufacturers also are required to provide in their operator's manuals a discussion on the effects of lossy compression on image quality. Data from laboratory tests are required as a premarket notification only when the medical device uses new technologies and asserts new claims, however. The 1993 PACS guidance document from the FDA allows manufacturers to use lossy coding techniques to report the normalized mean-square error (NMSE) of their communication and storage devices. This measure was chosen because it has often been used by the manufacturers themselves and there is some objective basis for comparisons. However, as discussed in Section 6.5, NMSE does not provide any local information regarding type of loss (e.g., spatial location or spatial frequency). The development of a better, and general, method for characterizing compression losses is urgently needed and should be a *high priority research topic* in medical imaging.

6.8.3 Image Postprocessing

The effect of lossy compression on image postprocessing software has received little attention. Postprocessing image software includes filtering (e.g., smoothing, edge enhancement, and morphological operations), mensuration algorithms (e.g., surface and volume determinations), and image feature extraction (e.g., identification of lung nodules and breast cancer microcalcifications). The postprocessing of lossy images is seldom used because the physician would not need to apply these techniques. On the other hand, for storing large image data for transmitting images to a referring physician at a remote location, such as in a PACS image database, and for performing certain kinds of examination, such as cine-type examinations, postprocessing is desirable. The basic position of the FDA on lossy image postprocessing is to have the developers demonstrate that the software will function with the chosen level of compression and submit test data to support their claims.

6.8.4 Legal Standards for Compression

Presently there is no legal standard for radiologic image compression. The absence of such a standard means that there is no objective clinical reference for courts to use in judging malpractice cases that involve the use of medical devices incorporating lossy algorithms. To be acceptable, a compression algorithm requires thorough clinical validation tests, carried out on a large number of images and involving many clinicians, to assure that diagnostic accuracy is not jeopardized by lossy compression. This approach could conceivably comprise a "reasonable" standard before the courts. Such a task would be difficult, though not impossible, to carry out for measuring the image quality of a wide variety of modalities available. Currently, when a misdiagnosis is the subject of a legal trial, radiologists testifying for the plaintiff and for the defense will argue image quality before the jury, and the judge will give instructions regarding reasonableness as related to the issue of the defendant's duty owed to the plaintiff as well as image quality. We then let a jury decide whether there was a breach of duty to provide reasonable image quality. One obvious question is: Should courts dictate compression schemes? Our position is that it is the clinical and engineering professionals who should dictate clarity in legal compression standards, not the judiciary.

The regulation of the federal government shifts the responsibility to the user. The aim is to reduce the chance of misinterpretation of lossy images by ensuring that imaging equipment has the desired features and by providing the user with enough information to make a decision. But, there is no clear specification on which the user may formulate an objective judgment of using lossy schemes. A standard also would be important for teleradiology applications, where there is less control of the medical devices used at both ends than at a single site. The derivation of a legal standard should not depend on a court decision, but should be a task, albeit difficult, that is undertaken with the assistance of expert medical imaging professionals.

6.8.5 Product Liability

A plaintiff who feels that he has been injured as a result of degradation of image quality during a radiological operation may bring a suit against a vendor under product liability theory. This legal theory, which originated in California, has been in place for a number of years: it holds the vendor liable for any physical harm caused by a defective product that is "unreasonably" dangerous to the user even if the seller has made an effort in good faith to use all possible care in its preparation. This situation is even more complex in teleradiology, since an image may be subjected to lossy compression on one system, transmitted to another for reconstruction, and retransmitted to yet a third for viewing. There is the unsettled question of who should bear the responsibility—the company whose device applies the compression, the manufacturer of reconstruction software, or the developer of the viewing workstation. The current federal policy, which requires that images subjected to lossy compression be labeled with a caution, can help only to some extent. Thus, manufacturers and developers must invest time in examining the response of their image processing algorithms, and physicians should be aware of problems which can be introduced by lossy compression.

6.9 SUMMARY AND RESEARCH DIRECTIONS

Despite rapid progress in mass storage density and computer network performance, the demand for transmission bandwidth and storage space in the digital radiology environment continues to outstrip the capabilities of available technologies. To overcome these two stumbling blocks, research in radiologic image compression aims to achieve a high compression ratio in representing digital images of various modalities while maintaining an acceptable image quality for clinical use.

Many studies done in the field of medical imaging indicate that it is conceivable to compress a radiologic image to 10:1 or even higher without losing diagnostic quality. Because of the legal and medical implications of permanent loss of image quality, reversible compression is the currently acceptable way to compress medical images. Nevertheless, the promise of using high performance irreversible compression to solve data storage and transmission problems has enticed medical imaging researchers and developers for years. The recent formation of certain industrial standards, such as ACR-NEMA and DICOM, and the emerging market for PACS and teleradiology, help to trigger a marked increase in the development of medical devices that use lossy coding algorithms.

The choice of a compression scheme is a complex trade-off of system and clinical requirements. Discrete cosine transform coding, as in other digital imaging fields, is the most common approach to lossy compression in medical imaging today. Since the characteristics of radiologic images vary with modalities and applications, our discussion reveals that there are also many strong candidates in subband coding techniques, such as the wavelet transforms. Recent results using wavelet transforms demonstrate the possibility of achieving compression ratios up to 20–30 in projectional radiography without compromising image diagnostic quality. This accomplishment raises the possibility of using wavelet transforms as the future standard for image compression.

Although significant progress has been made in radiologic image compression since its beginning in the last decade, many research challenges remain. First, the coming of a digital radiology environment, especially PACS and teleradiology, will continue to test the limits of disk storage and transmission bandwidth. Further improvement on existing compression techniques thus are necessary.

Second, large 2-D image files (e.g., digital mammography files with 160 Mbyte per examination) will push the urgency of implementing image compression in the clinical environment. Acquisitions of 3-D and 4-D medical image sequences are becoming more usual nowadays, especially in the case of dynamic studies performed with modalities such as MRI, fast XCT, ultrasonography, nuclear medicine, or PET. Thus, another challenge is to enable multidimensional medical image coding but still provide fast response time and affordable disk space. For these new applications, special hardware design and parallel processing technology offer a solution to the problems inherent in manipulating and processing the significantly increased data volume. Existing image compression algorithms are optimized for sequential computing, although the literature contains reports of sporadic attempts to explore parallel compression techniques, such as the full-frame DCT and the parallel digital video interface compression using dedicated hardware. As the price of parallel computers is dropping, we anticipate that more effort will be spent in developing parallel compression techniques for medical applications.

It is worth noting that medical imaging scanners typically have adequate local memory space and dedicated hardware to acquire images efficiently. The critical issue of medical imaging applications is how to transmit and display the archived images promptly on request. Hence, the focus of parallel radiologic image compression is on image decoding. This differs from other digital imaging applications, such as satellite imaging (which emphasizes fast data encoding to process the rapid arrival of satellite signals) and teleconferencing (which concerns both encoding and decoding processes).

Third, it is important to develop a large and comprehensive image database that contains image sets for various modalities and diseases. The image set of each disease will cover a wide spectrum of standardized diagnostic images for that disease, with various degrees of diagnostic difficulty. This database must be established by a national committee and could be used as a universal tool for one evaluation of any image compression devices submitted to the FDA for marketing clearance.

Finally, the development of a better, and general, method for characterizing compression losses of radiologic images is urgently needed. The availability of lossy compression raises several important legal and regulatory issues that remain to be settled. For the lossy compression technology to be put into the clinical environment, one crucial task is to define an objective measure of image quality so as to set a legal standard for lossy compression. The traditional noise and compression ratio measurements are insufficient. They do not provide any information regarding the type of loss (e.g., the spatial location or spatial frequency) that causes image unsharpness. On the other hand, besides being costly and time-consuming to perform, ROC studies are too specific to cover the wide range of medical imaging modalities and applications. Developing such a measure of radiologic imaging is not trivial: it would require the cooperative efforts of imaging scientists, manufacturers, and clinicians to define a general means of classifying, measuring, and evaluating the quality of radiologic images, covering not only global parameters, such as noise and compression ratio, but also local parameters, such as texture and sharpness. The standardization of an image database for radiologic image compression, augmented by recent advances in the area of *perception coding*, would shed some light on this subject.

CHAPTER 7

Picture Archiving and Communication System Components and Industrial Standards

7.1 PACS COMPONENTS

A picture archiving and communication system (PACS) consists of image and data acquisition, PACS controller and archive, and display subsystems integrated by digital networks as shown in Figure 1.1 (see p. 4). This section introduces these components, which are discussed in more detail in subsequent chapters.

7.1.1 Data and Image Acquisition Component

PACS requires images and related patient data to be sent from imaging modalities (devices) to the PACS controller and archive. The most troublesome PACS issues to date have been the reliability and timely acquisition from a radiologic imaging modality of images and associated study support text (information on patients, description of the study, and parameters of acquisition and image processing).

This bottleneck exists mainly because many manufacturers of imaging equipment are not prepared to follow the industry standards developed by, for example, the ACR-NEMA (American College of Radiology–National Electrical Manufacturers Association), and DICOM (Digital Imaging and Communications in Medicine), as discussed later (Section 7.3). To circumvent these difficulties, an acquisition gateway computer can be placed between the imaging modality(s) and the rest of the PACS network to isolate the radiologic imaging modality host computer from the PACS. Isolation is necessary because traditional imaging device computers lack the necessary communication and coordination software that is standardized in the PACS infrastructure. Furthermore, they lack general PACS system knowledge that enables the PACS computers to cooperatively recover from various error conditions. The acquisition gateway computer has three primary tasks: it acquires image data from the radiologic imaging devices, converts the data from manufacturer's specifications to the PACS standard format (header format, byte-ordering, matrix sizes) that is compliant with the ACR-NEMA/DICOM data formats, and forwards the image study to the PACS controller (Section 7.1.2) or display workstations.

Connecting general-purpose PACS acquisition gateway computers and radiologic

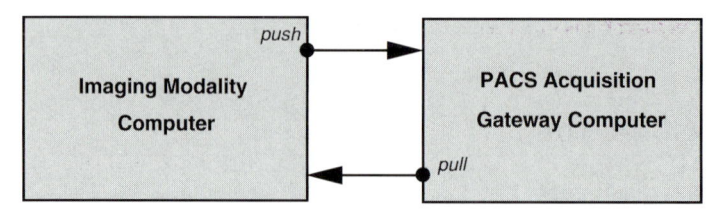

Figure 7.1 Peer-to-peer network interface between an imaging device computer and a PACS acquisition gateway computer: Push, from the modality computer; Pull, from the gateway computer.

imaging modalities are interfaces of two types. With peer-to-peer network interfaces, which use the TCP/IP (transmission control protocol/Internet protocol) Ethernet protocol, image transfers can be initiated either by the radiologic imaging modality (a "push" operation) or by the destination PACS acquisition gateway computer (a "pull" operation). The pull mode is advantageous because if an acquisition gateway computer goes down, images can be queued in the radiologic imaging modality computer until the gateway computer becomes operational again, at which time the queued images can be pulled and normal image flow resumed. Assuming that sufficient data buffering is available on the imaging modality computer, the pull mode is the preferred mode of operation because an acquisition computer can be programmed to reschedule study transfers if failure occurs (to itself or to the radiologic imaging modality). If a delay in acquisition is not acceptable, images from examinations can be rerouted to a designated backup acquisition gateway computer or to a workstation on the network when the primary acquisition gateway computer is unavailable. Figure 7.1 illustrates the concept of the "push" and "pull" operations.

The second interface type is a master/slave device-level connection such as the de facto industry standard, DR-11W. This parallel-transfer direct memory access connection is a point-to-point, board-level interface. Recovery mechanisms again depend on which machine (acquisition gateway computer or imaging modality) can initiate a study transfer. If the gateway computer is down, data may be lost. An alternative image acquisition method must be used to acquire these images (e.g., the technologist manually sends individual images stored in the imaging modality computer after the gateway computer has been brought back up, or the technologist digitizes the digital hard copy film image). These interface concepts are described in more detail in Chapter 8.

7.1.2 PACS Controller and Archive

Imaging examinations along with pertinent patient information are sent from the acquisition gateway computer, the hospital information system (HIS), and the radiology information system (RIS) to the PACS controller. The PACS controller is the engine of the PACS consisting of high end computers or servers; its two major components are a database server and an archive system. Table 7.1 lists operations of a PACS controller. Some of the basic functions of the PACS database server are illus-

TABLE 7.1　Operations of a PACS Controller

Receives images of a study from acquisition computers
Extracts text information describing the received studies
Updates a network-accessible database management system
Determines the destination workstations to which the newly generated studies are to be forwarded
Automatically retrieves necessary comparison images from a distributed cache storage or optical disk library archive system
Automatically corrects the orientation of computed radiographic images
Determines optimal contrast and brightness parameters for image display
Performs image data compression
Archives new studies onto optical disk library
Deletes images that have been archived from acquisition gateway computers
Services archive retrieval requests from workstations and other PACS controllers

trated in Figure 7.2. The archive system consists of short-term, long-term, and permanent storage. These components are explained in detail in Chapter 10.

7.1.3 Display Workstations

PACS display workstations should fully use the resources and processing power of the entire PACS network. A workstation includes communication, database, display, resource management, and processing software. The fundamental workstation operations are listed in Table 7.2.

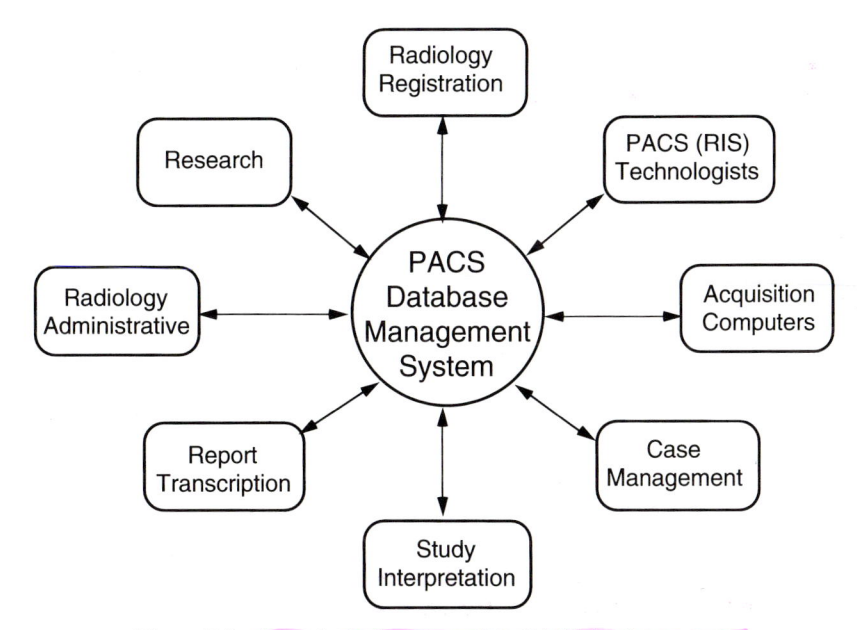

Figure 7.2　Some basic functions of the PACS database server.

TABLE 7.2 Major Functions of a PACS Workstation

Function	Description
Case preparation	Accumulation of all relevant images and information belonging to a patient examination
Case selection	Selection of cases for a given subpopulation
Image arrangement	Tools for arranging and grouping images for easy review
Interpretation	Measurement tools for facilitating the diagnosis
Documentation	Tools for image annotation, text, and voice reports
Case presentation	Tools for a comprehensive case presentation

There are four types of display workstation: (1) high resolution (2.5K × 2K) monitors for primary diagnosis at the radiology department, (2) medium resolution (1.5K × 1K) monitors for primary diagnosis of sectional images and at the hospital wards, (3) physician desktop workstations (512 monitor), and (4) hard copy workstations for printing images on film and paper. At primary diagnostic workstations, current and historical images are stored on local high speed magnetic disks for fast retrieval. Access to the global PACS database is provided if needed for retrieving longer term historical images. Chapter 12 elaborates on the concept and applications of workstations.

7.1.4 System Networking

A basic function of any computer network is to provide a path by which end users (e.g., radiologists and clinicians) at one geographic location can access information (e.g., images and reports) at another location. The important networking data needed for system design include location and function of each network node, frequency of information passed between any two nodes, cost for transmission between nodes with various speed lines, desired reliability of the communication, and required throughput. The variables in the design include the network topology, communication line capacities, and flow assignments.

At the local area network level, digital communication in the PACS infrastructure design can consist of low speed (10 Mbit/s signaling rate) Ethernet, medium speed (100 Mbit/s) fiber distributed data interface (FDDI), or fast Ethernet, and high speed asynchronous transfer mode technology (ATM: 155–622 Mbit/s and up) or Gbit/s Ethernet (gigabit Ethernet). In a wide area network, various digital service (DS) speeds can be used, ranging from DS-0 (56 Kbit/s) and DS-1 (T1, 1.544 Mbit/s) to DS-3 (45 Mbit/s), and ATM (155–622 Mbit/s). There is a trade off between transmission speed and cost.

The network protocol used should be standard, for example, TCP/IP. A low speed network is used to connect the imaging modalities (devices) to the acquisition gateway computers because of the time-consuming processes during imaging acquisition. Several segmented local area Ethernets may be involved in transferring data from imaging devices to acquisition gateway computers. The decision to use a medium or high speed network is based on the balance of data throughput requirements and costs.

A faster image network is used between acquisition gateway computers and the PACS controller because several acquisition computers may send large image files to the controller at the same time.

Process coordination between tasks running on different computers connected to the network is an extremely important issue in system networking. This coordination of processes running either on the same computer or on different computers is accomplished by using interprocessor communication methods with socket-level interfaces to TCP/IP. Commands are exchanged as American Standard Code for Information Interchange (ACSII) messages to ensure standard encoding of messages. Various PACS-related job requests are lined up into disk-resident priority queues, which are serviced by various computer system daemon (agent) processes. The queue software can have a built-in job scheduler that is programmed to retry a job several times by using either a default set of resources or alternative resources if a hardware error is detected. This mechanism ensures that no jobs will be lost during the complex negotiation for job priority among processes. Communications and networking are presented in more detail in Chapter 9.

7.2 PACS INFRASTRUCTURE DESIGN CONCEPT

Four major ingredients in the PACS infrastructure design concept are system standardization, open architecture and connectivity, reliability, and security.

7.2.1 Industry Standards

The first important rule in building a PACS infrastructure is to incorporate as many industry de facto standards as possible that are consistent with the overall PACS design scheme. The philosophy is to minimize the development of customized software. Furthermore, using industry standard hardware and software increases the portability of the system to other computer platforms. For example, the following industry standards should be used in the PACS infrastructure design: UNIX operating system, Windows NT operating system, TCP/IP and DICOM communication protocols, SQL (Structured Query Language) as the database query language, ACR-NEMA and DICOM standards for image data format, C and C++ programming languages, X Windows user interface, ASCII text representation for message passing, and HL7 for health care database information exchange.

The implications of using standards in PACS implementation are several. First, implementation of all future PACS components and modules is straightforward. Second, system maintenance is easier because each module looks similar to others, if not physically, then logically. Moreover, defining the PACS primitive operations serves to minimize the amount of redundant computer code in the PACS, which in turn makes the code easier to debug, understand, and search. It is self-evident that using standardizing industrial terminology, data format, and communication protocols in PACS design facilitates system understanding and documentation among all levels of PACS developers. Among all standards, HL7 and DICOM are the most impor-

182   PICTURE ARCHIVING, COMMUNICATION SYSTEM COMPONENTS

tant: the former allows the interfaces between PACS and HIS/RIS [HL7]; the latter, interfaces images among various manufacturers (see Section 7.3). [DICOM]

7.2.2 Connectivity and Open Architecture

If two PACS modules in the same hospital cannot communicate with each other, they become two isolated systems, each with its own images and patient information, and can never be combined with other systems to form a total hospital-integrated PACS.

Open network design is essential, to allow a standardized method for data and message exchange between heterogeneous systems. Because computer and communications technology changes rapidly, a closed architecture would hinder system upgradability. For example, suppose an independent imaging workstation from a given manufacturer would, at first glance, make a good addition to an MR or a CT scanner for viewing images. If the workstation has a closed proprietary architecture design, however, no components except those specified by the same manufacturer can be installed to augment the system. Potential overall system upgrading and improvement are limited, and perhaps other changes as well. Considerations of connectivity are important even when a small–scale PACS is planned. To be sure that a contemplated PACS is well designed and will allow future connectivity, the following questions should be considered:

> Can we transmit images from this PACS module to other systems and vice versa?
> Does this module use a standard data and image format?
> Does the computer in the module use a standard communication protocol?

7.2.3 Reliability

Reliability is a major issue in a PACS for two reasons. First, a PACS has many components; the probability of component failing is high. Second, because the PACS manages and displays critical patient information, extended periods of downtime cannot be tolerated. In designing a PACS, it is therefore important to use fault-tolerant measures, including error detection and logging software, external auditing programs (i.e., network management processes that check network circuits, magnetic disk space, database status, processes status, and queue status), hardware redundancy, and intelligent software recovery block. Some recovery mechanisms that can be used include automatic retry of failed jobs with alternative resources and algorithms, and intelligent bootstrap routines (software blocks executed by a computer when it is restarted) that allow a PACS computer to automatically continue operations after a power outage or system failure. Improving reliability is costly; however, it is essential to maintain high reliability of a complex system.

7.2.4 Security

Security is an important consideration because of medicolegal issues, including particularly the need for patient confidentiality. Data security is subject to violations mainly of the following kinds: physical intrusion, misuse, and behavioral. Physical intrusion relates to facility security, which can be handled by building management. Misuse and behavioral violations can be minimized by account control and privilege control. Most sophisticated database management systems have identification and authorization mechanisms that use accounts and passwords. Application programs may supply additional layers of protection. Privilege control refers to granting and revoking a user's access to specific tables, columns, or views from the database. These security measures provide the PACS infrastructure with a mechanism for controlling access to clinical and research data. With these mechanisms, the system designer can enforce policy as to which persons have access to clinical studies. In some hospitals, for example, referring clinicians are granted image study access only after a preliminary radiology reading has been performed and attached to the image data.

An additional security measure is encryption during image and data communication. If implemented, this feature increases the system software overhead, but data transmission through open communication channels is more secure.

7.3 TWO HEALTH CARE INDUSTRY DATA AND IMAGE STANDARDS

Imagery and textual communications among health care information systems have always been difficult because these components vary with platforms, modalities, and manufacturers. With the emergence of industry standards, it becomes feasible to integrate all these heterogeneous, disparate medical images and textual data. Interfacing two devices requires two ingredients, a common data format and a communication protocol. Some major health care industry standards are Health Level 7 (HL7) for textual data and ACR-NEMA and DICOM for image data. HL7 is a standard textual data format, whereas ACR-NEMA and DICOM include data format and communication protocols. In conforming to the HL7 standard, it is possible to share medical information between the hospital information systems, radiology information systems, and PACS. When the ACR-NEMA/DICOM standards are adopted, it becomes possible to convert medical images generated from a variety of modalities and manufacturers to the standardized data format. The conversion can use the data dictionary defined in the ACR-NEMA and DICOM documents.

7.4 THE HEALTH LEVEL 7 (HL7) STANDARD

7.4.1 Health Level 7

Health Level 7 (HL7), established in March 1987, was organized by a user–vendor committee to develop a standard for electronic data exchange in health care environments, particularly for hospital applications. The common goal is to simplify the interface implementation between computer applications from multiple vendors. This standard emphasizes data format and protocol for exchanging certain key textual data among health care information systems, such as HIS, RIS, and PACS.

HL7 addresses the highest level (level 7) of the Open System Interconnection (OSI) model of the International Standards Organization (ISO), but does not conform specifically to the defined elements of the OSI's seventh level (see Section 9.1). It conforms to the conceptual definitions of an application-to-application interface placed in the seventh layer of the OSI model. These definitions were developed to facilitate data communication in a health care setting by providing rules to convert abstract messages associated with real-world events into strings of characters comprised in an actual message.

7.4.2 An Example

Consider the three popular computer platforms used in HIS, RIS, and PACS, namely, the IBM mainframe computer running VM operating system, VAX file server running open VMS, and, Sun SPARC workstations running UNIX. Interfacing involves the establishment of data links between these three operating systems via TCP/IP communication protocol (Section 9.1) with HL7 data format at the application layer.

When an event occurs, such as a patient admission, discharge, or transfer (ADT), the IBM computer in the HIS responsible for tracking this event initiates an unsolicited message to the remote VAX file server in the RIS that takes charge of the next event. If the message is in HL7 format, the VAX parses the message, updates its local database automatically, and sends a confirmation to the IBM. Otherwise, a rejected message is sent instead.

In HL7 standard, the basic data unit is a message. Each message comprises multiple segments in a defined sequence. Each segment contains multiple data fields and is identified by a unique, predefined three-character code. The first segment is the message header segment with the three-letter code MSH, which defines the intent, source, destination, and some other relevant information, such as message control identification and time stamp. The other segments are event dependent. Within each segment, related pieces of information are bundled together based on the HL7 protocol. A typical message, such as patient admission, may contain the following segments:

	MSH	Message header segment
	EVN	Event type segment
	PID	Patient identification segment
	NK1	Next of kin segment
	PV1	Patient visit segment

In this patient admission message, the patient identification segment may contain the segment header and other demographic information, such as patient identification, name, birthdate, and gender. The separators between fields and within a field are defined in the message header segment. Here is an example of transactions of admitting a patient for surgery in HL7:

1. Message header segment

   MSH||STORE|MISSION|MIME|LAUREL|199801181007|security|ADT|MSG00201|||<CR>

2. Event type segment

   EVN|01|199801181005||<CR>

3. Patient identification segment

   PID|||PATID1234567||Doe^John^B^II||19470701|M||C|
   371 MAIN AVE^SAN FRANCISCO^CA^94122-0619
   ||415-681-2888|||||||<CR>

4. Next of kin segment

   NK1|Doe^Linda^E||wife|<CR>

5. Patient visit segment

   PV1|1|I|100^345^01||||00135^SMITH^WILLIAM^K|||SUR|ADM|<CR>

Combining these five segments, these messages translate to:
"Patient John B. Doe, II, male, Caucasian, born on July 1, 1947, lives at 371 Main Avenue in San Francisco, was admitted on January 18, 1998, at 10:05 A.M. by Doctor William K. Smith (#00135) for surgery. The patient has been assigned to Room 345, bed 01 on nursing unit 100. The next of kin is Linda E. Doe, wife. The ADT message 201 was sent from system STORE at the Mission site to system MIME at the Laurel site on the same date two minutes after the admit."

The vertical line "|" is the data file separator. If no data are entered in a field, a blank will be used followed by another "|" symbol.

The data communication between a HIS and a RIS is event driven. When an ADT event occurs, the HIS would automatically send a broadcast message, confined in HL7 format, to the RIS. The RIS would then parse this message and insert, update, and organize patient demographic data in its database according to the event. Similarly, the RIS would send an HL7-formatted ADT message, the examination reports, and the procedural descriptions to the PACS. When the PACS had acknowledged and verified the data, it would update the appropriate databases and initiate any required follow-up actions.

For example, the HIS at UCSF, which consists of an IBM main frame computer and 11 other computer systems, uses a custom-built interface engine called MIMP (mediware information message processor) to distribute ADT data. It generates HL7 bundled messages and transfers them over the local area network to RIS. IDXrad, the application running on RIS, uses the programming language environment Digital Standard MUMPS (DSM version 6.3) for the interface. This interface works for point-to-point communication. Upon receiving HL7 messages from HIS, IDXrad triggers appropriate events and transfers patient data over the network to the PACS controller (Sun SPARC). After conversion to the HL7, the message can be transmitted between HIS, RIS, and PACS with a communication protocol—most commonly, TCP/IP through a network. (See Section 9.1.) In Chapter 11 we present the mechanism of interfacing PACS with HIS and RIS using the HL7 standard.

7.5 THE ACR-NEMA STANDARD

7.5.1 ACR-NEMA and DICOM

ACR-NEMA, formally known as the American College of Radiology and the National Electrical Manufacturers Association, created a committee to draft a set of standards to serve as the common ground for various medical imaging equipment vendors in developing instruments that can communicate and participate in sharing medical image information, in particular in the PACS environment. The committee, which focused chiefly on issues concerning information exchange, interconnectivity, and communications between medical systems, began work in 1982. The first version, which emerged in 1985, specifies standards in point-to-point message transmission, data formatting, and presentation, and includes a preliminary set of communication commands and data format dictionary. The second version, ACR-NEMA 2.0, published in 1988, was an enhancement to the first release. It included both hardware definitions and software protocols, as well as a standard data dictionary. Networking issues were not addressed adequately in either version. For this reason, a new version aiming to include network protocols was released in 1992. Because of the magnitude of the changes and additions, it was given a new name: Digital Imaging and Communications in Medicine (DICOM 3.0). The latest version was released in 1996, consisting of 13 published parts. Each DICOM document is identified by title and standard number in the form: PS 3.X-YYYY where "X" is the part number, and "YYYY" is the year of publication. Thus, PS 3.1–1996 means DICOM 3.0 preliminary specification document part 1 (Introduction), released in 1996, and PS is an internal ACR-NEMA code. Although the complexity and involvement of the standards were increased by manyfold, DICOM remains compatible with the earlier ACR-NEMA versions. The two most distinguishing new features in DICOM are adaptation of the object-oriented data model for message exchange and utilization of existing standard network communication protocols.

Although the standard committee is influential in the medical imaging community, in the beginning, medical imaging equipment manufacturers were slow to respond and comply with the ACR-NEMA standards. As the specifications of DICOM 3.0 becomes widely accepted, the manufacturers have taken a very cooperative manner and have begun to develop new versions of software and equipment totally based on this standard.

Modalities that do not conform with the DICOM standard, either follow the ACR-NEMA standard or have their own format. To accommodate the former, a conversion from ACR-NEMA to DICOM should be developed. And for the latter, a translator is needed to convert the manufacturer's specifications to either the ACR-NEMA or DICOM standard. A set of software modules, collectively called the encoder library, is needed for these purposes. A well-developed encoder library should have the following characteristics:

1. Generic for multimodalities and various vendor's imaging equipment.
2. Portability to various hardware platforms.
3. Software architecture based on the top-down and modular prinicples.
4. Standard programming language, such as C.

7.5.2 The ACR-NEMA Standard

The ACR-NEMA standard consists of image format and point-to-point communication standard. Since point-to-point communication has been completely replaced by DICOM network protocols, we will not consider it further. Instead, we focus on its data format, as many existing PACS systems and components are still using ACR-NEMA format standard. Let us use an encoder to explain how images are converted from a manufacturer's modality to ACR-NEMA format standard.

According to the ACR-NEMA 2.0 data dictionary, each image should contain two parts: a command group and a data set. The data set can be further divided into information groups: identifying, patient, acquisition, relationship, image presentation, overlay, and image pixel data. The data in these groups, when transmitted across equipment, constitutes a message.

When an image is generated from an imaging modality by a manufacturer, it consists of an image header that describes the nature of the image, and the image pixel values. Since the image header has no standard, its content is pretty much up to the manufacturer. For this reason, not every piece of header information from a modality will have a corresponding group-element category specified in the ACR-NEMA format. On the other hand, not every element defined in the ACR-NEMA dictionary will cover data types included in the image headers of various equipment vendors. Therefore, a minimum set of groups and a minimum set of elements within those groups as the core data structure should first be defined (see Table 7.3). In other words, all images, regardless of modality and manufacturer, should bear this minimum set once it has been formatted. Additional groups and elements are then defined based on the header information provided by the specific modality and the manufacturer. Additional information can be defined in two shadow groups: display shadow group and a raw header shadow group. The display shadow group stores the information that is vital to support workstation display and provide fast access. The raw

TABLE 7.3 Required Groups and Elements in the ACR-NEMA Conversion

Group	Element
0000	0000 (Command Group)
	0001
	0010
	0800
0008	0000 (Identifying Group)
	0001
0009	0000 (Display Shadow Group)
	0001
0010	0000 (Patient Information)
0019	0000 (Raw Header Shadow Group)
	0000
7fe0	0000 (Pixel Data Group)
	0010

header group retains the entire header information to permit the retrieval of data items not formatted, should it become necessary.

Additional groups and elements, such as acquisition information (group 0018), relationship information (group 0020), image presentation (group 0028), and overlay (group 6000-601E; even numbers only) will be applied depending on the type of information provided by the manufacturers.

Dependent on the modality, the numbers of groups and elements to be formatted differ considerably. To provide a systematic way for an encoder program to extract and map data from the image header to the ACR-NEMA format, a configuration file, which describes the included groups and elements, is needed for each modality. The encoder of a modality reads in a specific configuration file and calls various modules in its program to convert image data to the ACR-NEMA format. The last data group to be converted should be the pixel data group (7fe0), which is attached to the end of the message. In addition, for each modality, these encoders are grouped in a library with all the necessary modules for encoding. This library resides in the acquisition gateway computer to perform the data conversion once the image data has been received from the imaging modality.

The general algorithm of converting raw image data into ACR-NEMA format is as follows. First, an image is acquired from a modality. If it is not in the ACR-NEMA format upon arrival at the acquisition gateway computer, it goes through the encoding process and is converted to the standard format. After that, the formatted image is sent to the PACS controller for archiving, and subsequently, is transmitted to display workstations.

7.6 THE DICOM 3.0 STANDARD

The DICOM 3.0 standard provides several major enhancements of the earlier ACR-NEMA versions. Among these are [see DICOM 1994]:

1. DICOM 3.0 is applicable to a networked environment.
2. It specifies how devices claiming conformance to the standard react to commands and data being exchanged.
3. It provides guidelines on levels of conformance.
4. It structures as a multiple-part document. (see Section 7.5.1).
5. It uses information objects to describe entities (images, graphics, studies, reports, etc.).
6. It uses the entity-relationship model for uniquely identifying any information objects.

The major differences between the ACR-NEMA 2.0 and the DICOM 3.0 Standard are given in Table 7.4.

Two fundamental components of DICOM are the information object class and the service class. Information objects define the contents of a set of images and their re-

TABLE 7.4 Differences Between ACR-NEMA 2.0 and DICOM 3.0 Standards

ACR-NEMA 2.0	DICOM 3.0
Based on an intuitive information model	Based on an explicit information model
Services provided are built into commands and described fully in service classes	Services supported are descriptions of their use
Defines a minimum for conformance, but does not describe how a claim of conformance is structured	Includes a detailed specification about how to describe conformance
Supports point-to-point communication; if it is used and over networks, network interface equipment (NIE) is required to support the network protocol	Supports network communications
Supports a single image per message	Supports a folder capability for multiple images per message (by value or by reference)
Defines unique commands	Makes use of existing standards to define the new commands

lationship, and the service classes describe what to do with these objects. The service classes and information object classes are combined to form the fundamental units of DICOM, called service–object pairs (SOPs). This section describes these fundamental concepts and provides some examples.

7.6.1 Object Class and Service Class

In the DICOM 3.0 standard, there are two classes of information: object classes and service classes. The former defines objects (e.g. patients, modalities, studies), whereas the latter describes services (image storage, print, query, retrieval, etc.). Each class has a dictionary defining the attributes for proper encoding. Tables 7.5 and 7.6 list some service classes and some object classes.

TABLE 7.5 DICOM Service Classes

Service Class	Description
Image storage	Provides storage service for data sets
Image query	Supports queries about data sets
Image retrieval	Supports retrieval of images from storage
Image print	Provides hard copy generation support
Examination	Supports management of examinations (which may consist of several series of management images)
Storage resource	Supports management of the network data storage resource(s)

TABLE 7.6 DICOM Information Object Classes

Normalized
- Patient
- Study
- Results
- Storage resource
- Image annotation

Composite
- Computed radiograph
- Computed tomogram
- Digitized film image
- Digital subtraction image
- MR image
- Nuclear medicine image
- Ultrasound image
- Displayable image
- Graphics
- Curve

7.6.1.1 Object Classes

DICOM object classes consist of normalized objects and composite objects. Each normalized information object class includes the attributes inherent in the real-world entity represented. Let us consider two of the normalized object classes listed in Table 7.6: study information and patient information. Study date and image time are attributes in the study information object class because these attributes are inherent whenever a study is performed. On the other hand, patient name is not an attribute in the study information object class. Rather, because the patient's name is inherent in the patient information object class on which the study was performed, not the study itself, this attribute belongs in the patient object class. The use of information object classes permits objects encountered in medical imaging applications to be identified more precisely and without ambiguity. For this reason, objects defined in DICOM 3.0 are very precise.

However, sometimes it is advantageous to combine normalized object classes to form composite information object classes for facilitating operations. For example, the computed radiography image information object class is a composite because it contains attributes from the study information object class (image date, time, etc.) and patient information object class (patient's name, etc.). Table 7.6 also lists some composite information object classes. ACR-NEMA describes images obtained from different modalities based on the concept of composite information. Although it is not as precise as the normalized object classes in DICOM, the earlier standard has certain advantages during daily routine operation. Because it allows for backward compatibility between the two standards, and the decoding of a composite object is less time-consuming, composite objects from the ACR-NEMA complex data structure are retained in DICOM.

DICOM uses a unique identifier (UID) 1.2.840.10008.X.Y.Z to identify a specific part of an object, where the numerals are called the organizational root, and X, Y, Z are additional fields to identify the parts. Thus, for example, the UID for the DICOM explicit values representing little endian transfer syntax is 1.2.840.10008.1.2.1. Note that UID is used to identify a part of an object; it does not carry information.

7.6.1.2 DICOM Services

DICOM services are used for communication of imaging information objects within a device, and for the device to perform a service for the object, (e.g., to store the object, to display the object, etc.). A service is built on top of a set of "DICOM message service elements" (DIMSE). These DIMSEs are computer software programs written to perform specific functions. There are two types of DIMSE, one for the composite objects and the other for the normalized objects, given in Tables 7.7 and 7.8, respectively. Each composite DIMSE is paired in the sense that a device issues a command request and the receiver responds to the command accordingly. These commands are backward compatible with the earlier ACR-NEMA versions. The composite commands are generalized, whereas the normalized commands are more specific.

DICOM services are referred to as "service classes" because of the object-oriented nature of the information structure model. If a device provides a service, it is called a service class provider; if it uses a service, a service class user. Thus, for example, "magnetic disk" in the PACS controller is a service class provider for the controller to store images. On the other hand, a CT scanner is the service class user of the mag-

TABLE 7.7 Composite DICOM Message Service Elements (DIMSEs)

Command	Function
C-ECHO	Verification of connection
C-STORE	Transmission of an information object service-object pair (SOP) instance
C-FIND	Inquiries about information object instances
C-GET	Transmission of an information object instance via third-party application processes
C-MOVE	Similar to C-GET, but end receiver is usually not the command initiator

TABLE 7.8 Normalized DICOM Message Service Elements (DIMSEs)

Command	Function
N-EVENT-REPORT	Notification of information object-related event
N-GET	Retrieval of information object attribute value
N-SET	Specification of information object attribute value
N-ACTION	Specification of information object-related action
N-CREATE	Creation of an information object
N-DELETE	Deletion of an information object

netic disk in the PACS controller to store images. Note that a device can be either a service class provider or a service class user or both, depending on how it is asked to function. For example, in its routing process that receives images from the scanners and distributes these images to the workstations, the PACS controller takes on the roles of both storage service class provider and storage service class user. As a service class provider, it accepts images from the scanners by providing a storage service for these images. On the other hand, the PACS controller is a service class user when it sends images to the workstations by issuing service requests to the individual workstations for storing these images.

7.6.2 DICOM Communication

DICOM uses existing network communication standards based on the International Standards Organization Open Systems Interconnection (ISO-OSI, see Section 9.1 for details) for imaging information transmission. The ISO-OSI consists of seven layers from the lowest physical layer (cables) to the highest application layer. When imaging information objects are sent between layers in the same device, the process is called a service. When objects are sent between two devices, it is called a protocol. When a protocol is involved, several steps are invoked in two devices, and we say that two devices are in "association" using DICOM. Therefore, to send an image object from a CT scanner to a workstation with DICOM would invoke the following steps:

1. The CT scanner encodes all images into a DICOM object.
2. The scanner invokes a set of DIMSEs to move the image object from a certain level to the physical layer in the ISO-OSI model.
3. The workstation uses a counterset of DIMSEs to receive the image object through the physical layer and move it up to a certain level.
4. The workstation decodes the DICOM image object.

This movement of the image object from the CT scanner to the workstation uses communication protocols, the most commonly used is the TCP/IP. Figure 7.3 illustrates the movement of the CT images from the scanner to the workstation.

If an imaging device transmits an image object with a DICOM 3.0 command, the receiver has to use a DICOM 3.0 command to receive the information. On the other hand, if a device transmits a DICOM 3.0 object with a TCP/IP communication protocol through a network without invoking the DICOM communication, any device connected to the network can receive the data with the TCP/IP protocol. A decoder is needed to convert the DICOM 3.0 object for proper use. Figure 7.4 shows the procedure of converting a generic image format from a modality to the ACR-NEMA and DICOM standards.

7.6.3 DICOM Conformance

Part Two of the DICOM document PS 3.2–1996, instructs manufacturers how to conform their devices with the DICOM standard. In the conformance statement the manufacturer describes exactly how the device or its associated software conforms to the

THE DICOM 3.0 STANDARD   193

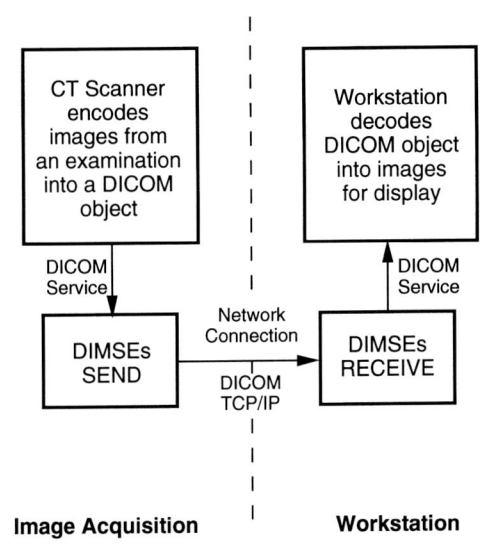

Figure 7.3 Movement of a set of CT images from the scanner to the workstation.

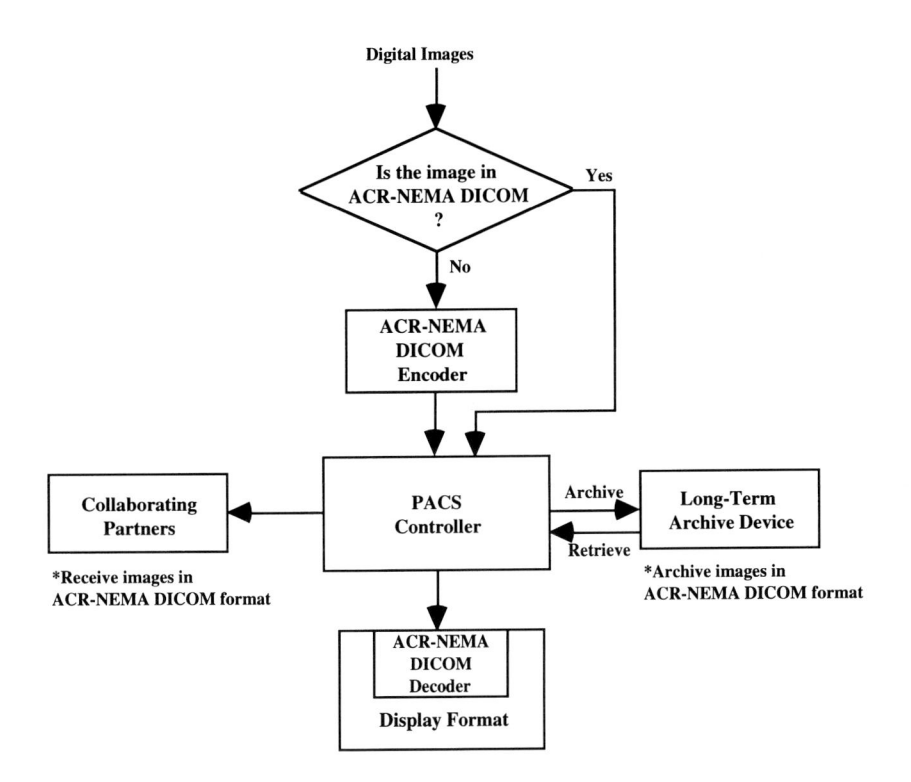

Data Encoding/Decoding to ACR-NEMA and DICOM Standards

Figure 7.4 Procedure of converting image format to the ACR-NEMA and DICOM standards.

standard. A conformance statement does not mean that the subject device follows every detail required by DICOM, it only means that the device follows a certain subset of DICOM. The extent of the subset is described in the conformance statement. For example, a laser film digitizer needs to conform only with the minimum requirements for the digitized images to be in DICOM format, and the digitizer should be a service class user to send the formatted images to a second device (e.g., a magnetic disk), which is a service class provider. Thus, if a manufacturer claims that its imaging device is DICOM-conforming, any system integrator who follows the manufacturer's conformance document should be able to interface this device with other DICOM-compliant components from other manufacturers.

In general, the contents of the conformance statement include [see DICOM 1994]:

1. The implementation model of the application entities (AEs) in the implementation and how these AEs relate to both local and remote real-world activities.
2. The proposed (for association initiation) and acceptable (for association acceptance) presentation contexts used by each AE.
3. The SOP classes and their options supported by each AE, and the policies with which an AE initiates or accepts associations.
4. The communication protocols to be used in the implementation.
5. A description of any extensions, specializations, and publicly disclosed privatizations to be used in the implementation.
6. A description of any implementation details that may be related to DICOM conformance or interoperability. [DICOM PS3.2-1996]

7.6.4 Examples of Using DICOM

Two most important DICOM services are sending and receiving images, and querying and retrieving images. In this section, we use two examples to explain how DICOM accomplishes these services. Note that the query and retrieve service is built on top of the send and receive services.

7.6.4.1 Send and Receive

Let us consider the steps involved in using DICOM to send a CT examination with multiple images from the scanner to the PACS controller. Each individual image is transmitted from the CT scanner to the PACS controller utilizing DICOM's C-STORE service. In this transmission procedure, the scanner takes on the role of a client as the C-STORE service class user (SCU) and the PACS controller has the role of a server as the C-STORE service class provider (SCP). The following steps illustrate the transmission of a CT examination with multiple images from the scanner to the PACS controller (Fig. 7.5).

0. The CT scanner and the PACS controller first establish the connection through DICOM communication "association request and response" commands.

1. The invoking scanner (SCU) issues a C-STORE service request to the PACS controller (SCP).
2. The PACS controller receives the C-STORE request and issues a C-STORE response to the invoking scanner.
3. The CT scanner sends the first data packet of the first image to the PACS controller.
4. The PACS controller performs the requested C-STORE service to store the packet.
5. Upon completion of the service, the PACS controller issues a confirmation to the scanner.
6. After receiving confirmation from the PACS controller that the storing of the packet has been completed, the scanner sends the next packet to the PACS controller.
7. Processes 4 to 6 repeat until all packets of the first image have been transmitted.
8. The scanner issues a second C-STORE service request to the PACS controller for transmission of the second image. Steps 1 to 7 repeat until all images from the study have been transmitted.
9. The scanner and the PACS controller issue the DICOM communication command "dropping association request and response" to disconnect.

7.6.4.2 Query and Retrieve

Using C-STORE to invoke the send and receive service class is relatively simple compared with the query/retrieve service class. Let us consider a more complicated example, in which the workstation queries the PACS controller to retrieve a historical CT examination to compare with a current study available at the workstation. Note that this composite service class involves three DIMSEs: C-FIND, C-MOVE (Table 7.7), and C-STORE, described, in Section 7.6.4.1. In performing the Query/Retrieve SOP service, there is one user and one provider in each of the workstations and the PACS controller as follows:

	Workstation	PACS Controller
Query/Retrieve	User	Provider
C-STORE	Provider	User

Thus, the workstation takes on the roles of Query/Retrieve (Q/R) SCU and C-STORE SCP, whereas the PACS controller has the roles of Q/R SCP and C-STORE SCU. Refer to Figure 7.6. After the association between the workstation and the PACS controller has been established, the following steps are accomplished.

1. The workstation's Q/R application entity (AE) issues a C-FIND service request to the PACS controller.

196 PICTURE ARCHIVING, COMMUNICATION SYSTEM COMPONENTS

```
           CLIENT                                              SERVER
         CT SCANNER                                       PACS CONTROLLER
        (C-STORE SCU)                                       (C-STORE SCP)

   Requests for         (0)      Association Request
establishing association   ───────────────────────────►  (0) Association granted
                           ◄───────────────────────────
                                 Association Response

                                    C-STORE Request
       Requests for      (1)   ───────────────────────►  (2) C-STORE
      C-STORE service         ◄───────────────────────   (2) service granted
                                   C-STORE Response

                         (3)      First Data Packet       (4)
      Sends image data   (6)   ───────────────────────►      Receives image data
                              ◄───────────────────────   (5)
                                     Confirmation
         (1) - (7)
                                          ●
                                          ● (7)
                                          ●

                                   Last Data Packet
      Sends image data         ───────────────────────►  (7) Receives image data
                              ◄───────────────────────
                                     Confirmation
          (8)

       Requests for       (9)   Dropping Association Request
    dropping association      ───────────────────────►    (9) Drops association
                              ◄───────────────────────
                                Dropping Association Response
```

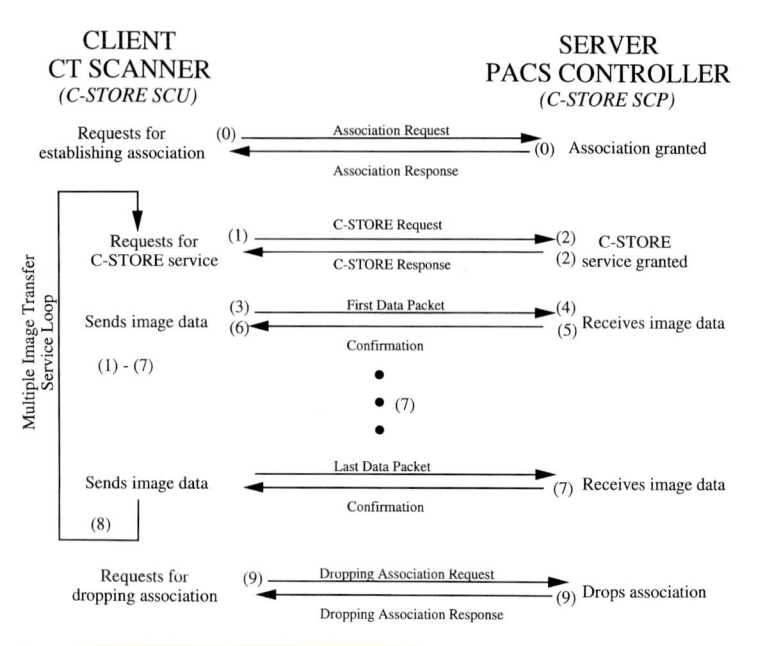

Figure 7.5 DICOM send and receive operations. Numerals designate steps described in text.

2. The PACS controller's Q/R AE receives the C-FIND request from the querying workstation (2a), performs the C-FIND service (2b) to look for studies, series, and images from the PACS database, and issues a C-FIND response to the workstation (2c).
3. The workstation's Q/R AE receives the C-FIND response from the PACS controller. The response is a table with all the requests.
4. The workstation selects interesting images from the table (4a) and issues a C-MOVE service request for each individual selected image to the PACS controller (4b).
5. The PACS controller's Q/R AE receives the C-MOVE request from the workstation (5a) and issues an indication to the PACS controller's C-STORE SCU (5b).
6. The PACS controller's C-STORE SCU retrieves the requested images from the archive device.
7. The PACS controller's C-STORE SCU issues a C-STORE request to the workstation's C-STORE SCP.
8. The workstation receives the C-STORE request and issues a C-STORE response to the PACS controller. From this point on the C-STORE SOP service is identical to the example given in Figure 7.5.
9. When the workstation has retrieved the last image, it issues a "dropping association request" and terminates the association.

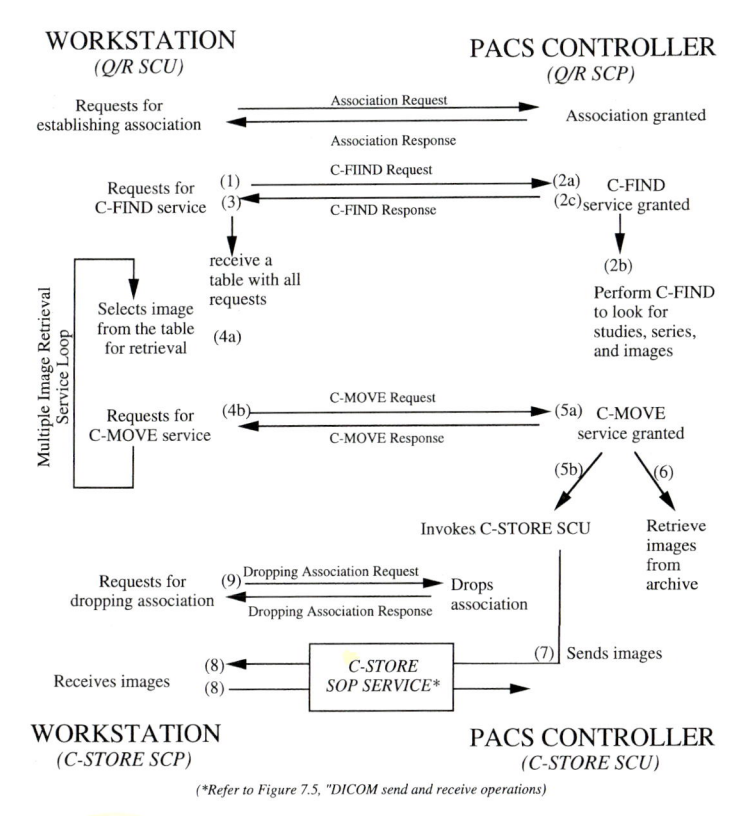

Figure 7.6 DICOM query/retrieve operation. Numerals designate steps described in text.

7.7 OTHER STANDARDS

The four industrial standards used commonly in PACS are described in Sections 7.7.1 to 7.7.4

7.7.1 UNIX Operating System

The first UNIX operating system (System V) was developed by AT&T and released in 1983. Other versions of UNIX from different computer vendors include BSD (Berkeley Software Distribution by the University of California at Berkeley), Solaris (Sun Microsystems), HP-UX (Hewlett-Packard), Xenix (Microsoft), Ultrix (Digital Equipment Corporation), AIX (International Business Machines), and A/UX (Apple Computers).

Despite its many varieties, the UNIX operating system provides an open system architecture for computer systems to facilitate the integration of complex software systems within individual systems and between different computer systems. UNIX offers great capability and high flexibility in networking, interprocess communication, multitasking, and security, which are essential to medical imaging applications. UNIX is mostly used in the server, PACS controller, gateway, and high end workstations.

7.7.2 Windows NT Operating System

The Microsoft Windows New Technology (Windows NT) operating system runs on desktop personal computers (PCs) and is a derivative of the University of California at Berkeley's BSD UNIX. Windows NT, like UNIX, supports TCP/IP communications and multitasking, and therefore provides a low cost software development platform for medical imaging applications in the PC environment. Windows NT is mostly used in workstations and single task environments.

7.7.3 C and C++ Programming Languages

The C programming language was introduced by Brian Kernighan and Dennis Ritchie in 1970. The simple, flexible language soon became one of the most popular programming languages in computing. C++, built on top of the C programming language, was created by Bjarne Stroustrup in 1980. C++ is an object-oriented language, which allows programmers to organize their software and process the information more effectively than is possible with most other programming languages.

7.7.4 Structured Query Language

Structured query language (SQL) is an industry standard data manipulation language adopted by most database management systems. SQL allows a user or an application to select, insert, update, and delete data from the databases.

CHAPTER 8

Image Acquisition Gateway

8.1 BACKGROUND

The image acquisition gateway computer, with a set of software programs, serves the purpose of acquiring images from different imaging modalities and PACS modules for the PACS controller (server) to archive and the workstation to display. The gateway can be a stand-alone computer, or it may share a computer with other PACS components. In this chapter, the terms *acquisition gateway computer, gateway computer,* and *acquisition gateway* have the same meaning. The functions of a good acquisition gateway are as follows:

1. Preserve the integrity of image data transmitted from the imaging device
2. Totally or highly automatic
3. Deliver images in a timely manner to the archive and workstations
4. Transparent to the users

Establishing a reliable acquisition gateway in the PACS is the most difficult task compared with other components for the following reasons. First, an acquisition gateway must interface with many imaging modalities and PACS modules made by other imaging manufacturers. Such interfacing is difficult because these modalities and modules have their own image formats and communication protocols. Even when some devices follow the DICOM standard, the PACS integrator may have to negotiate several DICOM conformance statements (see Section 7.6.3) for a successful interface. Second, performing examinations with an imaging device requires human input (entering patient's name, identification, and accession number, transmitting images, etc.). During this process, the occurrence of human error is unavoidable. However, a very minor error from input may have a severe impact on the data integrity of the PACS data. We will discuss this issue in later sections and in Chapter 16 on PACS pitfalls and bottlenecks. Third, ideally the acquisition gateway should be 100% automatic, for efficiency and to minimize system errors. To achieve a totally automatic component with much human interaction and equipment from varied manufacturers is very challenging. The degree of difficulty and the cost necessary to achieve are widely debated in the PACS design community.

Automated image acquisition from imaging devices to the PACS controller plays an important role in a PACS infrastructure. The word "automatic" is important because the need to rely on labor-intensive manual acquisition methods would defeat the purpose of the PACS. However, there is no single means of enabling automated data acquisition from existing digital medical imaging systems. Based on existing manufacturers' pre-DICOM imaging devices, we categorize the interface methods into five architectural models: sequential chain, direct interface, memory access, shared disk, and interconnected network. We discuss the methodology, cost, rate of data transfer, and ease of implementation of each model in Section 8.2. An important measure of the success of an automatic acquisition system is its effectiveness in ensuring the integrity and availability of patient images in a PACS. For this reason, automated fault tolerance design in the image acquisition gateway is required. We discuss in Section 8.3 common scenarios that cause an acquisition to fail and techniques to automatically restart the operations under these circumstances. These techniques include recovery from errors and traps of the acquisition process, image acquisition gateway computer downtime, and shutdown of the medical imaging system. Section 8.4 explores the interface method of the DICOM conformance imaging device based on the DICOM query/retrieve service. An automatic image recovery scheme forDICOM conformance imaging devices is presented in Section 8.5, along with an experiment to measure its performance. Very often, the acquisition gateway has to accept images from other PACS modules, Section 8.6 is devoted to this topic.

An imaging acquisition gateway also performs certain image preprocessing functions. Section 8.7 considers some image preprocessing functions commonly used in PACS. When the acquisition gateway has to deal with DICOM formatting, communication, and many image preprocessing functions, multiple-level processing with a queuing mechanism is necessary. In Scction 8.8 we discuss the concept of multilevel adaptive processing control, which ensures the reliability of the acquisition gateway as well as image integrity.

8.2 AUTOMATED IMAGE ACQUISITION INTERFACE METHODS FOR PRE-DICOM DEVICES

Generally speaking, the PACS image acquisition system consists of three major components: a medical imaging system, a computer system that acquires images from the imaging system (i.e., an acquisition computer), and an interface mechanism (hardware and software) between the imaging system and acquisition computer, as shown in Figure 8.1. Although manufacturers have gradually conformed to the DICOM standard during the past two years, there are still many imaging devices in the field that do not use DICOM. For this reason, it is necessary to consider how to connect a non-DICOM device to the image acquisition gateway. Within the interface mechanism, the non-DICOM-conforming devices can be further categorized into five models: sequential chain, direct interface, memory access, shared disk, and interconnected network. Sections 8.2.1 to 8.2.5 illustrate the interface mechanism of each model by using manufacturers' imaging systems as examples. Each model's costs, data transfer rate, and ease of implementation are discussed.

AUTOMATED IMAGE ACQUISITION INTERFACE METHODS FOR PRE-DICOM DEVICES 201

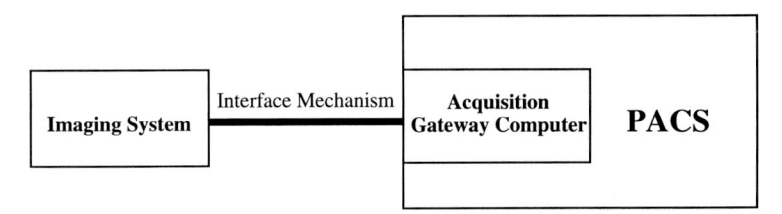

Figure 8.1 Schematic showing the PACS image acquisition, with an interface mechanism connecting the imaging device to the acquisition gateway computer.

8.2.1 Sequential Chain Model

In the sequential chain model, the PACS acquisition computer links a medical imaging system through a chain of interface devices provided by a manufacturer. An example of the sequential chain model is the IDNET-1 (Integrated Diagnostics Network, version 1.0) solution provided in the late 1980s by General Electric Medical Systems (GEMS) for acquiring CT images from the GE-9800 CT scanners. Figure 8.2 shows the schematic diagram of IDNET-1 in the total PACS context. The parallel peripheral interface (PPI) board, residing in the scanner system, functions as a virtual magnetic disk driver that reads the data from the disk of the scanner to one of the network interface equipment (NIE) units, which is separate from the scanner system. At the NIE-1 node (see Fig. 8.2), the image data and associated text data are encoded into the ACR-NEMA format and transmitted to the NIE-2 by means of a proprietary GE data transfer protocol and a dedicated, Ethernet-based GEMS network.

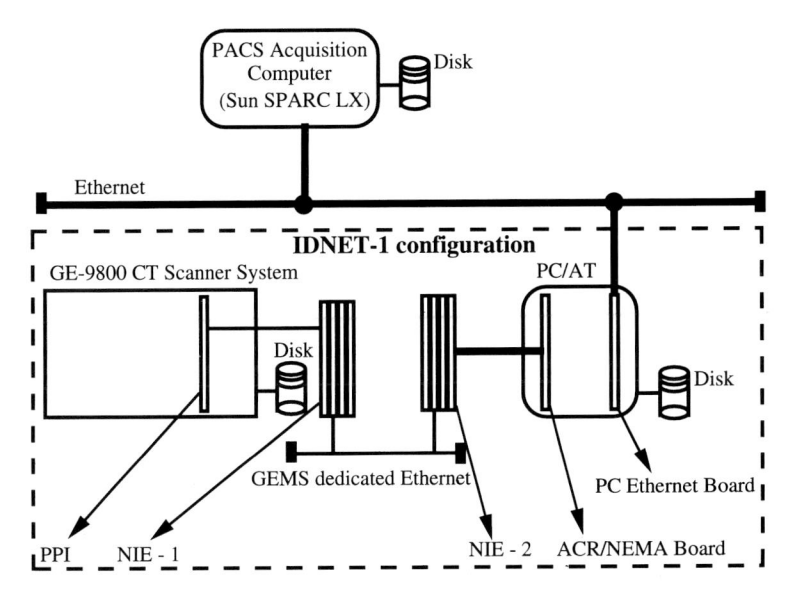

Figure 8.2 Example of the sequential chain model: image data are propagated from the scanner through the PPI, the NIE-1, the GEMS dedicated Ethernet, the NIE-2, the PC/AT, and the PACS acquisition computer.

The second node in the GEMS network, NIE-2, and has a standard ACR-NEMA output (50-pin connector) to an ACR-NEMA interface board, which resides in a PC/AT computer. The PC/AT transmits the image data to the acquisition computer through the Ethernet with a PC Ethernet board.

Since this configuration requires several interface units, the cost of the interface is high (approximately $40,000) and the connectivity is complicated. Implementation of this configuration requires several man-months. Furthermore, it is difficult to measure the data elapse time in each interface unit, which in turn makes it hard to determine the data transfer performance precisely. Field data demonstrate that the data transfer rate between the PC/AT and the PACS acquisition computer is the most time-consuming component; between a PC/AT and a Sun minicomputer 3/260 (Sun Microsystems, Mountain View, CA), for example, this rate is about 50 Kbyte/s. The sequential chain model has the disadvantages of being costly and complex, with a low data transfer rate. Until GEMS introduced the IDNET-2, however, it was the only means available for the automatic acquisition of images from the GE-9800 CT scanners to the PACS. The interface configuration of IDNET-2 is simpler than that of IDNET-1. We categorize the IDNET-2 as the shared disk model.

8.2.2 Direct Interface Model

The direct interface model is composed of an acquisition computer connected to a medical imaging system through a set of standard electronic interface boards. An example of this model is the small-computer systems interface (SCSI) of the Array Corporation (formerly Abe–Sekkei Inc., Tokyo, Japan) film laser digitizer (see Section 3.2.2). Figure 8.3 shows the configuration of this model, the DR11-W interface, in which the image data from the scanner are buffered in the DR11-W interface board and transmitted to the PACS acquisition computer. The buffer size in this application is 32 Kbyte. Whenever the buffer is full, the data are archived to the disk of the PACS acquisition computer through the DR11-W host adapter. Other examples of this model are the SCSI data acquisition system manager (DASM) of the Fuji computed radiography (CR) system (Fuji Medical Systems, U.S.A. Inc., Stamford, CT, see Section 4.1) and the SCSI interface of the Lumiscan digitizer (Lumisys, Inc., Sunnyvale, CA).

The advantages of this model are several: the interface units are commercial products, the connectivity is simple, the cost is affordable, and data throughput is fast. Integration takes approximately 2 man-weeks. The price of this type of interface device ranges from $2000 to $8000. The transfer rate between the Array film laser scanner and the SCSI disk of a Sun SPARC LX computer shown in Figure 8.3 is greater than 1.2 Mbyte/s.

8.2.3 Memory Access Model

In the memory access model, a PACS acquisition computer connects to a medical imaging system through a dual-port RAM. The interface product called MegaLink, which transmits images from the Imatron Cine CT scanner (Imatron Company, Oyster Point, CA, see Section 5.2.3) to the PACS acquisition computer, belongs to this

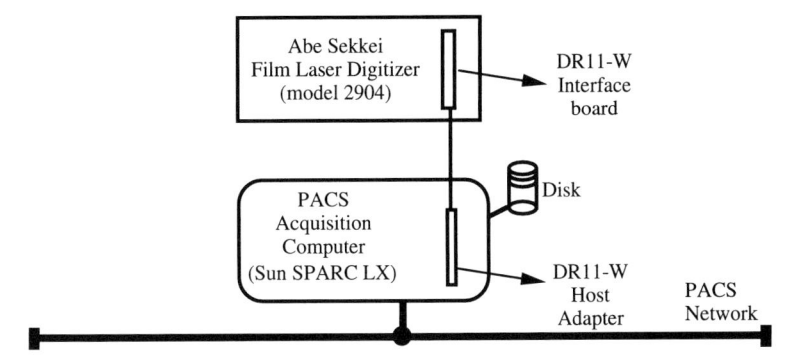

Figure 8.3 The direct interface model showing the DR11-W interface between the Abe–Sekkei film laser digitizer and the PACS acquisition computer.

category. In Figure 8.4, two MegaLink bus adapter boards are linked by a pair of 25-foot ribbon cables (one for signal acknowledgment and one for data transfer). The adapter board installed in the Fast Reconstruction System (FRS) of the Imatron CT scanner contains 1 Mbyte of dual-ported RAM. The memory is accessible by both the FRS and the PACS acquisition computer. The FRS stores the header and reconstructed image data in this RAM, which can be accessed by the PACS acquisition computer via the MegaLink bus adapter board using the direct memory access mechanism. Simple semaphore-based interlock protocol software is used to synchronize the data transfer between the two computer systems.

The direct memory access model provides fast data throughput because the data transfer is very similar to the scenario of writing data from the CPU memory of a computer to its own disk. Field measurement for the configuration shown in Figure 8.4 is greater than 1 Mbyte/s. Since the interface devices consist of RAM memory, the cost

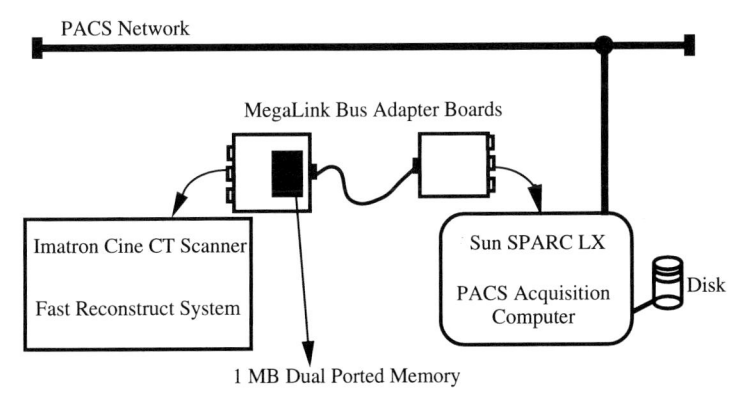

Figure 8.4 The memory access mode demonstrates the MegaLink connecting the Imatron Cine CT scanner and the acquisition computer. The acquisition computer can access the image data through the dual-ported memory.

is high (approximately $15,000). Implementation of the automatic image acquisition from the Imatron CT scanner takes about 6 man-weeks.

8.2.4 Shared Disk Model

The shared disk model makes a disk accessible by both the PACS acquisition computer and a medical imaging system. The Seimens Medical Systems, (Iselin, NJ) MR scanners (both Impact and Vision models) are examples. The Siemens MR scanner can be interfaced by using the network file system (NFS) protocol. The local disk of the imaging system can be remotely mounted by the acquisition computer through a network accessible by both computers, as shown in Figure 8.5. Thus, whenever images are available in the local disk of the imaging system, they are also available in the acquisition computer.

Of all interface architectural models, the shared disk model has the best image data availability in the sense that no image data propagation is required. In addition, the NFS-based shared disk model is a very low cost and easily implemented configuration because the NFS feature is commonly available in most of computer systems today. It takes about one man-week to complete the physical connections. The NFS-based shared disk model has a drawback, though. Any interaction between the imaging system and the acquisition computer during data transfer requires the network and disk input/output operations at the imaging computer system. Frequent I/O operations of peripheral devices, however, may cause noticeable performance slowdown of the imaging system. Any such interruption to the operation of the imaging system is undesirable, especially when the system is in heavy use.

8.2.5 Interconnected Network Model

The interconnected network model consists of a PACS acquisition computer and the medical imaging system host computer, which are connected in a network and com-

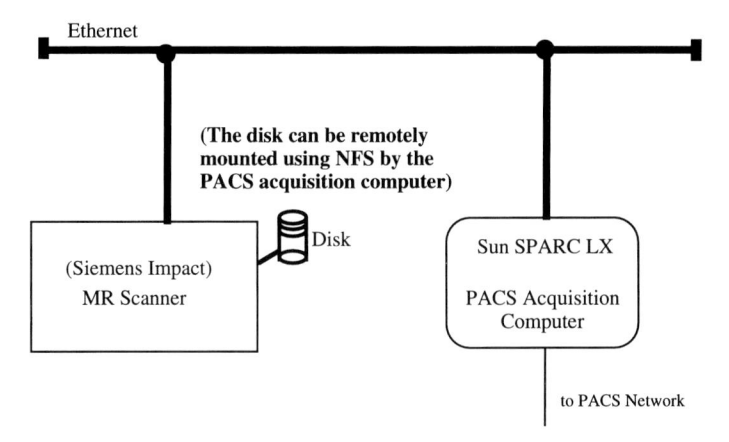

Figure 8.5 Example of the shared disk model. The Sun computer using the network file system (NFS) protocol remotely mounts the disk, which is physically connected to the MR scanner. As a result, the acquisition computer can access the image data in the remote disk.

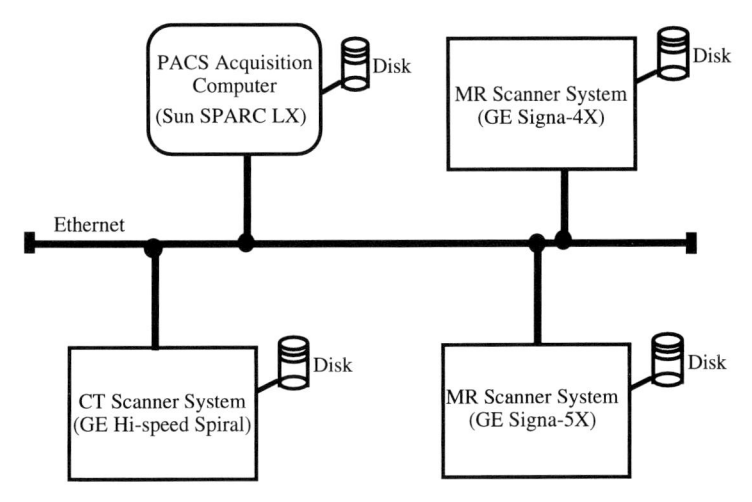

Figure 8.6 The interconnected network model. The acquisition computer acquires images from the CT and MR scanners through a standard network (Ethernet) and standard communication protocols (TCP/IP) or DICOM upper layer protocols TCP/IP.

municate through standard communication protocols. GEMS's newer CT and MR scanners, such as the Hi-speed Spiral CT and Signa 5x MR scanners (see Sections 5.2.2 and 5.6.1) are designed based on this model. Figure 8.6 shows the configuration of a GE imaging medical system's interconnected network. The network follows the ISO's Open System Interconnection standard layers (see Section 9.1.2). The physical and data link layers are Ethernet, the network layer is Internet protocol (IP), and the transport layer is transmission control protocol (TCP). For the application layer, the GEMS proprietary communication programs are based on TCP/IP and a file transfer protocol (FTP). Other application layer software is the Central Test Node (CTN) software developed by Electronic Radiology Laboratory, Mallinckrodt Institute of Radiology (St. Louis, MO) based on the DICOM 3.0 standard.

Since the interconnected network model follows the industrial standards, its advantages include affordable cost, portable components, and easy implementation. The hardest part of configuring this model is laying down the network infrastructure. For an existing networking environment, this interface model can be configured with minimal effort ($<$ 1 man-week). The image data transmission performance (disk-to-disk) of this interface model ranges from 100 to 400 Kbyte/s. The range is so wide because its choice depends on type of computer systems used (both the imaging system and acquisition computer), type of system disks, utilization of the network, and workload of the computer systems.

Table 8.1 summarizes the five interface models according to three parameters: costs, rate of data transfer, and time required for implementation. For each model, an example imaging system is given, as well as the associated interface mechanism.

PACS is an essential ingredient for the realization of digital radiology in the hospital environment. One crucial task is to integrate image scanners and modalities of various types into the open system PACS network. Most existing scanners, however,

TABLE 8.1 Summary of the Five Pre-DICOM Interface Models

Parameters	Sequential Chain	Direct Interface	Direct Interface Access	Shared Disk	Interconnected Network
Cost	<$40,000	<$8,000	<$15,000	$0	$0
Rate of data transfer	50 KByte/s	>1 MByte/s	>1 MByte/s	N/A	100–400 KByte/s
Time required for implementation, man-weeks	>24	2	6	11	12
Example					
Imaging system	GE CT-9800	Microscope Abe-Sekkei Film Digitizer	Imatron CT	Siemens MR Impact	GE MR Signa 5x
Interface	IDNET-1	SCSI or DR11-W	MegaLink	NFS	Ethernet and CTN

were developed based on "closed" architectural design and do not communicate with one another.

Open systems interoperability has been acknowledged to be an important feature in a digital medical imaging system. It can be attained only by following the standards. For this reason, the direct interface model and the interconnected network model are more favorable for pre-DICOM imaging devices.

8.3 FAULT TOLERANCE METHODS FOR AUTOMATED IMAGE ACQUISITION

Many factors can cause an automated image acquisition system to fail. For this reason a mechanism must be designed to detect and recover from downtime during automated acquisition. If the period of downtime is too long, the limited amount of disk space may cause the images in the imaging system to be purged before they can be acquired by the acquisition computer. In the absence of a backup system to store the data, such images may be lost forever. To ensure the integrity and availability of patient images in a PACS system, automatic recovery from faults is a crucial component in the image acquisition design. In this section, we describe the major software programs involved in the acquisition computers, the common scenarios causing the acquisition process to fail, and methods for automatically recovering the operation.

8.3.1 Image Acquisition Software

In general, the image acquisition task consists of four programs (Fig. 8.7). The acquiring program receives images from the imaging system to the acquisition gateway

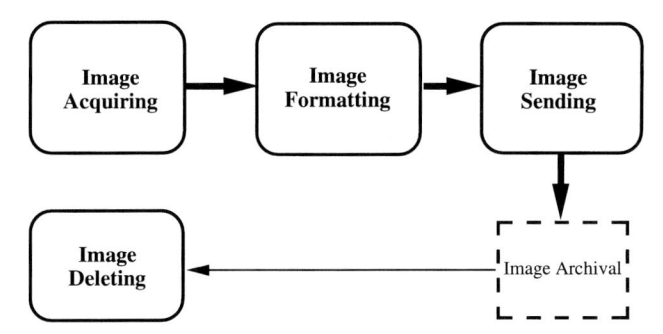

Figure 8.7 Four major software programs in the PACS acquisition computer, which complete the chain in an image acquisition task.

computer. The formatting program organizes the acquired images and the associated text information based on a standard format (e.g., DICOM). The sending program transfers the formatted image to another component of the PACS (see Fig. 8.1). This component is usually an image archiving system, but depending on the PACS architectural design, it may be an image display system as well. After the formatted image has been properly archived in the PACS controller, the deleting program erases the acquired images from the gateway computer to free up the storage space. These four programs complete the chain of image acquisition data flow. If the chain is broken, the image acquisition task will fail to function. For simplicity, we use the term "acquisition process" to represent these four programs in the following discussions.

8.3.2 Acquisition Process Recovery from Errors

The acquisition process can be ended prematurely if certain fatal error conditions are encountered. Examples include I/O errors of peripheral devices and not enough CPU memory in the acquisition gateway computer. A monitoring process is required to recover the acquisition task from faults of this type. The monitoring process should possess three functions: activation at periodic alert times, examination of the status of designated processes, and restart of the designated processes if necessary. If, for example, the monitoring process wakes up at a given time and detects that the acquisition process has been terminated, it must restart acquisition automatically. Usually, if the computer system has a clock daemon utility available, the periodical wake-up feature of the monitoring process can be replaced by the clock daemon. In this way, the user can be sure that the monitoring program will be executed periodically as long as the acquisition computer is in operation.

8.3.3 Acquisition Process Recovery from Traps

Occasionally, the acquisition process is terminated immediately after it has been launched by the monitoring process. If this situation occurs repeatedly (i.e., if the acquisition process is trapped), human intervention will be necessary. In the most com-

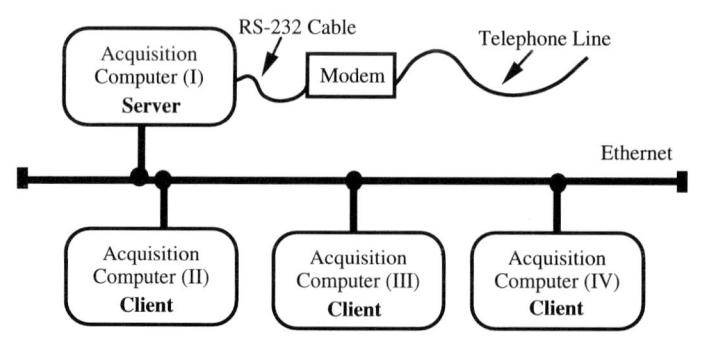

Figure 8.8 The configuration of the central dial-up and paging scheme for recovery from traps during acquisition failure. The modem is configured with the server that connects the clients with the PACS network. The clients send messages to the server through the PACS network whenever the image acquisition is trapped. The server then sends the messages to service personnel through the modem via a pager.

mon example of this problem, no space is left on the acquisition computer's disk. This is a fatal error and must be addressed at once. Thus there is a need for a centralized dial-up and paging scheme to alert service personnel automatically. A typical hardware configuration of the central dial-up scheme is shown in Figure 8.8; software implementation is required, as well.

The hardware involves a computer system to be configured with a modem device that is connected to a telephone line. This central dial-up computer can be in any component in the PACS, provided it is networked with the acquisition computers and others. From the task-oriented point of view, the central dial-up computer is the server and the acquisition computers are the clients.

The software required in the server and clients mainly includes four modules: (1) sending of the service request, (2) receiving of the service request, (3) automatically dialing the pager number of the designated troubleshooter, and (4) checking the availability of the computer system network. Consider our earlier example: no disk space in the acquisition computer is available, the acquisition process is trapped, and human intervention has become necessary. In this situation, the message "no disk space" is sent from the client to the server through a network. The message contains the client computer name, the process name, and the service engineer's pager number. The computer name and the process name can be represented by numbers. Each pair of numbers is then coded to become a callback number. In this way, the dial-up software module delivers the message to the engineer on call based on the pager number and the coded callback number. Besides the function of receiving request from the clients, the software checks the availability of the clients via the network. This feature is helpful because when a computer goes down, it is not available to other computers through the network.

8.3.4 Acquisition Computer Recovery from Downtime Occurrence

The acquisition process cannot proceed if the acquisition computer goes down. There are two possibilities: either the computer can reboot itself or it cannot. If the computer can reboot itself, then it can initiate an operating system kernel program, check the configured peripheral devices, and execute necessary system processes during the computer rebooting. Since the system processes can be started up in the rebooting procedures, the image acquisition programs can be launched as well. If the computer cannot reboot itself—for example, because of a power outage—then the dial-up and paging scheme can be used to request operator service.

8.3.5 Handling Imaging System Shutdown

When the technician who manages the imaging system is obliged to observe its operational procedure and maintenance schedule irrespective of the ongoing acquisition process, the imaging system may shut down while image data are being transferred from the imaging system to the acquisition computer. An acquisition process that required special care whenever the technician turned the imaging system on or off would be unacceptable. Thus, the acquisition process must be transparent to the technician. To meet this requirement, the software in the image acquisition computer is designed to handle such an abrupt shutdown event. That is, code is written to impart to the system the ability to manage such error events as a broken network connection, a dropped network connection, or a connection time-out. If one of these events is detected, the acquisition process resets the uncompleted task to initial status, thus allowing the task to be processed from the beginning in the next execution. This scheme may repeatedly handle the same uncompleted task if the imaging system remains in down status. However, this mechanism ensures that the acquisition process will continue in operation whenever the imaging system is turned back on.

The integrity and availability of patient images in a PACS system very much depend on the uptime of the image acquisition process. To optimize the system uptime probability during image acquisition, automatic recovery schemes from faults must be implemented in the image acquisition software design. This section has presented some common scenarios that cause the acquisition task to fail and the methods used to automatically recover the operation.

8.4 INTERFACE USING DICOM

8.4.1 Introduction

DICOM conformance (compliance) among manufacturers is a major factor contributing to the interoperability of different medical imaging systems in a hospital environment. We described the DICOM standard in Chapter 7 noting that it defines the basis of the interface mechanism allowing different manufacturers' digital imaging systems to communicate images. With the standardized interface mechanism, the task of acquiring images from the DICOM compliance imaging systems is simpler than from those with a "closed" architectural design described in Section 8.2.

When the DICOM standard is used to transmit images, one image is transmitted at a time; the order of transmission does not necessarily follow the order of scan, series, nor study. The image device's job queue priority, which dictates what job needs to be processed next, is always in favor of scanning and image reconstruction. For this reason, if an image waiting in the queue to be transmitted next is bumped, it will lose its priority and may spend a long period of time in the lower priority waiting queue, without being discovered. The result is a temporary loss of images in a series and in a study. If such a failure to transmit is not discovered early enough, the images may be lost permanently as a result of various system conditions; (e.g., a system reboot, disk maintenance, premature closing of the patient image file at the acquisition gateway) Neither temporary nor permanent loss of images is acceptable in PACS operation. In Section 8.3 we emphasized that the design of the PACS image acquisition task must consider automatic recovery from failures. A failure may be a hardware malfunction, a software error, a temporary loss of images, or a manual interruption during the PACS acquisition process. In the case of acquiring images from a DICOM-compliant imaging device, we also must consider a similar error recovery mechanism, in particular, to recover images that are temporarily lost.

8.4.2 Concept of DICOM-Based PACS Image Acquisition

8.4.2.1 Database Management in the Acquisition Gateway Computer

The most complicated data structure in imaging acquisition is from MR in which the hierarchical data structure is patient study, image series, and images, in that order. Let us use Figure 8.9 to demonstrate the concept of DICOM-based image acquisition of MR images. The DICOM MR imaging device on the left served as the C-STORE client, and the image acquisition gateway on the right functioned as the C-STORE server. They are connected by an Ethernet running the DICOM TCP/IP protocols. Regardless of whether a "push" from the scanner or a "pull" operation from the gateway is used (see Section 7.6.4), one image is transmitted at a time, and the order of transmission depends on the database architecture of the scanner. After these images have been received, the gateway computer must know how to accumulate them accordingly, to form series and studies without compromising the integrity of the image data.

In the gateway acquisition computer, a database management system serving three functions is used for the following purposes. First, it supports the transaction of each individual image received by the acquisition computer. Second, it monitors the sta-

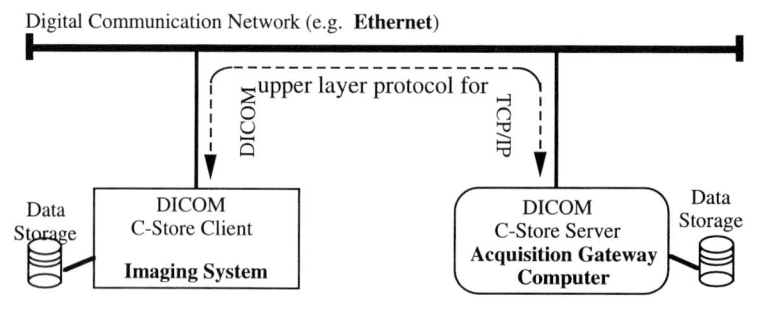

Figure 8.9 Schematic showing the DICOM C-STORE server and client programs developed according to the DICOM upper layer protocol for TCP/IP.

tus of the patient studies and their associated series during the transmission. Third, it provides the basis for the automatic image recovery scheme to detect unsuccessfully transferred images. Three database tables are used: study, series, and image. Each table contains a group of records, and each record contains a set of useful data elements. For the study and series database tables, the study name and the series name are the primary keys for searching. In addition, the following major data elements are also recorded: (1) patient name and hospital identification number, (2) dates and times when the study and series were created in the imaging device and acquired in the gateway, (3) number of acquired images per series, (4) acquisition status, and (5) the DICOM unique identification (UID) value for the study and series.

8.4.2.2 Determination of the End of an Image Series

If DICOM transmits images one by one, but not necessarily in order, from the scanner to the gateway, how does the gateway computer know when a study is completed and when it should close the study file for archive or display? The images of a series or study can be grouped together by the formatting process only when the end of the series or study has been determined by the image receiving process. To algorithmically determine the end of a series in a manner both accurate and efficient is not trivial. We present two methods used for determining the end of series and discuss the advantages and drawbacks of each as follows.

Presence of the Next Series   The first method for detecting the end of a series is based on the presence of the next series. This method assumes that the total number of images for the current series will be transferred to the acquisition gateway computer before the next series begins. In this case, the presence of the first image slice of the next series indicates the termination of the preceding series. The success of this method depends on the following two premises: the imaging device transfers the images to the acquisition computer in order, and no images are lost during the transfer. Note that the first assumption depends on the specific implementation of the image transfer by the imaging system. If the imaging system transmits the image slices in sequence (e.g., General Electric Medical Systems MR Signa 5.4), this method can faithfully group the images of a series intact. On the other hand, if the imaging system transfers the image slices in a random fashion (e.g., Siemens MR Vision), this method may identify the end of a series incorrectly. Even though one could verify the second assumption by checking the order of the image, whether the last image has been transferred remains unknown to the gateway computer. Another drawback of this method relates to the determination of the last series of a particular study that is based on the presence of the first image of the next study. The time delay for this determination could be lengthy because the next study may not begin for hours.

Constant Number of Images in a Time Interval   The second method for determining the end of a series is based on a time interval criterion, since it is assumed that an image series should be completed within a certain period of time. With this method, the end of a series is determined when the acquisition time of the first image plus a designated time interval has elapsed. This method is obviously straightforward and simple, but a static time interval criterion is not practical in a clinical environment. Thus, an alternative recourse uses the concept of the constant number of images in a time interval.

This method requires recording the number of acquired images for a given series at two different times, say time t_1 and time $t_2 = t_1 + \Delta t$, for some predetermined constant Δt. By comparing the number of images acquired at time t_1 versus the number of images acquired at time t_2, a premise can be constructed for determining whether the series is complete. If, for example, the number of images is a constant, we conclude that the series is complete; otherwise, the series is not yet complete. This process (time interval with image verification) is iterated until a constant number of images has been reached.

Next, let us consider how to select Δt. Should it be a static number, or dynamic? A short Δt may result in missing images, whereas a long Δt may result in a lengthy and inefficient image acquisition. Usually, the first Δt chosen for this method is empirical, depending on the imaging protocols used by the imaging system. For example, if the imaging protocols frequently used in a scanner generate many images per series, then the Δt should be long, otherwise, a shorter Δt is preferred. However, it is possible that for a shorter Δt this method may conclude a series prematurely. This is because in some rare cases the technologist or clinician may interrupt the scanning process in the middle of a series to conduct a patient position alignment or to inject a contrast agent. If the time required for such procedures is longer than the Δt, then the images scanned after the interruption will not be grouped into the current series. For a careless PACS design, this could result in a severe problem—missing images.

Should Δt be dynamic during the iteration? One thought is that the number of images transferred from the imaging device to the gateway computer decreases while the iteration cycle increases. Therefore, it seems reasonable to suggest that Δt may be reduced proportionally to the number iterations. On the other hand, the number of images transferred to the acquisition gateway computer may vary with time depending on the design of the imaging device. For example, an imaging device may be designed to transfer images according to the imaging system workload and priority schedule. If the image transfer process has a low priority, then the number of images transferred during a period when the system workload is heavy will be less than when it is light. In this case, Δt is a variable.

Combination of Both Methods (COMBO) Based on our experience, a **com**bination of **bo**th methods seems to be the best. The COMBO can be implemented in three stages: (1) identify and count the acquired images for a particular series, (2) record the time stamp whenever the number of acquired images has changed, and (3) update the acquisition status of the series. The acquired images can be tracked as follows, by means of a transaction table designed in association with the series database table discussed above. We start with the time interval method.

Whenever an image is acquired from the imaging device, a record of the image is created in the transaction table, identified by the modality type, the imaging system ID, the study number, the series number, and the image number. A tracking system can be developed based on these records. Three major events during the current iteration are recorded in the transaction table: (1) the number of acquired images, (2) the t_2 value, and (3) the acquisition status (declaring the series as standby, ongoing, completed, or image missing). Here, the information regarding the number of acquired images and acquisition status is useful for the maintenance of the image receiving process. If the series is ongoing, the comparison time is updated for the verification of the number of images during the next iteration.

When the interval method detects the end of a series, this result can be further verified by the presence of the next series method. If the next series exists in the series database table or the next study exists in the study table, the image series is determined to be complete. Otherwise, one more iteration is given and the series remains in standby status. In this case, the series will be held to be complete after the next iteration, regardless of the existence in the queue of another series or study. In general, Δt can be set at 10 minutes. In this way, the completeness of an image series is verified by both methods and the potential lengthy time delay problem of the first method is minimized.

8.5 AUTOMATIC IMAGE RECOVERY SCHEME FOR DICOM CONFORMANCE DEVICE

8.5.1 Missing Images

Images being transmitted from the imaging device may be missing at the acquisition gateway computer. As an example, consider an MR scanner using the DICOM C-STORE client transferring images by means of one of the following three modes: autotransfer, autoqueue, or manual transfer. Only one transfer mode can be in operation at a time. The autotransfer mode transmits an image whenever one is available; the autoqueue mode transfers images only when the entire study has been completed; and the manual transfer mode allows the transfer of multiple images, series, or studies. Under normal operation, the autotransfer mode is routinely used; and the manual transfer mode is used only when a retransmission is required. Once the DICOM communication between the scanner and the gateway computer has been established, if the technologist changes the transfer mode for certain clinical reasons during the transmission, some images will be lost temporarily. In the next section, we discuss an automatic recovery method for these images.

8.5.2 Automatic Image Recovery Scheme

8.5.2.1 Basis for the Image Recovery Scheme

The automatic image recovery scheme includes two tasks: identifying the missing studies, series, or images, and recovering them accordingly. These two tasks can be accomplished by using the DICOM Query/Retrieve service class in conjunction with the acquisition gateway database described in Section 8.4.2.1. The operation mechanism of the Query/Retrieve service involves three other DICOM service classes: C-FIND, C-MOVE, and C-STORE (see Section 7.6.4.2). The task of identifying missing studies is performed through C-FIND by matching one of the image grouping hierarchies, such as study level or series level, between the gateway database and the scanner database. The recovering task follows the missing study detection and is carried out by the C-MOVE and C-STORE service classes. The Query/Retrieve operation is performed via a server process at the MR scanner, and a client process at the acquisition gateway computer, respectively.

8.5.2.2 Design of the Image Recovery Scheme

Figure 8.10 shows the flow diagram of the automatic image recovery scheme. First, consider the recovery of missing studies. In the beginning, the Query/Retrieve client

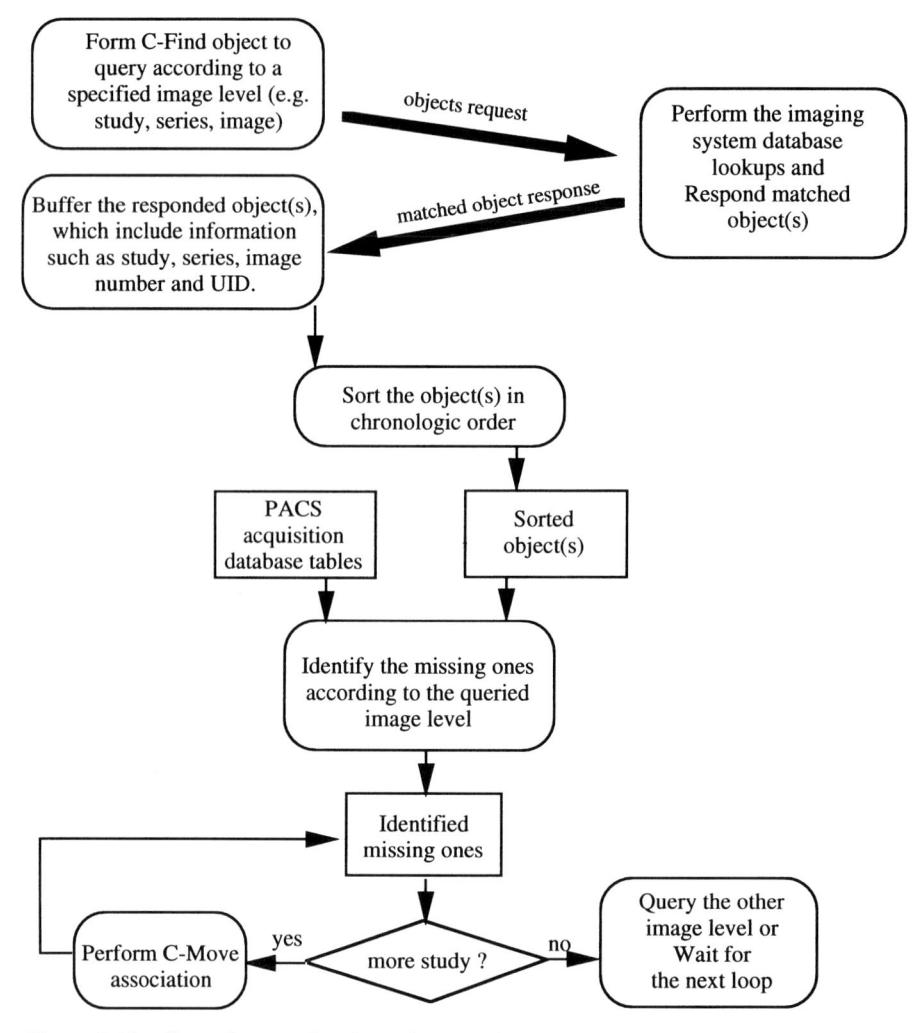

Figure 8.10 General processing flow diagram of the automatic DICOM query/retrieve image recovery scheme. The scheme starts by the acquisition computer issuing a C-Find command (upper left). The recovery starts by a C-Move command (lower left). Both commands are received by the scanner Q/R server.

encodes a C-FIND query object containing the major information elements such as image study level and a zero-length UID value defined by the DICOM standard. The zero-length UID prompts the Query/Retrieve server to return every single UID for the queried level. Then, the Query/Retrieve server responds with all the matching objects in the scanner database according to the requested image study level. The content of each responded object is mainly information such as a study number and the corresponding study UID. The information of each responded object is then compared with the records in the gateway database. Any study numbers that are in the responded objects but not recorded in the PACS acquisition computer database are considered to represent missing studies. Each of them can be retrieved by issuing a C-MOVE object, which is equivalent to an image retrieval request. Since the retrieval is study specific, the study UID must be included explicitly in the C-MOVE object. In the scanner, after the C-MOVE object has been received by the Query/Retrieve server, it relays the retrieval request to the C-STORE client. As a result, the image transfer is actually conducted by the C-STORE client and server processes.

The tasks of identifying and recovering missing series or images are performed with the same recovery operation mechanism following the study level. The difference between the study level and the series level in this recovery scheme is that a specific study UID must be encoded in the C-FIND query object for the series level or the image level, as opposed to a zero-length UID for the study level.

The records of available images in the scanner database and the gateway database may not synchronize. This situation can be encountered during a current study when its associated series and images are being generated in the scanner but have not yet been transferred to the gateway computer. Such asynchronization can result in an incorrect identification—that is, the image recovery process may mistake the current study listed in the scanner database as a missing one. To avoid an error of this type, the responded objects from the Query/Retrieve server are first sorted in chronological order by study creation date and time. If the study in question was created within a period shorter than a predefined time interval (measured with respect to the current time), it is considered to be part of the study being generated by the scanner. Thus, the image recovery process will not identify the most recent study as a missing study.

8.5.2.3 Some Results and the Extension of the Recovery Scheme

Figure 8.11 shows an experiment connecting an acquisition gateway computer to an existing clinical CT and MR network running DICOM communication protocols. Consecutive daily clinical image data are collected before and after the implementation of the recovery scheme. Table 8.2 compares the results. With the recovery scheme implemented, of 259 studies, human intervention error at the scanner sites caused 49 completely missing and 9 partially missing studies; all 58 were automatically recovered successfully.

Our discussion of the recovery scheme has concentrated on missing images due to human intervention at the scanner site. This concept can be extended to missing images due to hardware and software malfunctions during DICOM communications as

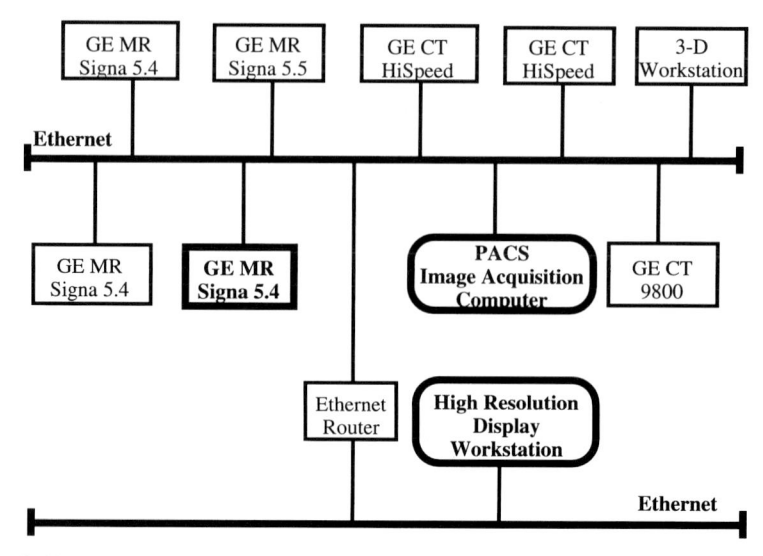

Figure 8.11 Schematic of the network connection for evaluation of the DICOM automatic image recovery scheme. Data are taken from one GE MR Signa 5.4 (bold) and validated at the high resolution workstation (bold). Results are shown in Table 8.2.

well. The reason is that missing images from these equipment malfunctions have no characteristic difference from those created by the human intervention.

8.6 INTERFACE WITH A PACS MODULE

In Sections 8.2.5 and 8.4 we discussed the networked and DICOM interface. These methods can be used to interface a PACS module with an acquisition gateway computer. A *PACS module* is loosely defined as a self-contained PACS that has connections to some imaging devices, a short-term archive, a database, some display workstations, and a communication network linking these components together. In practice, the module can function alone as an individual unit in which the display workstations show images from the imaging devices.

An example of a PACS module is the US PACS, in which several US scanners are connected to a short-term archive for up to 1–2 days of examinations. The display workstations can show images from all US scanners with display format tailored for US images. There are certain advantages to connecting the US PACS module to a hospital integrated PACS (HI-PACS). First, US images can be appended into the same patient's image and data folder to form a complete file, then sent to the PACS database for long-term archiving. Second, US images can be shown with other modality images in the PACS general display workstations for cross-modality comparisons. Third, some other modality images can also be shown in the US module's specialized workstations. In this case, care has to be taken because the specialized workstation (e.g., US workstation) may not have full capability for displaying images from other

TABLE 8.2 Performance of the DICOM Automatic Image Recovery Scheme

Recovery Scheme	Total Number of Studies Conducted	Number of Missing Studies Due to Human Intervention Errors		Number of Missing Studies Manually Recovered	Number of Missing Studies Automatically Recovered	Number of Series Missing Images Due to Grouping Process
		Completely	Partially			
Before	475	133 (28%)	29 (6.1%)	162	0	0
After	259	49 (19%)	9 (3.5%)	0	58	0

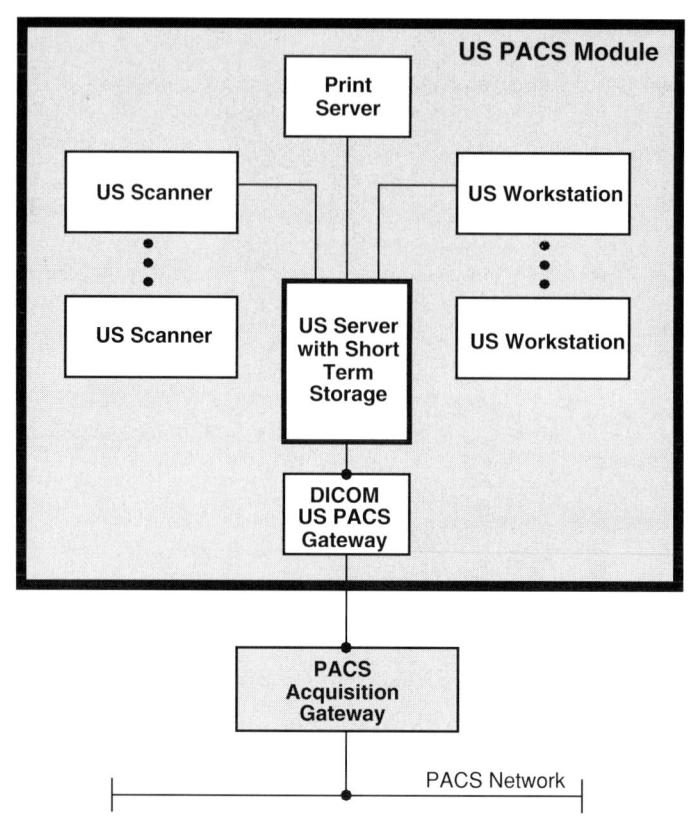

Figure 8.12 Interface of a PACS module to an acquisition computer: this example features a US PACS module.

modalities. For these reasons, there are advantages to integrating the US PACS module into a hospital-wide PACS. A preferred method for interfacing a PACS module to the HI-PACS is to treat the module as an imaging acquisition device and use the interconnected network model for the linkage. We use the US PACS module as an example.

Figure 8.12 shows the general connection of the US PACS module to a PACS acquisition gateway computer via a DICOM gateway. Each patient image file in the US server contains the full-sized color or black and white images (compressed or original), thumbnail (quarter-sized) images for indexing, and image header information for DICOM conversion. In the DICOM gateway, several processes are running concurrently. The first one is a daemon constantly checking for new US examinations arriving from scanners. When one is found, the device sends it to a second process to convert the file to the DICOM format. Because a color US image file is normally large (see Sections 5.5.4 and 6.7.3), a third process compresses it to a smaller file, normally with a 3:1 ratio. The gateway generates a DICOM *send* command to transmit the compressed DICOM file to the acquisition computer, using DICOM TCP/IP protocols.

In the acquisition gateway computer, several daemons are running concurrently also. The first is a DICOM gateway routine that checks for the DICOM *send* command from the gateway. Once the *send* has been detected, the second daemon checks the proper DICOM format and saves the information in the gateway computer. The third daemon queues the file to be stored by the PACS controller's long-term archive.

To request other modality images from a US workstation, the patient's image file is requested from the PACS long-term archive. The archive transmits the file to the gateway computer, which sends it to the US PACS gateway. The US gateway computer transmits the file to the US workstation.

Other important PACS modules that can be interfaced to the HI-PACS are the Nuclear Medicine PACS module and the Emergency Room PACS module. The requirement for the interface of these modules is a built-in DICOM gateway in the respective module with DICOM commands for communication and DICOM format for the image file.

8.7 IMAGE PREPROCESSING

In addition to receiving images from imaging devices, the acquisition gateway computer must perform certain image preprocessing functions before images are sent to the PACS controller or workstations. There are two categories of preprocessing functions. The first is related to the image format—for example, a conversion from the manufacturer format to DICOM. This type of preprocessing involves mostly data format conversion and was described in Section 7.6. The second type of preprocessing prepares the image for an optimal viewing at the display workstation. To achieve optimal display, an image should have proper size, good initial display parameters (i.e., a suitable lookup table), and proper orientation; any distracting background should be removed. Preprocessing function is modality specific in the sense that each imaging modality has a known set of preprocessing requirements. Some preprocessing functions may work well for certain modalities but poorly for others. In Sections 8.7.1 to 8.7.4 we discuss preprocessing functions according to modality.

8.7.1 Computed Radiography (CR)

8.7.1.1 Reformatting

A CR image can have three different sizes (given here in inches) depending on the type of imaging plates used: $L = 14 \times 17$, $H = 10 \times 12$, or $B = 8 \times 10$. These plates give rise to 1760×2140, 1670×2010, and 2000×2510 matrices, respectively. There are two methods of mapping a CR image to monitor of a given size. First, since display monitor screens vary in pixel sizes, a reformatting of the image size from these three plate dimensions may be necessary to fit a given monitor. In the reformat preprocessing function, since both the image and the monitor size are known, a mapping between the size of the image and the screen is first established. We use as an example two of the most commonly used screen sizes: 1024×1024 and 2048×2048. If the size of an input image is larger than 2048×2048, the reformatting takes two steps. First a two-dimensional bilinear interpolation is performed to shrink the image at a

5:4 ratio in both directions; this means that an image size of 2000 × 2510 is reformatted to 1600 × 2008. Second, a suitable number of blank lines is added to extend the size to 2048 × 2048. If a 1024 × 1024 image is desired, a further subsampling ratio of 2:1 from the 2048 image is performed.

For imaging plates that produce pixel matrix sizes smaller than 2048 × 2048, the image is extended to 2048 × 2048 by adding blank lines and then subsampling (if necessary) to obtain a 1024 × 1024 image.

The second method is to center the variable-sized CR images on the screen without altering its size. For smaller image sizes, the screen is filled with blank pixels and lines. For image sizes larger than screen, only a portion of the image is displayed; a scroll function is used to roam the image (see Section 12.3.2.1).

8.7.1.2 Background Removal

The second CR preprocessing function is to remove the image background due to X-ray collimation. In pediatric work and in extremity images, collimation can result in the inclusion of significant white background that should be removed to reduce the amount of unwanted background light in the image during soft copy display. This topic was discussed extensively in Section 4.1.6, with results shown in Figures 4.8 to 4.12.

After background removal, the image size will be different from the standard *L, H, B* sizes. To center an image such that it occupies the full monitor screen, it is sometimes advantageous to automatically zoom and scroll the background-removed image for an optimal display. Zoom and scroll functions are standard image processing functions and are discussed later (Section 12.3.2.1).

8.7.1.3 Automatic Orientation

The third CR preprocessing function is automatic orientation. "Properly oriented" means that the image displayed on a monitor appears in the conventional way expected by a radiologist about to read the hard copy image from a light box. Depending on how the imaging plate is placed under the patient, there are eight possible orientations (Fig. 8.13). An image can be oriented correctly by rotating 90° clockwise, 90° counterclockwise, or 180°, or it can be *y*-axis-flipped.

The algorithm first determines from the image header the body region contained in the image. Three commonly examined body regions are the chest, abdomen, and extremities. Let us first consider the automatic orientation of the anterior–posterior (AP) or PA chest images.

For AP or PA chest images, the algorithm searches for the location of three characteristic objects: spine, abdomen, and neck or upper extremities. To find the spine and abdomen, horizontal and vertical pixel value profiles (or line scans), evenly distributed through the image, are taken. The average density of each profile is calculated and placed in a horizontal or a vertical profile table. The two tables are searched for local maxima to find a candidate location. Before a decision is made regarding which of the two possible (horizontal or vertical) orientations marks the spine, however, it is necessary to search for the densest area that could belong to either the ab-

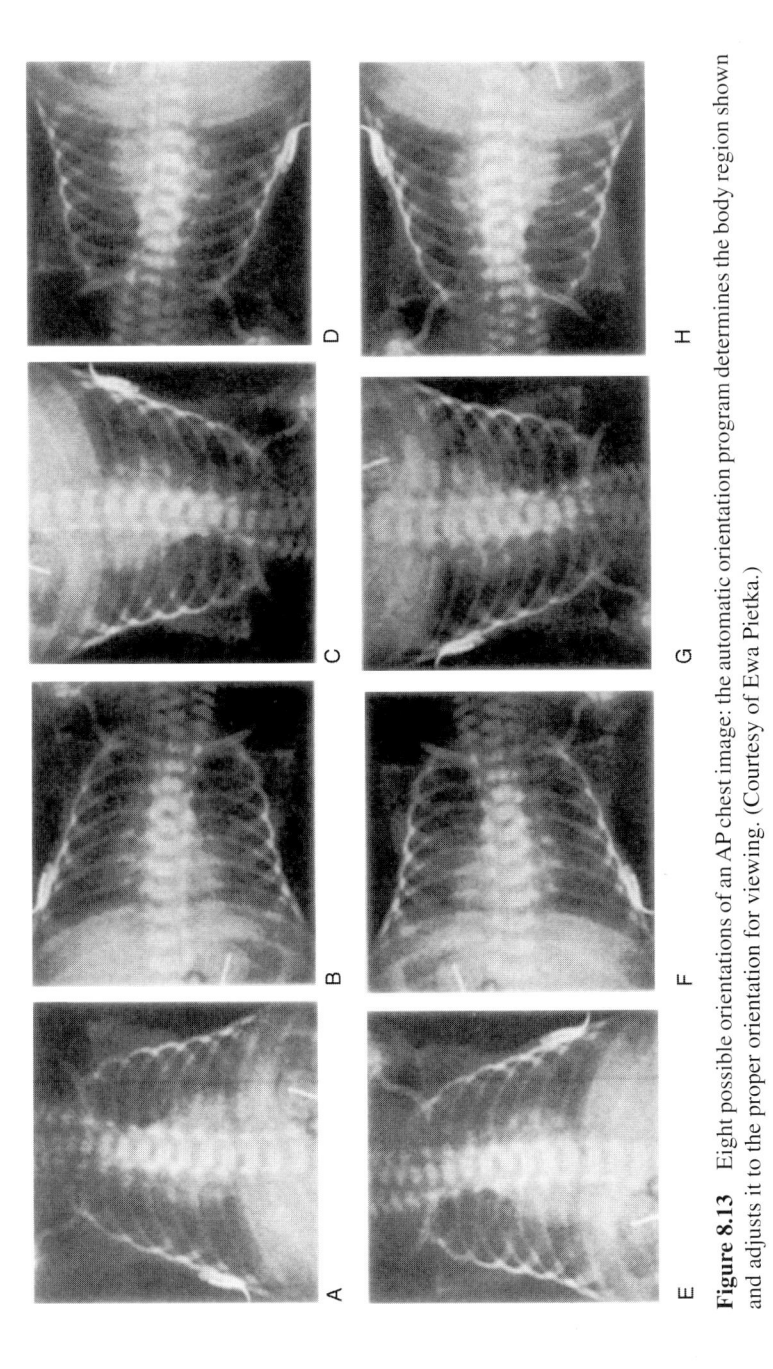

Figure 8.13 Eight possible orientations of an AP chest image: the automatic orientation program determines the body region shown and adjusts it to the proper orientation for viewing. (Courtesy of Ewa Pietka.)

domen or the head. To find this area, an average density value is computed over two consecutive profiles taken from the top and bottom of both tables. The maximum identifies the area to be searched. From the results of these scans and computations, the orientation of the spine is determined to be either horizontal or vertical.

A threshold image (threshold at the image's average gray value) is used to find the location of the neck or upper extremities along the axis perpendicular to the spine. The thresholding marks the external contours of the patient and separates them from the patient background (area that is exposed, but outside the patient). Profiles of the threshold image are scanned in a direction perpendicular to the spine (identified earlier). For each profile, the width of the intersection between the scan line and the contour of the patient is recorded. Then the upper extremities for an anterior–posterior (AP) or posterior–anterior (PA) image are found on the basis of the ratios of minimum and maximum intersections for the threshold image profiles. This ratio also serves as the basis for distinguishing between AP (or PA) from lateral views.

The AP and PA images are oriented on the basis of the spine, abdomen, and upper extremity location. For lateral chest images, the orientation is determined by using information about the spine and neck location. This indicates the angle that the image needs to be rotated (0°, 90° counterclockwise, 180°, or y-axis-flipped).

For abdomen images, again there are several stages. First the spine is located by using horizontal and vertical profiles, as before. The average density of each profile is calculated, and the largest local maximum defines the spine location. At the beginning and end of the profile marking the spine, the density is examined. Higher densities indicate the subdiaphragm region. The locations of the spine and abdomen determine the angle at which the image is to be rotated.

For hand images, the rotation is performed on a threshold image: a binary image in which all pixel values are set at zero if they are below the threshold value and at one, otherwise. To find the angle (90° clockwise, 90° counterclockwise, or 180°), two horizontal and two vertical profiles are scanned parallel to the borders. The distances from the borders are chosen initially as one-fourth of the width and height of the hand image, respectively. The algorithm then searches for a pair of profiles: one that intersects the forearm and a second that intersects at least three fingers. If no such pair can be found in the first image, the search is repeated. The iterations continue until a pair of profiles (either vertical or horizontal), meeting the above-mentioned criteria, is found. On the basis of this profile pair location, it is possible to determine the angle at which the image is to be rotated.

8.7.1.4 Lookup Table Generation

The fourth preprocessing function for CR images is the generation of a lookup table. The CR system has a built-in automatic brightness and contrast adjustment; since CR is a 10-bit image, however, it requires a 10- to 8-bit lookup table for mapping onto the display monitor. The procedure is as follows. After background removal, the histogram of the image is generated. Two numbers, the minimum and the maximum, are obtained from the 5 and the 95% points on the cumulative histogram, respectively. From these two values, one computes the two parameters in the lookup table: level

= (maximum + minimum)/2, and window = (maximum − minimum). This is the default linear lookup table for displaying the CR images. Note that a background-removed CR image always yields a better representative histogram, and hence a better representative lookup table, than one with the background in place.

For CR chest images, preprocessing at the imaging device (or the exposure itself) sometimes results in images that are too bright or lack contrast, or both. For these images, several piecewise-linear lookup tables can be created to adjust the brightness and contrast of different tissue densities of the chest image. These lookup tables are created by first analyzing the image gray level histogram to find several key breakpoints, which serve to divide the image into three regions: background (outside the patient, but still within the radiation field), radiographically soft tissue region (skin, muscle, fat, and overpenetrated lung), and radiographically dense tissue region (mediastinum, subdiaphragm, and underpenetrated lung).

From these breakpoints, different gains can be applied to increase the contrast (gain or slope of the lookup table > 1) or reduce the contrast (gain or slope < 1) of each region individually. In this way, the brightness and contrast of each region can be adjusted dependent on the application. If necessary, several lookup tables can be created to enhance the radiographically dense and soft tissues, with each having different levels of enhancement. These lookup tables can be easily built in and inserted into the image header and applied at the time of display to enhance different types of tissue.

8.7.2 Digitized X-Ray Images

Digitized X-ray images share some preprocessing functions with the CR: reformatting, background removal, and lookup table generation, for example. Each of these algorithms requires some modifications, however. Most X-ray film digitizers are 12 bits and allow the user to specify a field in the film to be digitized; as a result, the digitized image differs from the CR image in three aspects. First, the size of the digitized image can have various dimensions instead of just three; for reformatting, the mapping algorithm should be modified for multiple input dimensions. Second, there will be no background in the digitized image because the user can effectively eliminate it by positioning the proper window size during digitizing. No background removal is necessary, although the zoom and scroll functions may be still needed to center the image and occupy the full screen size. Third, since the image is 12 bits instead of 10 bits, the lookup table parameters are computed from 12 instead of 10 bits. Note that no automatic orientation is necessary, since the user will have oriented the image properly during the digitizing.

8.7.3 Digital Mammography

A digital mammogram size is $4K \times 5K \times 12$ bits, with a lot of background outside the breast contour. For this reason, image preprocessing is necessary to optimize the presentation of both the spatial resolution and gray level on the monitor. Three types of preprocessing function are of important. The first function is to perform a background removal outside the breast. The concept is similar to that discussed in Section 8.7.1.2. In this case, the background removal is simpler because the separation between the breast tissues and the background is quite distinct. An edge detection algorithm can automatically delineate the boundary of the breast. The background is replaced by an average grey level of the breast tissues (see Figure 6.3).

The second function is to optimize the default brightness and contrast of the digital mammogram presented on the monitor. A preprocessing algorithm determines the histogram of the image. The 5 and 95% cumulative histogram values are used to generate the initial mean and window for the display of the image.

The third function is to automatically correct the orientation of the mammogram based on left versus right side as well as specific mammography projection.

8.7.4 Sectional Images: CT, MR, and US

In sectional imaging, the only necessary preprocessing function is lookup table generation. The two lookup table parameters, window and level, can be computed from each image (either 8 or 12 bits) in a sectional examination similar to that described in the case of the CR image. The disadvantages of taking this approach are twofold: inspection of many images in a sectional examination can turn out to be a very time-consuming process, and a lookup table is needed for each image. The requirement for separate lookup tables will delay the multiple image display on the screen because the display program must perform a table lookup for each image. A method to circumvent the drawback of many lookup tables is to search the corresponding histograms for the minimum and maximum gray levels of a collection of images in the examination and generate a lookup table for all images. For US, this method works well because the US signals are quite uniform between images. In CT, several lookup tables can be generated for each region of the body for optimal display of lungs, soft tissues, or bones. This method in general works well for CT. However, for MR, even though a series of images may be generated from the same pulse sequence, the strength of the body or surface coil can vary from section to section, creating variable histograms for each image. Thus, automatic generation of a lookup table for a set of MR images would perform poorly, and the problem remains a challenging research topic.

8.8 MULTILEVEL ADAPTIVE PROCESSING CONTROL IN THE IMAGE ACQUISITION GATEWAY

The application of multilevel adaptive processing control in the image acquisition gateway will improve the reliability and efficiency of the PACS image acquisition component.

8.8.1 Concept of Multilevel Adaptive Processing Control

At the acquisition gateway computer, many sequential operations of intertwined computational processes are in progress. These include functions like image reformatting, automatic background recognition and removal, orientation correction, automatic lookup table adjustment, image encoding, and communications, as discussed in this chapter. Because most of these functions are normally processed in a sequential manner, slower processes will cause computational bottlenecks, which result in delays in the transmission of other images in the queue from the gateway to the PACS controller and workstations. In addition, a crash in any one of these processes due to certain errors may even stop the image transmission chain from the imaging device to the acquisition gateway. Such serious errors include illegal input parameters, software bugs, or system errors. The concept of multilevel adaptive process control is a method of circumventing problems of this type. We use CR acquisition as a demonstration of this concept.

8.8.2 Data Flow of CR Images in PACS

Figure 8.14 lists seven important computational processes involved in the acquisition and preprocessing of CR images. The functions of these processes are as follows:

1. *DASM_server:* acquires images from a CR system.
2. *Communication:* transfers data between computers in CR, acquisition gateway, and PACS controller.
3. *Reformatting:* converts and formats the acquired image from different sizes to specifications.
4. *Automatic background recognition and removal:* eliminates background signals.
5. *Automatic orientation correction:* aligns and rotates the CR image to an orientation suitable for viewing in the workstation.

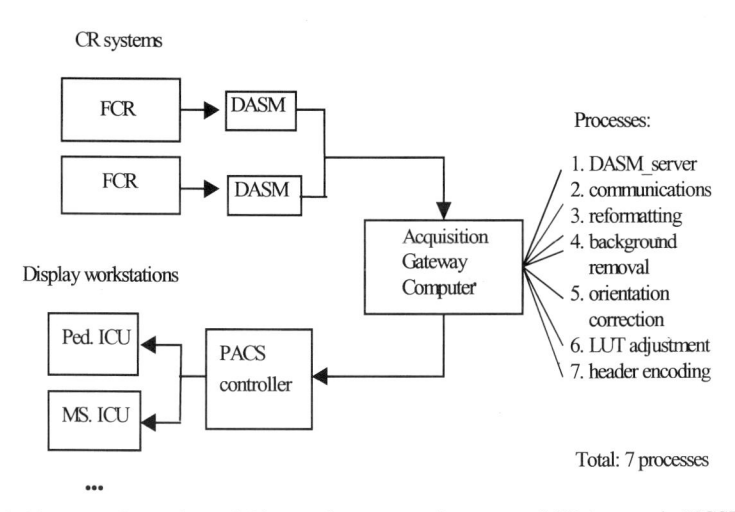

Figure 8.14 Data flow of acquisition and preprocessing steps of CR images in UCSF PACS and ICUs. Seven processes are needed.

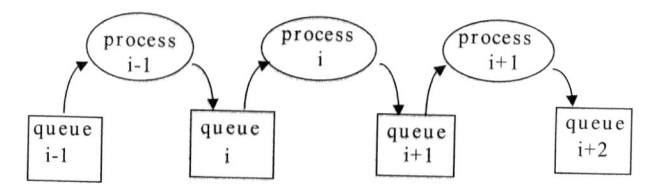

Figure 8.15 Single level process structure in CR image preprocessing procedure.

6. *Lookup table (LUT) adjustment:* modifies the default lookup table to enhance the visual quality after the background removal.
7. *Header encoding:* converts the image header from CR format to the ACR-NEMA or DICOM standard.

These seven processes are independent programs running in the background at the gateway computer. Processing of a CR image is sequential through these processes and in that order, and it follows the FIFO model (first in, first out). Conventional method of executing these processes using a single level model is illustrated in Figure 8.15.

Each computational process takes a job from its input queue file, which is a partially processed CR image from previous processes. When the job is done, the process puts it into its output queue file and removes it from the input queue file. Thus, in Figure 8.15, the input and output queue files for process i, are denoted by queue i and queue $i+1$, respectively. This single level processing structure suffers many drawbacks. First, it creates a bottleneck as a result of various computing speeds and unevenly distributed workloads among the computational processes. For slow computational processes, the jobs may be piled up in their input queue file. Meanwhile, faster processes are wasting the computer's CPU cycles when there is no work in process while the system is waiting for new jobs to arrive. Second, the system often crashes because of images with incorrect input parameters, software bugs, and system errors. For example, an illegal patient ID may cause a reformatting process crash that suspends the image preprocessing of all images waiting in the queue.

A multilevel adaptive process control structure consists of the following components: a process control theory to minimize the preprocessing time, a fault tolerance algorithm to improve the system reliability, and a multilevel adaptive process control monitoring mechanism to combine the control theory and the fault tolerance. These topics are discussed in following sections.

8.8.3 Process Control Theory

Process control theory can be used to optimize the acquisition and preprocessing time of CR images. This theory is based on the fact that all seven processes described earlier have equal priority in accessing the multitasking CPU. Let f_0 represent the CPU frequency, and S_i the number of CPU cycles required to complete process i. Suppose that each process i running in the CPU shares a portion of the CPU frequency, f_i. Then it can be derived from control theory [Zhang97] that the minimum time T to process one CR image is given by

$$T = \frac{\left(\sum_{i=1}^{m}\sqrt{S_i}\right)^2}{f_0} \quad (8.1)$$

where $m = 7$, is the total number of processes, and

$$\frac{n_i}{n_j} = \frac{\sqrt{S_j}}{\sqrt{S_i}} \quad (8.2)$$

where n_i is the number of jobs needed to be performed by the ith process.

Equations (8.1) and (8.2) can be used to attain the statistical minimum of the total processing time required by all processes to handle CR images waiting to be processed. This can be achieved by controlling the ratios of the number of jobs done between every process specified by Eq. (8.2). Controlling the ratios of the numbers of jobs for every process can be implemented by the client/server model described in Section 8.8.5.

8.8.4 Fault Tolerance Algorithm

In CR image acquisition, two factors can undermine the system reliability. The first factor, encountered infrequently, is an imaging device error that may cause the operation of the CR to cease. Device errors can be detected by periodically checking the communication states of every process with a monitor process running in the gateway computer. If any error occurs in the device computer, the monitor process in the gateway computer immediately pages the system administrator for system service through a telephone.

The second factor is due to illegal parameters entered by the operator and software bugs; both can result in crashing the process. These errors can be minimized by periodic service training and software refinement. However, in certain unpredictable situations, some defective inputs (e.g., an image with an illegal character in the header) may still crash the process regardless of the software's robustness. In image preprocessing, a process crash means that the process (1) cannot finish its assigned job, (2) cannot remove the job from its input queue file, and (3) cannot get the next job from its input queue file. Once an image has crashed the process, it will continue crashing it regardless of how many times the process is attempted. This will result in poor CR image acquisition and preprocessing system performance. Algorithms can be developed to keep track of a job that has crashed the system before. Once identified, the process removes this job from its input queue file permanently and gets the next job from the queue. In this way, all jobs are processed no more than once in every process. Therefore any image that has crashed a process will not be processed again.

8.8.5 Combining the Control Theory and Fault Tolerance

In the client/server model shown in Figure 8.16, the **monitor_server** controls ratios of the numbers of jobs n_i between all client processes (Eq. 8.2). All clients, in this case, all the processes, have to make a request to the monitor_server after they get a job from their respective input queue file. The monitor_server returns a message according to the ratio calculated from Eq. (8.2) in order to notify the client (process) whether to process the job. The client begins to perform a function only when it gets permission from the monitor_server; otherwise, it turns to the sleep state and repolls the monitor_server at regular intervals (e.g., 2–3 seconds).

The fault tolerance algorithm described in Section 8.8.4 can be implemented by means of multilevel adaptive process controls for all seven processes. Each process can be split into a parent process and a child process. Figure 8.17 shows the original process, the child and the parent process, and the functional diagram of a child process.

The major tasks for a parent process are as follows: (1) check the input queue file to detect whether there is a job available; (2) generate a child process to perform a desired image preprocessing function; and (3) monitor the processing time of the child process. If the child takes longer than normal to process a job, the parent will realize that something is wrong and kill the child process during the processing of the image. Since all these tasks in the parent process are independent of image data, illegal parameters or software bugs that may be present will not crash the parent process.

Every child process is composed of two parts as shown in Figure 8.17c. The first is the fault tolerance algorithm described in the Section 8.4.4, and the second is the image preprocessing functions. A child process has five tasks. First, after being generated by its parent, it gets a job from its input queue file and applies the fault tolerance algorithm to this image. If the algorithm fails (i.e., if the image had been processed before but not completed), the child process removes this job from its input queue file with an error message and then exits. Second, the child process identifies the image in a special file in order to correlate it with the next job. Third, it performs the assigned image preprocessing function. Fourth, upon completion of the processing, the child moves the job into its output queue file. Finally, it deletes the job from its input queue file with a successful message and then exits.

The merit of this child/parent architecture is that any error causing the crash of a child process will not prevent the parent process from completing the CR image ac-

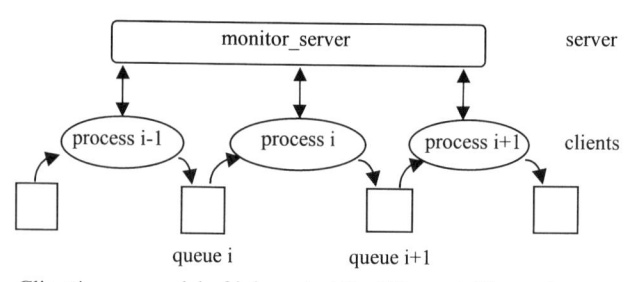

Figure 8.16 Client/server model of job control for CR acquisition and preprocessing.

MULTILEVEL ADAPTIVE PROCESSING CONTROL IN THE IMAGE ACQUISITION GATEWAY

quisition and the image preprocessing chain. This results in improving system reliability.

8.8.6 Event-Driven Multilevel Adaptive Process Control Structure

The job control algorithm and the fault tolerance algorithm can be incorporated into an event-driven multilevel processing structure as shown in Figure 8.18. There are three process levels: monitor_server, parent, and child. In addition to tasks and functions described in Figure 8.17, they have the following functions in the event-driven multilevel process control structure.

The monitor_server, apart from controlling the number of jobs of each process, also monitors parent processes and the system environment. For example, it makes sure that all parents are alive and that there is enough memory space for parents to generate children. It receives results from child processes and transfers error messages to the **central_monitor** (see Fig. 8.19) to notify the system administrator that service is required. It also accepts communication checking events sent from the central_monitor. In other words, the monitor_server is a server for all parents and chil-

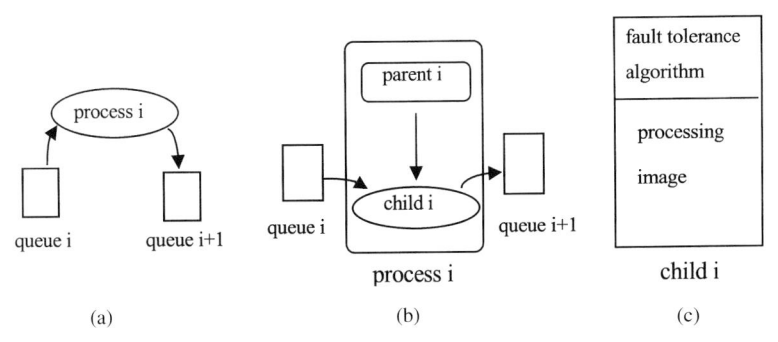

Figure 8.17 Diagrams of child and parent processes as well as child process functions: (a) the original process, (b) the parent and the generated child, and (c) functional diagram of a child process.

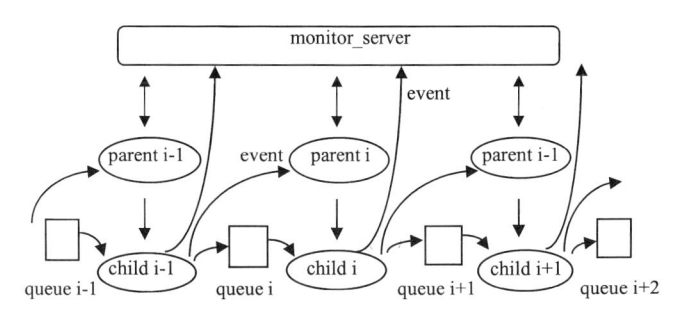

Figure 8.18 Event-driven multilevel process structure implemented with the control theory and fault tolerance algorithm.

```
                    ○ monitor_server
                   ↗
                  ↗   ○ parent 1
        ┌─────────┐↗
        │ Central_│↔  ○ parent 2
        │ monitor │↘
        └─────────┘  ....
                  ↘    ·
                    ○ parent m
```

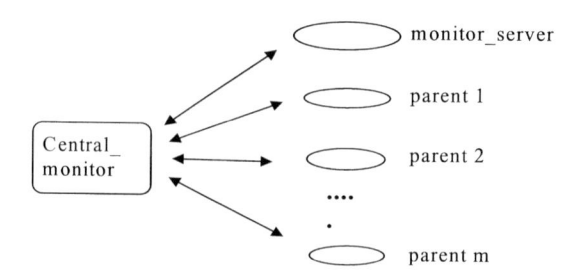

Figure 8.19 Communication between the central_monitor, the monitor_server, and the parents.

TABLE 8.3 Summary of Client/Server Relationship in the Event-Driven Multilevel Process Structure

Process Type	Client/Server Relations
Central—monitor	Server of monitor—server, clients of parents
Monitor—server	Server of parents and children, client of central—monitor
Parent processes	Client of monitor—server, server of central—monitor and children
Child processes	Client of monitor server

dren, but a client of central_monitor. Figure 8.19 gives the communication relationship between the central_monitor, the monitor_server, and the parents.

New functions for each parent are receiving trigger events sent from the preceding child, and receiving communication checking events sent from the central_monitor. The new functions for each child are sending to the monitor_server and the succeeding parent commands such as "job start," "job end," and "trigger," as well as any abnormal events. Table 8.3 summarizes the client/server relationships of various process types in the event-driven multilevel processing structure.

8.8.7 Some Results

The CR image acquisition and preprocessing processes with a fault tolerance algorithm and event-driven multilevel process control structure described here were implemented in the hospital-integrated PACS environment at UCSF (Zhang, 1997a). All interprocess communications use TCP/IP protocols. Results demonstrate that CR image acquisition and preprocessing become more efficient, and their performance is very acceptable in the PACS environment. More importantly, event-driven multiple process control does not crash the communication between the CR systems and the acquisition gateway computer, whereas the single level process control structure does, and often.

Figure 8.20 compares 20 randomly monitored consecutive CR images by means of the single level structure and the multilevel structure. The average processing time for one CR image required by all processes with the single level process structure is

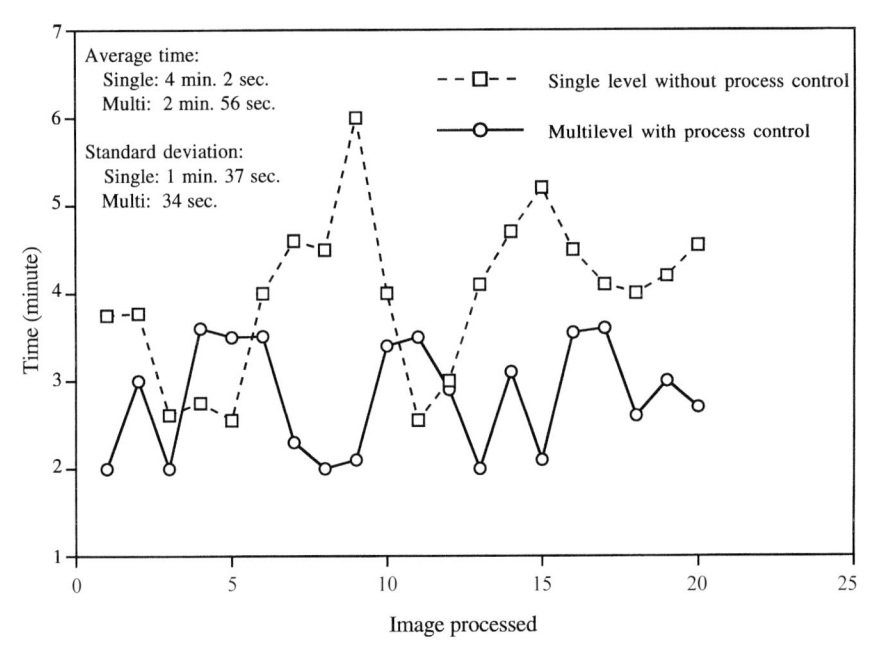

Figure 8.20 Time required for processing one CR image: single level without process control versus multilevel with process control structure.

4 minutes 2 seconds; standard deviation is 1 minute 37 seconds. The average time for one CR image with event-driven, multilevel processing structure is 2 minutes 56 seconds; standard deviation is 34 seconds. Hence, the processing time for one image with the controlled, multilevel structure is over 25% faster than the traditional single level structure.

We use CR as an example to emphasize the importance of multilevel process control, which includes speeding up processing time, reducing system downtime, improving system reliability, and decreasing user intervention time. The principle of adaptive multilevel process control can be applied to acquisition gateways of any image modality where heavy image preprocessing is required.

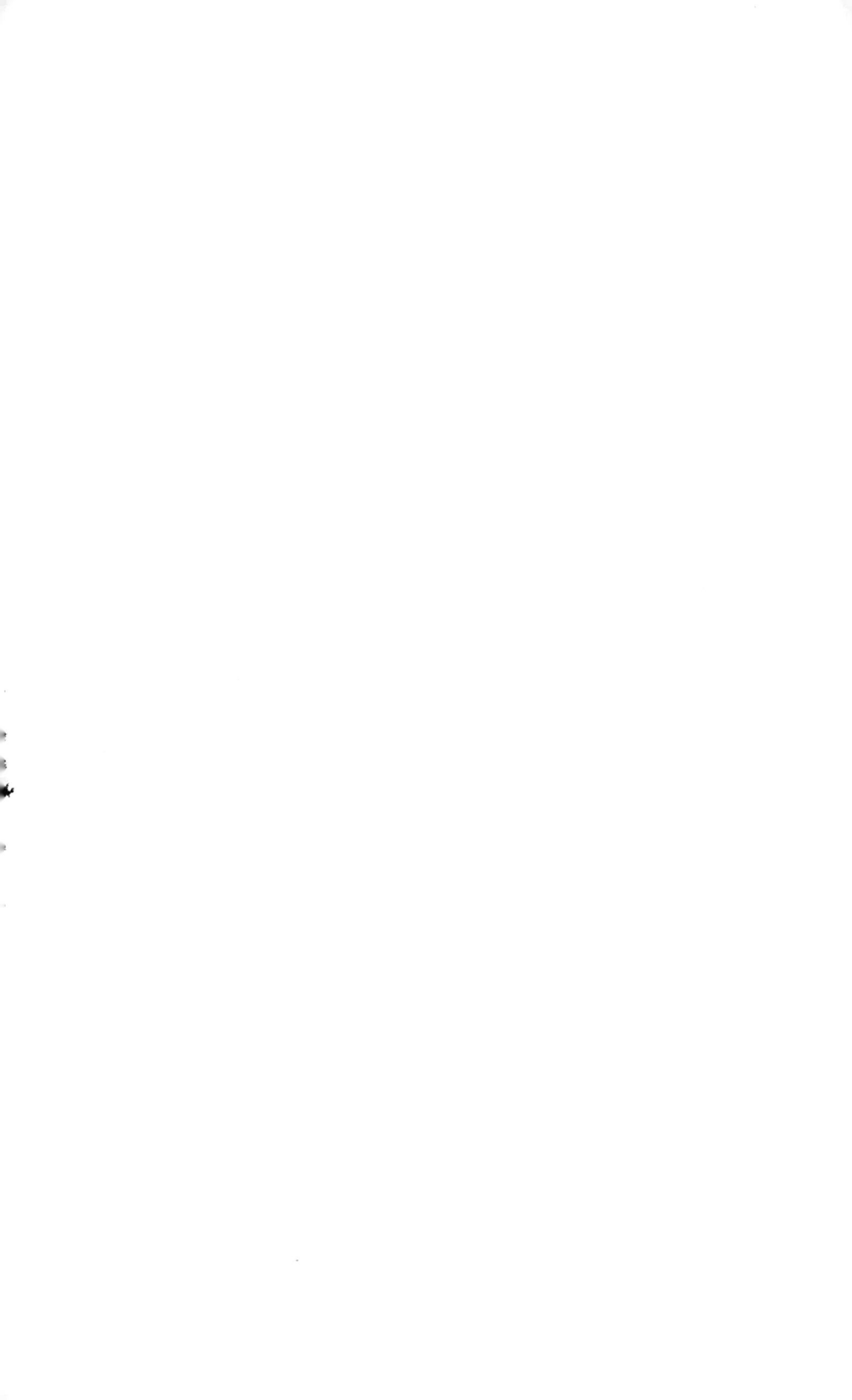

Chapter 9

Communications and Networking

9.1 BACKGROUND IN COMMUNICATIONS AND NETWORKING

9.1.1 Terminology

Communication is the movement of information from one place to another, usually by way of media of some type. Media may be either bound (cables) or unbound (broadcast). *Analog* communication systems encode the information into some continuum (video) of signal (voltage) levels. *Digital* systems encode the information into two discrete states ("0" and "1") and rely on the collection of these binary states to form meaningful data. A communication standard encompasses detailed specifications of the media, the explicit physical connections, the signal levels and timings, the packaging of the signals, and the high level software necessary for the transport. A video communication standard describes the characteristics of composite video signals including interlace or progressive scan, frame rate, line and frame retrace times, number of lines per frame, and number of frames per second. In a PACS, the soft copy display is video signals; depending on the types of monitor used, these video signals also follow certain standards.

In digital communications, the packaging of the signals to form bytes, words, packets, blocks, and files is usually referred to as a communication protocol. *Serial* data transmission moves digital data, one bit at a time, over a single wire or pair of wires. This single bit stream is reassembled into meaningful byte/word/packet/block/file data at the receiving end of a transmission.

On the other hand, *parallel* data transmission uses many wires to transmit bits in parallel. Thus, at any moment in time, a serial wire has only one bit present, but a set of parallel wires may have an entire byte or word present. Consequently, parallel transmission effects an n-fold increase in transmission speed, where n is the number of wires used.

In applications that call for maximum speed, *synchronous* communication is used. That is, the two communication nodes share a common clock and data are transmitted in a strict way according to this clock. *Asynchronous* communication, used when simplicity is desired, relies on start and stop signals to identify the beginning and end of data packets. Accurate timing is still required, but the signal encoding allows a wide variance in the timing on the different ends of the communication line. We discuss the asynchronous transfer mode (ATM) technology in Section 9.1.3.3.

In digital communication, the most primitive protocol is the RS-232 asynchronous

TABLE 9.1 Five Commonly Used Network Topologies

Topology	In PACS Applications	Advantages	Disadvantages
Bus	Ethernet	Simplicity	Difficult to trace problems when a channel fails
Tree	Video broadband head end	Simplicity	Bottleneck at the upper level
Ring	Fiber distributed data interface (FDDI); high speed ATM SONET ring	Simplicity; no bottleneck	In a single ring, the network fails if the channel between two nodes fails
Star (hub)	High speed Ethernet switch, ATM switch	Simplicity; simple to isolate a fault	Bottleneck at the hub or switch; single point of failure at switch
Mesh		Immunity to bottleneck failure	Complicated

standard for point-to-point communication, promulgated by the Electrical Industry Association (EIA). This standard specifies the signal and interface mechanical characteristics, gives a functional description of the interchange circuits, and lists application-specific circuits. This protocol is mostly used for peripheral devices (e.g., the trackball and mouse in a display workstation). Current digital communication methods are mostly networking. Table 9.1 lists the five popular network topologies and Figure 9.1 shows their architecture. The Bus, ring, and star architectures are most commonly used in PACS applications. A network that is used in a local area (e.g., within a building or a hospital) is called a local area network, or LAN. If provides service beyond a local area, it is called a metropolitan area network (MAN) or wide area network (WAN), depending on the area covered. The term MAN is not used often now, and such networks are grouped under WAN.

9.1.2 Network Standards

The two most commonly used network standards in PACS applications are the DOD standard developed by the U.S. Department of Defense, and the OSI (Open Systems Interconnect) developed by the ISO (International Standards Organization). As shown in Figure 9.2, the former has four-layer protocol stacks and the latter with seven layer stacks. In the DOD protocol stack, the FTP and the TCP/IP are two popular communication protocols used widely in the medical imaging field. The seven layers in the OSI protocols are defined in Table 9.2.

We now discuss an example of how data can be sent from a node to another node

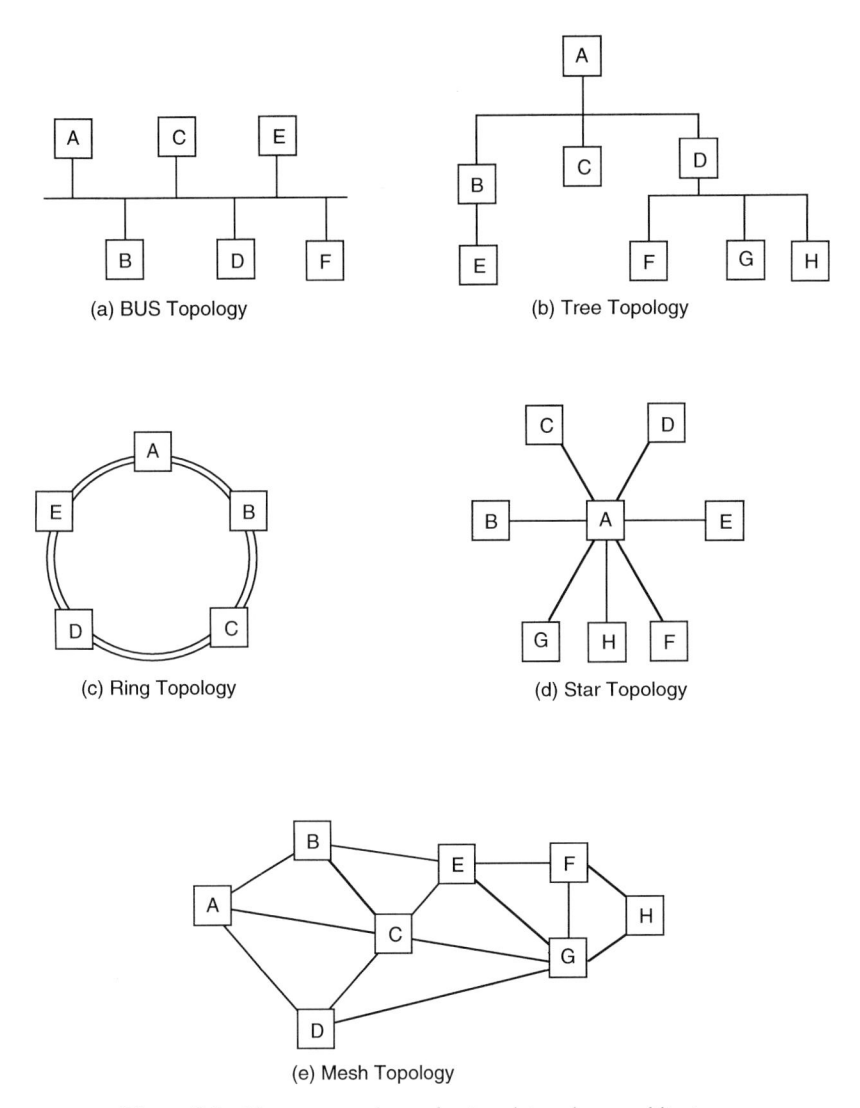

BACKGROUND IN COMMUNICATIONS AND NETWORKING   235

(a) BUS Topology

(b) Tree Topology

(c) Ring Topology

(d) Star Topology

(e) Mesh Topology

Figure 9.1   Five commonly used network topology architectures.

in a network through the DOD TCP/IP protocol. Figure 9.3 shows the procedure: the steps by which a block of data is transmitted with protocol information are listed at the left. First, the block of data is separated into segments (or packets) of data, whereupon each segment is given a TCP header, then an IP header, and finally a packet header. The packet of encapsulated data is then sent, and the process is repeated until the entire block of data has been transmitted. The encapsulated procedure is represented by the boxes on the right. In the TCP/IP protocols, the overheads in transmission are the TCP header, the IP header, and the packet header.

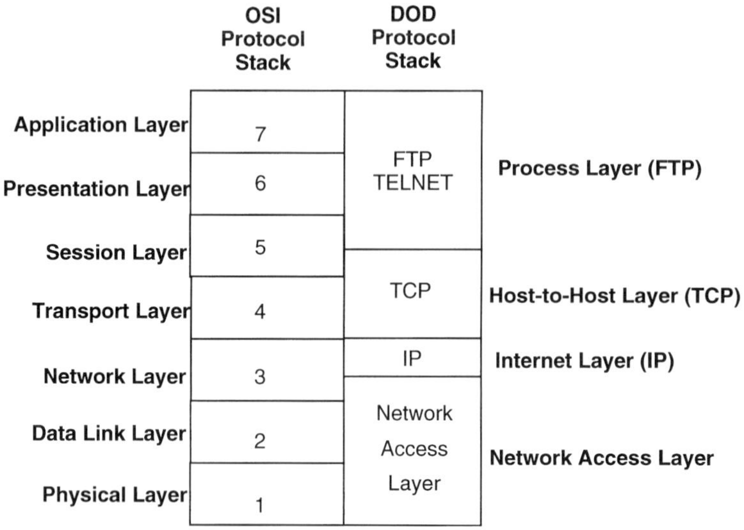

OSI Protocol Stack vs DOD Protocol Stack

OSI Layer	#	DOD Stack	DOD Layer
Application Layer	7	FTP / TELNET	Process Layer (FTP)
Presentation Layer	6	FTP / TELNET	Process Layer (FTP)
Session Layer	5	TCP	Host-to-Host Layer (TCP)
Transport Layer	4	TCP	Host-to-Host Layer (TCP)
Network Layer	3	IP	Internet Layer (IP)
Data Link Layer	2	Network Access Layer	Network Access Layer
Physical Layer	1	Network Access Layer	Network Access Layer

Figure 9.2 Correspondences between the seven-layer OSI and the four-layer DOD communication protocols.

9.1.3 Network Technology

Now we turn to three commonly used network technologies in PACS applications: the Ethernet, fiber distributed data interface (FDDI), and asynchronous transfer mode (ATM), which are used for low speed, medium speed, and high speed communications, respectively. In addition, we discuss the fast and gigabit Ethernet server switch-

TABLE 9.2 The Seven-Layer Open Systems Interconnect (OSI) Protocols

Layer	Protocol	Definition
7	Application layer	Provides services to users
6	Presentation layer	Transforms data (by means of encryption, compression, reformatting)
5	Session layer	Controls applications running on different workstations
4	Transport layer	Transfers of data between end points with error recovery
3	Network layer	Establishes, maintains, and terminates network connections
2	Data link	Medium access control: network access (collision detection, token passing) and network control. Logical links control: sends and receives data messages or packets
1	Physical layer	Hardware layer

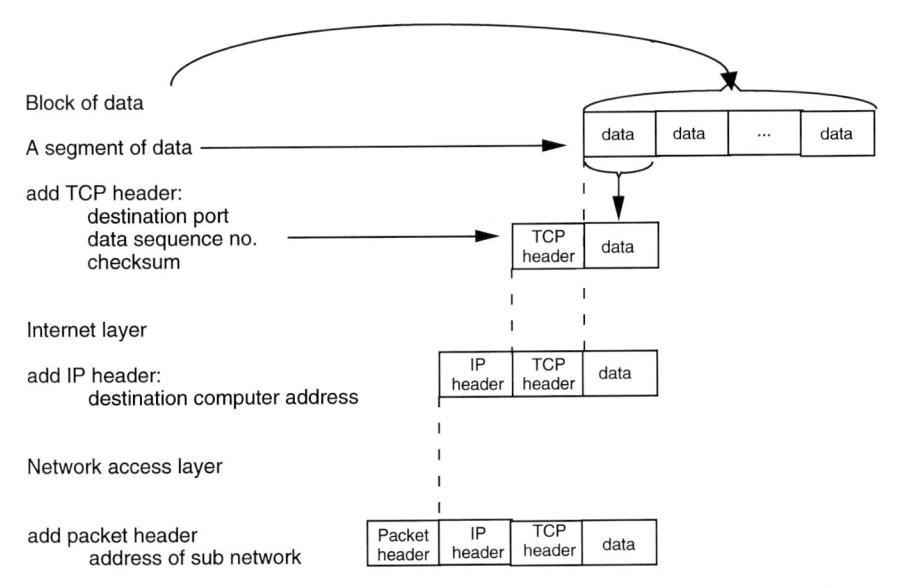

Figure 9.3 Example of sending a block of data from one network node to another with the TCP/IP protocol.

es, a recent advance in Ethernet technology. All these technologies can run on TCP/IP communication protocols.

9.1.3.1 Ethernet

The standard Ethernet (luminiferous ether), which is based on IEEE Standard 802.3, Carrier Sense Multiple Access with Collision Detection (CSMA/CD), uses the bus topology (see Fig. 9.1). It operates at 10 Mbits/s either on a half-inch coaxial cable, twisted-pair wires, or fiber-optic cables. Data are sent out in packets to facilitate the sharing of the cable. All nodes on the network connect to the backbone cable via Ethernet taps. New taps can be added anywhere along the cable, and each node possesses a unique node address that allows routing of data packets by hardware. Each packet contains a source address, a destination address, data, and error detection codes. In addition, each packet is prefaced with signal detection and transmission codes that ascertain status and establish the use of the cable. For twisted-pair cables, the Ethernet concentrator acts as the backbone cable.

As with all communication systems, the quoted operating speed or signaling rate represents the raw throughput speed of the communication channel—in this case, a coaxial cable with a base signal of 10 Mbits/s. The Ethernet protocol calls for extensive packaging of the data. Since a package may contain as many as 1500 bytes, a single file is usually broken up into many packets. This packaging is necessary to allow proper sharing of the communication channel. It is the job of the Ethernet interface hardware to route and present the raw data in each packet to the necessary destination computer. Dependent on the type of computer and communication software used, the performance of a node at a multiple connection Ethernet can deteriorate from 10 Mbit/s to as slow as 60 Kbyte/s. For this reason, in PACS applications, Ethernet is best for transmitting images from an imaging device to the acquisition gateway computer and for the complete system backup purposes. Not only is the very mature, low cost Ethernet technology ideal as a backup system, but high speed is not required to transmit images to the acquisition gateway computer because the process of imaging acquisition is slow.

A recent development is the concept of high speed Ethernet, in which all Ethernet connections go through an Ethernet switch instead of the Ethernet backbone cable or concentrator. The early Ethernet switch has the capacity to process each connection with 10 Mbit/s. As a result, each node can experience a true 10 Mbit/s specification throughput. Most conventional Ethernet using the bus topology has gradually changed to the 10 Mbit/s switch. In Section 9.1.3.5 we come back to the fast and gigabit Ethernet switches after a discussion of the ATM switch.

9.1.3.2 Fiber Distributed Data Interface (FDDI)

FDDI is a fiber-optic token ring LAN running at 100 Mbit/s. The FDDI runs on two rings, one transmitting in the clockwise direction and the other counterclockwise. The second ring is used as a backup. Figure 9.4a shows the double FDDI ring. In case one connection fails, the double ring can revert to a single ring and the FDDI can continue operating (Fig. 9.4b). FDDI can be used as a medium speed communication application—for example, from the gateway computer to the PACS controller.

FDDI is an established technology and is found in most large-scale hospital information systems developed in the late 1980s or early 1990s. Its innovations, at that time, were relatively higher speed than the conventional Ethernet, the double ring architecture for fail-safe, and the utilization of fiber-optic cables for longer distance and less noise during the transmission. Lately, FDDI has been losing its edge as a competitive network technology compared with the Ethernet switch and ATM for reasons of performance, cost, and lack of continuous research and development efforts by the industry. Since, however, many large-scale hospital information systems still rely on this technology for transmitting patient-related records, the PACS network design has to consider integration with existing FDDI setups.

9.1.3.3 Asynchronous Transfer Mode (ATM)

Both Ethernet and FDDI are designed for LAN applications. The current concept in radiologic image communication is that no physical or logical boundaries should exist between LANs and WANs. For this reason, ATM for both LANs and WANs has become the emerging technology. ATM is a method for transporting information that splits data into fixed-length cells, each one consisting of 5 bytes of ATM transmission protocol header information and 48 bytes of data information. Based on the virtual circuit–oriented packet-switching theory developed for telephone circuit-switching applications, ATM systems are designed on the star topology, in which an ATM switch serves as a hub. The basic signaling rate of ATM is 51.84 Mbit/s, called

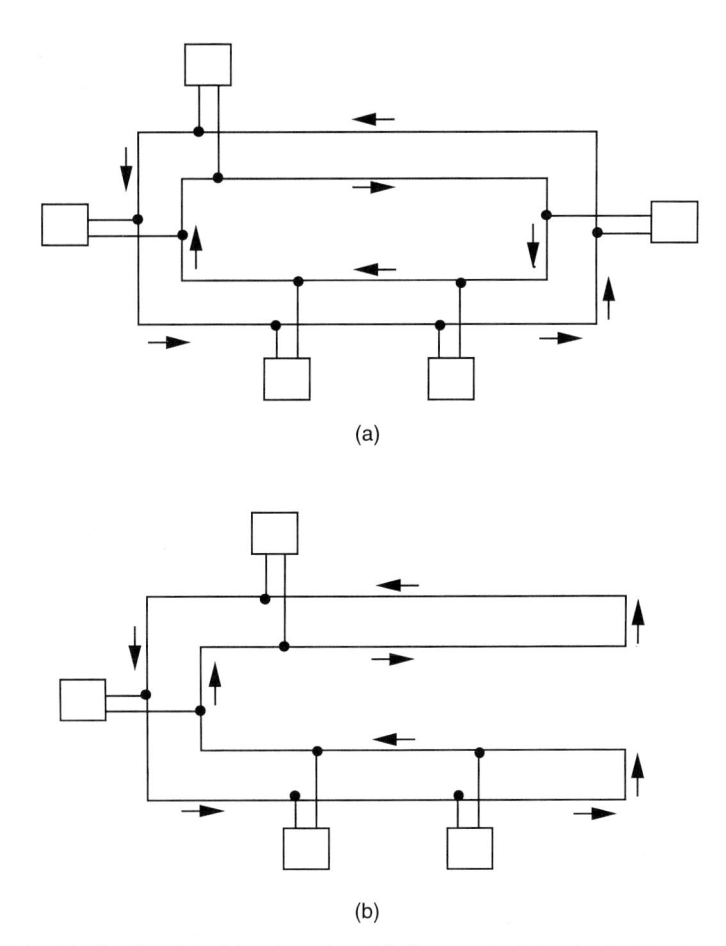

Figure 9.4 (a) The FDDI double token ring. (b) If one node fails, the double ring reverts to a single ring and the FDDI can continue operating.

optical carrier level 1 (OC-1). Others are multiples of OC-1: for example, OC-3 (155 Mbit/s), OC-12 (622 Mbit/s), and potentially to OC-48 (2.5 Gbit/s). Imaging applications can use the standard TCP/IP for both LAN and WAN, or application software containing TCP/IP, like the DICOM 3.0 standard.

In Figure 17.1, we will discuss a SONET (**s**ynchronous **o**ptical **net**work) ATM ring, which can be used as a high speed WAN supporting multiple campuses.

9.1.3.4 Examples of ATM Performance

Since ATM can be used for both LAN and WAN, it is ideal for PACS applications. In this section we present four examples on the ATM performance. The first example shows how to set up a simple experiment to measure the ATM performance, the second details the parameters affecting the ATM LAN performance in a PACS, and the

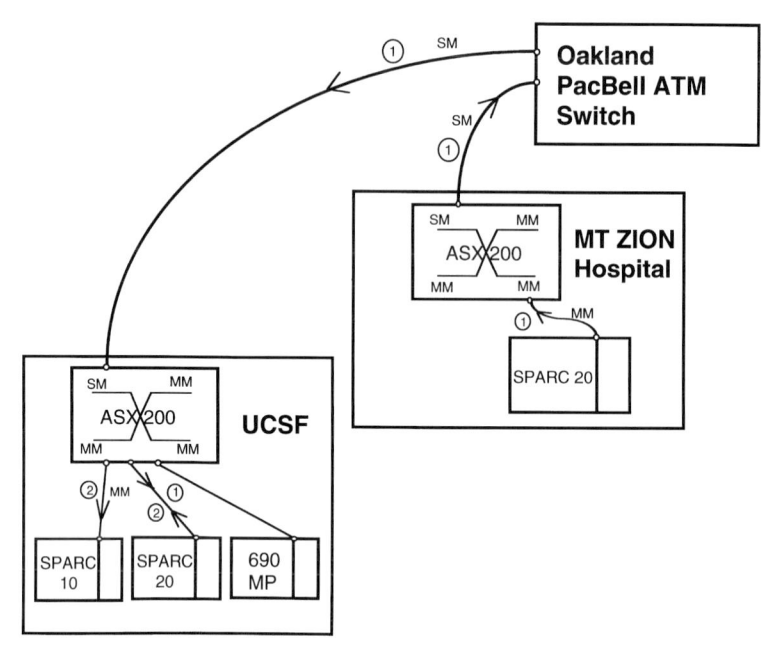

Figure 9.5 Experimental setup using multimode (MM) and single mode (SM) fibers for the asynchronous transfer mode (ATM) (OC-3 specification, 155 Mbit/s transfer rate) wide area network (WAN) and local area network (LAN) throughput test between University of California, San Francisco, and Mount Zion Hospital, using the ATM switch of Pacific Bell (PacBell) in Oakland, CA. Path 1 is for WAN performance measurement, path 2 for LAN performance measurement; for both WAN and LAN measurement, paths 1 and 2 are combined.

third measures the actual clinical ATM LAN and WAN performance. The fourth example pinpoints the performance of the ATM OC-12.

Example 1   Set Up an ATM LAN and WAN   Figure 9.5 shows an example of the use of an ATM switch to achieve both WAN and LAN communication.

At Mount Zion Hospital (MZH), two miles away from the University of California at San Francisco (UCSF), an ASX 200 ATM switch (FORE, Warrendale, PA) is connected to a SPARC 20 computer (Sun Microsystems) with an S-bus ATM adapter board (FORE) using two multimode optical fibers (see Section 9.2.1). This ASX 200 ATM switch is connected to the ATM main switch at Pacific Bell in Oakland, via single-mode optical fibers.

At UCSF, another ASX 200 ATM switch (Fig. 9.5, bottom) is connected to SPARC 10, 20, and 690 multiprocessor (MP) computers using multimode optical fibers. A SPARC 20 computer was used to simulate the acquisition gateway computer at Mount Zion Hospital; SPARC 20, 10, and 690 MP computers were used to simulate the display workstation computers and the PACS controller computer at UCSF, respectively. During the experiment, connection(s) were turned on and off as needed. The ATM WAN and LAN throughputs were measured under various conditions.

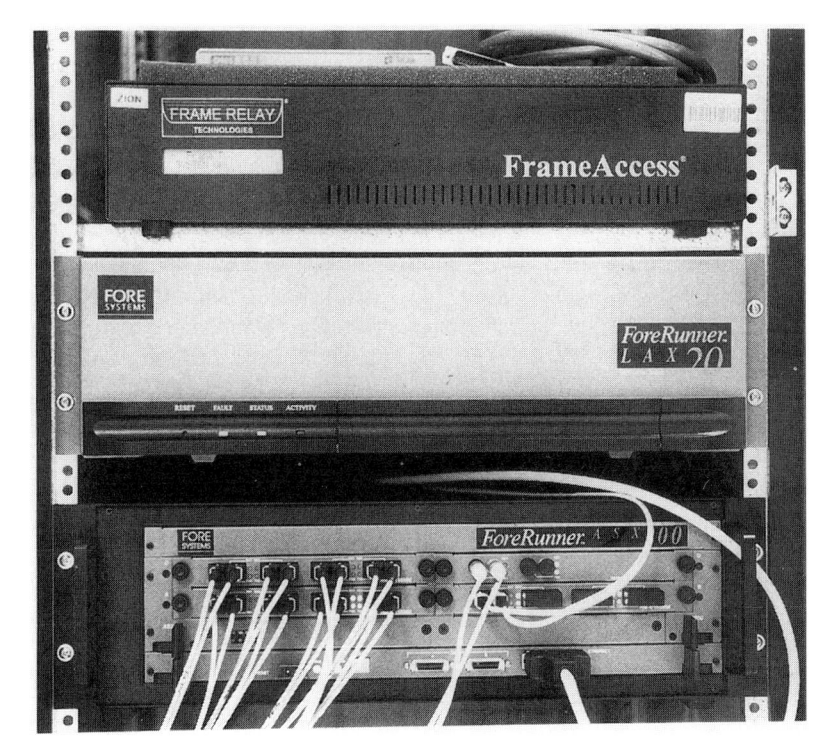

Figure 9.6 Stacked WAN and LAN components: *top,* frame access for T1; *middle,* LAX20, ATM to Ethernet LAN; *bottom,* ASX200, ATM WAN.

The ATM WAN performance can be measured by activating only the path marked with a 1 in Figure 9.5. ATM LAN performance can be measured by activating only the path marked 2 in Figure 9.5. The performance of both networks can be measured by activating paths 1 and 2 simultaneously. The simulation used the following parameters: image buffer size of 128Kbyte; measurement from computer memory to computer memory; data set size, 256 Mbyte; communication protocol, TCP/IP.

Table 9.3 shows that the ATM WAN performance is about 60.64 Mbit/s, and for

TABLE 9.3 Asynchronous Transfer Mode Optical Carrier Level 3 (OC-3) Performance Statistics

	Network Performance (Mbit/s)		
	WAN	LAN	Aggregate (%)
Path 1: From Mount Zion Hospital SPARC 20 (Sun Microsystems) to UCSF SPARC 20	60.64		60.64
Path 2: From UCSF SPARC 20 to Mount Zion Hospital SPARC 10		66.64	66.64
Paths 1 and 2 concurrently	28.16	48.80	76.96

the ATM LAN it is 66.64 Mbit/s (or close to 40% of the 155 Mbit/s signaling rate). When the WAN and the LAN are combined concurrently, performance decreases to 28.16 and 48.80 Mbit/s, respectively, but the aggregate performance reaches 77 Mbit/s.

Example 2 Parameters Affecting LAN ATM Performance   Our second example describes the ATM performance in LAN connected with workstations using computers and operating systems of different types. Refer to Figure 9.7, which shows the ATM PACS network in a daily routine clinical mode at UCSF as of January 1997. To measure the ATM performance in a clinical environment, additional TCP/IP communication processes were inserted in six workstations using different Sun computers connected to the network. Each workstation had its own specific functions in the PACS and was running different operating systems. One megabyte of image data was transmitted memory-to-memory, continuously, between two workstations. Transmission rates for both sending and receiving were measured separately at each workstation. The transmission rate is defined as the time elapsed between sending and receiving the data. Table 9.4 shows the results from point-to-point connections. The workstations shown in each row represent the sending sites, while workstations in the columns are the receiving sites. Thus, for example, matrix (1,2) = 1.35 Mbyte/s means that the performance was measured by sending images from SPARC 5 running Solaris 2.3 operating system and received by SPARC 20 running Solaris 2.4.

Thus for memory-to-memory transmission under normal clinical loads, Table 9.4 shows the following:

1. The ATM LAN can achieve over 9.0 Mbyte/s between two SPARC 20s.
2. The performance differs for a given pair of workstations if the order of sending and receiving is reversed. This can be explained as follows: in TCP/IP protocols, the receiving site is responsible for managing the incoming flow of data. Therefore, a lower performance computer used in the receiving workstation will result in a poorer transmission rate than that obtained when the same unit is used for sending.
3. The performance depends on the type of workstation and the operating system used.

Example 3 Performance of ATM LAN and WAN in an Actual Clinical Environment

Experimental Setup. This example shows how to measure the performance of ATM LAN and WAN under actual clinical environments. The intensive care unit PACS

Figure 9.7 Detailed ATM LAN and WAN connections between UCSF, MZH, and SFVAMC. AUI/UTP: attachment unit interface/unshielded twisted pair. The components in the top row are all image acquisition devices, dashed lines extend to components not yet connected; the second-row components are image acquisition computers. The components in the shaded box, and the ICU module in the lower part of the figure are used for the measurements of ATM LAN and WAN performance. See also Figure 9.8.

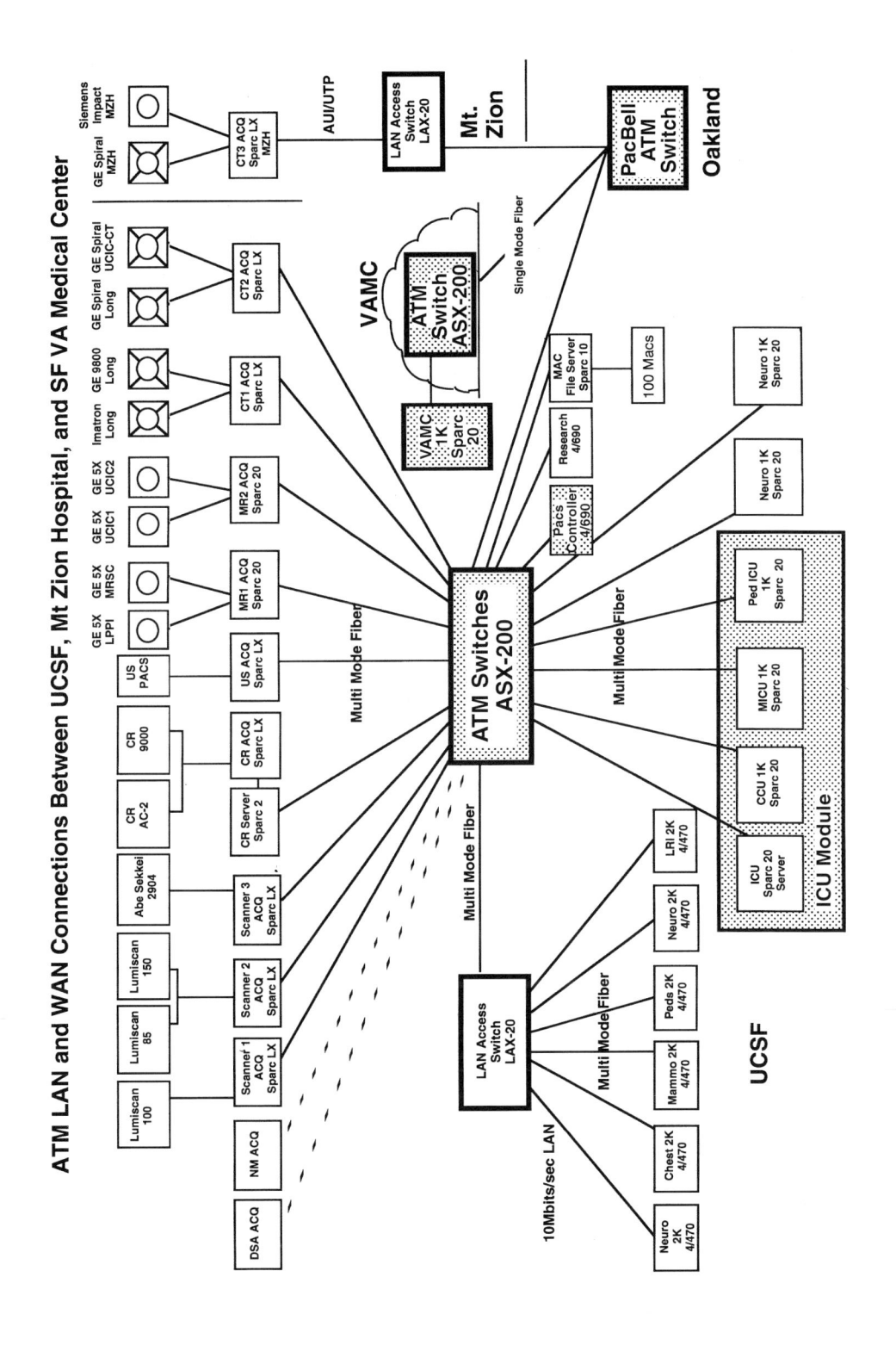

ATM LAN and WAN Connections Between UCSF, Mt Zion Hospital, and SF VA Medical Center

TABLE 9.4 Performance of ATM LAN from Point-to-Point Connections* (Mbyte/s)

REC Sending	SPARC 5 (Solaris 2.3)	SPARC 20 (Solaris 2.4)	SPARC 20 (Solaris 2.3)	SPARC 20 (SunOS 4.1.3)	SPARC 20 (Solaris 2.4)	SPARC 20 (Solaris 2.4)	Function of the WS in PACS
SPARC 5 (Solaris 2.3)		1.35	4.72	4.45			isg.ucsf
SPARC 20 (Solaris 2.4)	0.25		9.07	5.50	4.63	4.54	ICU 1
SPARC 20 (Solaris 2.3)	0.30	1.57		7.29	1.72	1.76	isg.nr
SPARC 20 (SunOS 4.1.3)	0.05	2.60	9.47			4.76	mr2.acq
SPARC 20 (Solaris 2.4)		4.17	9.59			5.39	ICU 2
SPARC 20 (Solaris 2.4)		4.22	9.65	9.75	5.45		ICU 3
	isg.ucsf	ICU 1	isg.nr	mr2.acq	ICU 2	ICU 3	

*isg.ucsf, ICU quality assurance workstation; isg.nr, neuroradiology workstation; mr2.acq, MR2 acquisition computer; ICU 1,2,3, three ICU workstations.

module shown in Figure 9.7 (bracket in the lower row) was used. Figure 9.8 illustrates the ATM WAN connection between UCSF and the San Francisco VA Medical Center (SFVAMC), and Figure 9.9 details the connection of workstations used in this example. The ICU module at UCSF with three workstations and one server had been in clinical operation for over three months before the experiment. Since SFVAMC did not have an ICU workstation, a fourth workstation was installed there for four weeks during the measurement. This example measures both the LAN and WAN performance in asynchronous transfer mode. For other hardware and software used in the experiment, see Huang.

ATM performance depends on the workstations and their operating systems (see results from Example 2), as well as the storage devices used. Four common storage devices used in PACS are local SCSI magnetic disk, remote SCSI magnetic disk, redundant array of inexpensive disks (RAID), and computer memory. For this reason, four types of measurement were obtained: local disk to remote disk, local disk to remote RAID, local RAID to remote memory, and local memory to remote memory. The measured total transmission time, **TOTAL,** is in general, a combination of five different times required during the transmission:

$$\text{TOTAL} = T_1 + T_2 + T_3 + T_4 + T_5 \tag{9.1}$$

where T_1 = sender disk (or RAID) to local memory
T_2 = sender local memory buffering
T_3 = ATM transmission time
T_4 = receiver local memory buffering
T_5 = receiver local memory to disk (or RAID)

Since the local disk input/output speed (about 4 Mbyte/s) is slower than that of the ATM OC-3 (155 Mbit/s- about 19.3 Mbyte/s), the transmission rate between two workstations, either both with magnetic disks, or one with a magnetic disk and the other with RAID, was dominated by T_1 and/or T_5. Therefore the measurement did not truly reflect the ATM performance. The I/O speeds of RAID to memory (about 24 Mbyte/s) and memory to memory (24 Mbyte/s) are in the same range or faster than the ATM signaling rate. Therefore, the measurements between workstations from RAID-to-memory or memory-to-memory trials would be a better measure of the ATM performance.

Experiment 1: Magnetic Disk–Magnetic Disk with ATM and Ethernet. The first experiment was to measure the ATM performance from disk to disk and compare the result with that of the conventional Ethernet network (10 Mbit/s). Figure 9.10a shows the configuration. During regular clinical hours, we measured the disk-to-disk transmission rates of CR images from the PACS controller's disks via (1) the Ethernet and (2) the ATM to the ICU image server's disks. The ICU server received two copies of each individual image, one over the Ethernet and the other over the ATM, from the PACS controller.

The transmission rate for the PACS controller to send CR images to the ICU serv-

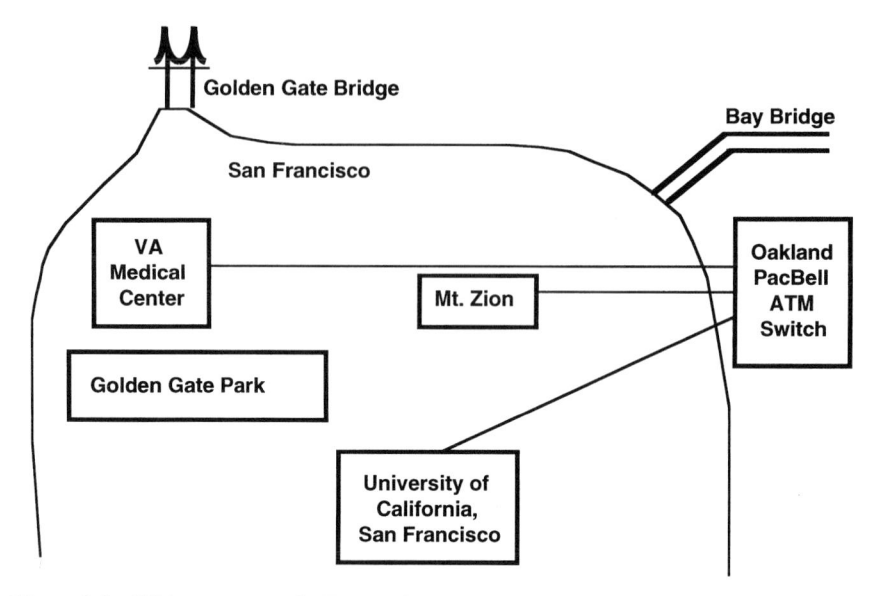

Figure 9.8 Wide area network (WAN) with ATM OC-3 (155 Mbit/s) technology connecting UCSF, MZH, and SFVAMC in a star architecture.

er were measured on a 24 h/day, 7 days/week basis. Approximately one month of transaction data was analyzed. The performance measurements, of 1247 and 452 Kbyte/s for ATM and for Ethernet, respectively, indicate that even with the constraint of slow disk input/output speed, the ATM is almost three times faster than the Ethernet.

Experiment 2: Magnetic Disk–RAID with ATM. The second experiment was performed using the configuration shown in Figure 9.10b. The setup is almost identical to that of experiment 1 except that the receiving site at the ICU server uses the RAID. The average transmission rate is 1500 Kbyte/s. Results from experiments 1 and 2 demonstrate that the ATM performance from disk to RAID is only about 20% better than from disk to disk. This smaller improvement is due to the limitation of the regular disk I/O speed, which dictates the transmission rate despite higher I/O performance of the RAID.

Experiment 3: RAID-to-Memory Transmission. In the third and fourth experiments, five ICU workstations using Sun SPARC 20 computers were interconnected via two ASX-200 ATM switches (Fig. 9.9). The ICU server distributed CR images in ATM to ICU display workstations in the Pediatrics, Medical Surgery, and Cardiac Care Departments) at UCSF, and a workstation at SFVAMC. This image server uses a 30 Gbyte RAID for all ICU images. In this environment, the three ICU workstation connections are in the LAN, whereas the SFVAMC workstation is in the WAN.

RAID-to-memory transmission rates were measured for transferring 80 CR images, each 8 Mbyte in size, from the image server's RAID over ATM to individual

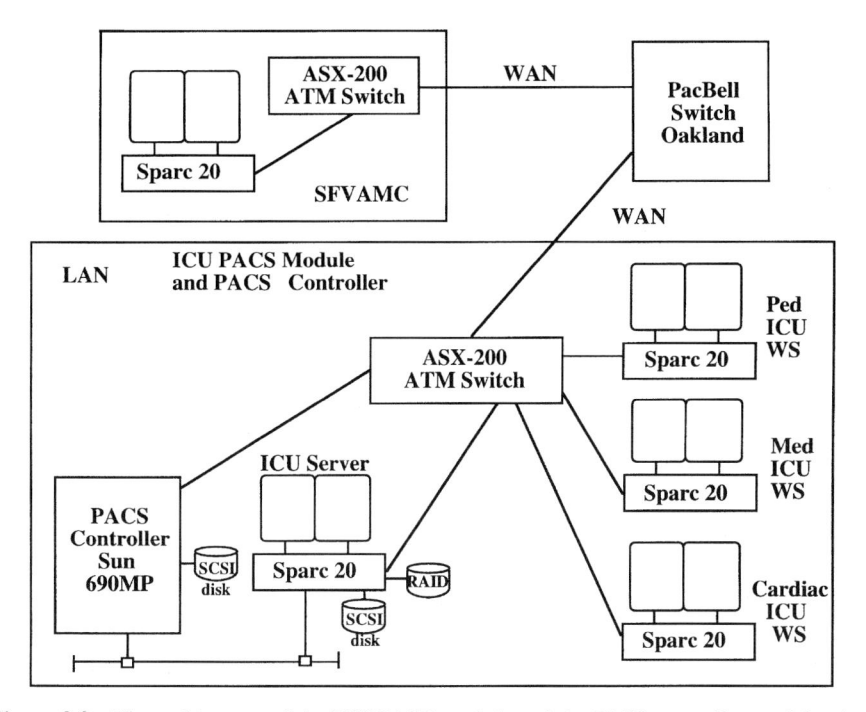

Figure 9.9 The architecture of the ICU PACS module and the PACS controller used for the ATM LAN and WAN measurements. Five dual-monitor, 1600 × 1280 resolution display workstations running ICU applications were used with two ASX200 ATM switches. The ICU server has a 30 Gbyte RAID disk. The workstation at SFVAMC was connected to UCSF via Pacific Bell's ATM switch in Oakland. During the experiment, the PACS controller acquired images from all acquisition devices and transmitted to the ICU server through the ASX200 ATM switch and the Ethernet.

Sun SPARC 20 system memory of the workstations. The communication processes allocated a 64 Kbyte TCP window size and 128 Kbyte image buffer size for the data transfers.

Table 9.5 shows the results from point-to-point and concurrent transmissions of data over the LAN and the WAN. The average point-to-point transmission rate be-

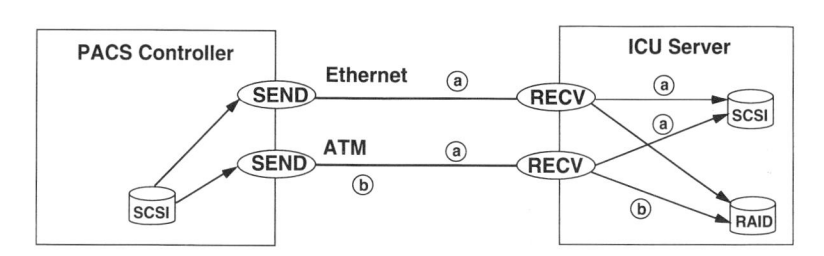

Figure 9.10 Configurations used for ATM performance measurements: (a) magnetic disk–magnetic disk, ATM and Ethernet and (b) magnetic disk–RAID, ATM only.

TABLE 9.5 RAID-to-memory Transmission Rates (Mbyte/s)

Number of Concurrent Processes	Sender*	Receiver			
		VA	Pediatric	Medical Surgery	Cardiac
1 WAN	5.2	5.2			
1 LAN	5.8		5.8		
1 WAN 2 LAN	6.98	3.31	3.68		
1 WAN 4 LAN	7.3	1.8	1.8	1.9	1.9

*In terms of server aggregate throughput.

tween the ICU server at UCSF was 5.8 Mbyte/s and to SFVAMC was 5.2 Mbyte/s. These transmission rates correspond to transferring an 8 Mbyte CR image in less than 2 seconds. When the server had to send images to all workstations simultaneously, the rates deteriorated to about 1.8 Mbyte/s. In all these measurements, the standard deviations computed were less than 2%, insignificant to affect the accuracy of the average values.

Experiment 4: Memory-to-Memory Transmission. Memory-to-memory transmission rates were measured for transferring 2000 data packets, each 128 Kbyte in size, from the image server's Sun SPARC 20 memory over ATM to the individual Sun SPARC 20 memory of the workstations. This amount of data is equivalent to 256 Mbyte or 32 CR images. Again, 64 Kbyte of TCP window size were used for the communication processes.

Results from point-to-point and concurrent transmissions of data over the LAN and the WAN are shown in Table 9.6. The average point-to-point transmission rate between UCSF and SFVAMC was 8.1 Mbyte/s and at UCSF was 9.8 Mbyte/s. These transmission rates correspond to sending a 40-image (about 20 Mbyte) CT examination over LAN or WAN in less than 3 seconds. When the server had to send images to all four workstations, the performance deteriorated to about 4 Mbyte/s.

From these experiments we can conclude that factors affecting the throughputs of an ATM network include (1) the computer and the operating system used in the workstation, (2) the number of simultaneous transmissions, (3) the processing overhead of the network protocols (e.g., TCP/IP), (4) the storage device used in the workstation, and (5) the data buffering arrangement in the computer system and the ATM switch. Among these factors, improvement of network transmission protocols and storage speed are two major determining parameters for optimization of ATM throughput performance.

Example 4 Performance of ATM OC-12 Performance tests of the ATM OC-12 (622 Mbit/s) also have been conducted at UCSF. For a two-node connection, the sys-

TABLE 9.6 Memory-to-Memory Transmission Rates (Mbyte/s)

Number of Concurrent Processes	Sender*	Receiver			
		VA	Pediatric	Medical Surgery	Cardiac
1 WAN	8.1	8.1			
1 LAN	9.8		9.8		
1 WAN 2 LAN	13.4	6.3	7.2		
1 WAN 4 LAN	16.0	3.7	4.0	4.1	4.3

*In terms of server aggregate throughput.

tem can achieve 360–380 Mbit/s with the following hardware and software components:

200 MHz Ultra SPARC 2
Sun ATM OC-12 adapter board
FORE-Runner ASX-200BX ATM switch
Solaris 2.5.1 operating system
Memory-to-memory transmission
64 Kbyte TCP window and 128 Kbyte buffer

The use of ATM for LAN has no other costs except purchasing the ATM switches and adapter boards, assuming the fiber cables are already in place. On the other hand, using ATM for WAN requires the user to pay a long-distance connection fee to a carrier. The price depends on the distance between the sites as well as the availability of optical fibers from carriers. Currently the charge from long-distance carriers for ATM is still prohibitively high, a major deterrent to the use of ATM in WAN applications. An alternative is to lease dark fibers from companies other than long-distance carriers. In this case, WAN becomes very much like LAN except that the cable distance is longer. The cost of ATM technology is decreasing very rapidly recently except for the use of long-distance cables.

9.1.3.5 Fast Ethernet and Gigabit Ethernet

In Section 9.1.3.1 we described the 10 Mbit/s Ethernet switch used in LAN as an alternate of the Ethernet bus topology to obtain 10 Mbit/s for every connection to the switch. Recent advances in the fast Ethernet switch (100 Mbit/s) and gigabit Ethernet (1.0 Gbit/s) allows very high speeds for every connection to the switch. Fast Ethernet is in the same performance bracket as the ATM OC-3, and the gigabit Ethernet has better performance than the ATM OC-12.

High speed Ethernet technology is a star topology very much like the ATM. Each

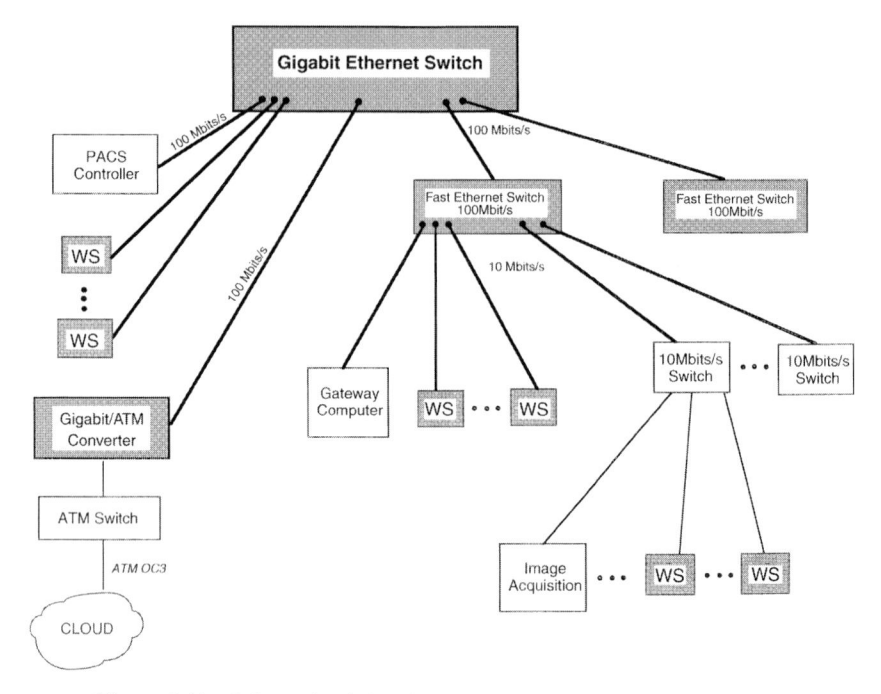

Figure 9.11 Schematic of gigabit Ethernet switch applications in PACS.

switch allows for a certain number of connections to the workstations through an adapter board in the workstation. A gigabit Ethernet switch can be branched out to 100 Mbit/s workstations and 100 Mbits/s Ethernet switches, which in turn can be stepped down to 10 Mbit/s switches and 10 Mbit/s workstations connections, as shown in Figure 9.11. Since Ethernet is used for LAN, and ATM can be used for both LAN and WAN, it is important to know that the gigabit Ethernet switch can also be used to connect to ATM OC-3 switches, providing a connection between these two technologies (Fig. 9.11). Currently, for a two-node connection, a Gbit/s Ethernet switch can achieve about 500 Mbit/s, which is sufficient for most medical imaging applications. Since gigabit Ethernet is a new technology, no large-scale sets of clinical data are yet available for evaluation of its actual performance. Figure 9.12 shows the market projection of various network technologies discussed in these sections.

9.1.4 Connecting Networks Together

Communication protocols set up standards to pass data from one node to another node in a network. To connect different networks, additional devices are needed, namely, repeaters, bridges, routers, and gateways.

A *repeater* passes data bit by bit in the physical layer. It is used to connect two networks that are similar but use different media; for example, a thinnet and a twisted-pair Ethernet (see Section 9.2.1) might be connected by means of hardware in layer 1 of the OSI standard. A *bridge* connects two similar networks (e.g., Ethernet to Ethernet or FDDI to FDDI) by both hardware and software in layer 2. A *router* directs

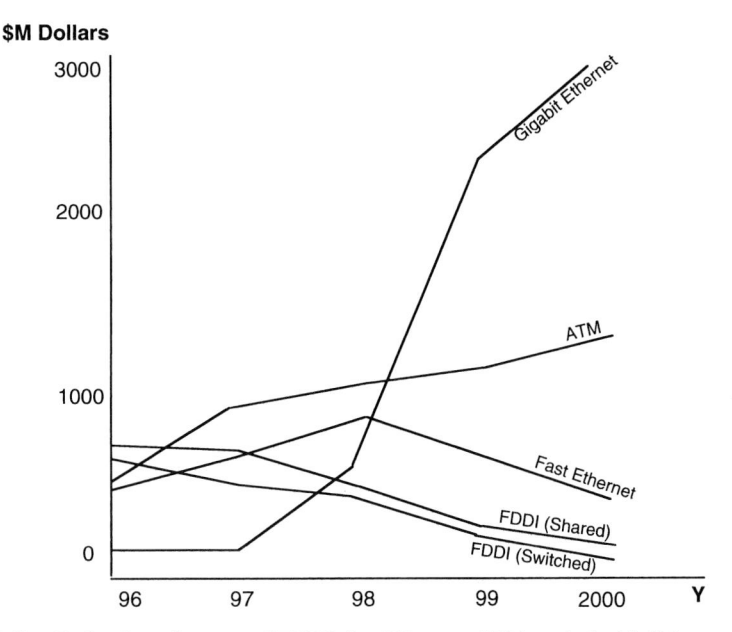

Figure 9.12 Technology forecast of FDDI, fast Ethernet, ATM, and gigabit Ethernet. (Diagram adapted from a technical brochure of Alteon Networks, San Jose, CA.)

TABLE 9.7 Communication Devices for Internetwork Connection

Device	Protocol Layer*	Network Connections
Repeater	Physical (1)	Similar network but different media
Bridge	Data link (2)	Similar network
Router	Network (3)	Similar or not similar network
Gateway	Application (7)	different network architecture

*Numbers in parentheses give OSI layer as defined in Table 9.2.

packets by means of network layer protocol (layer 3); it is used to connect two or more networks, similar or not (e.g., to transmit data between WAN, MAN, and LAN). A *gateway*, which connects different network architectures (e.g., RIS and PACS), uses the application level (level 7) protocol. A gateway is usually a computer with dedicated communication software. Table 9.7 compares these four communication devices.

9.2 CABLE PLAN

9.2.1 Types of Network Cable

This section describes several types of cable used for networking. The generic names have the form "10 BaseX," where 10 means 10 Mbit/s, and X represents media type as specified by IEEE Standard 802.3, because some of these cables were developed for Ethernet use.

10 Base5, also called thicknet or thick Ethernet, is a coaxial cable terminated with N series connectors. 10 Base5 is a 10 Mhz, 10 Mbit/s network medium with a distance limitation of 500 m. This cable is typically used as a Ethernet trunk or backbone path of the network. Cable impedance is 50 ohms (Ω).

10 Base2, also called thinnet or Cheaper net, is terminated with BNC connectors. Also used as a Ethernet trunk or backbone path for smaller networks, 10Base2 is a 10 MHz, 10 Mbit/s medium with a distance limitation of 185 m. Cable impedance is 50 Ω.

10 BaseT, also called UTP or unshielded twisted pair, is terminated with AMP 110, or RJ-45 connectors following the EIA 568 standard. With a distance limitation of 100 m, this low cost cable is used for point-to-point applications such as Ethernet and copper distributed data interface (CDDI), not as a backbone. Categories 3, 4, and 5 UTP can all be used for Ethernet, but category 5, capable of 100 Mhz and 100 Mbit/s, is recommended for medical imaging applications.

100 BaseT is used for the fast Ethernet connection to support 100 Mbit/s.

Fiber-optic cables normally come in bundles of 1 to 216 fibers. Each fiber can be either multimode (62.5 μm in diameter) or single mode (9 μm). Multimode, normally referred to as 10 BaseF, is used for Ethernet, FDDI, and ATM (see Section 9.1.3.3).

The single mode is used for longer distance communication. 10 BaseF cables are terminated with SC, ST, SMA, or FC connectors, but usually ST. For Ethernet applications, single mode has a distance limitation of 2000 m and can be used as a backbone segment or in point-to-point setups. 10 BaseF cables are used for networking. Patch cords are used to connect a network with another network, or a network with an individual component (e.g., imaging device, image workstation). Patch cords usually are AUI (attachment unit interface—DB 25), UTP, or short fiber-optic cables with the proper connectors.

Air-blown fiber (ABF) is a recent technology that makes it possible to use compressed nitrogen to "blow" fibers as needed through a tube distribution system (TDS). Tubes come in quantities from 1 to 16. Each tube can accommodate bundles of 1 to 16 fibers, either single mode or multimode. The advantage of this type of system is that fibers can be blown in as needed once the TDS has been installed.

Video cables are used to transmit images to high resolution monitors. For 2K monitors, 50 Ω cables are used: RG 58 for short lengths or RG 214U for distances up to 150 feet. RG 59, a 75 Ω cable used for 1K monitors, can run distances of 100 feet.

9.2.2 The Hub Room

A hub room contains repeaters, fanouts (one-to-many repeaters), bridges, routers, switches, and the gateway computer, as well as other networking equipment for connecting and routing/switching information to and from networks. This room also contains the center for networking infrastructure media such as thicknet, thinnet, UTP, and fiber-optic patch panels. Patch panels, which allow the termination of fiber optics and UTP cables from various rooms in one central location, usually are mounted in a rack. At the patch panel, networks can be patched or connected from one location to another or by installing a jumper from the patch panel to a piece of networking equipment. One of the main features of the hub room is its connectivity to various other networks, rooms, and buildings. Air conditioning and backup power are vital to a hub room to provide a fail-safe environment. If possible, semi-dust-free conditions should be maintained.

Any large network installation needs segmented hub rooms, which may span different rooms and/or buildings. Each room should have multiple network connections and patch panels that permit interconnectivity throughout the campus. The center or main hub room is usually called the network distribution center (NDC). The NDC houses concentrators, bridges, main routers, and switches. From this room it should be possible to connect via a computer to every network in the communication infrastructure. From the NDC, the networks span to a different building to a room called the building distribution frame (BDF). The BDF routes information from the main subnet to departmental subnets, which may be located on various floors in a building. From the BDF, information can be routed to an intermediate distribution frame (IDF), which will route or switch the network information to the end users.

Each hub room should have a predetermined path for cables entrances and exits. For example, four 3-inch sleeves (two for incoming and two for outgoing cables) should be installed between the room and the area the cables are coming from, to allow a direct path. Cable laddering is a very convenient way of managing cables throughout the room. The cable ladder is suspended from the ceiling, which allows the cables to be run from the 3-inch sleeves across the ladder and suspends the cables down to their end locations. Cable trays can also be mounted on the ladder for separation of coaxial, UTP, and fiber optics. In addition to backup power, access to emergency power (provided by external generators typically in a hospital environment) is necessary. The room should also have a minimum of two dedicated 20 A, 120 V quad power outlets—more may be required, depending on the room size. Figure 9.13 shows the generic configuration of hub room connections.

9.2.3 Cables for Input Sources

Usually, an imaging device is already connected to an existing network with one of the four media types: thicknet, thinnet, fiber optics, or twisted pair. A tap of the same media type can be used to connect a gateway computer to this network, or, the aid of a repeater may be required, as in the following example. Suppose a CT scanner is already on a thinnet network, and the acquisition gateway computer has access only to twisted-pair cables in its neighborhood. The system designer might select a repeater residing in a hub room that has an input of thinnet and an output of UTP to connect the network and the computer. When cables must run from a hub room to an image acquisition device area, it is always advisable at the time of installation to lay extra cables long enough to cover the diagonal of the room, and to run from the ceiling to the floor. This is easier and less expensive than pulling the cables later to clear the way for relocation or upgrade.

When installing cables from the IDF or BDF to areas housing acquisition devices planned for Ethernet use at a distance is less than 100 m, a minimum of one category 5 UTP per node and four strands of multimode fiber per imaging room (CT, MR, CR) is recommended. If a fiber-optic broadband video system (see Section 9.3) is also planned, an additional multimode fiber-optic cable should be allocated for each input

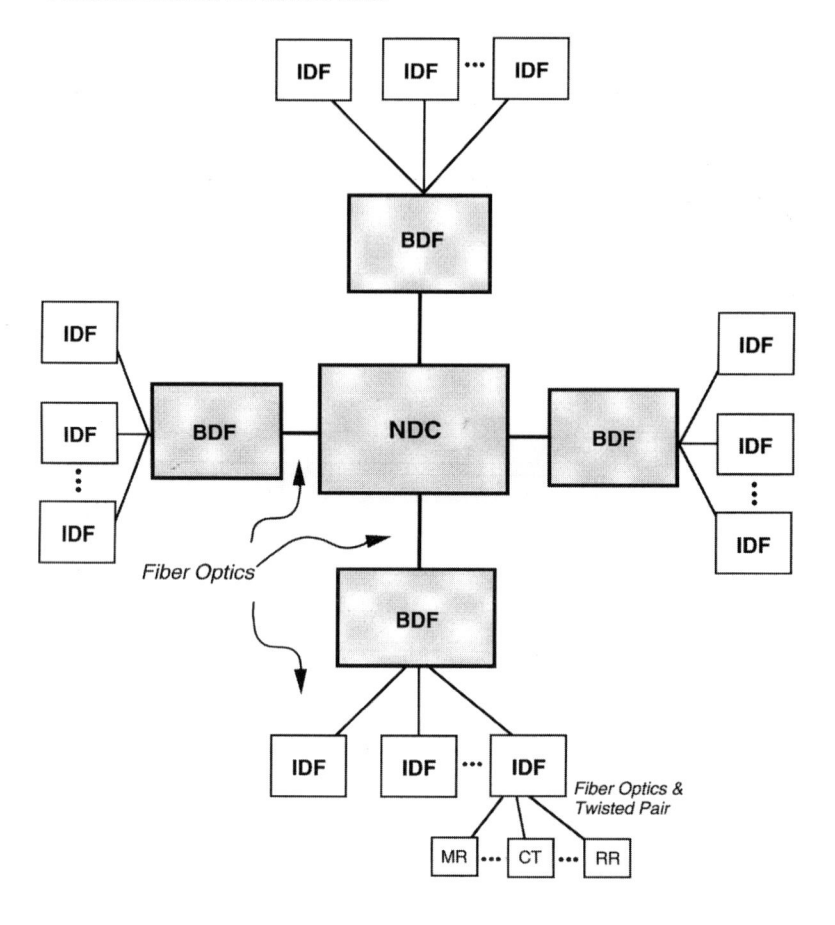

Figure 9.13 Generic configuration of hub room connections: the image acquisition devices and image workstations are connected from the IDF (see key in figure).

NDC: Network Distribution Center
BDF: Building Distribution Frame
IDF: Intermediate Distribution Frame
MR: Magnetic Resonance Imaging
CT: Computed Tomography Imaging
RR: Reading Room

device. With this configuration, the current Ethernet technology is fully utilized and the infrastructure still has the capacity to be upgraded to accept any protocols that may be encountered in the future.

9.2.4 Cables for Image Distribution

Cable planning for input devices and image distribution differs in the sense that the former is ad hoc—that is, most of the time the input device already exists, and there is not much flexibility in the cable plan. On the other hand, image distribution re-

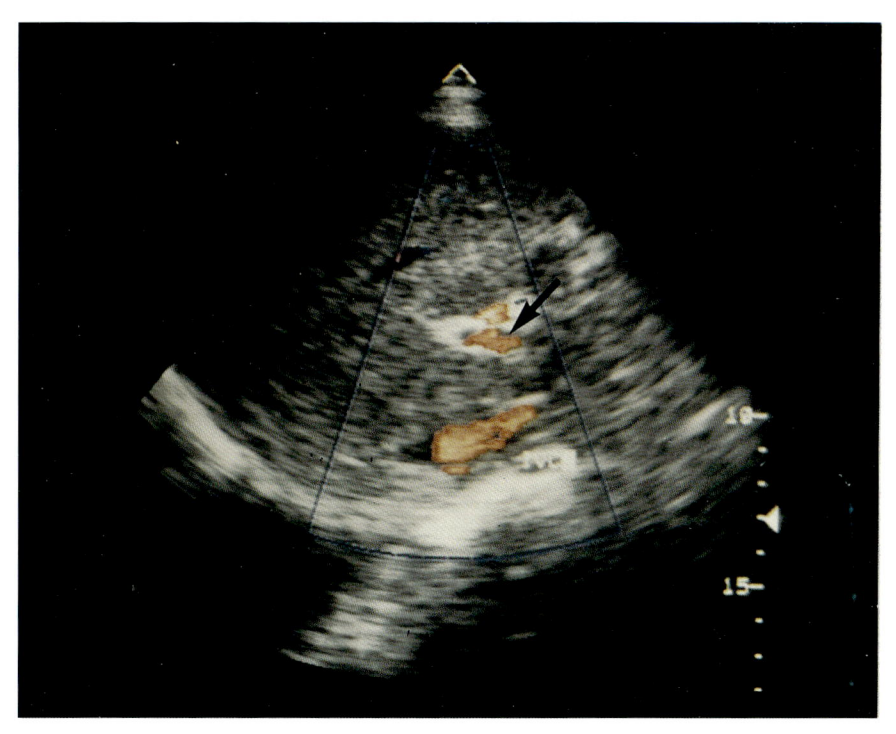

Figure 5.14 Color Doppler ultrasound image of the longitudinal section through the liver indicates that the flow in the inferior vena cava (IVC) is reversed: blood flow (in red) is directed toward the US scanning plane. Flow in the portal vein (arrow) is hepatopetal. (Courtesy of E. Grant.)

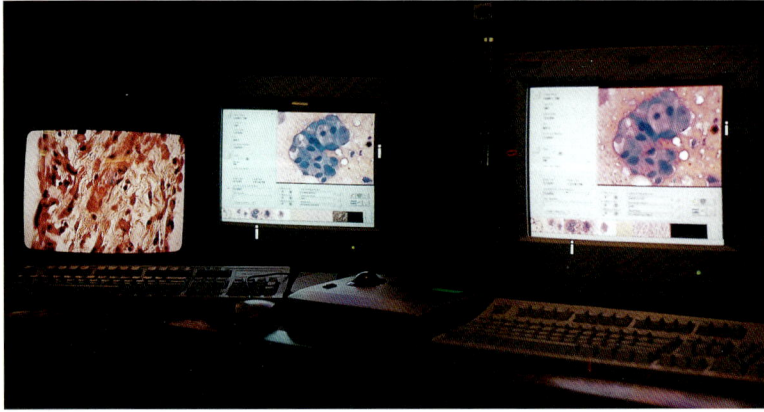

COLOR PLATES

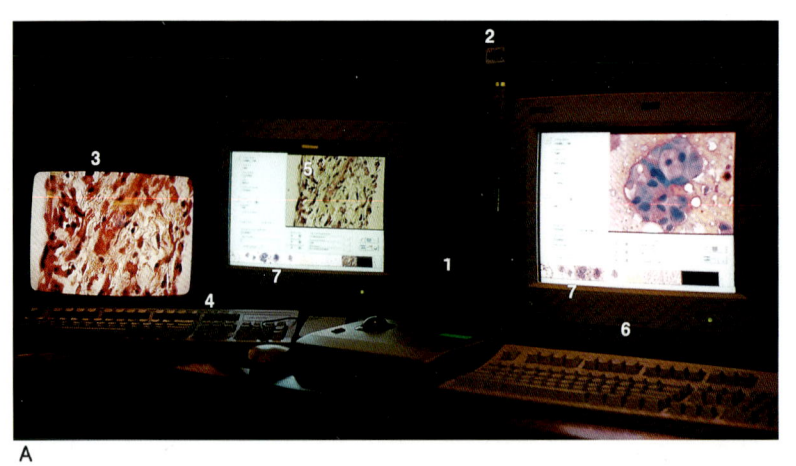

COLOR PLATES

D

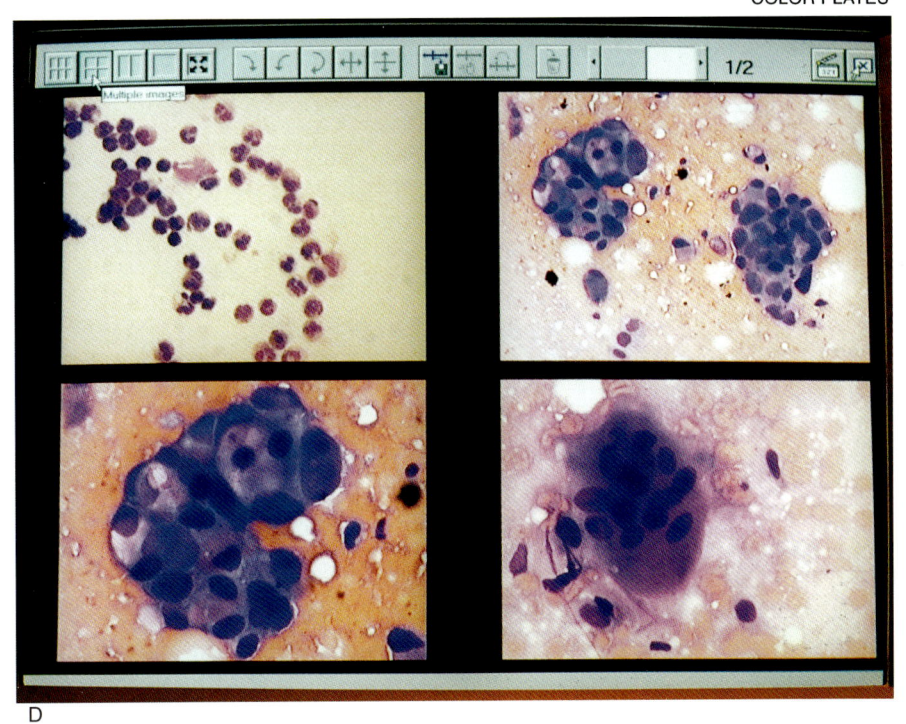

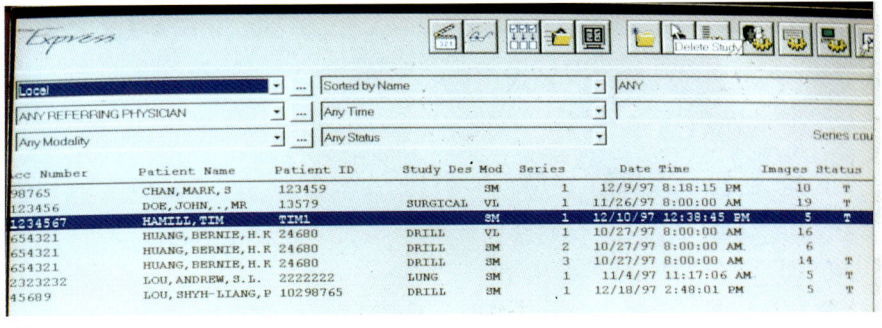

E

Figure 5.20 A digital telemicroscopic system. (A) *Left:* Image acquisition workstation, automatic microscope (1); CCD camera (2); video monitor (3); computer with an A/D converter attached to the CCD, an image memory, a database to manage the patient image file (4); the video monitor (3) showing a life image from the microscope, which is being digitized and shown on the workstation monitor (5). *Right:* Remote diagnostic workstation (6). Thumbnail images at bottom of both workstations are images have been captured and sent to the diagnostic workstation from the acquisition workstation (7). (B) Close-up of the acquisition workstation. Pertinent data related to the exam are shown in various windows. Icons on the bottom right (8) are six simple click-and-play functions: transmit, display, exit, patient information, video capture, digitize, and store. The last captured image (9) is shown on the workstation monitor. (C) Both the acquisition and the diagnostic workstations are displaying the same image for teleconsultation (i). (D) Four-on-one display format showing the first four thumbnail images (see b, bottom row) on one screen of the workstation. The top-row icons are simple image display, manipulation, and transmission functions. (E) Sample patient directory page. The top-row icons are basic user interface functions. [Prototype telemicroscopic imaging system at the Laboratory for Radiological Informatic Lab, UCSF. Courtesy of Drs. S. Atwater, T. Hamill, and H. Sanchez (images); and Nikon Research Corp. and Mitra Imaging, Inc. (equipment).]

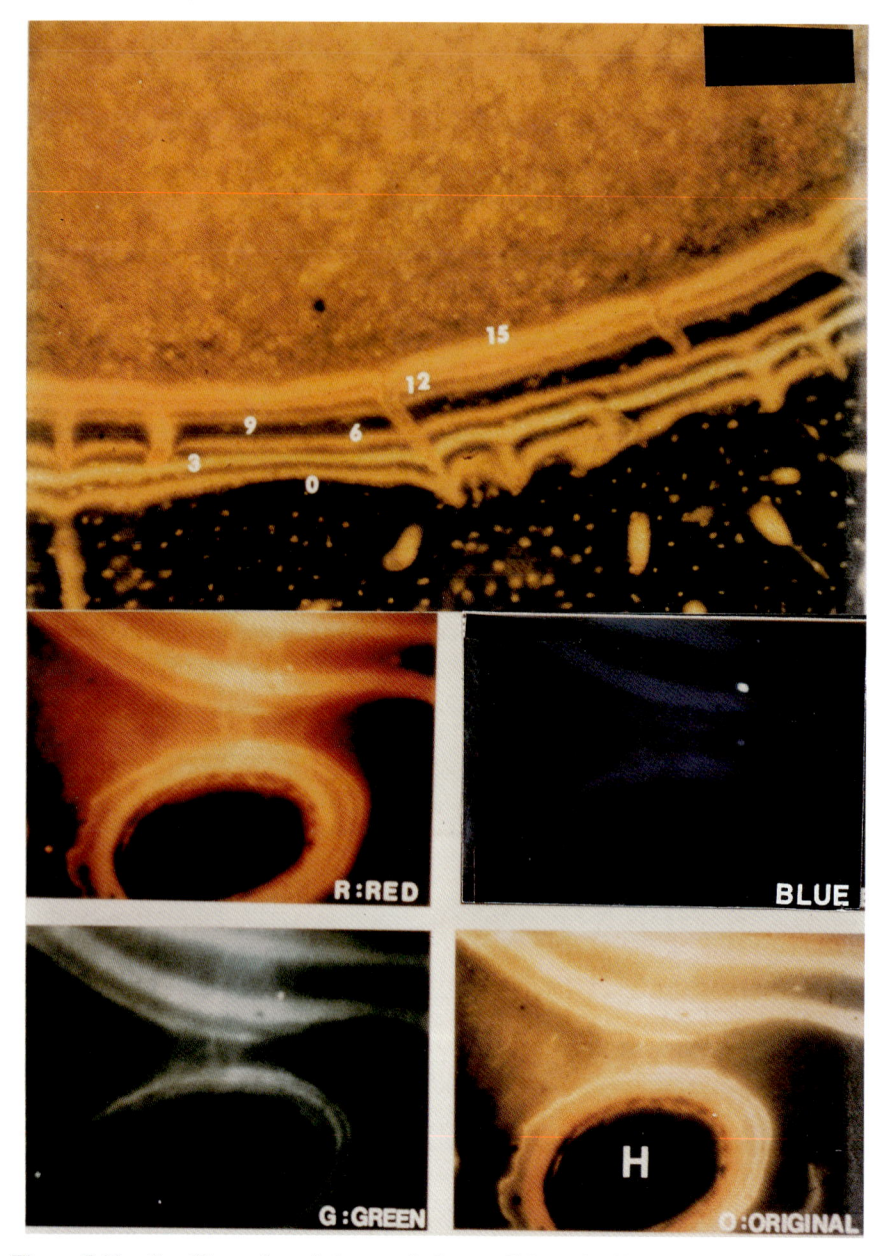

Figure 5.22 *Top:* Fluorochromic image of a bone cell from the tibia of a rat bone biopsy sample with tetracycline labels shown in orange-red. Each label has its own color characteristics: day 0, oxytetracycline label; day 3, DCAF; day 6, xylenol orange, 90 mg/kg; day 9, hematoporphyrin, 300 mg/kg (did not stain); day 12, doxycycline; day 15, alizarin red 5. The dose is 20 mg/kg. *Lower series:* Partial osteonal unit depicting the osteoid and the Haversian canal (H); one tetracycline label is shown in orange-red, the inside ring immediately adjacent to H. The three color images red, blue, and green are also shown.

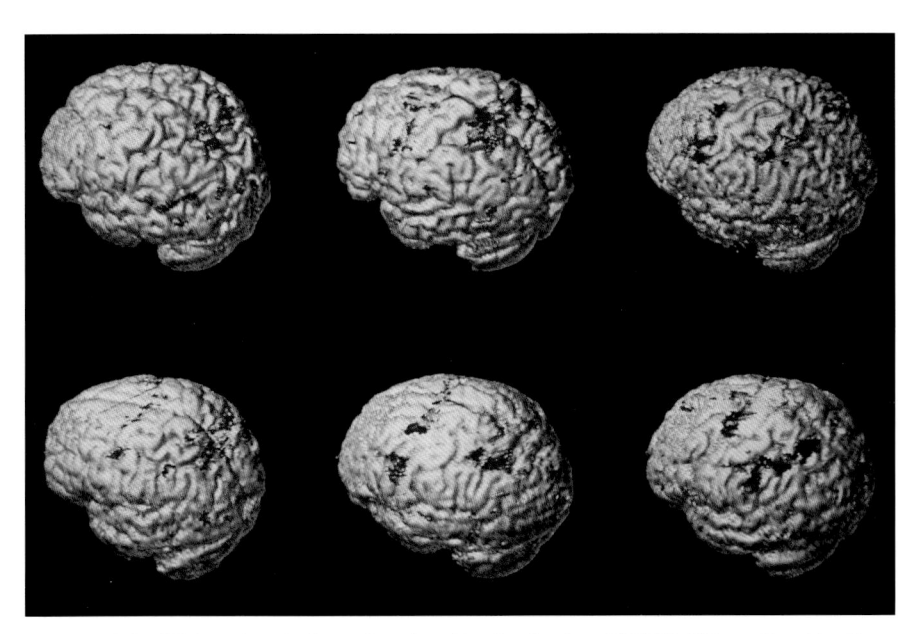

Figure 12.6 High end analysis workstation (Reality Station, ONYX, Silicon Graphics Computer Systems, Mountain View, CA) at UCSF showing 3-D rendering of MR (gray scale) and PET (red) fusion brain images. (Courtesy of K. Soo Hoo)

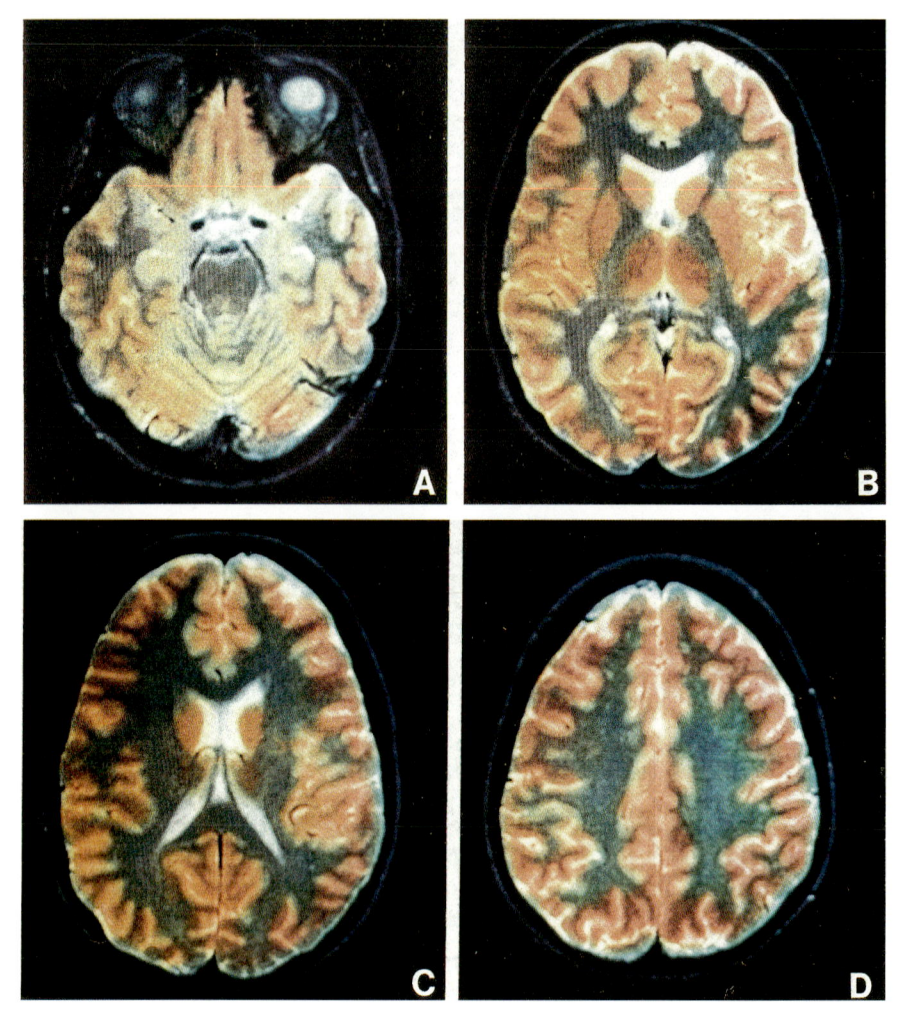

Figure 17.4 Mapping of 2-D brain function (PET, color) to anatomy (MRI, gray scale). Areas of high activity are colored red and orange, whereas lower activity are green and blue: (A) midbrain, (B) striatum, (C) head of the caudate, and (D) anterior pole of the cortex. (Courtesy of D. Valentino.)

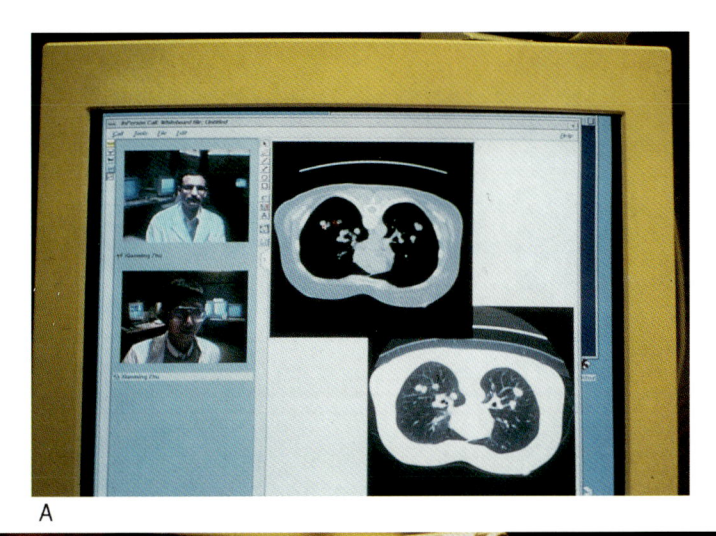

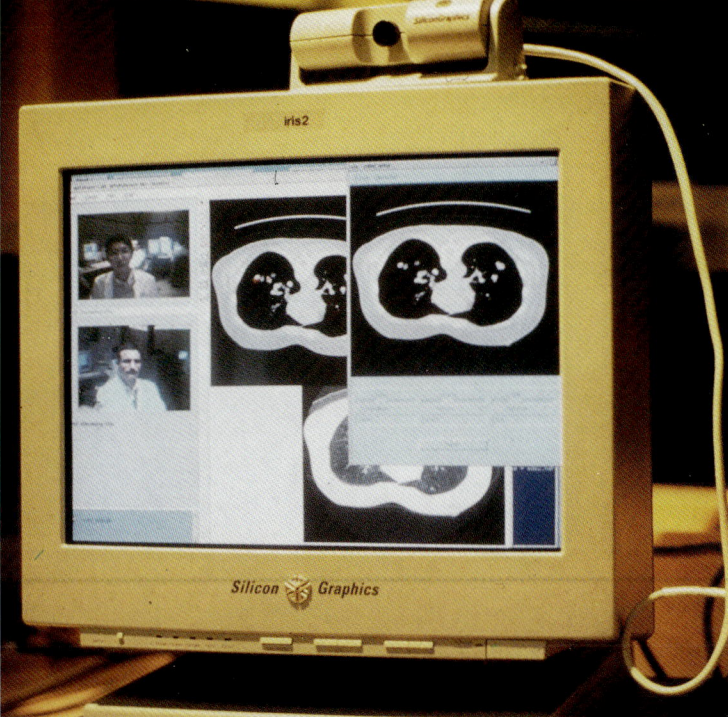

Figure 17.6 Video/image conferencing with PACS images at two workstations. (A) A video/image conferencing workstation with the left window showing two participants; right window shows two CT chest images with one active (controlled by this workstation) and one passive (controlled by the other workstation) arrows pointing to two lesions. CT images are shown with 8 bits/pixel without LUT capability. (B) The workstation at the other site with the participants in reverse positions. The two arrows are also in reversed positions. A third CT image has been requested by this workstation but it has not appeared in the first workstation yet. (Courtesy of Xiaoming Zhu.)

COLOR PLATES

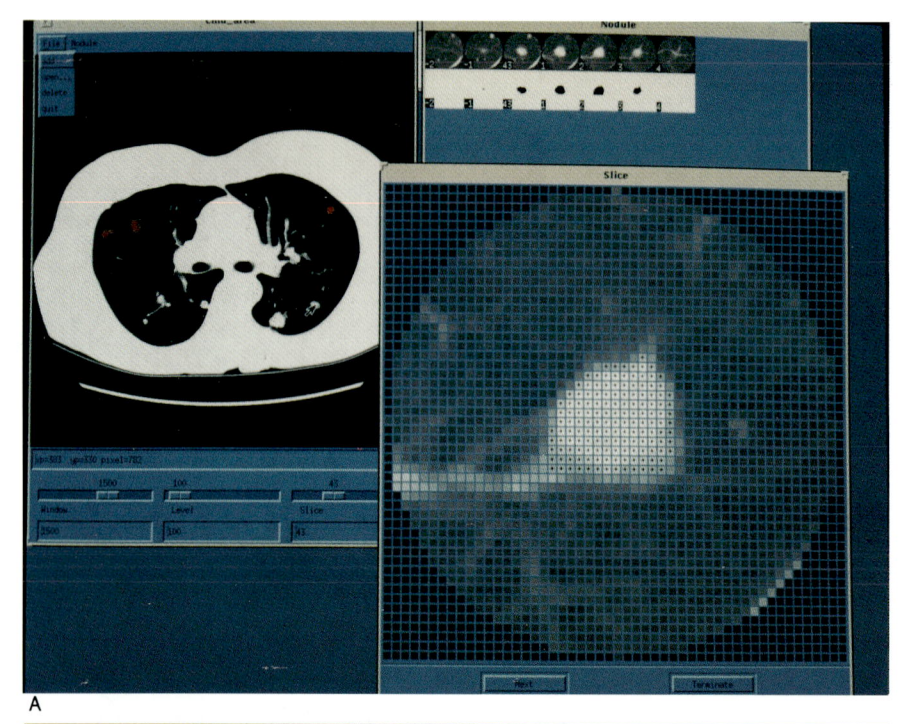

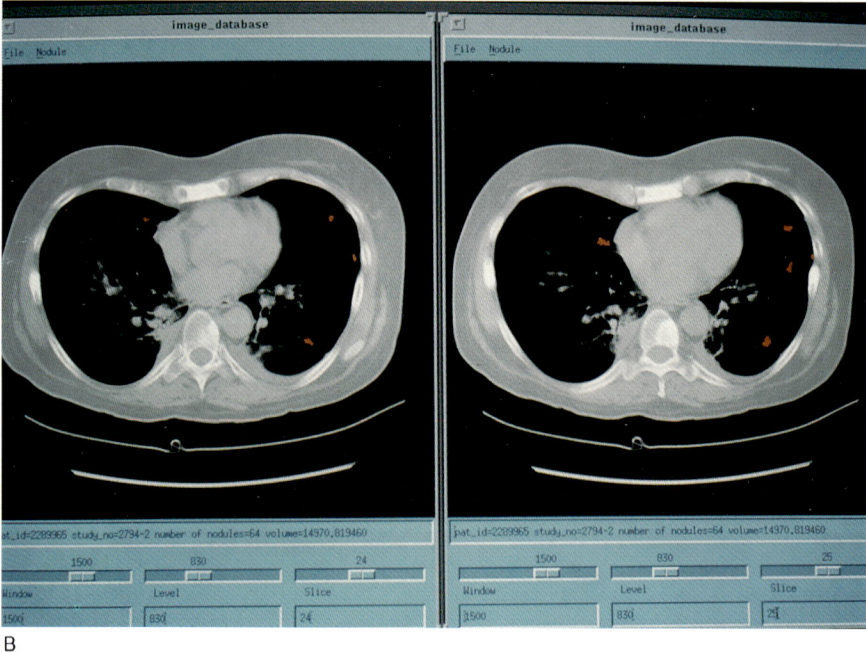

Figure 18.5 (A) Three windows in the graphic user interface. *Left:* a CT image. *Lower right:* an enlarged segmented nodule; + signs are the lesion pixels. *Upper right:* segmented nodules from CT scans stored in the chest image database. (B) Processed nodules in a CT image is turned "red" color to ensure that a nodule is not processed twice. Two consecutive sections are shown.

quires planning because the destinations usually do not have existing cables. In planning the cables for image distribution, the horizontal run and the vertical run should be considered separately. The vertical runs, which determine several strategical risers by taking advantage of existing telecommunication closets in the building, usually are planned first. From these closets vertical cables are run for the connection to various floors. Horizontal cables are then installed from the closets to different hub rooms, to NDC, to BDF, to IDF, and finally to the image workstation areas. All cables at the workstation areas should be terminated with proper connectors and should have enough cable slack for termination and troubleshooting.

Horizontal run cables should be housed in conduits. Since installing conduits is expensive, it is advisable whenever possible to put in a larger conduit than is needed initially, to accommodate future expansion. Very often, the installation of conduits calls for drilling holes through floors and fire walls (core drilling). Drilling holes in a confined environment like a small telephone cable closet in a hospital is a tedious and tricky task. Extreme care has to be exercised. It is important to check for the presence of any pipes or cables that may be embedded in the concrete. In addition, each hole should be at least three times the diameter of the cables being installed, to allow for future expansion and to meet fire code regulations. The following tips will also be useful when planning the installation of cables.

1. Always look for existing conduits and cables, to avoid duplication.
2. If possible, use Plenum cables (fire retardant) for horizontal runs.
3. When installing cables from a BDF to multiple IDFs or from IDF to various rooms, use fiber whenever possible. If the distance is long and if future distribution to other remote sites through this route is possible, install at least twice as many fibers as planned for the short term.
4. Label all cables and fibers at both ends with meaningful names that will not change in the near future (e.g., room numbers, building/floor number).

9.3 VIDEO BROADBAND COMMUNICATION TECHNOLOGY

9.3.1 Broadband Technology

A broadband video communication system employs single or double cables that can be tapped anywhere along the cable length for immediate two-way access to information. The term "broadband" refers to the transmission of information over a wide band of radio frequencies (RF). Information is encoded and modulated to the RF range (5–450 MHz), and demodulated and decoded at the receiving end, very much as in cable television technology.

In particular, a broadband communication system in the context of digital image networks uses a mix of modulation, encoding, and channel allocation to create a two-way communication system that allows both digital and analog information transfer. The capability of transmitting both digital and analog information in a single cable makes a broadband system very attractive to a digital radiology department.

9.3.1.1 Broadband Video

Video information is presented at the display monitor of an imaging device or a workstation as RS-170 analog signals. To place this baseband (base frequency, 30 frames of 525-line video per second) signal onto the broadband cable, the signal must first be frequency-modulated onto a broadband channel. Television channel names are simply numerical designators for particular frequency bands on a broadband system. Each channel actually occupies 6 MHz of radio frequency signal somewhere between 5 and 450 MHz. Only 4.2 MHz of the 6 MHz channel is used for video signal; the remaining 1.8 MHz serves as a buffer or guard between adjacent channels. Video modulators take the RS-170 signal and modulate it onto a broadband carrier operating within the specified band. This signal is then placed onto the broadband cable and mixed with the other channels present.

At the receiving end of the system, a television tuner (broadband demodulator) simply tunes to the appropriate RF channel and demodulates the video information back into RS-170 video, which can be displayed on a video monitor. Theoretically, video information can occupy the entire 5–450 MHz spectrum, thus yielding a total of 74 possible channels. The use of conventional broadcast video equipment allows the use of the predefined television channel system, resulting in a total of 60 available channels. Thus, as many as sixty $512 \times 512 \times 8$ images can be transmitted in a single cable at any instant of time.

9.3.1.2 Broadband Digital

Digital information travels in a broadband cable much as a video signal travels. In this case, the digital information is first encoded as voltage changes, then is modulated onto one or more video channels. Unlike video, a single digital signal requires a rather small band of the available channel. For example, a 19.2 Kbaud terminal theoretically requires only a 19.2 kHz channel; thus a 4.2 MHz video channel can accommodate the communication requirement of 200 terminals. Figure 9.14 shows the digital and video channel designations in a typical broadband communication system.

9.3.1.3 Two-Way Broadband Communication

Central to the design of a broadband system is the idea of a central retransmission facility (CRF: sometimes called the head end). This facility allows the use of a single cable broadband system or two-way communication. The CRF resides at one end of the cable system. The cable system branches out from the CRF in a tree pattern (see Fig. 9.1b) with the CRF at its root. Components such as taps and frequency dividers are designed to allow free flow of certain frequency ranges only in certain directions. Thus, the term *inbound* refers to signals moving toward the CRF and *outbound* refers to signals moving away from the CRF.

In a single cable system, the frequency spectrum is divided into a return band and a forward band, separated by a guard band (Fig. 9.14). Transmitting devices always transmit toward the CRF using the return band. A channel in the return band is received at the CRF, and its frequency is shifted by a frequency translator to a higher

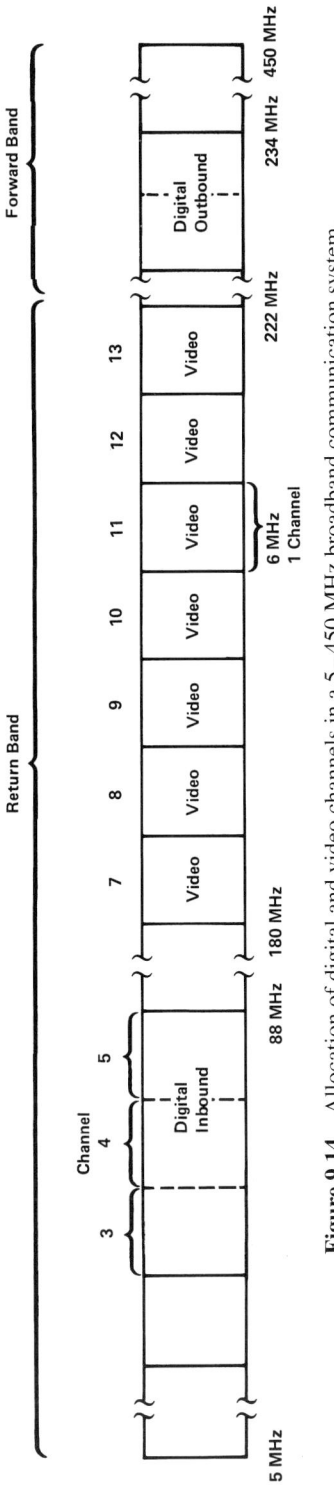

Figure 9.14 Allocation of digital and video channels in a 5–450 MHz broadband communication system.

frequency channel in the forward band. This frequency-shifted signal is then retransmitted outbound from the CRF in the forward band. The outband signals are available at any tap by a demodulator tuned to this higher frequency on the cable tree.

This split-frequency scheme for two-way communication can be applied to both video and digital information. Consider the RS-232 connection, which has both transmit and receive data lines. To use these connections on a broadband system, the RS-232 connector is plugged into a modulator/demodulator box (modem) that contains both transmit and receive electronics. Each modem has its own unique address and, when in operation, is logically connected to other modems via broadband cable. This logical connection is established by modem hardware or software switches. When a keypress is made on a broadband-connected terminal, the RS-232 signals go out the transmit line of the RS-232 cable to the modem. This signal is then packaged along with a source and destination address. The packet containing the data and the addresses is then encoded and modulated onto a low frequency carrier. The low frequency signal, in turn, is placed on the broadband cable, where it travels inbound and is received by the CRF. The frequency translator at the CRF adds a fixed-frequency offset to the signal (e.g., 216 MHz) and retransmits the higher frequency signal outbound. This outbound signal is received by all the modems on the network, but the packet source modem also listens to the message and verifies that it was retransmitted properly. This talk-low, listen-high strategy allows full-featured bidirectional communication. As mentioned, video information can be transmitted in a similar fashion except that no CRF is required if the transmission is unidirectional communication.

The discussion so far has concentrated on a single-cable system. Dual-cable systems are similar in architecture but have the advantage that one cable can be designated inbound and the other outbound. The CRF has only to amplify inbound signals and route them to the outbound cable, without recourse to frequency shifting. In this way, the effective bandwidth of the cable system is doubled (i.e., a full 450 MHz for inbound and 450 MHZ for outbound).

9.3.2 Fiber-Optic Broadband Video Communication System

9.3.2.1 Background

This section gives an example of how to utilize a fiber-optic broadband video communication system for real-time monitoring of patient CT/MR studies in a large imaging center with multiple CT and MR scanners. This system allows a technologist to transmit CT/MR images to a radiologist in real time for immediate consultation while the patient is being scanned. The radiologist, viewing the images generated during the examination without being physically in the scanner room, can instruct the technologist to continue, change the protocol, or abort the study. The radiologist can also monitor multiple scanners with the broadband system at the same time.

Traditional broadband systems use coaxial cable, which has high signal loss, a disadvantage that limits the distance between the input image source and the output viewing station. The fiber-optic broadband system minimizes the signal loss and can potentially connect scanners with a radius of 5.0 km.

9.3.2.2 Modeling

To design a fiber-optic broadband video network, we first derive a model to describe the signal loss characteristics due to various components in the communication system. The model

$$SL = F(B, D, M, C, W, TR) \qquad (9.2)$$

describes the signal loss SL of the image during the transmission as a function of the image bandwidth B, the distance between two nodes D, the mode of the fiber M, the fiber connector type C, the wavelength of the light source W, and the characteristics of the optical transmitter/receiver pair TR. As a first approximation, we assume that F is a linear combination of all these variables.

In this model, the losses associated with D, M, C, and W can be measured through the existing fiber-optic cables using an optical time domain reflectometer (OTDR). The CT/MR images output video signal have a known bandwidth, which is approximately 25 MHz with a horizontal scan rate of 33.36 kHz (1120 lines). The total video signal loss that is acceptable for a system in clinical use is -20 dB based on visual inspection. From this information the optical transmitter/receiver pair can be specified for this system. Unfortunately, the current "off-the-shelf" optical transmitter/receiver pair available can accommodate only a 10 MHz video signal bandwidth. Therefore, it is necessary to reduce the bandwidth of the transmitted video signal from 25 MHz to 10 MHz in two stages. First, the video signal is reduced from a 25 MHz to a 10 MHz; then the 10 MHz video signals are transformed to optical signals for transmission. This can be accomplished by using a fiber-optic laser transmitter tuned to 10 MHz (X285TV-V5, Meret, Inc., Santa Monica, CA). The result is equivalent to passing the image through a low pass filter; hence degradation of the image quality is minor.

9.3.2.3 Broadband Video Communication System

The multiplexed broadband video communication system is an established means of video image transmission. The term "multiplexed" refers to the method of modulating and combining multiple baseband (single video) signals into a composite broadband signal, effectively using a single broadband (relatively wide bandwidth) cable to transmit multiple-baseband (relatively narrow bandwidth) channels.

Real-time video images (10 MHz) are transmitted from CT/MR scanners to the head end, where they are converted to specific ranges of radio frequencies and distributed to receivers in a manner similar to that found in cable television technology. The communication medium used is either a multimode (shorter distance) or a single mode (longer distance) fiber-optic cable. The 512 × 512 × 8 (CT) and 256 × 256 × 8 (MR) pixel images can be assigned to a given channel (10 MHz in bandwidth) in the 5–450 MHz frequency range. The procedure of the operation is as follows (see Fig. 9.15):

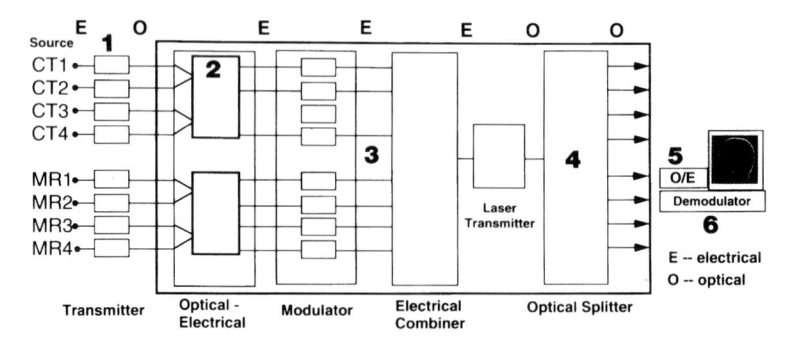

Figure 9.15 Detailed schematic diagram of a fiber-optic broadband system with a connection to eight CT/MR scanners and eight monitoring stations. The head end is the large rectangular box encompassing steps 2 to 4. Numerals designate steps described in text.

1. The video signal at the scanner is converted from an electrical to an optical signal before it is transmitted to a head end.
2. The video signal is received at the head end; it is converted back from an optical to an electrical signal.
3. The signal is multiplexed (modulated and combined) with the other scanner video signals, creating a multiplexed, broadband video signal.
4. The broadband signal is converted from an electrical to an optical splitter, where the signal is distributed to all monitoring stations.
5. At the monitoring station, the optical broadband signal is converted back to an electrical signal, demodulated (i.e., a channel is selected), and displayed on a viewing monitor.
6. Each monitor station consists of an optical receiver, a demodulator (channel selector), and a modified Conrac 1023-line, progressive scan, 8-bit video monitor (Duarte, CA).

Figure 9.15 shows the schematic of the video communication system for eight scanners and eight remote monitoring stations. Monitoring stations are placed in clinical locations such as the thoracic, neurological, abdominal, musculoskeletal, gastrointestinal, genitourinary, and pediatric radiology reading rooms. Figure 9.16A shows how a monitoring station can be connected with a high resolution video tape recording system for video image archive. Figure 9.16B illustrates displays on two remote monitoring stations: two different images from two MR scanners are shown simultaneously and in real time.

9.3.2.4 Clinical Operation

In any of the monitor stations, a radiologist/physician, by selecting the proper channel assigned to the scanner, can view a patient's CT/MR examination in real time while the study is being performed. The radiologist can communicate with the technologist by a telephone to monitor the examination.

VIDEO BROADBAND COMMUNICATION TECHNOLOGY   261

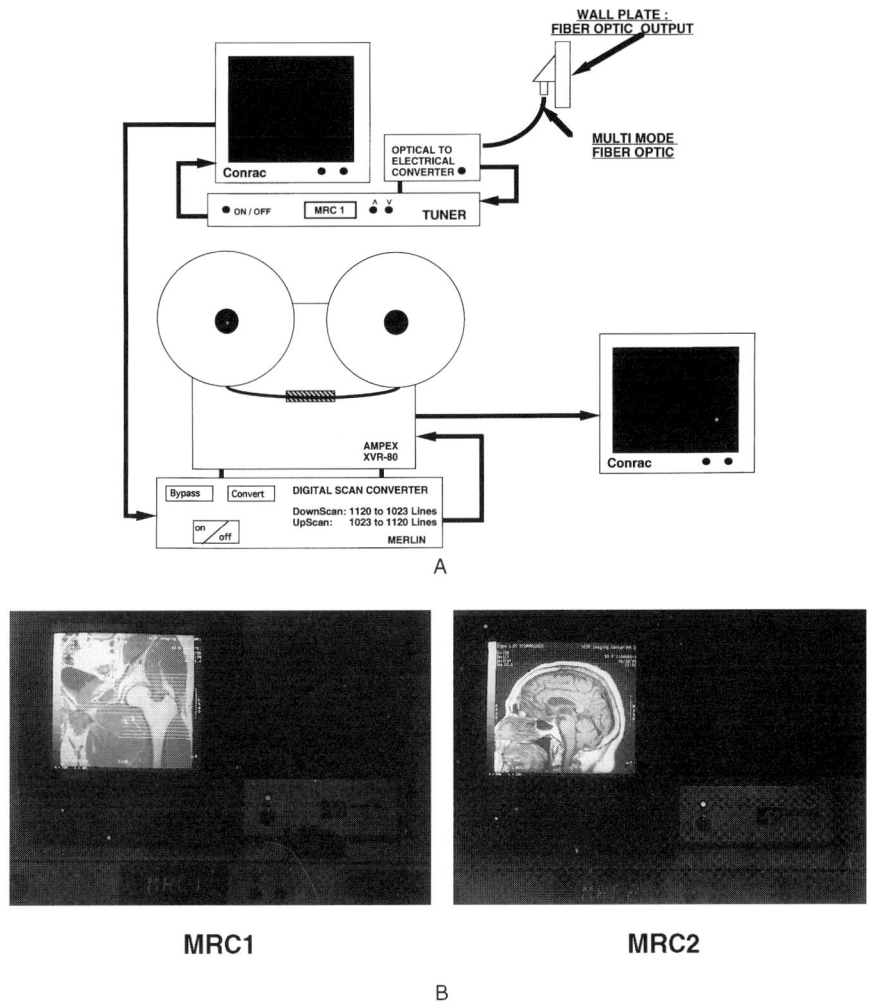

Figure 9.16 (A) A monitoring station tuned to the MR scanner (MRC1) is connected to a high resolution video tape recording system for archive. (B) Two monitoring stations at UCSF showing two different images from two MR scanners (MRC1, and MRC2), simultaneously and in real time. The stations are tuned to different channels.

This fiber-optic broadband communication system has the two advantages of being inexpensive and capable of transmitting images from many sources in real time. The system can be used primarily as a CT/MR examination monitoring system. The system also has some disadvantages, however. First, image quality may not be sufficient for primary diagnosis because the image transmitted to the video monitor is of a lower bandwidth. Second, images appearing on the monitor are volatile and therefore cannot be stored or retrieved later.

To obtain temporary image archiving, this system can be connected to a high resolution video tape recording system (Ampex XVR-80, San Fernando, CA). This video recorder coupled with a DownScan Converter from Merlin Engineering (Palo Alto, CA) can be connected to any of the monitoring stations to record images from any of the scanners. The resolution of the images saved in this video recorder is equivalent to what appeared on the monitor.

9.4 DIGITAL COMMUNICATION NETWORKS

9.4.1 Background

Within the PACS infrastructure, the digital communication network is responsible for transmission of images from acquisition devices to the PACS controller and then to display workstations. First, images are transmitted from imaging modality devices to image acquisition gateway computers, where the images are staged and reformatted. The reformatted images are sent to the PACS controller, where they are archived permanently and categorized in the PACS database. After images have been categorized, they are routed to workstations for display—either soft copy or hard copy. Many computers and processors are involved in this image communication chain: some have high speed processors and communication protocols and some do not. Therefore, in designing this network, a mixture of communication technologies must be used to accommodate the various computers and processors. The ultimate goal is to have an optimal image throughput in a given clinical environment.

Table 9.8 describes the image transmission rate requirements of PACS. Transmission from the imaging modality device to the acquisition gateway computer is slow because the imaging modality device is generally slow in generating images. The medium speed requirement from the acquisition computer to the PACS controller depends on the type of acquisition gateway computer used. High speed communication between the PACS controller and image display workstations is necessary because radiologists and clinicians must access images at a rapid rate. In general, 4 Mbyte/s, equivalent to transfer of a $2048 \times 2048 \times 8$ bit conventional digitized X-ray image in one second, is the average tolerable waiting time for the physician.

9.4.2 Design Criteria

The five design criteria for the implementation of digital communication networks for PACS are speed, standardization, fault tolerance, security, and component cost.

9.4.2.1 Speed of Transmission

Table 9.8 demonstrates that Ethernet should be used as the communication network (slow speed) between imaging devices and acquisition gateway computers. For image transfer between acquisition computers and the image archive servers, FDDI (medium speed) or ATM should be used if the acquisition computer supports the tech-

TABLE 9.8 Characteristics of Image Transmission in PACS

	Image Modality Device to Acquisition Gateway Computer	Acquisition Gateway Computer to PACS Controller	PACS Controller to Display Workstations
Speed requirement	Slow: 100 kbyte/s	Medium: 200–500 Kbyte/s	Fast: 4 Mbyte/s
Technology	Ethernet	Ethernet/FDDI/ATM/fast or gigabit Ethernet	ATM/fast or gigabit Ethernet
Signaling rate, Mbit/s	10	100, 155, 1000	100, 155, 1000
Cost per connection, units	1	1–10	10

nology; otherwise, Ethernet switch is acceptable. For image transfer between the PACS controller and an image display station, ATM or fast or gigabit Ethernet should be used.

9.4.2.2 Standardization

The throughput performance for each of the three networks described earlier (Ethernet, FDDI, and ATM) can be tuned through the judicious choice of software and operating system parameters. For example, the throughput of networks using TCP/IP can be increased by enlarging the TCP send and receive buffer within the UNIX kernel for Ethernet, FDDI, and ATM network circuits. Alternatively, transmission speed may be enhanced by increasing the memory data buffer size in the application program. The altering of standard network protocols to increase network throughput between a client/server pair can be very effective. The same strategy may prove disastrous in a large communication network, however, since it interferes with network standardization, making it difficult to maintain and service the network. All network circuits should use standard TCP/IP network protocols with a standard buffer size (e.g., 8192 bytes).

9.4.2.3 Fault Tolerance

Communications in the PACS infrastructure should have a backup. All active fiber-optic cables have a duplicate, as does the Ethernet backbone (thicknet and twisted pair). Since the standard TCP/IP protocol can be used over all three networks (Ethernet, FDDI, and ATM), in the event of failure of the higher speed network circuit (ATM, FDDI, fast Ethernet, gigabit Ethernet), the socket-based communications software immediately switches over to the next fastest network, and so forth, until all network circuits have been exhausted. The global Ethernet backbone, through which every computer on the PACS network is connected, is the ultimate backup for the entire PACS network.

9.4.2.4 Security

There are normally two cable systems in an imaging network. The first comprises the cables leased or shared with the campus or hospital, managed by the central network authority (CNA). In this case, users should abide by the rules established by the CNA. Once these cables have been connected, the CNA enforces its own security measures and provides service and maintenance.

The second cable system consists of the PACS cables, which are enclosed inside conduits with terminations at the hub rooms. The hub rooms should be locked, and no one should be allowed to enter without authorization from a departmental or PACS official.

The global Ethernet should be monitored around the clock with a LAN analyzer. The FDDI and ATM are closed systems and cannot be tapped in. Security should be set up such that authorized hospital personnel can access the network to view patient images displayed at a workstation, similar to the setup at a film library or film light box. Only authorized users are allowed to copy images and deposit information into the PACS database through the network.

9.4.2.5 Costs

The digital communication network is designed for clinical use and should be built as a very robust system with redundancy. Cost, although of importance, should not be compromised in the selection of components. Of the three network technologies mentioned, if we consider Ethernet to have a unit cost, then FDDI, ATM, and gigabit Ethernet would have a cost of 10 units for each computer connection.

9.5. PACS NETWORK DESIGN

PACS networks can be either external or internal. External networks have minimum security and are connected to other information systems, imaging devices, and workstations from the outside world. Internal networks, which have maximum security and are accessible only through layers of security measures, are networks connecting to components within the PACS controller. Another look at Figure 1.1 will emphasize that all networks except those inside the PACS controller are external networks.

9.5.1 External Networks

9.5.1.1 Manufacturer's Image Acquisition Device Network

Major image manufacturers have their own networks for connecting imaging devices for better image management. Examples are the General Electric Medical Systems Genesis network and Sienet of Siemens Medical Systems for connecting the respective vendors' CT and MR scanners. Most of these networks are Ethernet based; some use the TCP/IP protocols, and others use proprietary protocols for higher network throughput. If such a network is already in existence, the acquisition gateway computer must be connected to this manufacturer's acquisition device network before CT and MR images can be transmitted to the PACS controller (see Figs. 8.5 and 8.6). This network has no security with respect to the PACS infrastructure because every user with a password can have access to the network and obtain all information passing through it.

9.5.1.2 Hospital and Radiology Information Networks

Hospital and university campuses usually have a campus central network authority that operates the institutional network. Among the information systems that go through this network are the HIS and RIS. Since PACS requires data from both HIS and RIS, this portion of the PACS network is maintained by the campus network authority, over which the PACS network has no control. For this reason, as far as the PACS infrastructure design is concerned, the hospital network is an external network of the PACS.

9.5.1.3 Research and Other Networks

One major function of PACS is to allow users to access the wealth of the PACS database. A research network can be set up for connecting research equipment to the PACS. Research equipment should allow access to the PACS database for information query and retrieval but not to deposit information. In the PACS infrastructure design, this type of research network is considered an external network.

9.5.1.4 The Internet

A network carrying information from outside the hospital or the campus through the Internet is considered an external network in the PACS infrastructure design. Such a network carries supplemental information for the PACS, ranging from electronic mail and library information systems to data files available through FTP.

9.5.1.5 Display Workstation Networks

Sometimes it is advantageous to have display workstations of similar nature to form a subnetwork for the sharing of information. For example, workstations in a hospital intensive care unit can form an ICU network and neurology workstations can form a neuro network. These display workstation networks are open to all health care personnel to use, and therefore only a minimum security can be imposed. Too much in the way of restrictions would deter users from logging on. However, certain layers of priority can be imposed; for example, some users may be permitted to access the network but not to use it for deposit.

9.5.2 Internal Networks

A PACS internal network, on the other hand, has the maximum security. Data inside the internal network are considered to be clinical data to be archived; they cannot be corrupted. Both image and textual data from acquisition devices and other information systems coming from all the external networks just described except those of display workstations must go through a gateway computer, where data are checked and scrutinized for authenticity before they are allowed to be deposited in the internal network. Fire wall machines are sometimes incorporated into the gateway computer for this purpose. Only the PACS manager is authorized to allow data to be deposited to the archive through the internal network.

9.5.3 An Example

The PACS network at the University of California at San Francisco (as of January 1997: Fig. 16.1) is an example of a comprehensive PACS. In this architecture, there are several external networks: wide area network (WAN), campus network, departmental network, the Laboratory for Radiological Informatics (LRI) research network, the Internet, the PACS external network, and workstation networks.

9.5.3.1 Wide Area Network (WAN)

The WAN is used to connect UCSF main campus radiology department with radiology departments from affiliated hospitals and clinics in the San Francisco Bay area. The standard connection is the T1 line (Fig. 9.6 top: Frame access) with 1.5 Mbit/s and the ATM OC3 with a transmission rate of 155 Mbit/s (Fig. 9.6 bottom, ASX 200).

9.5.3.2 The Departmental Ethernet

The departmental Ethernet connects 150 Macintosh users in the department. This network is mainly for file transfer and electronic mail, and as a connection to the department image file server, which allows Macintosh users access to the PACS image database and the RIS database. This network is connected to the Laboratory for Radiological Informatics research network through a bridge that allows Macintosh users access to images generated from research equipment. Macintosh users can also have access to the Internet through the campus network. HIS, RIS, and digital voice information are transmitted to the PACS controller first through the campus network and then through the departmental network.

9.5.3.3 LRI Research Network

The Laboratory for Radiological Informatics research network connects all research equipment in the laboratory, including image acquisition devices, laser film scanners, laser film printers, image processing computers, research image file servers, display workstations, and the PACS image file server. It also connects to the departmental Ethernet through a bridge.

9.5.3.4 PACS External Network

The PACS external network connects all clinical digital image acquisition devices in the department, including CT, MR, and CR units, film digitizers, and the nuclear medicine PACS and US PACS modules. All 1K and 2K clinical viewing workstations are also connected through this network. The WAN ATM gateway and the T1 lines are connected to this network via a router and an ATM gateway computer.

9.5.3.5 PACS Internal Network

The PACS internal network is a secured network that connects the PACS controller and the PACS database to the PACS external network. The router and the fire wall machine protect the internal network by screening all incoming information to the PACS controller. The internal network transmits image files from the PACS image database to the 1K and 2K display stations for clinical use. Macintosh users can also access image files from the PACS controller through the departmental Mac image server.

Chapter 10
PACS Controller and Image Archive

The PACS central node, the engine of the PACS (see Figs. 1.1 and 9.17), has two components: the PACS controller and an image storage management system. The former, consisting of the hardware and software architecture, uses interprocess communication among major processes to direct the data flow in the complete PACS. The latter provides a hierarchical image storage management system for short-, medium-, and long-term image archiving. Section 10.1 describes the design concept and implementation strategy of the PACS central node and Section 10.2 presents the system software.

10.1 IMAGE MANAGEMENT DESIGN CONCEPT

Two major aspects should be considered in the design of the PACS image storage management system: data integrity, which promises no loss of images once received by the PACS from the imaging systems; and system efficiency, which minimizes access time for images at the display workstations. Now we turn to some major issues in storage management system design.

10.1.1 Local Storage Management Via PACS Intercomponent Communication

To ensure data integrity, the PACS always retains two copies of an individual image on separate storage devices until the image has been archived successfully to the long-term storage device (e.g., an optical disk or tape library). Figure 10.1 shows the various storage subsystems in the PACS. This backup scheme is achieved via the PACS intercomponent communication system, which can be broken down as follows:

- *At the radiologic imaging device.* Images are not deleted from the imaging device's local storage unless technologists have verified the successful archiving of individual images via the PACS connections. In the event of failure of the acquisition process or of the archive process, images can be re-sent from these imaging devices to the PACS.
- *At the acquisition gateway computer.* Images acquired in the acquisition gateway computer remain on its local magnetic disks until the archive subsystem has

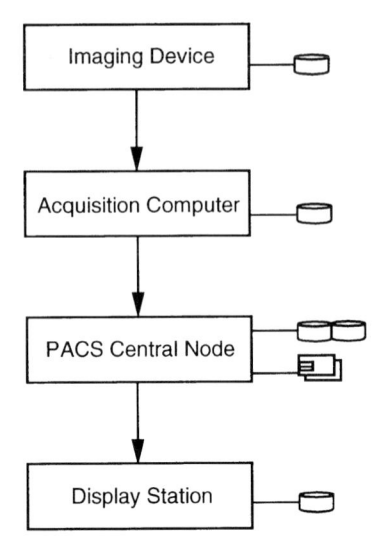

Figure 10.1 Various storage subsystems in the PACS to ensure data integrity. Until an individual image has been archived in the permanent storage (e.g., optical WORM, tape, CD-ROM), two copies of it are retained on separate storage (magnetic) devices.

acknowledged to the acquisition gateway computer that a successful archive has been completed. These images are then deleted from the magnetic disks residing in the acquisition computer, so that storage space from these disks can be reclaimed.

- *At the PACS central node.* Images arriving in the archive server from various acquisition nodes are not deleted until they have been successfully archived to the permanent storage. On the other hand, all archived images are stacked in the archive server's cache magnetic disks and will be deleted based on aging criteria (e.g., number of days ago an examination was performed; discharge or transfer of a patient).
- *At the display workstation.* Images stored in the designated display workstation will remain there until the patient is discharged or transferred. Images in the PACS archive can be retrieved from any display workstation via PACS intercomponent communication.

10.1.2 PACS Controller System Configuration

The archive system consists of four major components: an archive server, a database system, an optical disk library, and a communication network (Fig. 10.2). Attached to the archive system through the communication network are the acquisition computers and the display workstations. Images acquired by the acquisition computers from various radiologic imaging devices are transmitted to the archive server, from which they are archived to the optical disk library and routed to the appropriate display stations.

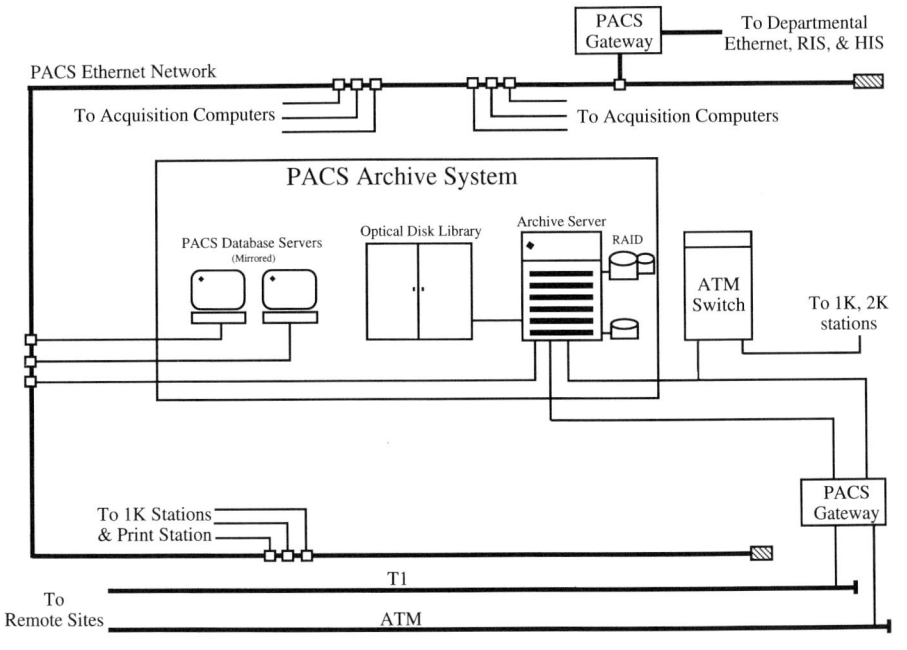

Figure 10.2 The configuration of the archive system and the PACS network. An optical disk library (ODL) for permanent storage is used as an example. The archive server is connected to the ODL and a pair of mirrored database servers. Patient, study, and image directories are stored in the database; images are stored in the ODL. A global Ethernet network interconnects all PACS components, and a high speed ATM network (as an example) connects the archive server to 1K and 2K display workstations, providing fast image display. In addition, the archive server is connected to remote sites via T1 and ATM, and to the hospital information system (HIS) and the radiology information system (RIS) via departmental and campus Ethernet.

10.1.2.1 The Archive Server

The archive server consists of powerful multiple central processing units (CPUs), small computer systems interface (SCSI) data buses, and network interfaces (Ethernet and ATM). With its redundant hardware configuration, the archive server can support multiple processes running simultaneously, and image data can be transmitted over different data buses and networks. In addition to its primary function of archiving images, the archive server acts as a PACS controller, mastering the flow of images within the entire PACS from the acquisition gateway computers to various destinations such as the display workstations or print stations.

The archive server uses its large capacity RAID or magnetic disks as a data cache (Section 10.3.1), capable of storing two weeks' worth of images acquired from different radiologic imaging devices. As an example, a 13.6 Gbyte disk storage, without using compression, can hold simultaneously up to 500 computed tomography, 1000 magnetic resonance, and 500 computed radiography studies. In this example, each CT or MR study consists of a complete sequence of images from one examination, and each CR study consists of one exposure. The calculation is based on the average study sizes in the field, in megabytes: CT, 11.68; MR, 3.47; CR, 7.46. The magnetic cache disks configured in the archive server should sustain high data throughput for the read operation, which provides fast retrieval of recent images from these RAID or magnetic disks instead of the slower optical disks.

10.1.2.2 The Database System

The database system comprises redundant database servers, running identical reliable commercial database systems, (e.g., Sybase, Oracle), with structured query language (SQL) utilities. A mirror database (i.e., two identical databases) can be used to duplicate the data during every PACS transaction involving the server. The data can be queried from any PACS computer via the communication networks. The mirroring feature of the system provides the entire PACS database with uninterruptible data transactions that guarantee no loss of data in the event of system failure or a disk crash.

Besides its primary role of image indexing to support the retrieval of images, the database system is necessary to interface with the radiology information system (RIS) and hospital information system (HIS), allowing the PACS database to collect additional patient information from these two health care databases (Chapter 11).

10.1.2.3 The Archive Library

The archive (optical disk, optical or digital linear tape, CD-ROM) library consists of multiple input/output drives [optical erasable, WORM (write once, read many) disk, optical or digital linear tape, or CD-ROM] and controllers, which allow concurrent archival and retrieval operations on all of its drives. The library needs to have a storage capacity of terabytes and to support mixed storage media. Redundant power supply is essential for uninterrupted operation.

The average overall throughputs for read and write operations between the magnetic disks of the archive server and the optical disks can reach 1.0 Mbyte/s.

10.1.2.4 Backup Archive

To build fault tolerance in the PACS server, a backup archive system can be used. Two copies of identical images can be saved through two different paths in the PACS network to two archive libraries, as described in Section 10.1.2.3. Ideally, the two libraries should be in two different buildings in case of natural disaster. To reduce the cost of redundant archiving, the primary unit can be an optical disk library and the backup an optical or digital linear tape library.

10.1.2.5 The Communication Network

The PACS archive system is connected to both the PACS local area network and the wide area network. The PACS LAN can have a two-tiered communication network composed of Ethernet and ATM or high speed Ethernet networks. The WAN provides connection to remote sites and can consist of T1 lines and ATM.

The PACS LAN uses the high speed ATM or Ethernet switch to transmit high volume image data from the archive server to 1K and 2K display workstations. Low cost standard Ethernet is used for interconnecting slower speed components to the PACS server, including acquisition gateway computers, RIS, and HIS, and as a backup of the ATM or high speed Ethernet. Failure of the high speed network automatically triggers the archive server to reconfigure the communication network so that images will be transmitted to the 1K and 2K display workstations over conventional Ethernet.

10.2 PACS CONTROLLER SYSTEM SOFTWARE

All software implemented in the archive server should be coded in a standard programming language—for example, C and C++ on the UNIX open systems architecture. In the archive server, processes of diverse functions run independently and communicate simultaneously with other processes using client/server programming, queuing control mechanisms, and job prioritizing mechanisms. Figure 10.3 shows the interprocess communications among the major processes running on the archive server and Table 10.1 describes the functions of these processes.

Major tasks performed by the archive server include image receiving, image stacking, image routing, image archiving, studies grouping, platter management, RIS interfacing, PACS database updating, image retrieving, and image prefetching. In this section, erasable optical disk and WORM are used as examples for illustration. The following subsections describe the functionality carried out by each of these tasks.

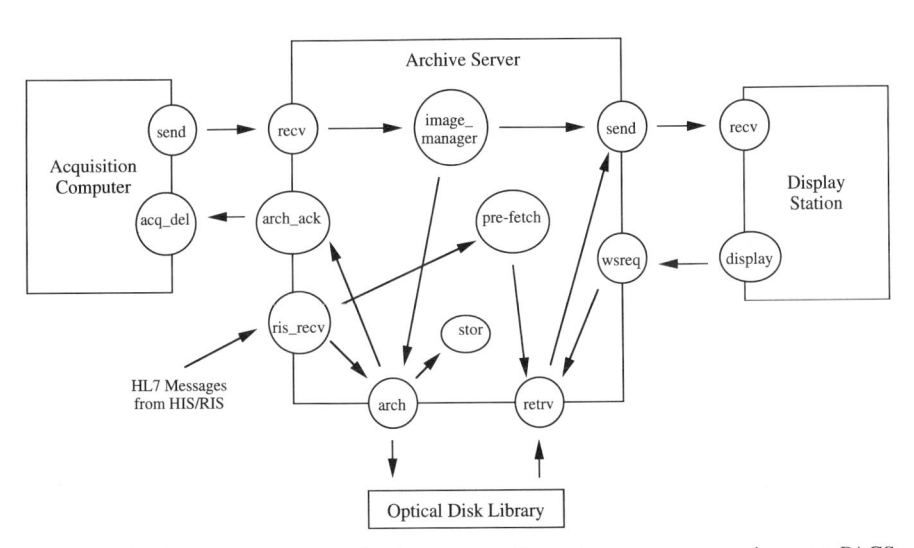

Figure 10.3 Interprocess communications among the major processes running on a PACS archive server: HL7, Health Level 7; other symbols defined in Table 10.1. This archive server does not support DICOM, comparing it with the DICOM-compliant server shown in Figure 10.10.

TABLE 10.1 Major Processes and Their Functions in the Archive Server (see Fig. 10.3)

Process	Description
arch	Copies images from magnetic disks to temporary archive (before patient discharge) and to permanent archive (at patient discharge); updates PACS database; notify *stor* and *arch_ack* processes for successful archiving
arch_ack	Acknowledges acquisition gateway computers for successful archiving
acq_del	Processes at acquisition gateway computers; deletes images from local magnetic disks
image_manager	Processes image information; updates PACS database; notifies *send* and *arch* processes
pre-fetch	Selects historical images and relevant text data from PACS data base; notifies *retrv* process
recv	Receives images from acquisition computers; notifies *image_manager* process
ris_recv	Receives HL7 messages (e.g., patient admission, discharge, and transfer; examination scheduling; impression; diagnostic reports) from the RIS; notifies *arch* process to group and copy images from temporary archive to permanent archive (at patient discharge), notifies *pre-fetch* process (at scheduling of an examination), or updates PACS data base (at receipt of an impression or a diagnostic report)
retrv	Retrieves images from permanent archive; notifies *send* process
send	Sends images to destination workstations
stor	Manages magnetic storage of the archive server
wsreq	Handles retrieve requests from the display process at the *display* workstations
display	Acknowledges archive server for images received

10.2.1 Image Receiving

Images acquired from various radiologic imaging devices in the acquisition gateway computers are converted into DICOM data format. From these acquisition computers, the reformatted images are then transmitted to the archive server via the Ethernet or ATM by using client/server applications over standard TCP/IP protocols. The archive server can accept concurrent connections for receiving images from multiple acquisition computers.

10.2.2 Image Stacking

Images arrived in the archive server from various acquisition computers are stacked in its local magnetic disks. The archive server holds as many images in its RAID or magnetic disks as possible and manages them on the basis of aging criteria. During a hospital stay, for example, images belonging to a given patient remain on the archive server's magnetic disks until the patient is discharged or transferred. Thus all recent images that are not already in a display workstation's local storage can be retrieved from the archive server's high speed magnetic disks instead of the low speed optical disks. This feature is particularly convenient for radiologists or referring physicians who must retrieve images from different display workstations.

10.2.3 Image Routing

Images that have arrived in the archive server from various acquisition computers are immediately routed to their destination display workstations. The routing process is driven by a predefined routing table composed of parameters including examination type, display workstation site, radiologist, and referring physician. All images are classified by examination type (1-view Chest, CT-Head, CT-Body, etc.) as defined in RIS, and the destination display workstations are classified by location (Chest, Pediatrics, CCU, etc.) as well as by resolution (1K or 2K). The routing algorithm performs table lookup based on the aforementioned parameters and determines an image's destination(s).

Images are transmitted to the 1K and 2K workstations over either Ethernet LAN or ATM, and to remote sites over dedicated T1 lines or the ATM WAN.

10.2.4 Image Archiving

Images arriving in the archive server from various acquisition computers are copied from temporary storage on magnetic disks to the erasable optical disks for longer term storage. When transfer to the erasable optical disks is complete, the archive server will acknowledge the corresponding acquisition computer, allowing that system to delete the image from its local storage and reclaim its disk space. In this way, the PACS always has two copies of an image on separate magnetic disk systems until the image is archived to the permanent storage.

Images that belong to a given patient during a hospital stay will be scattered across the erasable optical disks and will remain on these disks until the patient is discharged or transferred.

10.2.5 Studies Grouping

During a hospital stay, a patient may have different examinations on different days. Each of these examinations may consist of multiple studies. Upon discharge or transfer of the patient, images from these studies are grouped from the erasable optical disks and copied contiguously to a single WORM disk or to consecutive WORM disks for permanent storage. Once these images have been archived permanently, they are removed from the erasable optical disks, permitting storage space on the erasable disks to be reclaimed.

10.2.6 Platter/Tape Management

Studies grouping allows all images belonging to a patient during a hospital stay to be archived contiguously to one or more optical disks. Platter management, on the other hand, manages the storage space reserved on the WORM disks for future images in

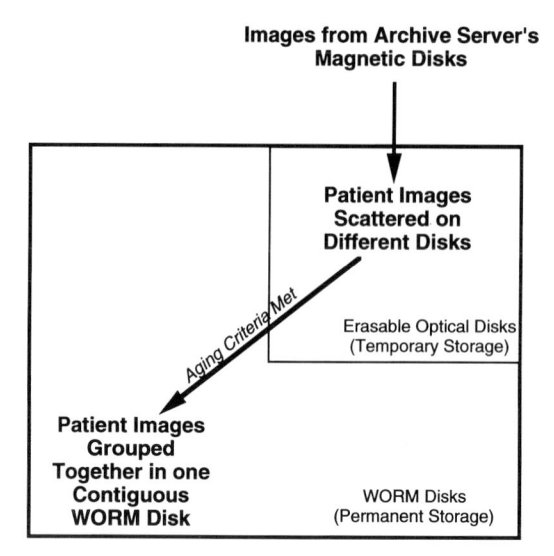

Figure 10.4 Studies grouping and platter management: current images are copied from the magnetic disks of the archive server to erasable optical disks; when an aging criterion is met (e.g., a given patient is discharged or transferred), images belonging to that patient are grouped and copied contiguously to WORM disks or tapes for permanent storage.

case a patient revisits or is readmitted. In this way, images of a patient from multiple hospital visits can be accumulated on a single WORM disk or on consecutive disks, reducing excess disk swapping and, consequently, minimizing retrieval time for these images. It is expensive, however, to preallocate storage space on an optical disk for a particular patient. To minimize the disk space preallocated for individual patients, the storage management software allows the PACS archive process to group multiple optical disks into one volume. In addition to saving disk space, logically grouping consecutive optical disks into one volume can reduce disk swapping time, hence speeding up the retrieval time for images resident on different disks in the same volume. Figure 10.4 illustrates the studies grouping and platter management mechanisms.

A similar concept can be applied to digital linear tapes if they are used for long term archive. In this case, patient images are grouped together before they are written on a tape.

10.2.7 RIS and HIS Interfacing

The archive server accesses the HIS/RIS through a PACS gateway computer. The HIS/RIS relays a patient admission, discharge, and transfer (ADT) message to PACS only when a patient is scheduled for an examination in the Radiology Department, or when a patient in the Radiology Department is discharged or transferred. Forwarding ADT messages to PACS not only supplies patient demographic data to the PACS but also provides knowledge the archive server needs to initiate the prefetch, studies grouping, and platter management mechanisms. Exchange of messages among these heterogeneous computer systems can use the Health Level 7 (HL7) standard data format running TCP/IP communication protocols on a client/server basis described in Section 7.4.

In addition to receiving ADT messages, PACS receives examination data and diagnostic reports from the RIS. This information is then used to update the PACS database, which can be queried and reviewed from any display workstation. Chapter 11 presents the RIS, HIS, and PACS interface in more detail.

10.2.8 PACS Database Updates

Data transactions performed in the archive server, such as insertion, deletion, selection, and update, are carried out using SQL utilities in the database. Data in the PACS database are stored in predefined tables, with each table describing only one kind of entity. For example, the patient description table consists of master patient records, which store patient demographics; the study description table consists of study records describing individual radiological procedures; the archive directory table consists of archive records for individual images; and the diagnosis history table consists of diagnostic reports of individual examinations. These tables are updated by individual PACS processes running on the archive server with information extracted from image headers or RIS interface to reflect any changes of the corresponding tables.

10.2.9 Image Retrieving

Image retrieval takes place at the display workstations. The display workstation is connected to the archive system through the communication networks. The archive library configured with multiple drives can support concurrent image retrievals from multiple optical disks or tapes. The retrieved data are then transmitted from the archive library to the archive server via the SCSI data buses.

The archive server handles retrieve requests from display workstations according to the priority level of these individual requests. Priority is assigned to individual display workstations and users on the basis of different levels of need. For example, highest priority is always granted to a display workstation that is used for primary diagnosis or is in a conference session or at an intensive care unit. Thus, in effect, a display workstation used exclusively for research and teaching purposes is compromised to allow "fast service" to radiologists and referring physicians in the clinic for immediate patient care.

The archive system supports image retrieval from 2K workstations for online primary diagnosis, 1K workstations for ICU and other primary care, and Macintosh/PC workstations for personal offices throughout the hospital. To retrieve images from the optical disk library, the user at a display workstation can activate the retrieval function and request any number of images from the archive system. Image retrieval is discussed in more detail in Chapter 12.

10.2.10 Image Prefetching

The prefetching mechanism is initiated as soon as the archive server detects the arrival of a patient via the ADT message from HIS/RIS. Selected historical images, patient demographics, and relevant diagnostic reports are retrieved from the optical disk library and the PACS database. Such data are distributed to the destination display workstation(s) prior to completion of the patient's current examination. The prefetch algorithm is based of predefined parameters such as examination type, disease category, radiologist, referring physician, location of display workstation, and the number and age of the patient's archived images. These parameters determine which historical images should be retrieved.

10.3 STORAGE MEDIA

The storage management system in the PACS central node can have storage media of different types: a redundant array of inexpensive disks (RAID) for immediate access of current images, magnetic disks for fast retrieval of cached images, erasable magneto-optical disks for temporary long-term archive, write once, read many (WORM) disks in the optical disk library, which constitute the permanent archive, read-only compact disks (CD-ROM) for low cost, low speed permanent archive, recently developed digital versatile discs (DVD-ROM) for low cost permanent archive, and digital linear tapes for backup storage. All local magnetic disks in radiologic imaging devices and acquisition gateway computers are used for storing newly acquired images. These images are deleted once they have been successfully archived to the permanent storage. Table 10.2 shows the configuration of these multiple-level storage media.

TABLE 10.2 Various Media Used in the PACS Storage Management System

	Storage Media	Location	Purpose	Optimal Capacity (Gbyte)
Level 1	Redundant array of inexpensive disks (RAID) (temporary storage)	PACS controller (archive server), workstations	Provides immediate access to both current and selected historical images	10–150
Level 2	Magnetic disks (temporary storage)	Archive subsystem (archive server)	Provides fast retrieval of current images	10
Level 3	Magneto-optical disks (temporary longer term storage)	Archive subsystem (optical disk library)	Provides retrieval of historical images	500
Level 4	Write once, read many disks (WORM), tapes, CD-ROM, DVD-ROM (permanent storage)	Archive subsystem (optical disk, tape, CD-ROM, DVD-ROM library)	Provides long-term archive and retrieval of historical images	1000–3000

Since magnetic and optical disks, CD-ROM, and magnetic tapes are established technologies, they will not be discussed further here. Instead, we will discuss RAID, optical tape cartridge, and DVD-ROM in more detail because certain features in each of these technologies are crucial for developing a more cost-effective PACS.

10.3.1 RAID

Low speed disk I/O has been a major obstacle to the quickly retrieval of high volume image data from PACS storage devices. Service delay at the display workstations due to access latency on images certainly reduces user confidence, hence diminishes acceptance of the PACS. A solution for improving data access from storage media is the RAID technology introduced in late 1980s. This technology uses a data striping technique to bind multiple disks so that data can be broken down into "chunks" and distributed evenly across the striped disks. Since RAID supports concurrent access to segmented data, their aggregate I/O performance improves.

RAID is a disk array architecture developed by Patterson, Gibson, and Katz at University of California, Berkeley. A RAID groups several magnetic disks as a disk array connected by a RAID controller. The RAID controller consists of multiple disk drive controllers for redundancy, and additional data paths to the disk drives to increase the data transfer rate of the disk array. In an array, some disks (or a portion of a disk) are used for data, others for parity checks for fault tolerance and for hot backup. For example, in a five-disk array, four disks will be used for data and one for parity checks. A RAID has two major advantages over a conventional magnetic disk, its I/O speed and the built-in fault tolerance feature. The I/O speed is important because data is striped (or distributed) over multiple disks through a RAID controller, which allows data to be read (or written) almost simultaneously through multiple paths onto these disks. For example, if each disk is capable of an 8 Mbyte/s data transfer rate, a four-data-disk RAID can have a theoretical rate of 32 Mbyte/s. The overhead of the RAID (i.e., redundant data) will reduce this rate to a percentage.

Data striping can be on a bit level or on a block level. Bit-level striping occurs in a multiples of 8 bits or one byte to and from each disk. The built-in fault tolerance is based on the fact that part of the storage capacity is used to store redundant information about the data so that the original data can be restored, should any one of the disks crash. However, if more than one disk crashes at the same time, original data cannot be rebuilt.

RAID can be categorized to levels 0, 1, 2, 3, 4, and 5, depending on the method of data striping and the amount of built-in redundancy. The two most popular RAIDs used in PACS applications are level 3 and level 5, shown in Figure 10.5b and 10.5c, respectively. The concept of data striping and redundancy can be explained from these two figures.

Consider a 2K × 2K CR image in the PACS controller to be stored in the RAID with five disks. The 2K image is first logically divided into blocks $D_1, D_2, \ldots,$ by the RAID controller: D_1 goes to disk one, D_2 to disk two, D_3 to disk three, D_4 to disk four. A parity byte based on the values of the corresponding byte in each of the four blocks is constructed and stored in the parity block of the fifth disk. If level 3 RAID

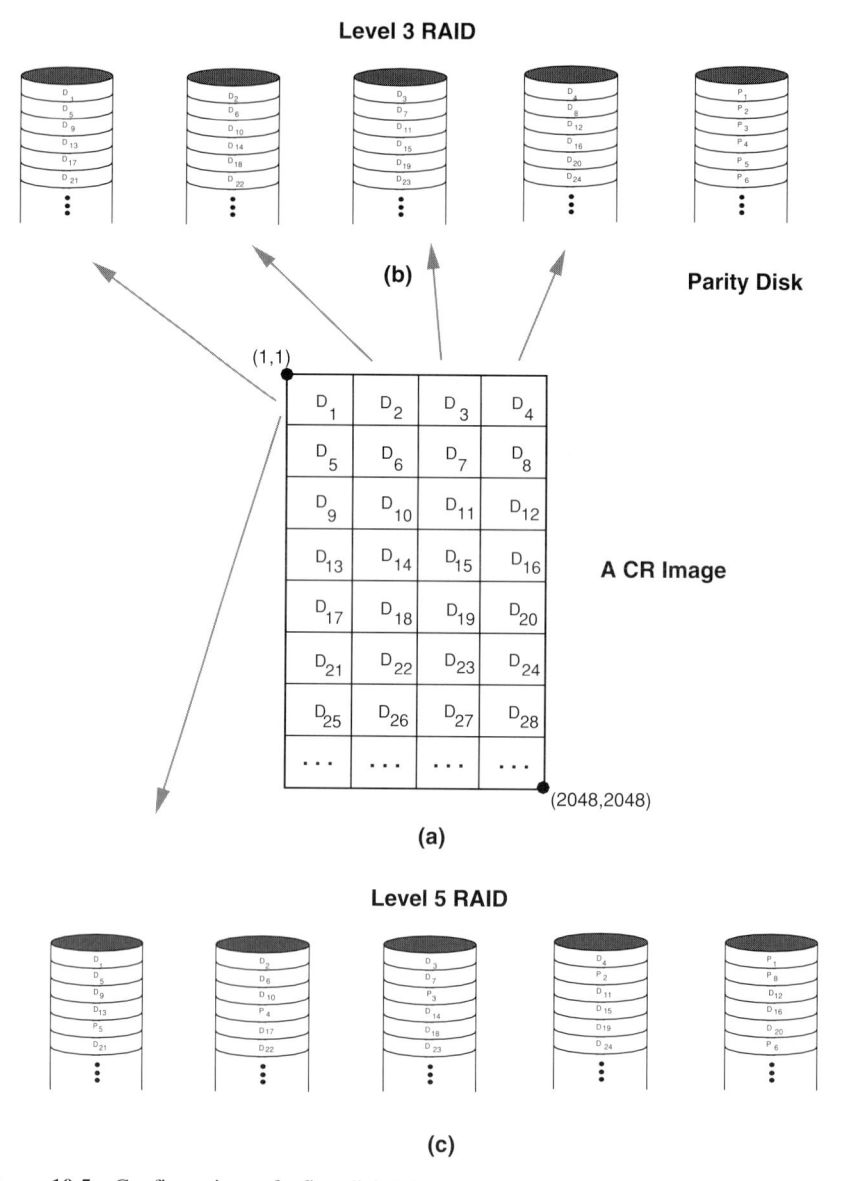

Figure 10.5 Configurations of a five-disk RAID.
(a) 2K × 2K CR image is striped in blocks (D_i) by the RAID controller and distributed to five disks. The parity check block (P_i) is constructed by the corresponding data block in the other four disks. (b) Level 3. (c) Level 5. The fifth disk in the level 3 configuration is the parity disk; whereas in level 5, the parity block is alternating among the five disks.

DISK NO.

Bit Order	1 8A (HEX)	2 01	3 2C	4 FF	5 58
8	1	0	0	1	0
7	0	0	0	1	1
6	0	0	1	1	0
5	0	0	0	1	1
4	1	0	1	1	1
3	0	0	1	1	0
2	1	0	0	1	0
1	0	1	0	1	0

(a)

XOR-Table

A	B	X
0	0	0
0	1	1
1	0	1
1	1	0

(b)

Figure 10.6 Built-in fault tolerance in RAID based on a parity check disk. (a) Example showing how a byte in a corrupted disk can be restored from the corresponding byte of the other four disks using the XOR table. (b) Logical exclusive OR (XOR) operation table.

is used, the parity block is always in the fifth disk. As a result, the fifth disk is the parity disk (Fig. 10.5b). If level 5 RAID is used, the parity block alternates among the five disks shown in Figure 10.5c. The parity byte is constructed based on a sequence of "exclusive or logical OR" operations shown in the XOR table in Figure 10.6b. If any one of the five disks crashes, the values of the crashed disk can be restored from the other four disks, byte by byte, block by block, from the XOR table. Figure 10.6a shows how a byte in any disk can be reconstructed from the corresponding byte from the remaining four disks. When any one disk fails in a RAID, it has to be restored immediately. Until the failed disk has been completely rebuilt, the RAID is vulnerable to another disk failure. For this reason, it is a good idea to have a hot backup disk in the RAID as an extra warranty at minimum cost.

RAID 5 is the preferred configuration of most computer manufacturers' off-the-shelf product because it is optimal for the overall application. For applications like PACS, which process large image files, RAID 3 has a distinct advantage in throughput because of the arrangement of the parity disk during write operations. Several manufacturers' market a RAID that uses this configuration in their PACS archive server.

10.3.2 Digital Optical Cartridge Tape

Digital optical cartridge tape uses a laser beam to write and to read, very similar to the optical disk technology. Current technology in digital optical tape drive has a sustained I/O rate of 5 Mbyt/sec, and a library can be of 80 Tbyte/ft^3 cartridge density. This large capacity in the tape library configuration and low medium cost is ideal for PACS applications in large archives or backup. The conventional magnetic tape has a drawback in large-scale applications requiring repeated read and write, namely, wear on the tapes due to the physical contact between these media and the tape drive's read/write head. Digital optical tape overcomes this problem because there is no physical contact between the tape and its read/write head.

10.3.3 DVD-ROM

DVD-ROM is a new technology being developed by several large industrial consortia, along with DVD-video and DVD-audio for video and audio player applications. It is a replacement of the CD-ROM mass market as a low cost computer peripheral storage device. DVD-ROM has the same data format as the CD-ROM and can be used in existing CD-ROM libraries. Current capacity of the DVD-ROM is 4.7 Gbyte/side. The read/write speed of the first-generation DVD-ROM, developed in mid-1997, defined as $1 \times$ s DVD-ROM, is already faster than that of the CD-ROM. Another advantage of the DVD-ROM over the CD-ROM is the slim-type model (17 mm, 20 times the CD-ROM speed) being developed, which will reduce the size of the storage device. Several PACS manufacturers that use the CD-ROM library as the long-term archive device will shift to the newer technology when it becomes mature in the not so distant future.

The next logical development after DVD-ROM is the DVD-RAM (or RW, rewritable). The first generation DVD-RAM has the capacity of 2.6 Gbyte/side, and the second-generation has 4.7 Gbyte/side. But no commercial product is available as of now. Figure 10.7 is a projection of the development of DVD-ROM and DVD-RAM to year 2000.

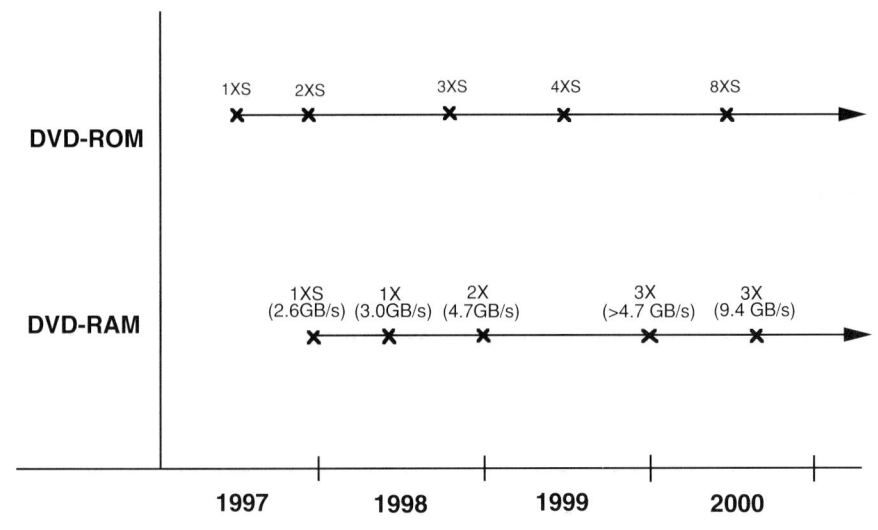

Figure 10.7 DVD-ROM and DVD-RAM product projection: 1 × s, one times speed of the first generation product; GB/S: gigabytes/side. (Modified from *DVD Communications,* No. 4, October 1997, Industrial Technology Research Institute, Taiwan.)

10.4 PACS SERVER SYSTEM OPERATIONS

The PACS server operates on a 24 hours a day, 7 days a week basis. All operations in a well-designed PACS should be software driven and automatic, requiring no manually operated procedures. Data disks removed from the library for reasons of overcapacity are managed by the PACS database and can be reinserted as needed for retrieval of older historical images. The only nonautomatic procedures are the addition of new optical disks and the removal of old ones (to make room for new disks from the optical disk library); such media must be manually inserted into or removed from the library.

A fault-tolerant mechanism in the archive system is used to ensure data integrity and to minimize system downtime. Major features of this mechanism include the following:

1. The uninterruptible power supply (UPS) system, which protects all archive components, including the archive server, database servers, and optical disk library, from power outages.
2. A mirrored database system, which guarantees data integrity.
3. Multiple optical drives and robotic arms, which provide uninterruptible image archival and retrieval in the event of operation failure of a single optical drive or robotic arm.
4. A central monitoring system, which automatically alerts quality control staff

via RS-232 terminals and pagers to salvage any malfunctioning archive components or processes.
5. Spare parts for immediate replacement of any malfunctioning computer components, which include network adapter boards, SCSI controllers, and the multi-CPU system board (archive server).
6. A 4-hour turnaround manufacturer's on-site service, which minimizes system downtime due to hardware failure of any major archive component.

10.5 CONCEPT OF DICOM-COMPLIANT PACS SERVER

10.5.1 Advantages of a DICOM-Compliant PACS Server

The Digital Imaging and Communications in Medicine (DICOM) standard described in Section 7.6 is intended to promote a generic communication method for heterogeneous imaging systems, allowing the transfer of images and associated information. By adapting the DICOM standard, a PACS becomes capable of interconnecting its individual components and the radiologic imaging devices to support image acquisition, archiving, and display. However, imaging equipment vendors often take different DICOM-compliant implementations (Section 7.6.3) for their systems, which leads to certain difficulties when these systems are required to interoperate. A DICOM-compliant PACS server holds the key for smooth system integration. Two mechanisms in the PACS server are essential to ensure system data integrity and to guarantee components interoperability. One mechanism is installed in the image acquisition gateway (IAG) computers and provides a reliable and efficient process for acquiring images from the radiologic imaging devices; the other is employed in the archive server, providing interoperability for multivendor imaging systems in the transfer of images. Both mechanisms can be incorporated in the DICOM-compliant PACS server.

We have described these two mechanisms in Chapters 5, 7, 8, and 9 in the context of components. In this section, we develop the mechanisms at the system level, based on the knowledge acquired in earlier chapters.

10.5.2 DICOM Communications in a PACS Environment

In Section 7.6.4 we discussed the two major DICOM communication service object pair (SOP) classes for PACS for images communication: the Storage service class (C-STORE) and the Query/Retrieve (Q/R) service class:

- Storage service class allows a PACS application running on vendor A's system (e.g., a CT scanner) to play the role of a storage service class user (SCU) that initiates storage requests and transmits images to vendor B's system (e.g., an image acquisition gateway computer), which serves as a Storage service class provider (SCP), accepting images into its local storage device.
- Q/R service class allows PACS applications running on vendor A's system (e.g., a display workstation) to play the role of a Q/R SCU that queries and retrieves

CONCEPT OF DICOM-COMPLIANT PACS SERVER 285

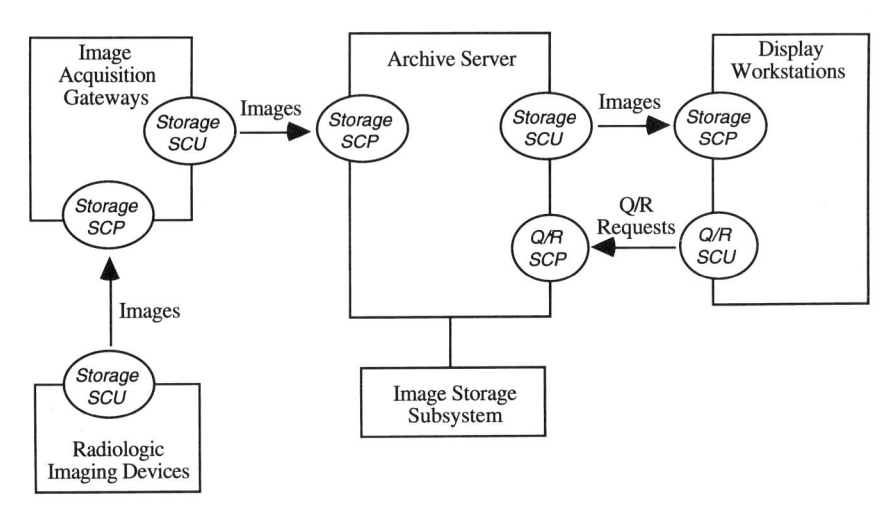

Figure 10.8 Image communication utilizing DICOM SOP services in PACS. Images generated from the radiologic imaging devices are acquired by the image acquisition gateway computers via the Storage SOP service. These images are then transmitted to the archive server, where they are routed to the permanent archive subsystem and display workstations. The archive server supports Query/Retrieve (Q/R) SOP service, handling all Q/R requests from the display workstations. Abbreviations: SOP, service object pair; SCU, service class user; SCP, service class provider.

images from vendor B's system (e.g., an archive server), which serves as a Q/R SCP processing query and retrieval requests.

Figure 10.8 illustrates the communication of images utilizing the Storage service class and Q/R service class in a PACS environment. These two service classes can be used to develop a DICOM-compliant PACS server.

10.5.3 DICOM-Compliant Image Acquisition Gateways

A DICOM-compliant image acquisition gateway (IAG) can be used to provide a reliable and efficient process for acquiring images from radiologic imaging devices. This section presents the hardware platform and software module of IAGs (see also Section 8.4).

10.5.3.1 IAG Hardware Platforms and Operating Systems

Two most popular hardware platforms used in an IAG are the UNIX-based workstations from Sun Microsystems and personal computers (PCs). Each IAG serves as an acquisition node for the PACS server and can be connected to one or more radiologic imaging devices for the acquisition of images. Software components in these two hardware platforms can include the following

Sun-Based IAG

- Solaris operating system
- C programming language
- ATM, high speed, and conventional Ethernet network interfaces
- UNIX socket communication over TCP/IP
- Mallinckrodt CTN-based DICOM communication software with modifications
- Informix local database

PC-Based IAG

- Windows NT operating system
- C and C++ programming languages
- ATM, high speed, and conventional Ethernet network interfaces
- WinSock communication over TCP/IP
- University of California, Davis's DICOM-based communication software with modifications
- Microsoft access local database

10.5.3.2 IAG Software Modules

The DICOM-compliant software running on an IAG should support two types of image acquisition: push-mode and pull-mode operations.

Push Mode Push-mode operation utilizes DICOM's Storage SOP service. An imaging device such as a CT scanner takes the role of a storage SCU initiating storage requests. The requesting IAG (storage SCP) accepts these requests and receives the images.

Pull Mode Pull-mode operation, on the other hand, utilizes DICOM's Q/R SOP service. An IAG plays the role of a Q/R SCU initiating query requests, selecting desired images, and retrieving images from an imaging device (Q/R SCP). Pull-mode operation requires the image acquisition process running on an IAG to incorporate IAG's local database to perform data integrity checks. This checking mechanism ensures that no images are lost during the acquisition process.

Figure 10.9 summarizes the characteristics of these two operations in DICOM (see also Fig. 7.1). The *ImgTrack* process in the IAG performs data integrity checks using the following procedures:

1. Query studies information from the scanners.
2. Generates acquisition status table.
3. Periodically checks acquisition status of individual image sequences.
4. Invokes *DcmPull* process to retrieve images from the scanners.

CONCEPT OF DICOM-COMPLIANT PACS SERVER

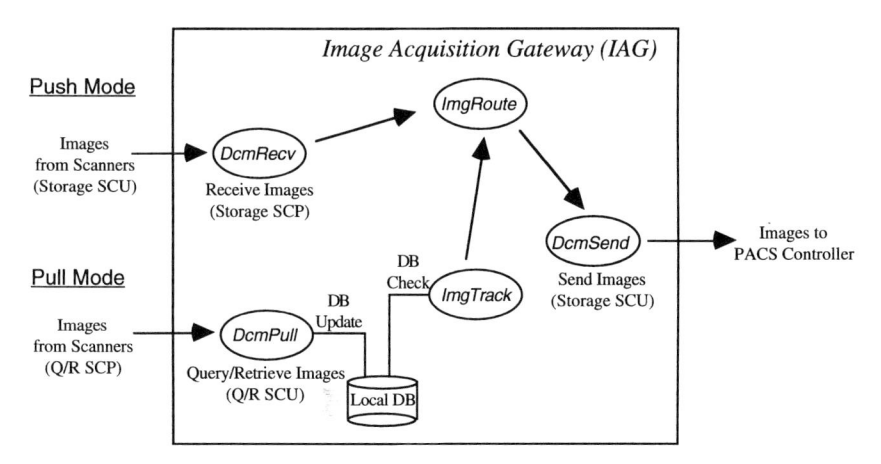

Figure 10.9 Interprocess communication among the major processes running on a DICOM-compliant image acquisition gateway (IAG). IAG supports both push and pull operations for acquiring images from the scanners. The *DcmPull* process incorporates IAG's local database to perform data integrity checking, ensuring that no images are missing from any image sequences during the acquisition process: Dcm, DICOM.

The *DcmPull* process, when invoked by *ImgTrack*, will retrieve desired images from the scanners and update the acquisition status table accordingly.

10.5.4 DICOM-Compliant PACS Server

For a DICOM-compliant PACS server to operate effectively, it should be integrated with DICOM-compliant IAGs and workstations. Assuming this to be the case, the PACS server can be developed using the properties described in the subsections that follow.

10.5.4.1 System Configuration

The DICOM-compliant PACS server should use a powerful UNIX server, such as Sun Microsystems Ultra Enterprise Series Multi-CPU server running the Solaris operating system. The server can be configured with the following components:

- Redundant array of inexpensive disks (RAID) cache storage
- Permanent archive systems like CD-ROM, tape, optical disk, DVD-ROM library long-term storage
- ATM and fast or gigabit Ethernet network interfaces
- Mallinckrodt CTN-based DICOM communication software with modifications
- Large database like Sybase or Oracle

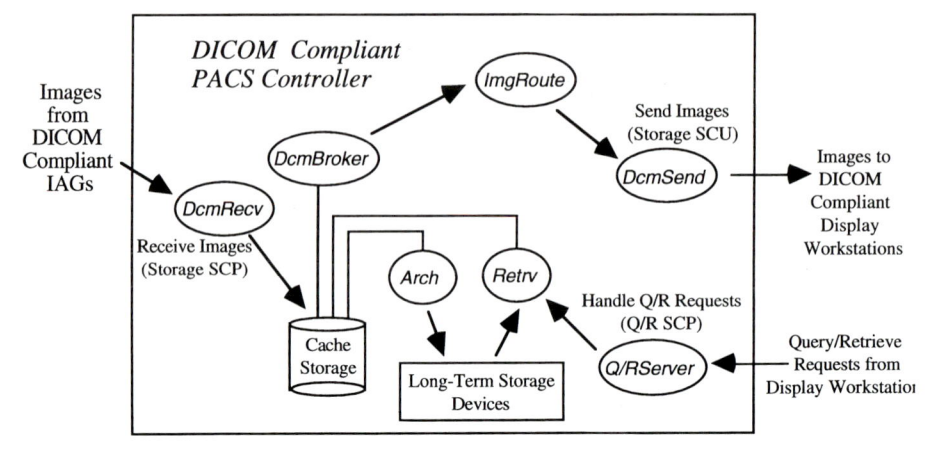

Figure 10.10 Interprocess communication among the major processes running on a DICOM-compliant PACS Controller. The *DcmBroker* serves as an arbitrator ensuring that images acquired from the radiologic imaging devices can be adequately distributed to the display workstations. Compare with the server shown in Figure 10.3.

10.5.4.2 PACS Server Software Modules

The DICOM-compliant PACS controller supports communication for images with the following DICOM implementations:

1. A Storage SCP that accepts images from the IAGs.
2. A Storage SCU that routes images to the display workstations.
3. A Q/R SCP that handles query and retrieval requests from the display workstations.

Figure 10.10 illustrates the management of images in the PACS controller. The *DcmBroker* process serves as an arbitrator ensuring that images acquired from the radiologic imaging devices can be adequately distributed to the display workstations. This process checks the individual images in the PACS controller's cache storage to determine whether any changes in their headers are necessary. The major tasks of *DcmBroker* include the following:

1. Correct any miscoded data in the existing elements.
2. Modify existing elements.
3. Add new elements or shadow groups.
4. Remove existing elements or shadow groups.

Most PACS manufacturers nowadays develop their systems with DICOM compliance. Three components in the compliace statements are the image acquisition gateway, PACS server, and workstations. Here we have discussed the architecture of the gateway and the server. Section 12.5 discusses the workstation component.

Chapter 11
HIS, RIS, and PACS Interface

PACS is an imaging management system that requires pertinent data from other medical information systems for effective operation. Among these contributing systems, the hospital information system (HIS) and the radiology information system (RIS) have the most important data. Many functions in the PACS controller or server described in Chapter 10 (i.e., image routing, prefetching, automatic grouping) rely on data extracted from both HIS and RIS. This chapter presents some HIS and RIS data that are important to the PACS operation and tells how HIS and RIS can be interfaced with PACS to obtain such data.

11.1 Hospital Information System

A hospital information system (HIS) is a computerized management system for handling three categories of tasks in a health care environment:

1. Support of clinical and medical patient care activities in the hospital.
2. Administration of the hospital's daily business transactions (financial, personnel, payroll, bed census, etc.).
3. Evaluation of hospital performances and costs, and projection of the long-term forecast.

Radiology, pathology, pharmacy, clinical laboratories, and other clinical departments in a health care center have their own specific operational requirements, which differ from those of general hospital operation. For this reason, special information systems may be needed in some health centers. Often, these subsystems are under the umbrella of the HIS, which maintains their operations. Others may have their own separate information systems, and some interface mechanisms are built to transfer data between these systems and the HIS. For example, the radiology information system (RIS) was originally a component of HIS. Later, an independent RIS was developed because of the limited support offered by HIS for the handling of special information required by the radiology operation.

Large-scale hospital information systems mostly use mainframe computers. These can be purchased through a manufacturer with certain customization software, or home-grown through the integration of many commercial products, progressively

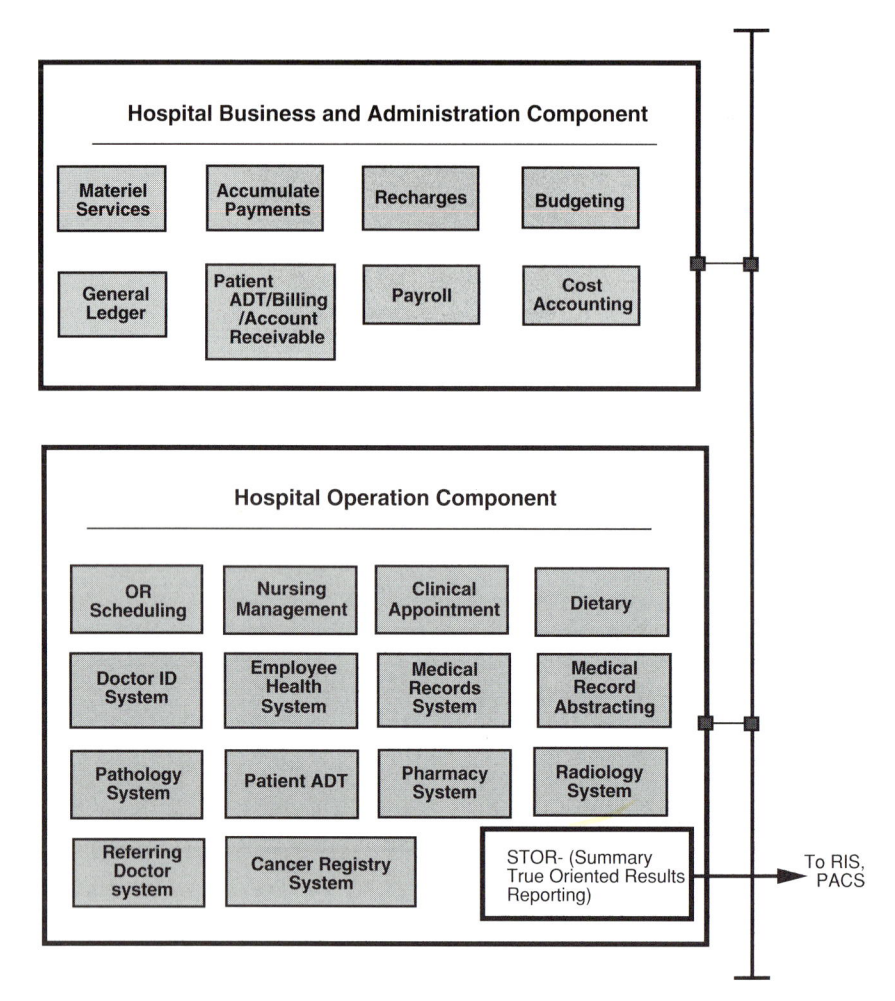

Figure 11.1 Major components in a typical HIS. The software package STOR provides a path for the HIS to distribute HL7-formatted data to the outside world.

throughout years. A home-grown system may contain many reliable legacy components, but with out-of-date technology. Therefore, in interfacing HIS to PACS, caution is necessary to circumvent the legacy problem. Figure 11.1 shows the major components in a typical HIS.

Consider the example of the HIS at UCSF, which is a MEDIPAC (HBO Corporation, Atlanta, GA) based on an IBM 3090/300 mainframe computer (IBM, Armonk, NY). The current system represents the integration of many components since 1969, and some older components have been replaced by newer ones over the years. The system supports the hospital business and administrative work. It provides automation for such events as patient registration, admissions, discharges, and transfers

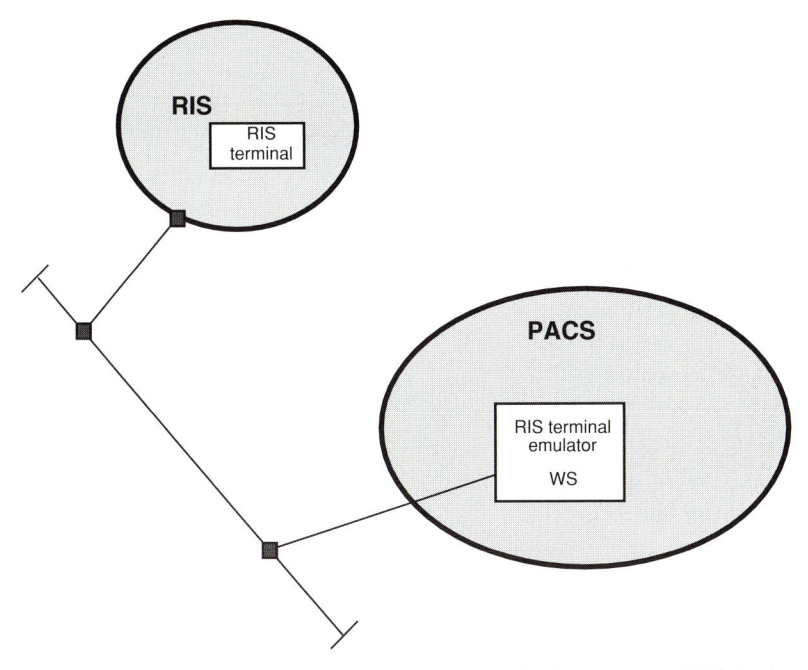

Figure 11.2 A workstation of PACS emulating a RIS terminal. It can access RIS data but cannot deposit to PACS.

(ADT), and patient accounting. It also provides online access to patient clinical results (e.g., laboratory, pathology, microbiology, pharmacy, radiology). The system broadcasts in real time the patient demographics and encounter information with HL7 standards to the RIS. Through this path, ADT and other pertinent data can be transmitted to the RIS and the PACS (see Fig. 11.2).

11.2 RADIOLOGY INFORMATION SYSTEM

RIS is designed to support both the administrative and the clinical operation of a radiology department, to reduce administrative overhead, and to improve the quality of radiological examination delivery. Therefore, RIS manages general radiology patient demographics and billing information, procedure descriptions and scheduling, diagnostic reports, patient arrival scheduling, film location, film movement, and examination room scheduling. The RIS configuration is very similar to the HIS except it is on a smaller scale. RIS equipment consists of a computer system with peripheral devices such as alphanumeric terminals, printers, and bar code readers. In most cases, an independent RIS is autonomous, with limited access to HIS. However, some HISs offer embedded RIS subsystems with a higher degree of integration.

For example, the RIS at UCSF, IDXrad (IDX, Burlington, VT), is based on a VAX 4000/500 (Digital Equipment Corp., Maynard, MA), which maintains many types of patient and examination-related information, including medical, administrative, patient demographics, examination scheduling, diagnostic reporting, and billing information. The major tasks of the system include the following:

- Process patient and film folder records.
- Monitor the status of patients, examinations, and examination resources.
- Schedule examinations.
- Create, format, and store diagnostic reports with digital signatures.
- Track film folders.
- Maintain timely billing information.
- Perform profile and statistics analysis.

The RIS interfaces to PACS based on the HL7 standard through TCP/IP over Ethernet on a client/server model using a trigger mechanism (Section 11.3.5.1). Events such as examination scheduling, patient arrivals, and examination begin and end times trigger the RIS to send previously selected information associated with the event (patient demographics, examination description, diagnostic report, etc.) to the PACS in real time.

11.3 INTERFACE PACS WITH HIS AND RIS

11.3.1 Background

There are three methods of transmitting data between information systems: through a terminal emulation, through database-to-database transfer, and by way of an interface engine.

11.3.1.1 Terminal Emulation

When a workstation of an information system is allowed to emulate a workstation of a second system, data from the second information system can be accessed by the first system. For example, a PACS workstation can be connected to the RIS with a simple computer program that emulates a RIS terminal. From the PACS workstation, the user can perform any RIS administration function such as scheduling a new examination, updating patient demographics, or recording a film movement, and view the diagnostic reports. This method has two disadvantages. First, there is no data exchange between RIS and PACS; and second, the user must know how to use both systems. Also, a terminal at RIS or HIS cannot be used to emulate a PACS workstation, since the latter is too specific for HIS and RIS to emulate. Figure 11.2 shows the mechanism of the terminal emulation method.

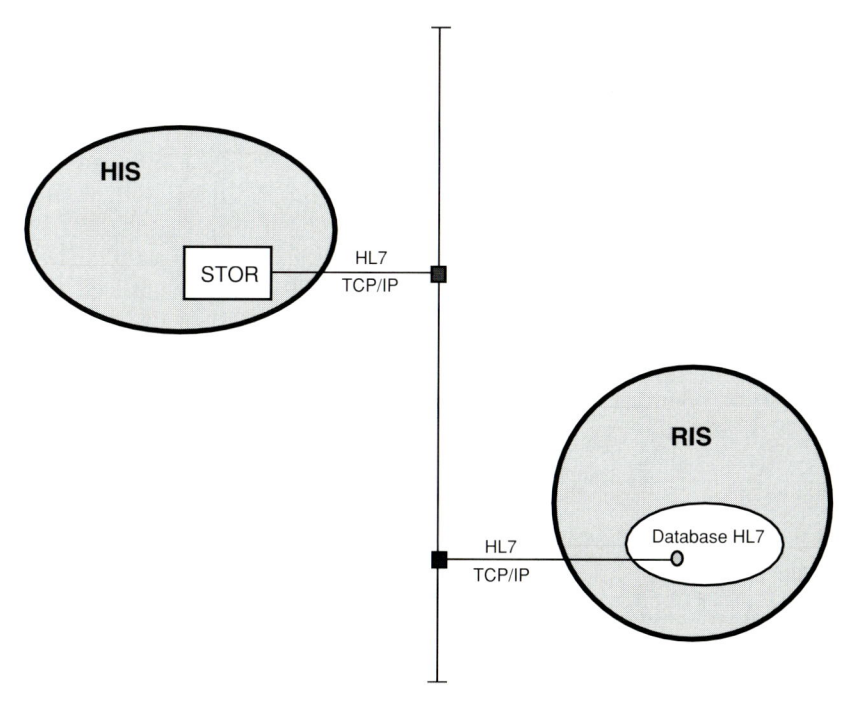

Figure 11.3 Database-to-database transfer using common data format (HL7) and communication protocol (TCP/IP). Data from HIS is accumulated periodically at STOR and broadcasted to RIS.

11.3.1.2 Database-to-Database Transfer

The database-to-database transfer method allows two or more networked information systems to share a subset of data by storing them in a common local area. For example, the ADT data from HIS can be reformatted to HL7 standard and broadcasted periodically to a certain local database in HIS. A TCP/IP communication protocol can be set up between HIS and RIS to allow HIS to initiate the local database and broadcast the ADT data to RIS through either a pull or a push operation. This method is most often used to share information between HIS and RIS, as shown in Figure 11.3.

11.3.1.3 Interface Engine

The interface engine provides a single interface and language to access distributed data in networked heterogeneous information systems. In operation, it appears as if the user is operating on a single integrated database from his or her workstation. In the interface engine, a query protocol is responsible for analyzing the requested information, identifying the required databases, fetching the data, assembling the results in a standard format, and presenting this information at the workstation. Ideally, all this processing is transparent to the user and does not affect the autonomy of

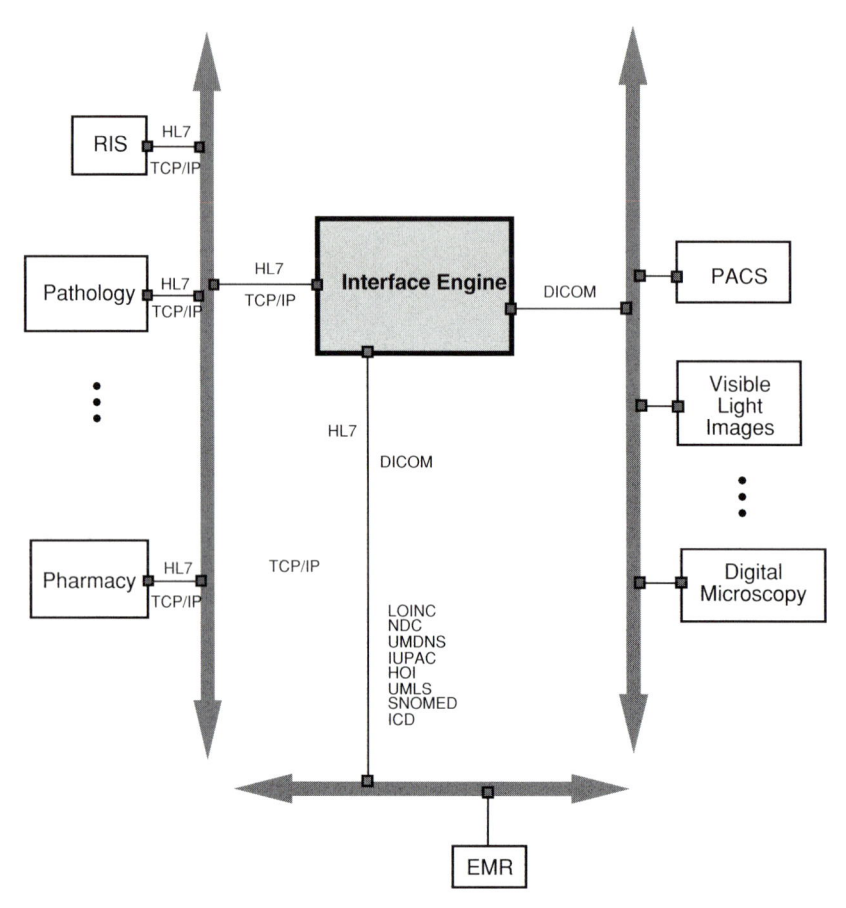

Figure 11.4 Principle of an interface engine. *Left*: HL7 textual data. *Right*: DICOM image data. *Bottom*: Electronic medical record (EMR, Section 11.5) can have image, textual, and messages. Message standards: LOINC, logical observation identifier names and codes; NDC, national drug codes; UMDNS, universal medical device nomenclature system; IUPAC, international union of pure and applied chemistry; HOI, health outcomes institute; UMLS, unified medical language system; SNOMED, systemized nomenclature of medicine; ICD, (ICD-9-CM: The International Classification of diseases, ninth revision, clinical modification).

any database system. To build a universal interface engine is not a simple task. Most currently available commercial interface engines are tailored to certain infromation systems. Figure 11.4 illustrates the concept of an interface engine for HIS, RIS, and PACS integration.

11.3.2 Reasons for Interfacing PACS with HIS and RIS

In a hospital environment, interfacing the PACS, RIS, and HIS has become necessary to enhance the diagnostic process, PACS image management, RIS administration, and research and training, as described in Sections 11.3.2.1 to 11.3.2.4.

11.3.2.1 Diagnostic Process

The diagnostic process at a PACS display workstation includes the retrieval not only of images of interest but also of pertinent textual information describing patient history and studies. Along with the image data and the image description, a PACS provides all related text information acquired and managed by the RIS and the HIS in a way that is useful to a radiologist during the diagnostic process. RIS and HIS information such as clinical diagnosis, radiological reports, and patient history are necessary at the PACS workstation to complement the images of the cases being viewed.

11.3.2.2 PACS Image Management

Some information provided by the RIS can be integrated into PACS image management algorithms to optimize the grouping and routing of image data on the network to the requesting locations (see Section 10.2). In the PACS database, which archives huge volumes of images, a sophisticated image management system is required to handle the depositing and distribution of this image data.

11.3.2.3 RIS Administration

Planning of a digital-based radiology department requires the reorganization of some administrative operations carried out by the RIS. For example, the PACS can provide the image archive status and the image data file information to the RIS. RIS administration operations would also benefit from the HIS by gaining knowledge about patient admission, discharge, and transfer.

11.3.2.4 Research and Training

Much research and teaching in radiology involves mass screening of clinical cases and determining what constitutes normal and abnormal conditions for a given patient population. The corresponding knowledge includes diverse types of information that must be correlated, such as image data, results from analyzed images, medical diagnosis, patient demographics, study description, and various patient conditions. Some mechanisms are needed to access and to retrieve data from the HIS and the RIS during a search for detailed medical and patient information related to image data. Cooperation between diverse medical database systems such as HIS, RIS, and PACS is therefore critical to the successful management of research and teaching issues in radiology.

11.3.3 Some Common Rules

To interface the HIS, RIS, and PACS, some common rules have to be followed.

1. Each system (HIS, RIS, PACS) remains unchanged in its configuration, in its data, and in the functions it performs.

296 HIS, RIS, AND PACS INTERFACE

2. Each system is hardware- and software-extended to allow communication with other systems.
3. Only data are shared; functions remain local. For example, RIS functions cannot be performed at the PACS or the HIS workstation. Keeping each system specific and autonomous will simplify the interface process, since database updates are not allowed at a global level.

Based on these common rules, successfully interfacing HIS, RIS, and PACS includes the following steps:

1. Identify the subset data that will be shared with the other systems. Access rights and authorization problems are solved during this process.
2. Convert the data to a standard form (i.e., HL7). This step, which consists of designing a high level presentation, solving data inconsistencies, and naming conventions, can be accomplished by using a common data model and data language, and by defining rules of correspondence between various data definitions.
3. Define the protocol of data transfer (e.g., TCP/IP or DICOM).

11.3.4 Common Data in HIS, RIS, and PACS

To archive images and associated data in permanent storage and distribute them to the display workstations in a properly and timely manner, the system software in the PACS archive server described in Section 10.2 requires certain data from HIS and RIS. Figure 11.5 illustrates information common to the HIS, RIS, and PACS. Table 11.1 describes the data definition, the origin and the destination, and the actions that trigger system software functions.

11.3.5 Implementation of RIS-PACS Interface

The RIS-PACS interface can be implemented by either the trigger mechanisms or the query protocol described in Sections 11.3.5.1 and 11.3.5.2, respectively.

11.3.5.1 Trigger Mechanism Between Two Databases

The PACS is notified of the following events in HL7 format when they occur in the RIS: ADT, order received, patient arrival, examination canceled, procedure complete, report approved. The application level of the interface software waits for the occurrence of one of these events and triggers the corresponding data to be sent. The communication level transfers the HL7 file to the PACS server using two processes: *send* (to PACS) and *recv* (from RIS). The PACS server receives this file and archives it in the database tables for subsequent use. Figure 11.6 shows the trigger mechanism interface. The trigger mechanism is used when a small amount of predefined information from RIS needs to be available in the PACS in a systematic and timely fashion. In addition to requiring storage overhead in both databases, this method is tedious for information updating; it is not suitable for user queries.

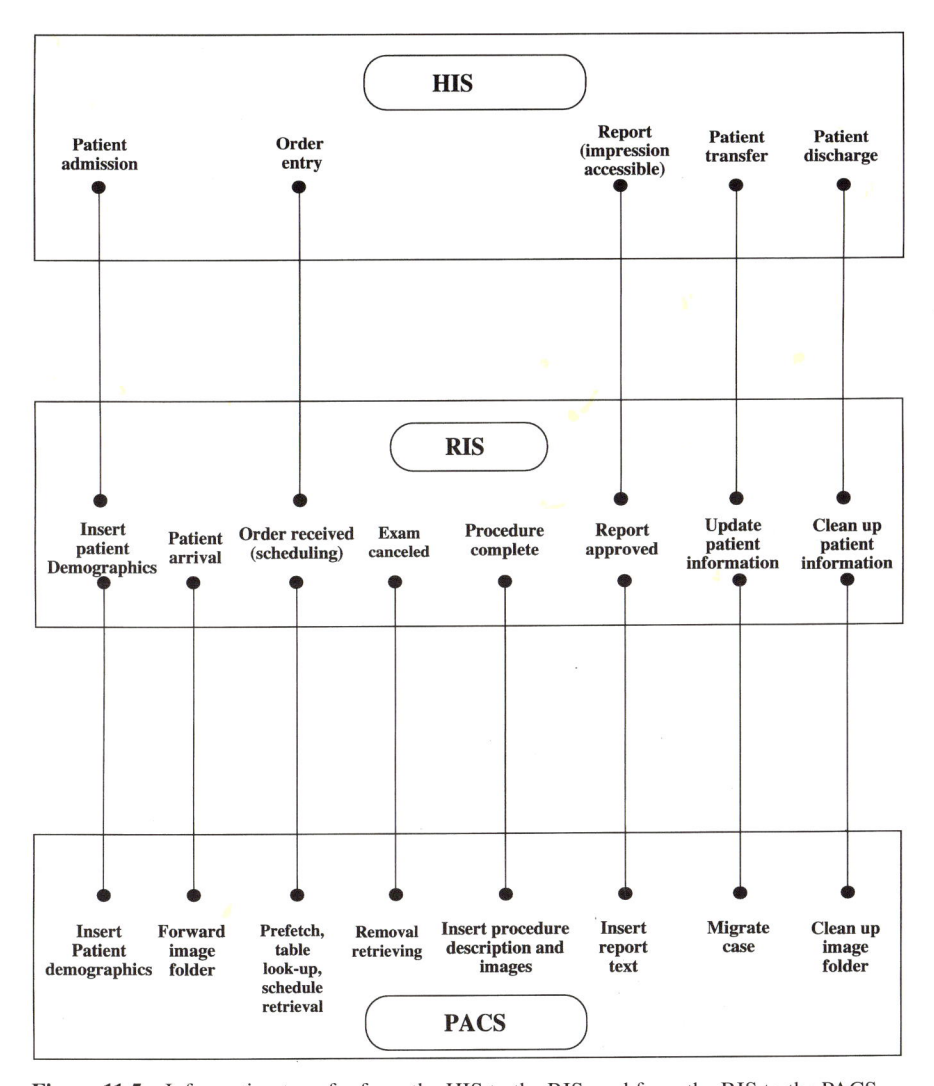

Figure 11.5 Information transfer from the HIS to the RIS, and from the RIS to the PACS.

11.3.5.2 Query Protocol

The query protocol allows access to information from the HIS, RIS, and PACS databases by means of an application layer software on top of these heterogeneous database systems. From a PACS workstation, users can retrieve information uniformly from any of these systems and automatically integrate them to one answer. Figure 11.7 illustrates the query protocol. The DICOM Query/Retrieve service class described in Section 7.6.4.2 is one method to implement such query mechanism. The application layer software utilizes the following standards:

- SQL as the global query language

TABLE 11.1 Information Transferred Between HIS, RIS, and PACS Triggering Events in the PACS Server

Events	Message	From	To	Action	Location
1. Admission	Previous images/reports	HIS/RIS	PACS server	Preselected images and reports transferred from permanent archive to workstations	WS at FL, RR
2. Order entry	Previous images/reports	RIS	PACS server, scanner	Check event 1 for completion	WS at FL, RR
3. Arrival	Patient arrival	RIS	PACS server, scanner	Check events 1 and 2 for completion	WS at FL, RR
4. Examination completed	New images	Scanner	RIS PACS server	New images to folder manager, WS	Temporary archive; WS at FL, RR
5. Dictation	"Wet" reading	RR	Digital dictaphone	Dictation recorded on DD, digital voice to folder manager and to WS	DD; WS at FL, RR
6. Transcript	Preliminary report	RR	RIS, PACS server	Preliminary report to RIS, temporary archive and to WS, dictation erased from DD	RIS; temporary archive: WS at FL, RR
7. Signature	Final report	RR	RIS, PACS Server	Final report to RIS, to WS, and to temporary archive; preliminary report erased.	RIS: temporary archive; WS at FL, RR
8. Transfer	Patient transfer	RIS	PACS Server	Transfer image files	WS at new location
9. Discharge	Images, report	HIS/RIS	PACS Server	Patient folder copied from temporary to permanent storage; patient folder erased from WS	WS at FL, RR; temporary and permanent storage

Key: DD, digital Dictaphone; FL, floors in the ward; RR, reading rooms in the Radiology Department; WS, workstations.

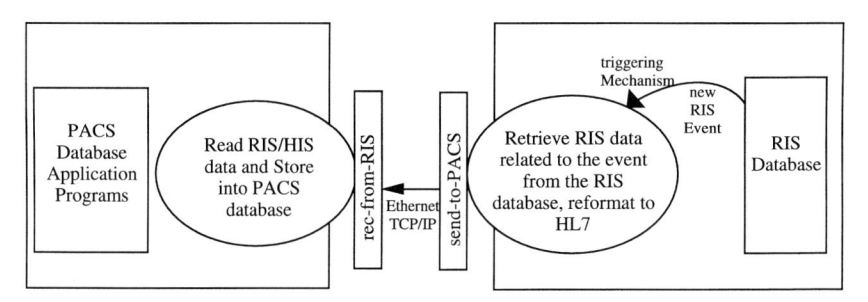

Figure 11.6 RIS-PACS interface architecture implemented using a database-to-database transfer with a trigger mechanism.

- Relational data model as the global data model
- TCP/IP communication protocols
- HL7 data format

11.4 INTERFACE PACS WITH OTHER MEDICAL DATABASES

11.4.1 Multimedia Medical Data

The many consultation functions of a radiology specialist in a large medical center include consulting with primary and referring physicians on the proper radiological procedures for patients, performing the procedures, reading images from the procedures, and dictating and confirming reports. Referring physicians review images with the radiologists and receive consultation. Based on these radiological images, reports, and consultations, the requesting physicians prescribe the proper treatment plan for

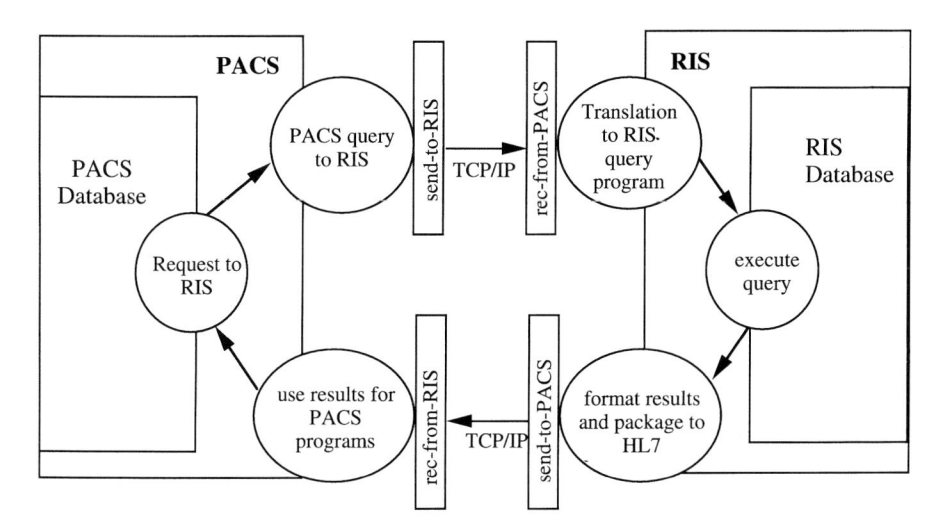

Figure 11.7 RIS-PACS interface with a query protocol.

their patients. The radiologists also use the images from the procedures and the corresponding reports to train fellows, residents, and medical students.

In their practice, the radiologists often request from medical records other necessary patient information (e.g., demographic data, laboratory tests, consultation reports from other medical specialists). Radiologists also review literature from the library information systems and give *formal rounds* to educate colleagues on radiological procedures and new radiological techniques. Thus, the practice of radiology requires integrating various types of information—voice, text, medical records, images, and video recordings—into proper files. These various types of information exist on different media and are stored in data systems of different types. The advance of computer and communication technologies allows the possibility of integration of these various types of information to facilitate the practice of radiology. We have already discussed two such information systems, namely, HIS and RIS.

11.4.2 Multimedia in the Radiology Environment

"Multimedia" has different meanings depending on the context. In the radiology environment, the term refers to the integration of medical information related to radiology practice. This information is stored in various databases and media either in voice form or as text records, images, or video loops. Patient demographic information, clinical laboratory test results, pharmacy information, and pathological reports are stored in the HIS. The radiological images are stored in the PACS permanent archive system, and its corresponding reports are stored in the reporting system of the RIS. The electronic mail and other files are stored in the personal computer system database. The digital learning files are categorized in the learning laboratory or the library in the department of radiology. Some of these databases may exist in a primitive way in the sense that the digital and communication technology used is primitive; others—PACS, for example—can be very advanced. Thus, the challenge of developing multimedia in the radiology environment is to establish infrastructure for the seamless integration of this medical information by means of blending different technologies, while providing an acceptable data transmission rate to various parts of the department and to various sites in the hospital. Once the multimedia infrastructure has been established, various units of medical information can exist as modules and be interfaced to this infrastructure. In the multimedia environment, radiologists (or their medical colleagues) can access this information through a user-friendly, inexpensive, efficient, and reliable interactive workstation.

RIS, HIS, electronic mail, and files involve textual information requiring from 1K to 2K bytes per transaction. For such a small data file size, although developing an interface to each information system is tedious, the technology involved is manageable. On the other hand, PACS contains image files that can be in the neighborhood of 20–40 Mbyte. The transmission and storage requirements for PACS are manyfold those of text information. For this reason, PACS becomes central in developing multimedia in the radiology environment. Figure 11.8 illustrates the concept of multimedia in the radiology environment. In Chapter 13 we describe the concept of medical image information infrastructure (MIII) as the foundation for the multimedia application.

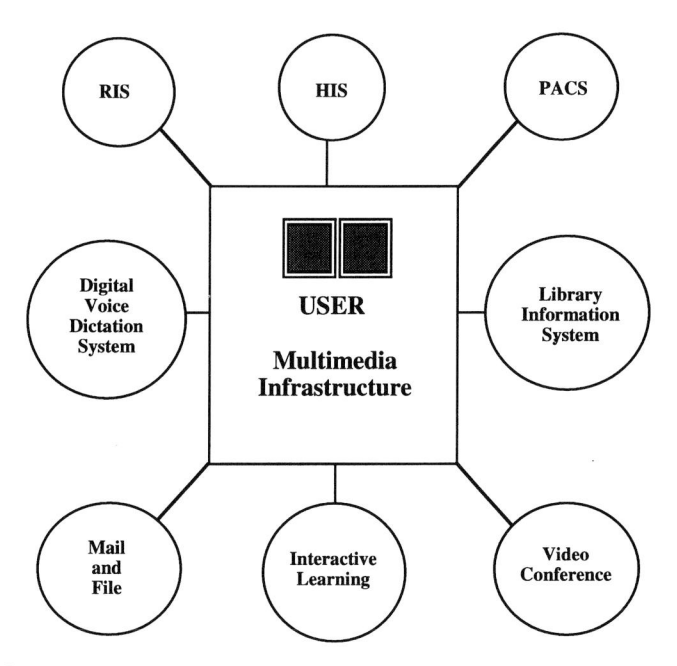

INTERFACE PACS WITH OTHER MEDICAL DIAGNOSES   301

Figure 11.8 Concept of multimedia in the radiology environment: user can use single or multiple monitors and access multiple databases at the desktop workstation.

11.4.3 Integration of Heterogeneous Databases

11.4.3.1 Other Related Databases

For multimedia to operate effectively in the radiology environment, at least five heterogeneous databases must be integrated, namely the HIS, RIS, PACS, electronic mail and file, and digital voice dictation systems. In Section 11.3, we described the HIS/RIS interface. In this section, we describe the digital voice system. Discussion of electronic mail and files is deferred until Chapter 13 (Section 13.2).

11.4.3.2 Digital Voice with PACS

Typically, radiological reports are archived and transmitted independently from the image files. They are first dictated by the radiologist and recorded on an audiocassette recorder, from which a textual form is transcribed and inserted into the RIS several hours later. The interface between the RIS and the PACS allows for sending and inserting these reports into the PACS database, from which a report can be displayed at the PACS workstation upon request by a user. This process is not efficient because the delay imposed by the need for transcription prevents the textural report from reaching the referring physician in a timely manner. The ideal method is to use a voice recognition system, which automatically translates voice into text. Although several such systems are available in the market, the accuracy of the voice recognition is still not high enough to merit widespread acceptance.

302 HIS, RIS, AND PACS INTERFACE

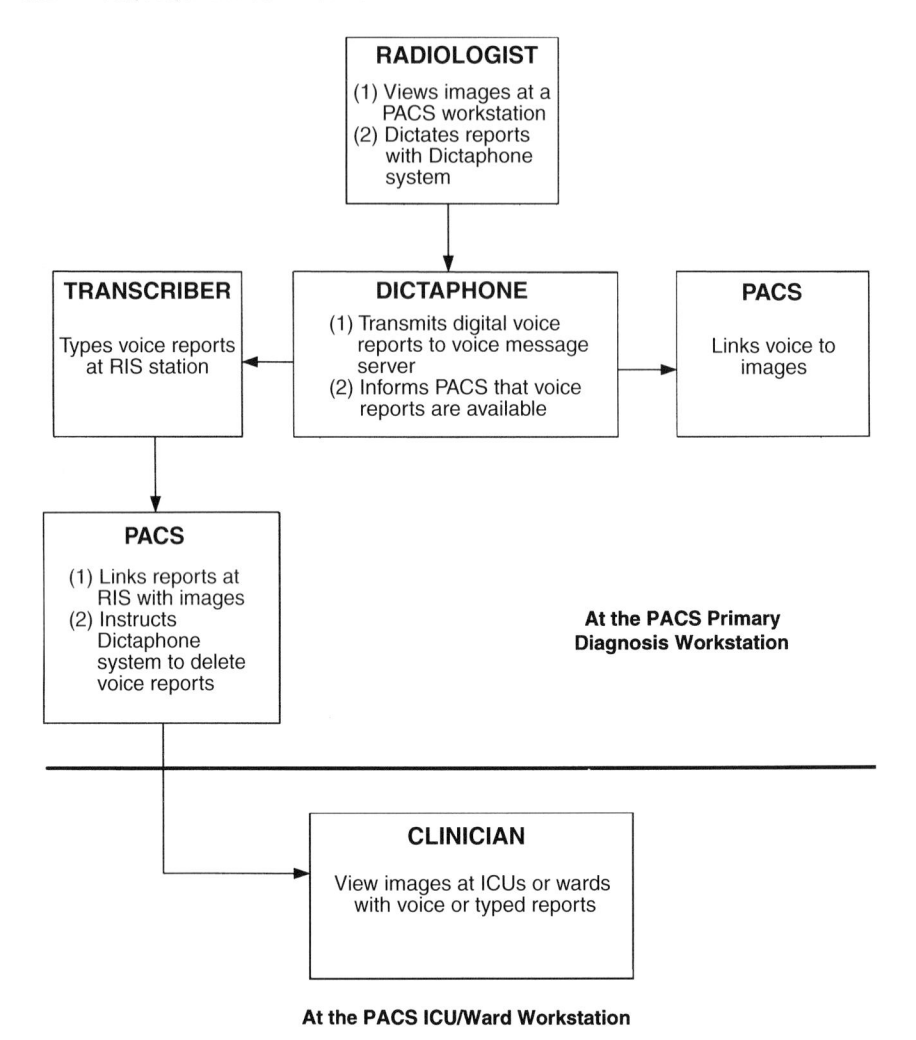

Figure 11.9 The operational procedure of a digital voice system connected with the PACS starts with the radiologist at the primary diagnosis workstation dictating a report with the digital Dictaphone system.

Figure 11.9 shows a method of interfacing digital voice system directly to the PACS database. The concept of interfacing these is to have the digital voice database associated with the PACS image database; thus before the written report becomes available, the referring physician can look at the images and listen to the report simultaneously. Following Figure 11.9, the radiologist views images from the PACS workstation and uses the digital Dictaphone system to dictate the report, which is then converted from analog signals to digital format and stored in the voice message server. The voice message server in turn sends a message to the PACS data server, which links the voice with the images. Thus, for example, the referring physicians at a workstation in an intensive care unit, can request to review certain images and at the same time listen to the voice report through the voice message server linked to the images. Later, the transcriber transcribes the voice using the RIS. The transcribed report is inserted into the RIS database server automatically. The RIS server sends a message to the PACS database server. The latter appends the transcribed report to the PACS image file and signals the voice message server to delete the voice message. Note that although the interface is between the voice database and the PACS database, the RIS database also comes into the picture.

11.5 ELECTRONIC MEDICAL RECORD

Electronic medical record (EMR) or electronic patient record (EPR) is the ultimate information system in a health care enterprise. One can consider EMR as the big picture of the health care information system of the future. Although the development of a universal EMR as a commercial product is still years away, its eventual impact on the health care delivery system should not be underestimated. An EMR consists of five major functions:

1. Accepts direct digital input of patient data.
2. Analyzes across patients and providers.
3. Provides clinical decision support and suggests courses of treatment.
4. Performs outcome analysis, and patient and physician profiling.
5. Distributes information across different platforms and health information systems.

HIS and RIS, which deal with patient non-imaging data management and hospital operation, can be considered to be a subset of EMR. An integrated HIS-RIS-PACS system, which extends the patient data to include imaging, forms the cornerstone of EMR.

Existing EMRs have certain commonalties. They have large data dictionaries with time stamped in their contents, and they can query and display data flexibly. Examples of successfully implemented EMRs are COSTAR (**c**omputer-**s**tored **a**mbulatory **r**ecord) developed at Massachusetts General Hospital (in the public domain), the Regenstrief Medical Record System at Indiana University, and the HELP (**h**ealth **e**valuation through **l**ogical **p**rocessing) system developed at the University of Utah and Latter-Day Saints (LDS) Hospital.

Like any other medical information system, however, EMR also faces several obstacles to its development: lack of a method for inputting patient examination and related data to the system, need to develop an across-the-board data and communication standard, need to ensure buy-in from manufacturers to adopt the standards, and need to gain acceptance by health care providers. An integrated HIS-RIS-PACS system provides solutions for some of these obstacles. First, it has adopted DICOM and

HL7 standards for imaging and text, respectively. Second, images and patient-related data are entered to the system almost automatically. Third, the majority of imaging manufacturers have adopted DICOM and HL7 as de facto industrial standards.

Therefore, in the course of developing an integrated PACS, one should keep in mind the big picture, the EMR. Anticipated future connections of the integrated PACS as a subsystem of EMR should be considered thoroughly. Figure 11.4 illustrates the concept of using an interface engine as a possible connection of the integrated PACS to EMR.

CHAPTER 12
Display Workstation

12.1 BASICS OF A DISPLAY WORKSTATION

The display workstation is the last component in the PACS data flow, where the user interprets the images along with relevant data. The interpreted results becomes the diagnostic report that feeds back to the hospital and radiology information systems as a permanent archive along with the images (Fig. 1.1). In this chapter, the terms *soft copy workstation, display workstation,* and *image workstation* are used interchangeably. The term *workstation* alone is reserved for a host computer: for example, a Sun SPARC station, that controls the image display.

The conventional method of reviewing radiologic images uses films hung on an alternator or a light box. Table 12.1 shows the characteristics of a typical alternator. Since the advantages of an alternator are its large surface area, high luminance, and convenience in use, the design of a soft copy display workstation should incorporate the function and convenience of the alternator.

An image workstation consists of four major hardware components: a host computer, an image display board, display video monitors, and local storage devices. A communication network and application software connect these components with the PACS controller, as described in Section 10.1. The computer and the image display board are responsible for transforming the image data for visualization on the monitors. Local storage devices that meet the high capacity, high performance requirements of the imaging display applications include magnetic disks and RAID described in Section 10.3.1. The communication network is used for transmitting images into and out of the display workstation. Figure 12.1 shows the schematic of a typical two-monitor display workstation based on an NT/PC computer. This section describes the image display board and the video monitor in more detail.

12.1.1 Image Display Board

The image display board has two components: a processing unit and image memory. The image memory is used to supplement the host computer memory to increase the storage capacity and to speed up the image display. There are two types of computer memory: the random access memory (RAM) and the video RAM (VRAM). RAM usually comes with the computer and is less expensive than VRAM, which has a very high input/output rate and is used to display images or graphics. A display worksta-

TABLE 12.1 Characteristics of a Typical Light Alternator

Dimensions (in.)		Table Height	Number of Panels	Viewing Capability				
Width	Height			Number of Visible Panels	Viewing Surface per Panel: Height × Width (in.²)	Average Luminance	Viewing height: From Tabletop to Top of Lower Panel	Time Required to Retrieve a Panel
72–100	78	30–32 in.	20–50	2 (upper and lower)	16 × 56 to 16 × 82	500	32 + 16 in.	6–12

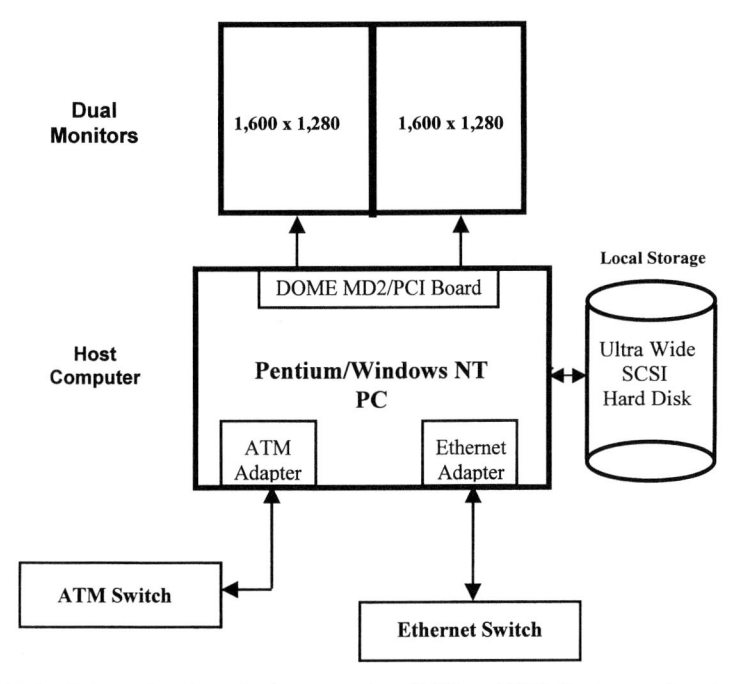

Figure 12.1 Schematic of a typical two-monitor (1600 × 1280) display workstation (WS). This WS is composed of a host computer (PC), a display board with image processing capability and image memory (DOME board), dual monitors, magnetic disk, and networking.

tion usually has more RAM than VRAM. Typical numbers are 128 Mbyte RAM and 10 Mbyte VRAM.

An image that comes to the display workstation from outside or from the internal disk is first stored in the RAM. If the RAM is not large enough to store the entire image, it is split between the RAM and the disk, an operation that calls for disk I/O swap. After certain operations, the image is moved to the VRAM; subsequently, it appears, in processed form, on the video monitor. RAM is used to increase the host memory size, to avoid I/O swapping between the magnetic disk and the computer memory. Insufficient memory would require the swapping of software programs and partial images to and from the magnetic disk, thereby slowing down the image display and manipulation. Figure 12.2 illustrates the concept of disk swapping due to insufficient memory. For example, if the image is 12 bits/pixel, it will take 2 bytes in the RAM to store one pixel. Since the VRAM is only 8 bits/pixel, a lookup table is required to map the 12 bits to 8 bits. The 8 bits/pixel image is then stored in the VRAM, and from there an analog-to-digital converter changes the 8-bit pixel value to an electrical signal to activate the phosphor of the video monitor forming a visual image. Figure 12.3 demonstrates the movement of an image from the magnetic disk to the video memory. For color images, such a transfer requires 24 bits/pixel; for graphic overlay, 1 bit/pixel is sufficient.

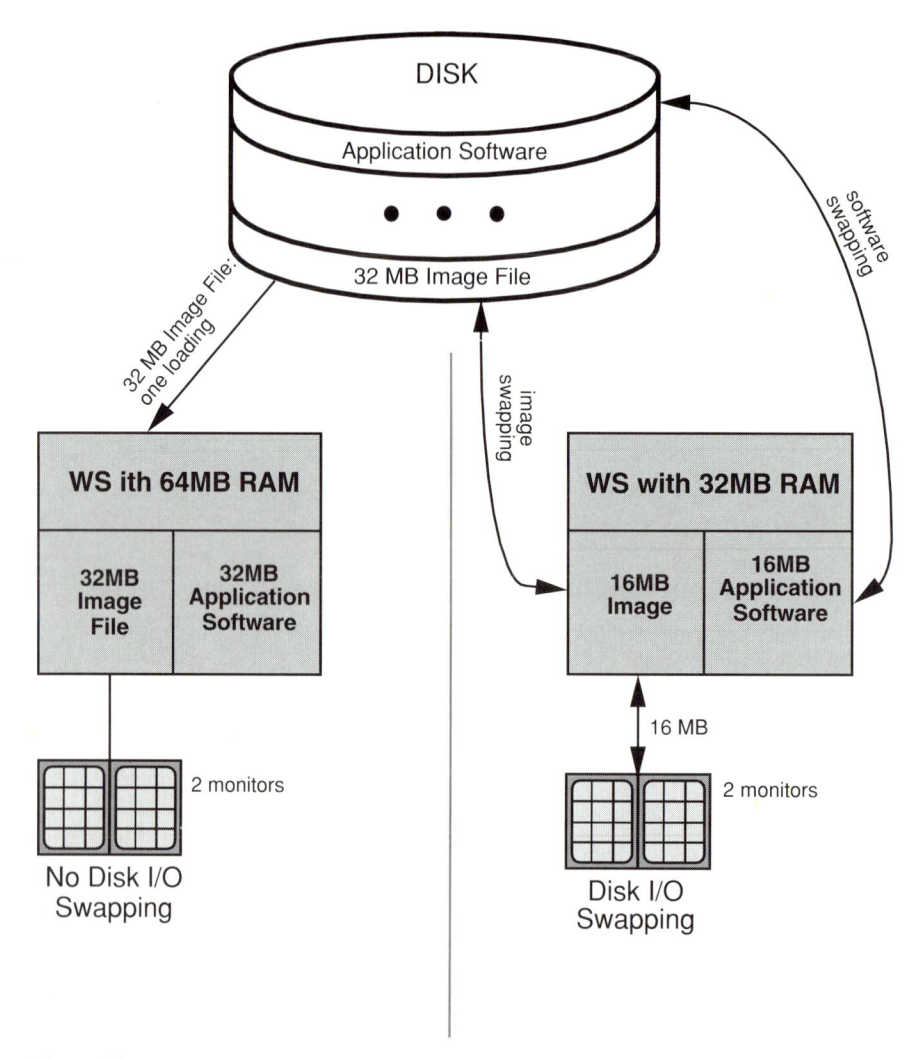

Figure 12.2 Insufficient RAM in the display workstation will require disk I/O swapping. Only a portion of the image file can be stored and processed in the RAM at a time, thereby slows down the image manipulation and display. *Left:* With sufficient memory. *Right:* Insufficient memory, requiring disk I/O swapping.

12.1.2 Video Monitor

Today, the cathode ray tube (CRT) monitor is still the predominant display device because of its overall superiority of image quality compared with other types of display like liquid crystal screens, light valves, and flat-panel display. Since the image quality of the visualized data can affect the interpretation of the data, the CRT display monitors play a crucial role in the formation of visual information. The characteristics of the video display monitor that affect the visual quality are video scanning,

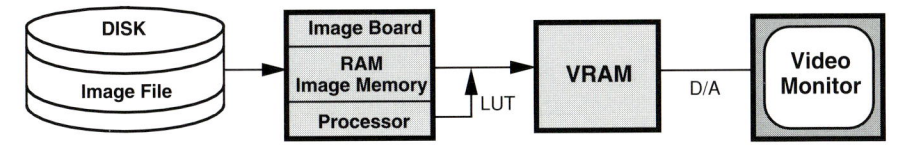

Figure 12.3 Dataflow of an image from the disk to the video monitor.

phosphor characteristics, resolution, luminance and contrast, human perception, and color display.

12.1.2.1 Video Scanning

CRT display utilizes the raster scanning method in which the electron beam scans the CRT screen in a fixed pattern of closely spaced parallel lines (see Section 3.2.1). These lines are usually horizontal, and scanning proceeds from the top to the bottom of the screen. The beam current is either "on–off" or continuous, to produce a monochrome or gray-scale picture, respectively. There are two modes of scanning: interlaced and progressive. An interlaced frame is displayed in two steps. For example, in the American standard, the even lines are painted (1/60 second), then the odd lines fill the gaps (1/60 second) to comprise a complete picture frame in a total of 1/30 second, or 30 Hz. The progressive scan consists of painting the image from left to right and top to bottom continuously. In progressive scans the trend is to use a monitor that is operating between 60 and 72 frames per second (Hz). It is commonly accepted now that to eliminate flicker, a 72 Hz progressive scan should be used in medical imaging applications.

12.1.2.2 Phosphor

Visible light is produced by the phenomenon called cathodoluminescence, in which high energy electrons excite phosphors deposited on a screen plate. As the excited electrons in the phosphor return to the ground state, light is emitted whose intensity is proportional to the electron beam current. More than 50 different types of phosphor are available and are listed in the P number register provided by the Electronic Industries Association (EIA). Crystalline materials most commonly used as phosphors are based on zinc sulfide, although recently there has been increasing usage of rare earth activated oxides and oxysulfides. The important factors to consider in the selection of phosphors are luminous conversion efficiency, decay time, color, and longevity. A large number of phosphors can convert 10–20% of electron beam energy into light. These efficiencies are remarkably high, with a magnitude of 10 or more times those used in display devices of other types, which is one of the reasons for the continued predominance of CRT technology.

Phosphor decay times may vary from less than a microsecond to a few seconds. The longer persisting phosphors can be used to reduce flicker by allowing significant integration of temporal variations in luminance. This practice works well for stationary images but causes smearing in dynamic images. Phosphors of almost any emis-

TABLE 12.2 Specifications of Three Popular Phosphors Used in Display Monitors

Phosphor*	Primary Color (%)			Decay Time (ms)	Efficiency (relative to P4)
	Red	Green	Blue		
P4	27	30	43	0.100	1.00
P40	26	33	41	>100.0	0.76
P164	27	29	44	>100.0	0.60

*From EIA registry.

sion color may be selected from the visible light spectrum. The conversion efficiency is degraded as the excitation increases. Most phosphors have a practical lifetime of several thousand hours. To prolong phosphor longevity, the screensaver feature (in which the electron beam is automatically shut off after a certain period of user input inactivity) is often installed in workstations.

Phosphor selection criteria involve the following considerations (see Table 12.2).

1. During excitation, the phosphor should acquire a slight blue tint (the phosphor steady state color), resemble the hue of the radiograph. The relative percentage of the primary colors presented in a given color can be found from the chromaticity diagram of the International Commission on Illumination (CIE).
2. Phosphors with light scintillation decay times shorter than the field refresh rate of an interlacing scan (16.7 ms), or the frame refresh rate of a progressive scan (33.3 ms), will cause an annoying flicker effect in the static image. To minimize flicker, the phosphor decay time should be longer than the scanning refresh rate.
3. Light output efficiency provides a scale of efficiency for a given input beam current. A phosphor with a low efficiency (relative to P4) needs a larger beam current to produce the same light output influence (intensity). A larger beam current, however, reduces the life expectancy of the electron beam in the monitor.

12.1.2.3 Coating of the Glass Tube

Some computer terminals use an antiglare coat or screen to minimize the glare due to the reflection from the glass tube. The currently available antiglare coating is not suitable for use in image display monitors, however, because it reduces resolution. Some removable antiglare screens are being tested to determine the trade-off between minimizing reflection and lowering resolution (see Section 12.2.1).

12.1.2.4 Resolution

The display screen contains a layer of phosphor 10 μm or less thick. The pixel size is limited by the spot size of the electron beam. The spot, which has a Gaussian-like current distribution over a cross-sectional area, is usually defined as the width between points at which the beam current has dropped to a certain fraction, such as $1/e$ ($\approx 37\%$) of its maximum value. The beam spot diameter increases linearly as the square root of the beam current. The minimum diameter to which this spot size can be reduced is dictated by the beam current required to produce acceptable phosphor brightness. Therefore, there is a trade-off between resolution and image brightness.

The resolution of a display monitor is most commonly specified in terms of number of scan lines. For example, a "1K monitor" has 1024 raster lines; "2K" means 2048 lines. In the strict sense of the definition, however, it is not sufficient to specify spatial resolution simply in terms of raster lines because the actual resolving power of the monitor may be less. Consider a digitally generated line pair pattern (black and white lines in pairs). The maximum displayable number of these line pairs on a 1K monitor is 512. If the electron beam spot is out of focus or the contrast/brightness is set too high, causing the adjacent raster lines to overlap, however, the monitor may not be able to resolve 1024 alternating black and white lines in the vertical direction. Horizontal resolution has no relation to the number of raster lines; rather, it is limited by the beam spot size and depends on how quickly the beam current changes according to the driving video signals (see Section 3.2).

Several techniques are available for the measurement of resolution. The simplest and most commonly used method employs a test pattern that consists of varying widths of line pair objects in vertical, horizontal, and sometimes radial directions (refer to Fig. 2.3A). It should be noted that this visual approach measures the resolution of the total display–perception system, including the visual acuity of the observer, and therefore it is prone to subjective variations.

Other techniques include the shrinking raster test, the scanning spot photometer, the slit analyzer, and measurement of the modulation transfer function (MTF) (Section 2.5.1.4). One additional noteworthy issue is that resolution is a function of location on the screen. In general, the defocusing effect increases as the electron beam moves away from the center of the screen. Therefore, resolution specification must be accompanied by data concerning where on the screen the measurement was taken, as well as the luminance of the screen.

12.1.2.5 Geometric Distortion

Soft copy display using a CRT monitor can create certain geometric distortions, such as the pincushion and barrel effects, nonlinearity, hook and flagging, line pairing, and ringing. Pincushion distortions, common in large screens, exhibited nonlinear inward edges. Barreling, or nonlinear outward edges, can be the result of overcorrection for pincushion distortion. Nonlinearity is noticeable when a large circle is displayed with flattening or stretching. Hooking or flagging is usually present as a bending of the upper left corner of the screen on the edge of the raster scan. Line pairing, a bunching of horizontal scan lines, which show up as bright and dark regions, happens most often in interlaced monitors. Ringing is seen at the left side of the screen as a series of dark and light shaded bands that disappear a small distance from the edge. Geometric distortion on a monitor does happen from time to time; it can be eliminated by means of calibration during preventive maintenance with a standard phantom (e.g., the SMPTE described in Fig. 2.3D).

12.1.2.6 Luminance and Contrast

Luminance measures the brightness in candelas per square meter (cd/m²) or in foot-lamberts (ft-L): 1 ft-L = 3.426 cd/m². Luminance is a function of the electron beam current and the conversion efficiency of the phosphor. There is more than one definition for contrast and contrast ratio. The one that is most often used for contrast, C, is the ratio of the difference between two luminances to one of the two luminances, usually the larger,

$$C = \frac{L_B - L_O}{L_B} \tag{12.1}$$

$$C = \frac{L_O - L_B}{L_O} \tag{12.2}$$

where L_O is the luminance of the object and L_B is the luminance of the background.

Contrast ratio C_r is frequently defined as the ratio of the luminance of an object to that of the background. This is expressed by:

$$C_r = L_{max} / L_{min} \tag{12.3}$$

where L_{max} is the luminance emitted by the area of the greatest intensity and L_{min} is the luminance emitted by the area of least intensity.

Because of the particular nature of the phosphors and their optical transparency, the screen acts as a high efficiency reflector that scatters 25–75% of the incident light. The light emitted from the phosphor is viewed against this reflected light. The contrast ratio, therefore, depends not only on the luminance of the CRT image but on the intensity of the ambient light as well. For instance, in bright sunlight the display surface can have an apparent luminance of 3×10^4 cd/m². To achieve a contrast of 10, the luminance of the cathodoluminescence must be 3×10^5 cd/m², which is extremely high even for a high efficiency phosphor.

12.1.2.7 Human Perception

Luminance of the CRT affects the physiological response of the eye in perceiving image quality (spatial resolution and subject contrast). Two characteristics of the visual response are acuity, or the ability of the eye to detect fine detail, and the detection of luminance differences (threshold contrast) between the object and its background. Luminance differences can be measured by using an absolute parameter, just noticeable differences (JNDs), or a relative parameter, threshold contrast (TC), related by:

$$\mathrm{TC} = \frac{\mathrm{JND}}{L_B} \qquad (12.4)$$

where L_B is the background luminance.

The relationship between the threshold contrast and the luminance can be described by the Weber–Fechner law. When the luminance is low (1 ft-L), in the double-log plot, the threshold contrast is a linear function of luminance, with a slope of -0.05 sometimes referred to as the Rose model.* When the luminance is high, the threshold contrast is governed by the Weber model, which is a constant function of the luminance, again in the double-log plot. In the Rose model region, when the object luminance L_o is fixed, the JND and the background luminance L_B are related by

$$\mathrm{JND} = k_1 L_o \, (L_B)^{1/2} \qquad (12.5)$$

In the Weber model region, we write

$$\mathrm{JND} = k_2 L_o \, (L_B) \qquad (12.6)$$

where k_1 and k_2 are constants.

In general, the detection of small luminance differences by the visual system is dependent on the presence of various noises that are measurable by their standard deviations, in particular:

- the fluctuations in the light photon flux
- the noise from the display monitor
- the noise in the visual system

Thus, the JND depends on L_o and L_B, which in turn are affected by the environment, the state of the display monitor, and the conditions experienced by the human observer.

12.1.3 Color CRT

Although the majority of radiographic images are monochromatic, Doppler US, nuclear medicine, and PET images use colors for enhancement. Also, recent developments in image-guided therapy and minimum invasiveness surgery use extensive color graphics superimposed on monochromatic images. The oldest and still most widely used design of color CRT is the shadow mask. It consists of three electron guns, a shadow mask with circular holes, and a phosphor screen. The phosphor screen has arrays of "triads," each consisting of the phosphors of the three primary emission colors, red, green, and blue. The guns are positioned in a triangular or delta form—the so-called delta gun. The geometrical relationship of delta gun, shadow mask, and screen is such that the beam from each gun strikes only one type of phosphor in the

---

* $\mathrm{TC} = -0.5 L_B$ in the double-log plot, or $\mathrm{TC} = k(L_B)^{-1/2}$ in the standard plot, where k is a constant.

triad. The other two types of phosphor are masked from the gun by the shadow mask. Since the beams are made larger than the holes, a beam will completely fill the hole to transfer the maximum energy to the phosphor. Three guns can independently modulate the beam current to produce the desired color mixture for each triad.

In the recent years, the shadow mask and gun design has been improved to meet the increasing demands of the high brightness, high resolution market in such applications as large-scale PC board design, detailed CAD/CAM, and computer graphics. The current trend is to place guns in line to achieve better tracking of the beam, thus improving the hit rate of the proper color phosphor. The shadow mask may be either slotted or circular to match with the corresponding screen, with color triads laid down as vertical stripes or as circular dots, respectively. To display a color image, three image memories (R, G, B) are needed. As shown in Section 5.7, composite video controller combines these three memories to form a color display (see Fig. 5.21).

12.1.4 Types of Image Workstation

Image workstations can be loosely categorized into six types based on their applications. Thus there are diagnostic, review, analysis, digitizing and printing, interactive teaching, and desktop workstations.

12.1.4.1 Diagnostic Workstation

A diagnostic workstation is used by the radiologists for making primary diagnosis. The components in this type of workstation must be of the best quality possible. If the workstation is used for displaying projection radiographs, multiple 2K monitors are needed. On the other hand, if the workstation is used for CT and MR images, multiple 1K monitors will be sufficient. A diagnostic workstation requires a digital Dictaphone to report the findings. The workstation provides software to append the report to the images. In addition to having all the image processing functions described in Section 12.3, the diagnostic workstation requires a rapid ($\approx$ 1–2 s) image retrieval. Figure 12.4 shows a two-monitor 2K display workstation at UCSF. The 2K workstation is based on the Sun SPARC server 470 computer and two 21-inch diagonal 2K portrait mode monitors (UHR-4820P MegaScan display system, E-Systems, Littleton, MA). The workstation has a parallel transfer disk (RAID) with 5.2 Gbyte formatted storage, which can display a 2048 × 2048 × 12-bit image in 1.5 seconds (Storage Concepts, Irvine, CA).

12.1.4.2 Review Workstation

A review workstation is used by radiologists and referring physicians to review cases in the hospital wards. The dictation or the transcribed report should be available, with the corresponding images. A review workstation may not require 2K monitors, since images might have been read by the radiologist from the diagnostic workstation, and the referring physicians will not be looking for every minute detail. Diagnostic and review workstations can be combined as a single workstation sharing both diagnos-

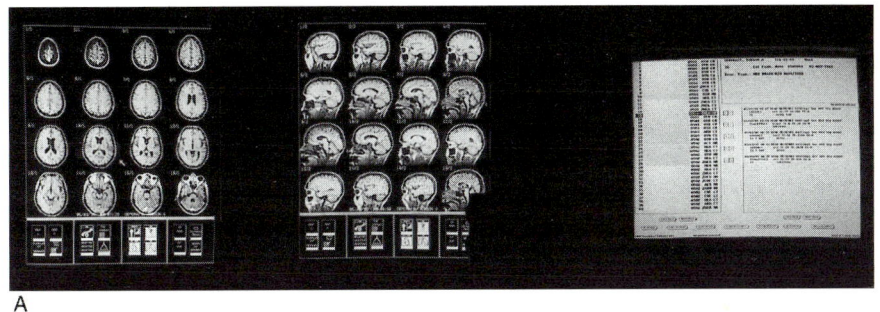

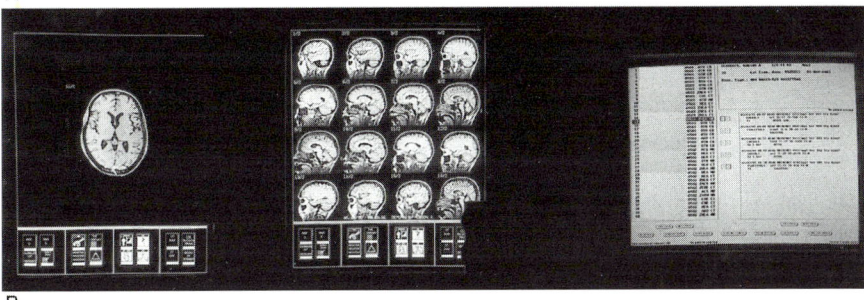

Figure 12.4 Two-monitor 2K display workstation showing two sets of MR neurological images. (A) The patient directory (left) and the study list (right) are shown on the text monitor. Image processing functions are controlled by the icons located at the bottom of the 2K monitor screens and by external knobs. (B) An enlarged image (left) appears during operation in cine mode; the right monitor display remains intact.

tic and review functions like an alternator. Figure 12.5 shows a two-monitor 1K (1600-line) display station used in the intensive care units at UCSF. This workstation consists of a Sun SPARC 20 workstation with 2 gigabyte magnetic disks, two GXTurbo video display boards, and two 1600×1024 display monitors.

12.1.4.3 Analysis Workstation

Analysis workstations differ from diagnostic and review workstations in that the former are used to extract useful parameters from images. Some parameters are easy to extract from a simple region of interest (ROI) operation, as described in Section 12.3; others (e.g., blood flow measurements from DSA, 3-D reconstruction from sequential CT images) are computation intensive and require an analysis workstation with a more powerful image processor and high performance software. Figure 12.6 shows an analysis workstation displaying a 3-D rendering PET brain image set fused with a corresponding MR image set.

12.1.4.4 Digitizing and Printing Workstation

The digitizing and printing workstation is for radiology department technologists or film librarians who must digitize historical films, and films from outside the depart-

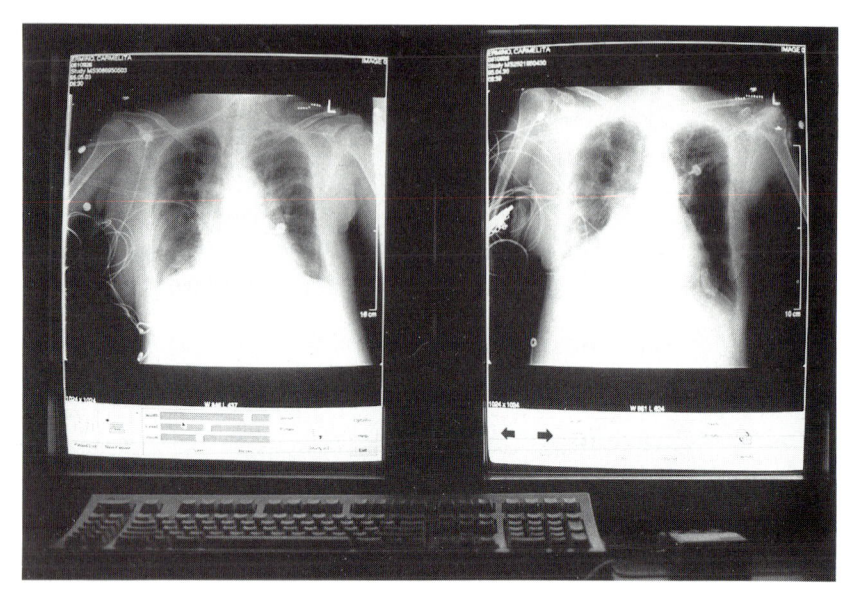

Figure 12.5 Two-monitor 1K (1600 lines) ICU display workstation showing two CR images. Left-hand monitor shows the current image; all previous images can be accessed within one second on the right-hand monitor by clicking the two lower icons (Previous and Next). Image processing functions are controlled by the icons located at the bottom of the screens.

ment. The workstation is also used for converting soft copy images to hard copy. In addition to the standard workstation components already described, this workstation requires a laser film scanner (see Section 3.2.2), a laser film imager (see Section 12.4), and a paper printer. The paper printer is used for pictorial report generation (see Section 12.1.4.6) from the diagnostic, review, and editorial and research workstations. A 1K display monitor for quality control purposes is sufficient for this type of workstation.

12.1.4.5 Interactive Teaching Workstation

A teaching workstation is used for interactive teaching. It emulates the role of teaching files in the film library but with more interactive features. Figures 12.7 and 12.8 show a digital mammography teaching workstation from VICOM (Fremont, CA), and the workstation architecture, respectively.

12.1.4.6 Desktop Workstation

The desktop workstation is for physicians or researchers to generate lecture slides, as well as teaching and research materials, from images and related data in the PACS database. This workstation uses everyday desktop computer equipment to facilitate the user's daily work. Sections 13.2 and 13.3 describe the architecture of a desktop workstation in more detail.

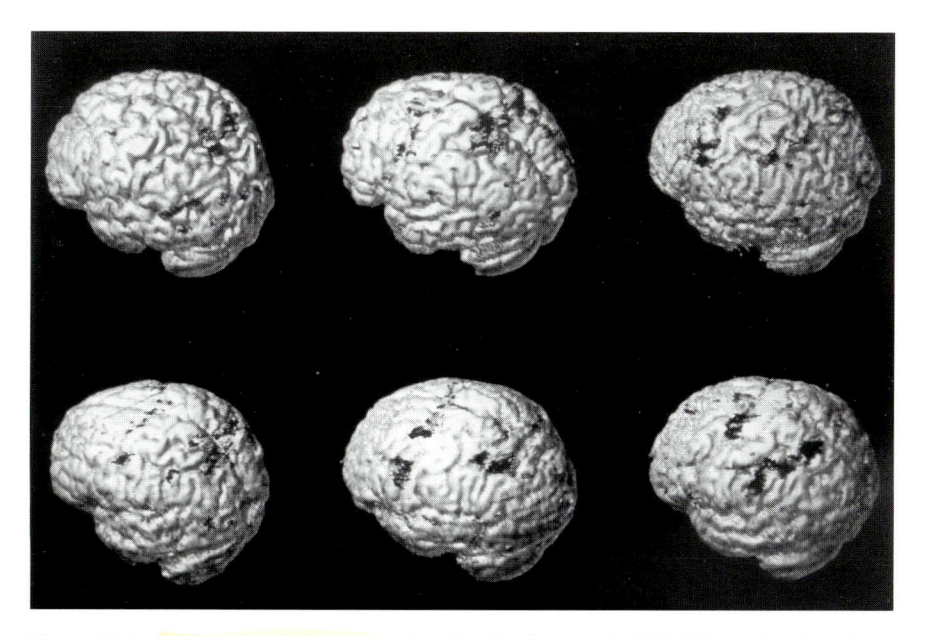

Figure 12.6 High end analysis workstation (Reality Station, ONYX, Silicon Graphics Computer Systems, Mountain View, CA) at UCSF showing 3-D rendering of MR (gray scale) and PET (red) fusion brain images. (Courtesy of K. Soo Hoo) (See color plate.)

Image workstations with which radiologists and physicians can directly interact are the most important and visible component in a PACS. To design them effectively, a thorough understanding of the clinical operation environment requirements is necessary.

12.2 ERGONOMICS OF IMAGE WORKSTATIONS

Among the factors in the ergonomics of an image workstation relating to perceived image quality are lighting conditions, glare, and acoustic noise due to hardware.

12.2.1 Glare

Glare, the most frequent complaint among the workstation users, is the sensation produced within the visual field by luminance that is sufficiently greater than the luminance to which the eyes are adapted to cause annoyance, discomfort, or loss in visual performance and visibility (see Section 12.1.2.6 on luminance and contrast).

Glare can be caused by reflections of electric light sources, windows, and light-colored objects including furniture and clothing. The magnitude of sensation of glare is a function of the size, position, and luminance of a source, the number of sources, and the luminance to which the eyes are adapted at the moment. It may be categorized according to its origin: direct or reflected glare. Direct glare may be caused by

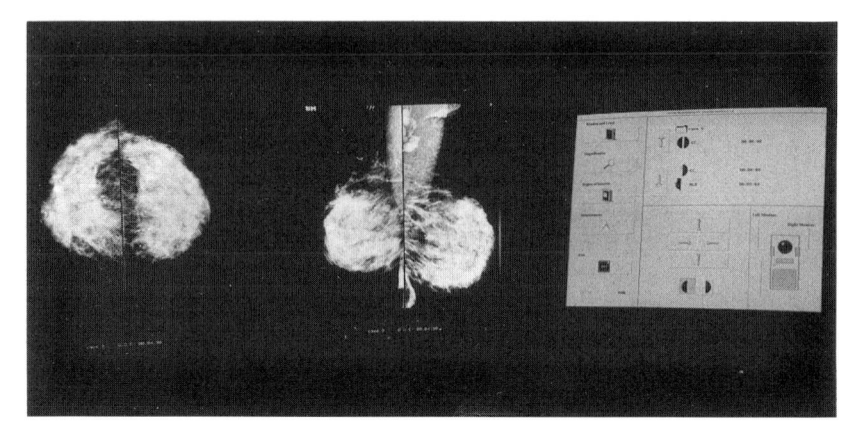

Figure 12.7 Four mammograms from a 2K digital mammography teaching workstation: *left:* left and right craniocaudal views; *middle:* left and right mediolateral oblique views; *right:* text monitor with icons for image display and manipulation at this workstation.

bright sources of light in the visual field of view (e.g., sunlight and lightbulbs). Reflected glare is caused by light reflected from the display screen (see Section 12.1.2.3 on coating of the glass tube). Diffuse reflections are referred to as veiling glare.

Image reflections are both distracting and annoying, because the eye is induced to focus alternately on the displayed and reflected images. The reflected glare can be reduced by increasing the display contrast, by wearing dark-colored clothing, by correctly positioning the screen with respect to lights, windows, and other reflective objects, and by adjusting the screen angle.

Further reduction of glare can be achieved by etching the screen glass, by treating the glass with antireflective coatings, or by superimposing on the screen antireflection filters such as micromesh, circular polarizers, and neutral density filters with antireflective coatings. Etching the glass reduces reflection by scattering the reflected light, thus giving reflected objects a more diffuse and less conspicuous appearance. Since the light emitted from the display phosphors is also dispersed, image sharpness may be compromised. Coating of the screen with a thin film of antireflective agent such as Lambda-4 usually does not diminish the image sharpness. Fingerprints, however, can easily and permanently smear the coating layer. Antireflection filters reduce the perceived glare by attenuating the reflected light more than the light emitted from the CRT, since the reflected light must pass through the filter twice. By means of an-

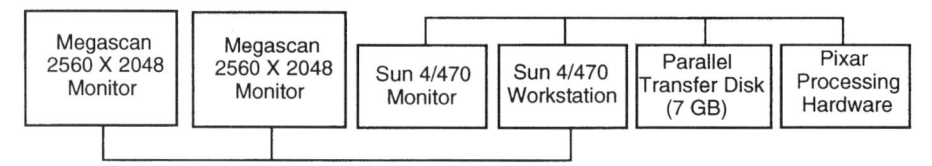

Figure 12.8 Architecture of the 2K digital mammography teaching workstation. In this design, the Sun 4/470 is the host computer and the Pixar is the image processor. The parallel transfer disk (RAID) setup allows 1–2 seconds display time for a 2K image.

tireflective techniques, objective methods can be derived to measure luminance, modulation transfer function, contrast, and glare, as well as subjectively evaluate brightness, sharpness, contrast, color, and glare. On the average, the order of preference of measures to reduce glare is as follows: gray antireflection filter, micromesh filter, circular polarizer, blue antireflection filter, etched plastic filter, and no filter.

12.2.2 Ambient Illuminance

An important issue related to the problem of glare is the proper illumination of the workstation area. Excessive lighting can increase the readability of documents but can also increase the reflected glare, while merely sufficient illumination can reduce glare but can make reading of source documents at the display workstation difficult.

Ergonomic guidelines for the traditional office environment recommend a high level of lighting: 700 lux (an engineering unit for lighting) or more (Cushman, 1987). A survey of 38 CAD operators who were allowed to adjust the ambient lighting at their workstations indicated that the median illumination level is around 125 lux (125 at keyboard, etc.) with 90% of the readings falling between 15 and 505 lux (Heiden, 1984). These levels are optimized for CRT viewing but certainly not for reading written documents. An illumination of 200 lux is normally considered inadequate for an office environment. Another study suggests a lower range (150–400 lux) for tasks that do not involve information transfer from paper documents. At these levels, lighting is sufficiently subdued to permit good display contrast in most cases. The higher range (400–550 lux) is suggested for tasks that require the reading of paper documents. Increasing ambient lighting (> 550 lux) reduces display contrast appreciably. If the paper documents contain small and low contrast print, however, 550 lux may not provide adequate lighting. Such cases may call for supplementary special task lighting directed at the document surface only. This recommendation is based on the conditions needed to read text, not images, on a screen. Another recommendation specifies the use of a level of ambient illumination equal to the average luminance of an image on the display workstation screen (Horii, 1992).

12.2.3 Acoustic Noise Due to Hardware

An imaging workstation often includes components like RAID, image processors, and other arrays of hardware that produce heat and require electric fans for cooling. These fans often produce an intolerably high noise level. Even a low noise host computer attached to the display workstation should be separated from the display workstation area to isolate the noise, which would affect the human performance.

As personal computers become more and more common, the computer, the terminal, and the display monitor meld into an integrated system insofar as they are connected by very short cables. Most imaging workstations utilize a personal computer as the host, however, and because of the short cabling, the host computer and the image processor wind up in the same room as the terminal, the display monitors, and the keyboard. Failure of the image workstation designer to consider the consequences of having all these units together creates a very noisy environment at the imaging workstation, and it is difficult for the user to sustain concentration during long working hours. Care must be exercised in designing the workstation environment to avoid problems due to acoustic noise from the hardware.

12.3 IMAGE PROCESSING AND DISPLAY FUNCTIONS

12.3.1 Image Enhancement Functions

Image processing is used at the display workstation to improve the diagnostic value of the images. This section discusses some commonly used image processing functions for enhancing radiology diagnosis. Image processing functions are different from preprocessing functions (see Section 8.7) in the sense that preprocessing does not alter the appearance of the image, whereas processing will.

12.3.1.1 Outlining

Let $f(x,y)$ be the gray level of a pixel located in (x,y). The absolute partial differences

$$|\Delta_x f| = K|f(x + 1,y) - f(x,y)| \qquad (12.7)$$

$$|\Delta_y f| = K|f(x,y + 1) - f(x,y)| \qquad (12.8)$$

measure the rate of change of gray level (or the gradient) at the pixel (x,y) in the horizontal and vertical directions, respectively, where K is a constant. An image sensitive to both horizontal and vertical directions can be measured by using the maximum absolute partial difference as follows:

$$\text{MAX } \Delta = \max(|\Delta_x f|, |\Delta_y f|) \qquad (12.9)$$

Figure 12.9 shows an example of applying Eqs. (12.7), (12.8), and (12.9) to a digitized chest radiograph (Fig. 12.9A). The results are shown in Figures 12.9B, C, and D, respectively. It should be pointed out that "outlining" only enhances the visual appearance of objects of interest in an image; it does not extract the boundary coordinates that are sometimes necessary to define a region of interest (ROI).

12.3.1.2 Boundary Detection

During an image review session it is sometimes desirable to measure some parameters (average gray level, shape, and geometry) of an object of interest in the image. To do so, we first extract the boundary of the ROI. When the region or object of interest has more than one boundary, the procedure is called *segmentation*.

Two steps are involved in boundary detection: determination of a cutoff gray level of the ROI and a boundary search. A cutoff gray level can be determined by using either the histogram method or an approach that is often more subjective, namely, defining the object boundary as one or more preset gray levels in an image.

In the histogram method, a CT head image (e.g., Fig. 12.10A) is analyzed to pro-

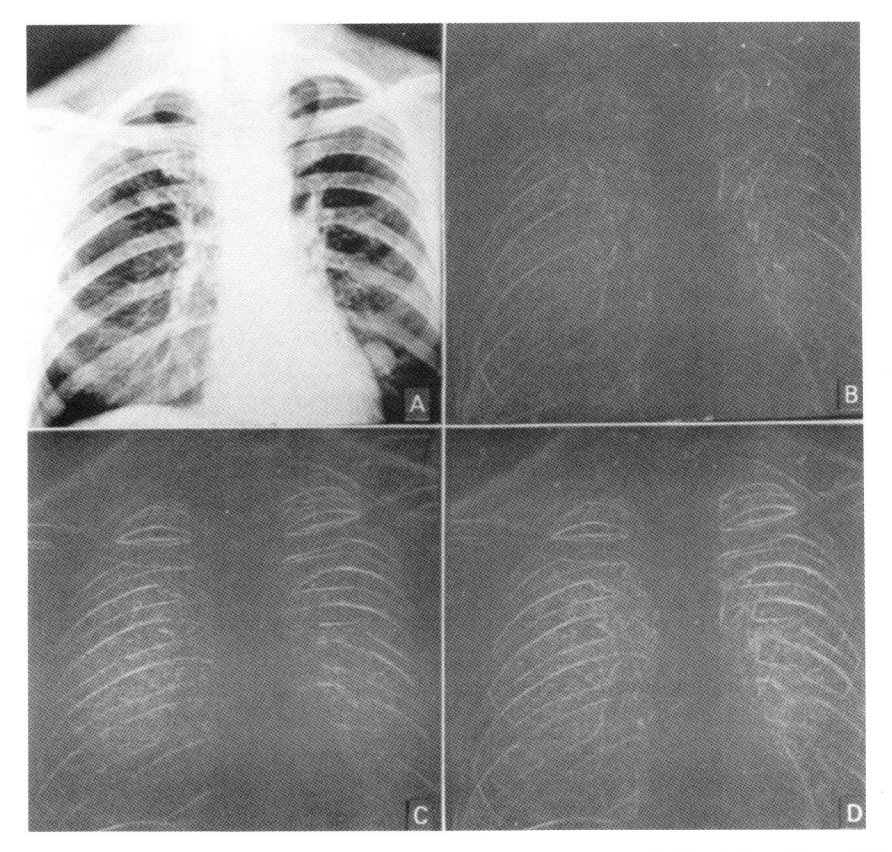

Figure 12.9 Example illustrating the principle of outlining: (A) digitized chest X-ray, (B) $\Delta_x f$, (C) $\Delta_y f$, and (D) MAX Δ.

duce a histogram (Fig. 12.10B), which includes the object of interest as well as the background. Boundary detection is initiated by defining the cutoff gray level of the ventricles and the brain (outlined in Fig. 12.10C) as the gray level value at the troughs: a and b in histogram of Figure 12.10B.

Once the cutoff gray level is known, the coordinates of the boundary can be obtained by a programmed search in the vicinity of the object of interest. The procedure starts with an automatic search of a pixel whose value is equal to the cutoff gray level value. Once identified, this pixel becomes the first boundary pixel of this ROI and its (x,y) coordinates are recorded. Its eight adjacent neighbors are searched systematically, one by one, to determine the best candidate for the next boundary pixel. The search follows the scheme:

$$
\begin{array}{ccc}
3 & 2 & 1 \\
4 & * & 8 \\
5 & 6 & 7
\end{array}
$$

where * is the current boundary pixel, and the numerals are the order of the search.

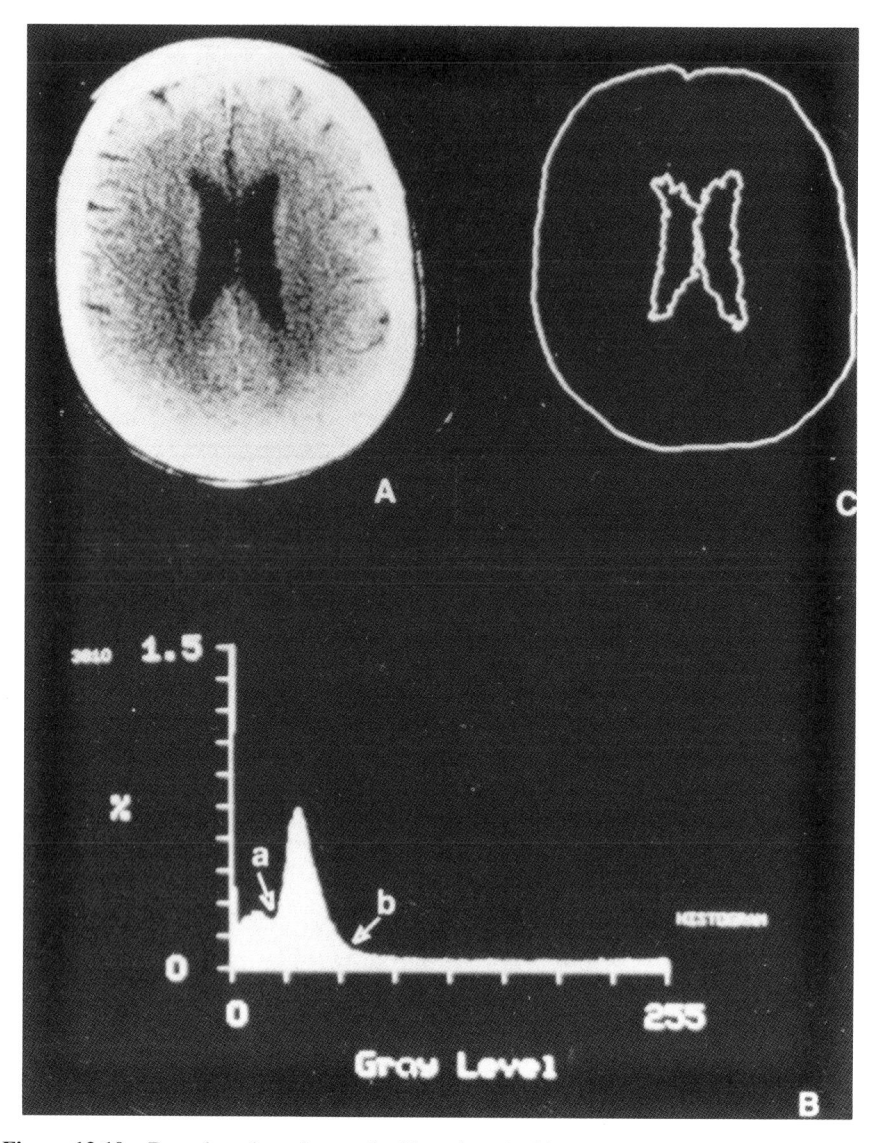

Figure 12.10 Boundary detection method based on the histogram of an image: (A) CT head image, (B) histogram of the CT head image, and (C) outlines of the brain and the ventricles using the boundary detection method.

The criteria used to determine the best candidate are closeness of pixel value to the cutoff boundary value and present status as a boundary pixel. The best candidate becomes the second boundary pixel, and the procedure is repeated until all the boundary pixels of the object have been located and recorded. In general, the boundary of an object of interest is a closed curve.

Deblurring Occasionally, an image is blurred as a result of an imperfection that comes about during the radiographic acquisition procedure. If the blur is not severe, it is possible to sharpen the image by using a deblurring procedure.

The most popular deblurring technique is based on the assumption that the picture has been blurred by a process that satisfies the two-dimensional diffusion equation. Thus to deblur the image, one can apply the following approximate equation:

$$f = 2\bar{f} - \bar{f}_{av} = (\bar{f} - \bar{f}_{av}) + \bar{f} \qquad (12.10)$$

where $\bar{f}$ is the blurred image, f is the deblurred image, and

$$\bar{f}_{av} = \frac{\nabla^2 \bar{f}}{5} + \bar{f} \qquad (12.11)$$

is the five-point average of $\bar{f}$, and

$$\nabla^2 \bar{f} = -4\bar{f}(x,y) + \bar{f}(x-1,y) + \bar{f}(x+1,y) + \bar{f}(x,y-1) + \bar{f}(x,y+1) \qquad (12.12)$$

is the Laplacian operator.

To obtain a sharper image f from an image $\bar{f}$, therefore, one can take the difference between this image $\bar{f}$ and its average image $\bar{f}_{av}$ and add the difference to $\bar{f}$. Intuitively, the difference between $\bar{f}$ and $\bar{f}_{av}$ yields the high frequency content of the original image f, which was lost during the acquisition of the imperfect image.

As an example, consider Figure 12.11A, which is the blurred image $\bar{f}$ obtained from Figure 12.9A using a Gaussian distribution filter (see Section 12.3.1.4). If one computes $2\bar{f} - \bar{f}_{av}$, the resulting deblurring image f is as shown in Figure 12.11B. It is seen immediately that the deblurred image (Fig. 12.11B) has better quality than the blurred image (Fig. 12.11A), but it is still not as good as the original image (Fig. 12.9A).

12.3.1.3 Noise Cleaning

Radiologic images often suffer from various types of noise. One common type is TV "snow" or "salt and pepper" noise, in which the gray levels of some points have been randomly increased or decreased. Such noise can be reduced by local averaging of the image using Eq. (12.11), but this process is undesirable because it produces a blurring effect. Instead, one can use a nonlinear process that replaces a point by the average of its neighbors, provided the point differs from most or all of its neighbors by a significant amount (i.e., above or below a threshold). If such a process still has a blurring effect on edges where the gray level is changing rapidly, one can use an edge-sensitive operator (i.e., the absolute partial difference: Eq. 12.9) to detect the presence of edges of objects of interest. And at edge points, one can average only the neighbors that lie in the direction along the edge detected by the edge-sensitive operator.

Figure 12.12A shows a chest image superposed by the salt-and-pepper noise. Fig-

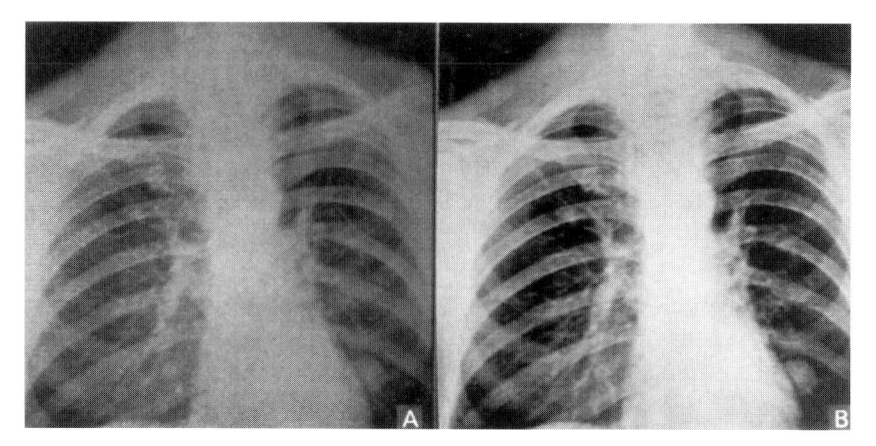

Figure 12.11 Example illustrating the deblurring process: (A) blurred image obtained from Figure 12.9A by using a Gausian smooth filter and (B) the image deblurred by means of Eq. (12.10).

ure 12.12B demonstrates how this noise can be minimized by using a median filter operation (see Section 12.3.1.4).

12.3.1.4 Filtering

Filtering can be used to smooth an image or to sharpen it, regardless of whether the image is represented in the spatial domain or in the frequency domain (see Section 2.4).

Spatial Domain Smoothing is usually performed to get rid of image noise. In the method for smoothing an image represented by Eq. (12.11), the image $\bar{f}$ is smoothed

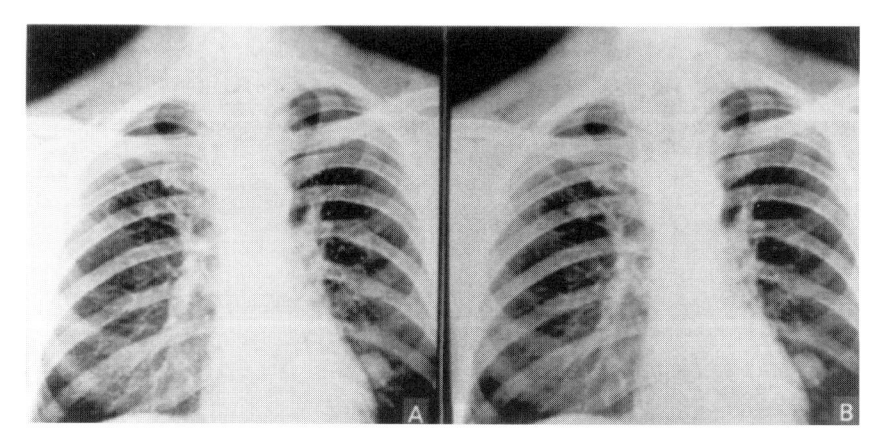

Figure 12.12 (A) Salt-and-pepper noise (small dots) is introduced in a chest pulmonary arteriogram randomly, (B) a 3 × 3 medium filter is used to minimize the salt-and-pepper noise (observe, however, that the image is not as sharp as the original image).

by replacing each pixel value with the average gray level of the four adjacent neighbor pixels and itself. The resultant image $\bar{f}_{av}$ is a smoother image than $\bar{f}$. Another smoothing filter in the spatial domain is the median filter, which replaces the pixel value by the median pixel value of certain neighbor pixels. The result shown in Figure 12.12B is an example. Still another useful smoothing filter is the Gaussian filter, which smoothes the image by convolving a Gaussian function with the image (see Section 5.1.3 for definition of convolution). Figure 12.11A illustrates the Gaussian smoothing of Figure 12.9A. Notice that the smoothing procedures described here are different from those described in Section 2.5.2. In the latter the smoothing is done with many images, whereas in this case the smoothing is performed on pixels within a neighborhood of an image.

The deblurring procedure described earlier in connection with Eq. (12.10) is a linear filtering technique used to sharpen an image. The difference $(\bar{f} - \bar{f}_{av})$ represents the sharper edges in the image, which are emphasized and added back to the original image $\bar{f}$. The image f appears to be sharper than $\bar{f}$.

Frequency Domain Filtering in the frequency domain is performed as follows. The image is first transformed to the frequency domain, and the amplitude of each frequency component of the image is modified (or filtered). The modulated image is transformed back to the spatial domain as the filtered image. Depending on how each frequency component is manipulated, the filtered image is either smoother or sharper than the original image.

The Fourier transform described in Section 2.4.2 is a method commonly used to perform the image transform. Recall from Eq. (2.5) that after $f(x,y)$ has been transformed, the real and imaginary components $R(u,v)$ and $I(u,v)$ of $F(u,v)$

$$F(u,v) = \frac{1}{N} \sum_{x=0}^{N-1} \sum_{y=0}^{N-1} f(x,y) \exp\left[\frac{-i2\pi(ux+vy)}{N}\right] \quad (2.5)$$

$$= R(u,v) + iI(u,v)$$

for $u, v = 0, 1, 2, \ldots, N-1$

can be modified for each frequency (u,v). In the process called low pass filtering, we write

$$\text{Re}(u,v) = 0 \quad \text{and} \quad \text{Im}(u,v) = 0 \quad \text{for} \quad (u^2 + v^2)^{1/2} \geq r \quad (12.13)$$

where r is some constant. That is, all frequency components with a radius greater than and equal to r are deleted, and only low frequency components remain. In high pass filtering, we have

$$\text{Re}(u,v) = 0 \quad \text{and} \quad \text{Im}(u,v) = 0 \quad \text{for} \quad (u^2 + v^2)^{1/2} < r \quad (12.14)$$

All frequency components with a radius less than r are deleted, and only high frequency components remain in the inverse transformed image. Figure 12.13 shows re-

Panel 1

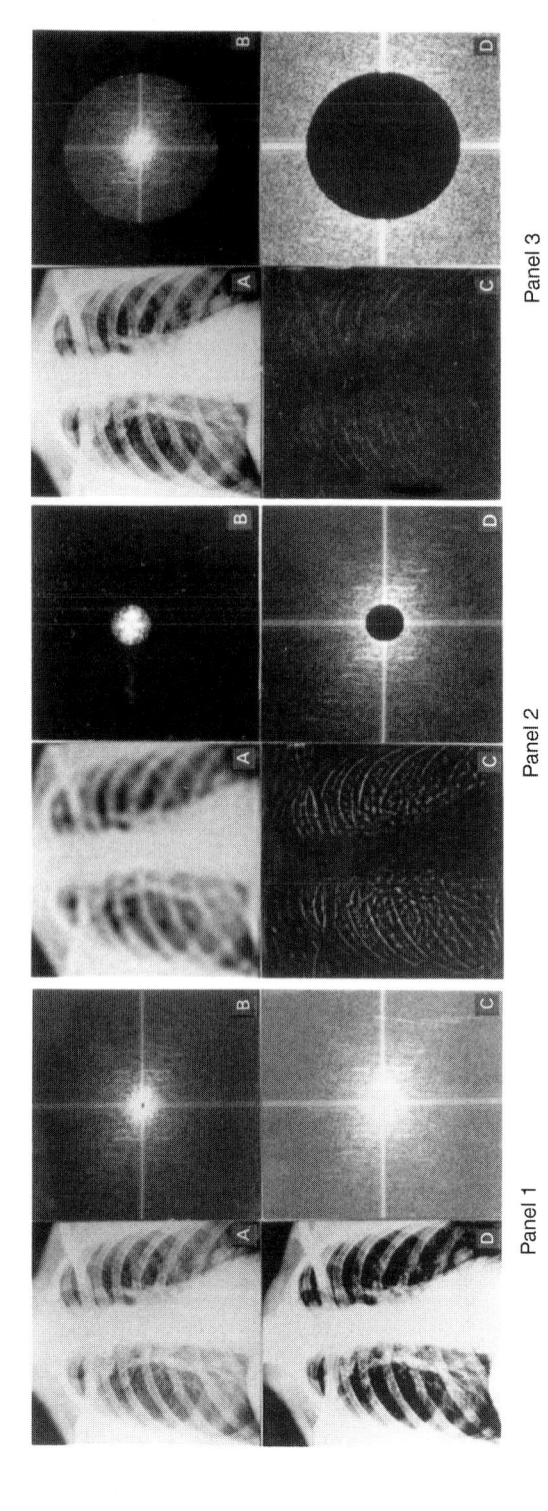

Panel 2

Panel 3

Figure 12.13 *Panel 1:* (A) Digitized chest x-ray. (B) Its Fourier transform, $N = 256$; the origin (0,0) of the display is at the center of the image, and the coordinates of the edges are ± 128. (C) The Fourier transform is modulated by an exponential filter for contrast enhancement. (D) The inverse modulated Fourier transform shows that it is higher contrast than (A). *Panel 2:* Upper row: Results from a low pass filter, Eq. (12.13), $r = (u^2 + v^2)^{1/2} \geq 20$ in the display coordinate system: (B) is the filtered transform image; the inverse filtered transform image, (A), has lost its sharpness. Lower row: Results from a high pass filter, Eq. (12.14), $(u^2 + v^2)^{1/2} < 20$. (D) is the filtered transform image; (C) is the inverse filtered transform image, (only the edges remained). By adding (A) and (C) together, we could have the original image (A, panel 1). *Panel 3:* Same as panel 2 except $r = 80$.

326

sults applying high pass and low pass filters on a chest radiograph for different values of *u* and *v*.

When Re(u,v) and Im(u,v) are modified for a given (u,v), the process is called a frequency emphasis. The inverse transformed image will emphasize the change of the particular frequency component (u,v).

12.3.2 Image Display and Measurement Functions

Although display workstations should have the image processing functions described in Section 12.3.1, it is not advisable to introduce these advanced image processing features into the clinical environment until the users thoroughly understand the consequences of such operations. Advanced features that are not well understood only cause confusion in the analysis of images. For these reasons, advanced image processing functions should be included in the analysis workstation and, as an option, in the diagnostic or review workstation. On the other hand, a set of easy-to-use image display and measurement functions should be included in the image workstation to assist users in diagnostic work. Sections 12.3.2.1 to 12.3.2.5 describe some of these functions.

12.3.2.1 Zoom and Scroll

Zooming and scrolling is an interactive command manipulated via a trackball or a mouse. The operator first uses the trackball to scroll about the image, centering the region of interest on the screen. The ROI can then be magnified by pressing a designated button to perform the zoom. The image becomes more blocky as the zoom factor increases, reflecting the greater number of times each pixel is replicated.

Although it is useful to magnify and scroll the image on the screen, the field of view decreases in proportion to the square of the magnification factor. Magnification is commonly performed via pixel replication or interpolation. In the former, one pixel value repeats itself several times in both the horizontal and vertical directions, and in the latter, the pixel value is replaced by interpolation of its neighbors. For example, to magnify the image by 2 by replication is to replicate the image 2×2 times.

12.3.2.2 Window and Level

The window and level feature allows the user to control the interval of gray levels to be displayed on the monitor. The center of this interval is called the *level value,* and the range is called the *window value.* The selected gray level range will be distributed over the entire dynamic range of the display monitor, and, thus, using a smaller window value will cause the contrast in the resulting video image to increase. Gray levels present in the image outside the defined interval are clipped to black or white (or both), depending on which side of the interval they are positioned. This function is also controlled by the user via a trackball or mouse. For example, moving the trackball in the vertical direction typically controls the window value, while the horizontal direction controls the level of which gray levels are displayed on the video moni-

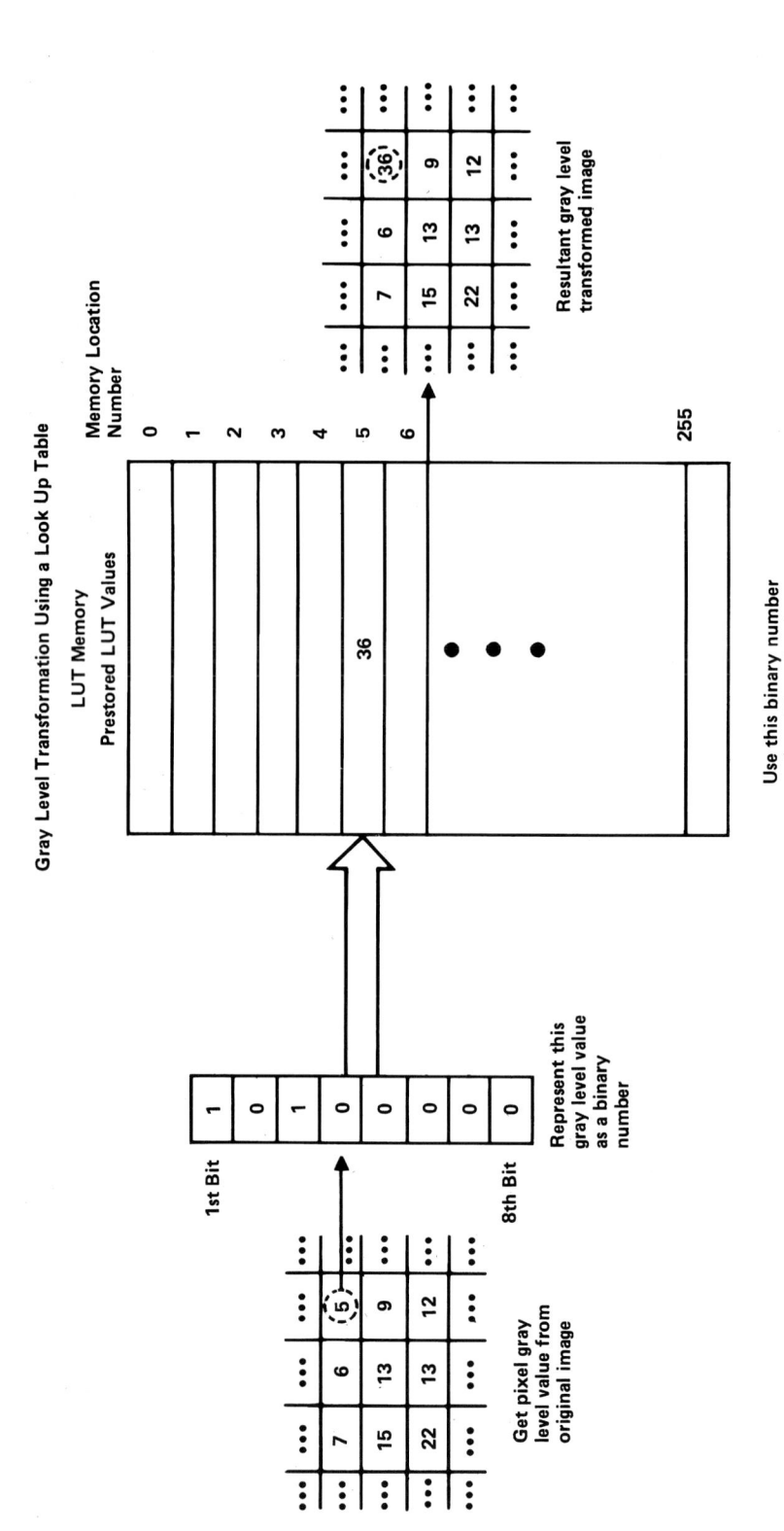

Figure 12.14 Concept of a lookup table (LUT). In this case, the pixel value 5 is mapped to 36 through a preset lookup table.

tor. Window and level operations can be performed in real time using an image processor with a fast access memory called a lookup table (LUT). A 256-value LUT inputs an 8-bit address whose memory location contains the value of the desired gray level transformation (linear scaling with clipping). The memory address for LUT is provided by the original data.

Figure 12.14 illustrates the concept of the LUT. Thus, for example, if one fixes a window value to 1 and changes the level value with the trackball one gray level at a time, the monitor will effectively display all 256 values of the image, one gray level at a time.

12.3.2.3 Histogram Modification

Another function that is useful for enhancing the display image is histogram modification. A histogram of the original image is first obtained, then modified by rescaling each pixel value in the original image. The new enhanced image that is formed will show the desired modification.

An example of histogram modification is histogram equalization, in which the shape of the modified histogram is adjusted to be as uniform as possible for all gray levels. The rescaling factor (or the histogram equalization transfer function) is given by:

$$g = (g_{max} - g_{min})P(f) + g_{min} \qquad (12.15)$$

where g is the output (modified) gray level, g_{max} and g_{min} are the maximum and minimum gray levels of the modified image, f is the input (original) gray level, and $P(f)$ is the cumulative distribution function (or integrated histogram) of f.

Figure 12.15 shows the concept of histogram equalization and an example of the modification of an overexposed (too dark) chest image using the histogram equalization method. In this example, the frequency of occurrence of some lower gray level values in the modified histogram has been changed to zero to enforce uniformity.

12.3.2.4 Image Reverse

A lookup table can be used to reverse the dark and light pixels of an image. In this function, the LUT is loaded with a reverse ramp such that for an 8-bit image; thus the value 255 becomes 0, and 0 becomes 255. Image reverse is used to locate external objects—for example, intrathoracic tubes in ICU X-ray examinations.

12.3.2.5 Distance, Area, and Average Gray Level Measurements

Three simple measurement functions are important for immediate quantitative assessment because they allow the user to perform physical measurement with the image displayed on the video monitor by calibrating the dimensions of each pixel to physical units, or the gray level value to the optical density.

The *distance calibration* procedure is performed by moving a cursor over the image to define the physical distance between two pixels. Best results are obtained when

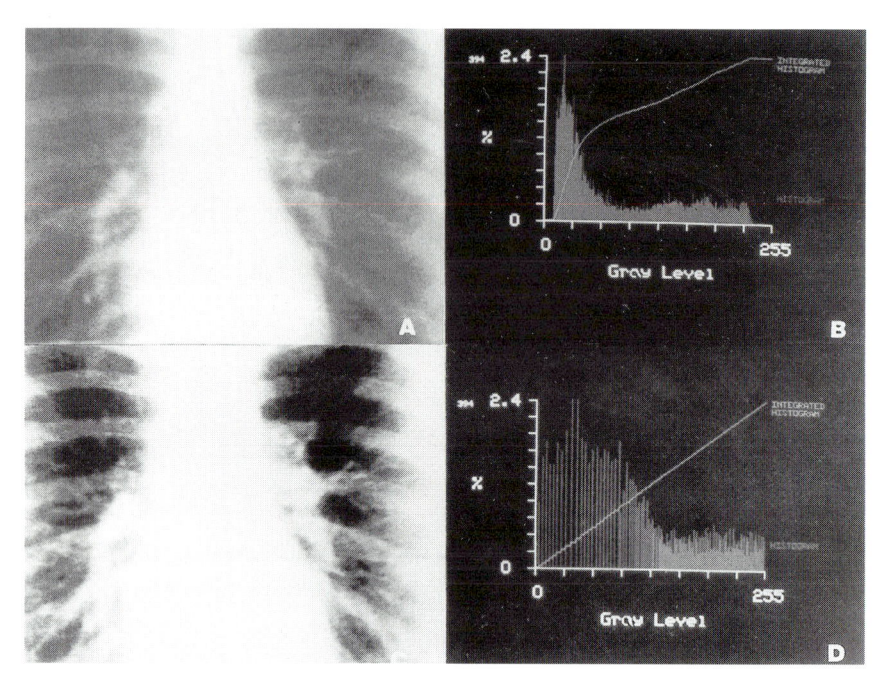

Figure 12.15 Concept of histogram equalization: (A) chest x-ray with lung region overexposed, showing relatively low contrast, (B) the histogram of the chest image, (C) lung region in the image enhanced using histogram equalization, and (D) the modified histogram.

the image contains a calibration ring or other object of known size. To perform *optical density* calibration, the user moves a cursor over many different gray levels and makes queries from a menu to determine the corresponding optical densities.

Finally, an interactive procedure allows the user to trace a region of interest from which the *area and average gray level* can be obtained.

12.3.3 Optimization of Image Perception in Soft Copy

There are three sequential steps in the optimization of an image for soft copy display: remove the unnecessary background, adjust for anatomical region, and correct for the gamma response of the video monitor. These steps can be implemented through properly chosen lookup tables. We discussed the importance of background removal in Section 4.16. Figures 12.16A and 12.16B show a CR image with background and the corresponding histogram, respectively. After the background of Figure 12.16A has been removed, the new histogram (Fig. 12.16D) has no values above 710. The new LUT based on this new histogram produces Figure 12.16C, which has a better visual quality than Figure 12.16A.

It is necessary to adjust for anatomical region because tissue contrast varies in different body regions. Thus, for example, in CT chest examinations, there are lung, soft tissue, and bone windows (LUT) to highlight the lungs, heart tissue, and the bone, re-

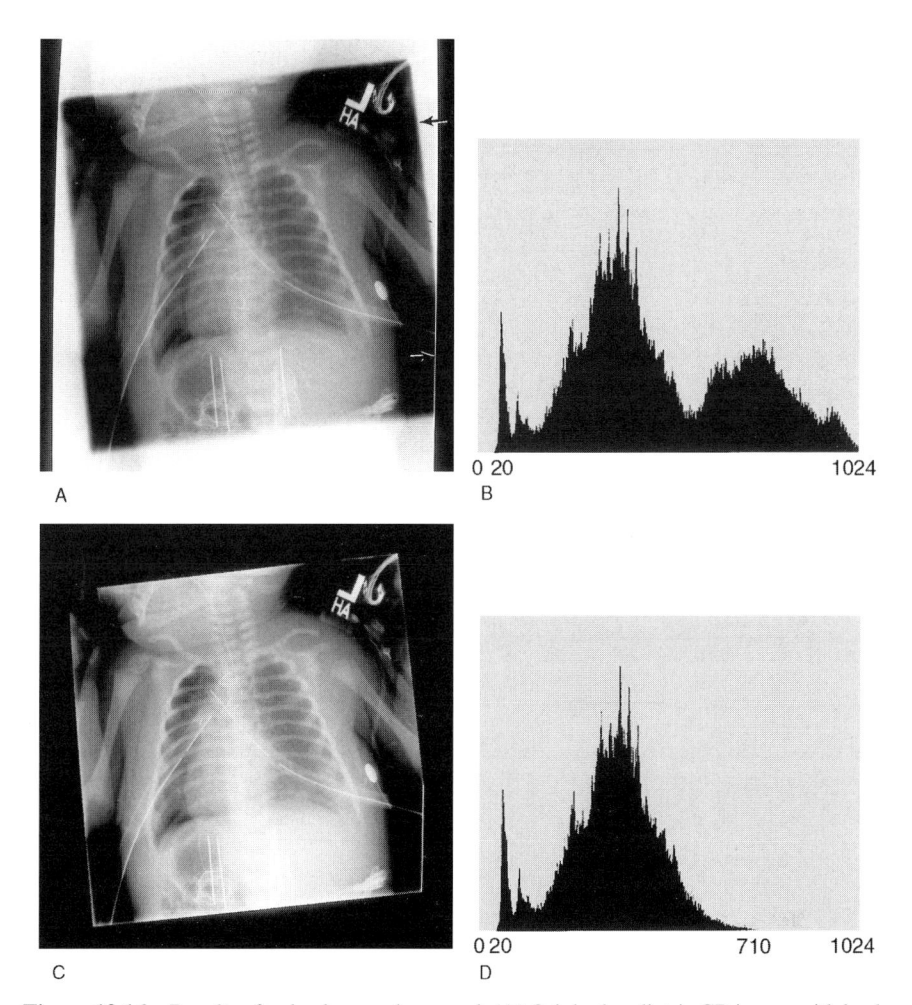

Figure 12.16 Results after background removal. (A) Original pediatric CR image with background (white). (B) Corresponding histogram. (C) Same CR image after background removal, displayed with a different LUT based on the new histogram shown in D. (D) Corresponding histogram of the background-removed CR image shown in C. All pixels with values greater than 710 had been removed. (Courtesy of Dr. J. Zhang.)

spectively. Figure 12.17 shows four curves used to adjust for the pixel values in the head, bone, chest, and abdomen regions in CR.

The pixel value versus its corresponding brightness in a video monitor is a nonlinear response which is a gamma curve different from monitor to monitor. An adjustment of this gamma curve to a linear curve will improve the visual quality of the image. A new monitor must be calibrated to determine this gamma curve, which is used to modify the LUT. Figure 12.18 shows the gamma curve from two different monitors and their linear correction. A monitor must be recalibrated periodically to maintain its performance.

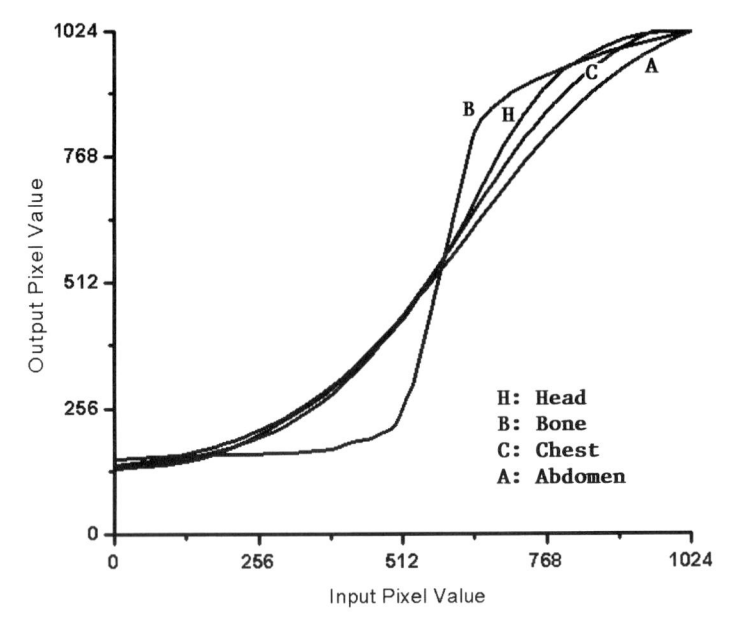

Figure 12.17 Pixel value adjustment for CR images in different body region: head (H), bone (B), chest (C), and abdomen (A). (Courtesy of Dr. J. Zhang.)

12.3.4 Montage

12.3.4.1 Overview

A montage represents a selected set of individual images from a CT, MR, US or any other multi-image modality series. Such groupings are necessary because only a few images from most series show the particular pathology or features of interest to the referring physicians or radiologists. For an average case, such as MR, where a half-dozen sequences may be done, averaging 30 images per sequence, 180 images typically are done for a given study on a patient. A typical montage contains 20 images, representing the significant features from the physician's point of view. So, typically, then, only 10% of the images taken in an examination are essential, and the rest are supplemental. Since it is difficult for the technologist to know at the time of the scanning what images will be the significant ones, a standard series is generally made covering the entire body region of interest. It is up to the radiologist/physician to select the images that will comprise the montage.

In the PACS display workstation, the montage feature allows the user to select and maintain in one file images of interest from all series. The montage file is then saved for future reference, and most subsequent reviews of prior studies can be done by simply referring to the montage file, which contains only the significant images, rather than retrieving all series that were done on a given examination.

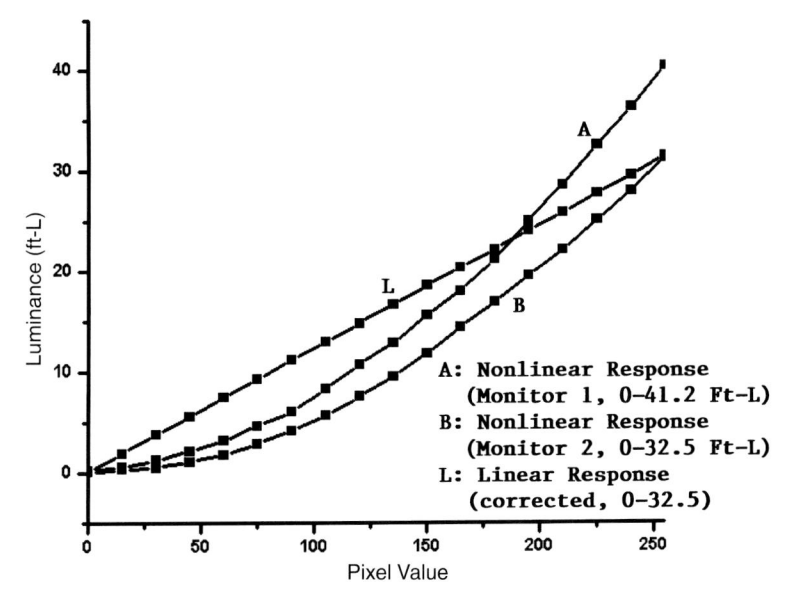

Figure 12.18 (A) and (B) Gamma curves of two monitors; (C) the linear response curve of both monitors after the gamma correction. (Courtesy of Dr. J. Zhang.)

12.3.4.2 Generic Montage Design

The following features are desirable in the design of a montage function:

1. The montage should be simple to use. The end users are radiologists/physicians who have little time to learn complex tools to perform functions they already do efficiently in a film-based operation system.
2. The function should be available on all image workstations currently used to view studies.
3. It should use selection methods similar to those familiar from the image workstation–user interface.
4. If the user elects not to impose a montage file name, the system can default to a standard name (i.e., patient name/date of exam/modality).
5. When a montage is displayed, each slice is displayed with its own correct window/level.
6. The user can use the workstation features (window/level, cine, zoom/scroll, etc.) to view the displayed montage.

One major issue regarding the internal aspects of montage designs must be resolved: Should the actual image pixel data be stored in the montage file, or should

334   DISPLAY WORKSTATION

the function simply use a pointer to the image data? The trade-off is between storage space and immediate access to images.

Storing the image data in the montage has the advantage of being the most efficient way to retrieve and display the images: since the data lie in one contiguous space, they will be easy to be loaded into the display workstation. The images will be duplicated in the database, however. Another disadvantage is that storing images in contiguous files makes editing the montage more difficult: deleting and inserting chunks of image data is much more CPU-intensive than moving pointers around.

Storing pointers to image data requires the smallest amount of additional storage space and has the advantage of ease of editing. Since, however, the actual image data are scattered throughout the PACS, recent image data will be in the display station local storage and older studies will be in the archive. To access montages stored in this fashion, each series containing a slice in the montage must be retrieved from the archive to local storage before the images can be loaded. In the worst case, 20 such retrievals may be necessary, meaning a delay of 10–20 minutes before a montage can be displayed.

Figure 12.19 shows a montage text file on a text monitor in a 2K workstation (see also Fig. 12.4), along with the MR montage images shown on the image display monitor. The montage images are selected from different MR sequences.

12.3.5   Basic Software Functions in a Display Workstation

Some of the basic software functions described in Sections 12.3.2 and 12.3.3 are needed in a display workstation to facilitate its operation. These functions should be easily used with a single click of the mouse, a turn of the dial knob, or a roll of the trackball through the patient's directory, study list, and image processing icons on the various monitors. The keyboard is used only for retrieving information not stored in the workstation's local disks. In this case, the user must input either the patient's name or ID, or a disease category, as the key for searching the long-term archive. Table 12.3 shows some basic software functions required for a display workstation. Table 12.4 shows the utilization of image processing functions obtained from an automatic log

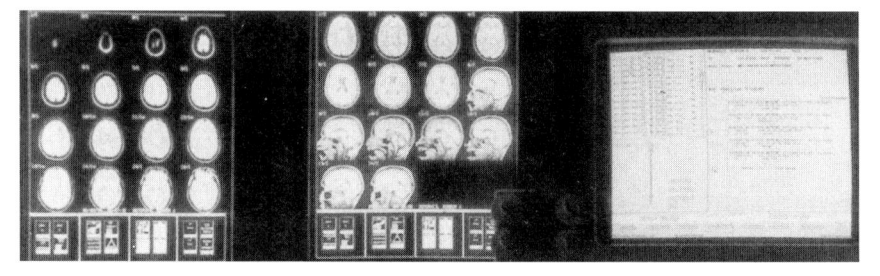

Figure 12.19   Example of a montage file: *right,* the text monitor shows the montage file at the left of the screen; *middle,* the right-hand 2K display monitor shows the montage images selected from different MR sequences mixing transverse and sagittal sectional images; *left,* the left-hand 2K monitor shows a standard transverse sectional study without the montage. Compare Figure 12.4.

TABLE 12.3 Software Functions for a Display Workstation

Function	Description
Directory	
Patient directory	Name, ID, age, sex, date of current exam
Study list	Type of exam, anatomical area, date studies taken
Display	
Screen reconfiguration	Reconfigures each screen for the convenience of image display
Monitor selection	Left, right
Display	Displays images according to screen configuration and monitor selected
Image manipulation	
Dials	Brightness, contrast, zoom, and scroll
LUT	Predefined lookup tables (bone, soft tissue, brain, etc.)
Cine	Single or multiple cine on multimonitors for CT and MR images
Rotation	Rotates an image
Negative	Reverses gray scale
Utilities	
Montage	Selects images to form a montage
Image discharge	Deletes images of discharged patients (a privileged operation)
Library search	Retrieves historical examinations (requires keyboard operation)
Report	Retrieves reports from RIS
Measurements	Linear and region of interest

program in two neuroradiology image workstations: one in the inpatient and the second in the outpatient reading area. It is seen from this table that of the 29 available functions in the image workstations, the seven most popular functions are select patient, sort patient directory, library search, select image, cine mode, zoom/scroll, and window and level.

12.4 THE LASER FILM IMAGER

Hard copy display is sometimes needed for sending a copy of the images to a remote site where a soft copy display system is not available. For a good quality hard copy, a laser film printer (imager) is used. The laser film imager uses a fine laser spot to write a digital image onto a red-sensitive film (8 in. × 10 in. or 14 in. × 17 in.). The spot moves from left to right, and the film advances to the next line after a complete line has been written. The intensity of the laser spot is modulated according to the gray level value of each pixel which, in turn, determines the optical density of the pixel on the film. For convenience of discussion, consider the schematic illustration of a laser imager shown in Figure 12.20. This system can write up to 2384 × 3050 × 8 bits on smaller film (8 in. × 10 in.) or 4288 × 5275 × 8 bits on a larger film (14 in. × 17 in.); each pixel corresponds to an area of 80 μm². The film advance speed is 16 mm/s. Table 12.5 lists the specifications of the laser imager.

TABLE 12.4 Neuroradiology WS Usage by Function at UCSF, August 1995

Function*	Inpatient	Outpatient
Patient Select	612	175
Sort Mode	110	29
Library Search	292	172
Report Select	9	4
Patient Search	45	24
Image Select 1	562	76
Image Select 2	906	176
Cine 1	357	54
Cine 2	603	101
Zoom/Scroll 1	37	2
Zoom/Scroll 2	107	9
Measure 1	9	
Measure 2	12	
Region of Interest (ROI) 1	7	
ROI 2	5	
Slice Select 1	1	8
Slice Select 2	3	3
Window/Level 1	175	24
Window/Level 2	435	49
CT brain	2	
CT liver	1	2
Bone	34	10
Lung	1	
Soft tissue	28	8
Lookup table (LUT) defaults	20	2
Negative	2	2
Globalize	22	13
Montage	5	1
WS main Start-Up	8	9

*1, 2, monitors 1 and 2.

12.4.1 The Block Diagram

To start, digital image data supplied by the host computer reach the imager's formatter module through a dedicated interface board. This data are sent through a programmable lookup table in the printer, which corrects for nonlinearities in the laser production of film density.

The lookup table is calibrated with the optical density—gray level transfer characteristics of the imager. The output signal from the lookup table is used to modulate the intensity of a 5 mW helium–neon laser beam using a lead molybdate ($PbM.O_4$) acousto-optic modulator such that the input data will be linearly mapped onto a range of optical densities on film. A conventional X-ray film processor is used to develop

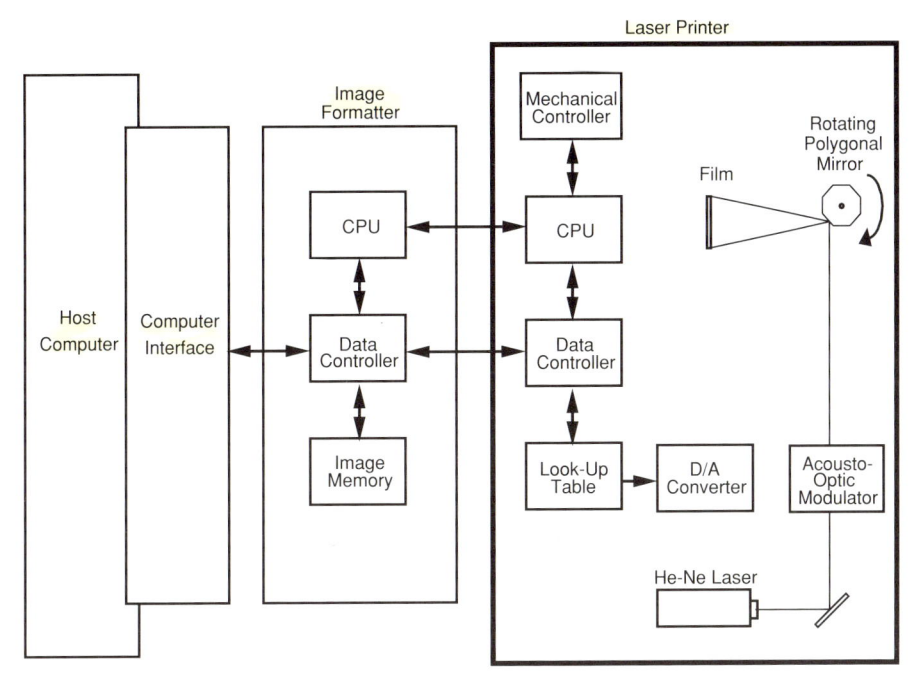

Figure 12.20 Schematic of a laser imager.

the exposed film. However, the red-sensitive film requires a green safe light in the darkroom.

12.4.2 Performance Characteristics of a Laser Film Imager

Several parameters are important in the determination of performance characteristics of a laser film imager: the transfer characteristics between the optical density and the gray level, the characteristics of the laser spot, including uniformity, and the imager's

TABLE 12.5 Specifications of a Laser Imager

Characteristic	Specification
Pixel size	80×80 μm
Density resolution	8 bits
Film size and corresponding matrix size	8×10 in.^{2} (2348×3050)
	14×17 in.^{2} (4288×5275)
Scan speed	16 mm/s
Magnification	$\times$ 0.5, 1, 2, 3, ..., 16
Image format	Up to 16 images/film
Laser power	5 mW

spatial resolution and spatial linearity. These parameters have to be measured periodically to maintain the optimal performance of the imager.

12.5 DICOM-BASED NT/PC DISPLAY WORKSTATION

In recent years, the Pentium-powered personal computer combined with the Windows NT operating system has become an attractive candidate in PACS workstation design for reasons of its high performance and reasonable price. We anticipate that workstations based on the NT/PC platform will be used extensively in PACS and in EMR environments. Thus, in this section we present the basic design of a DICOM-compliant NT/PC-based workstation developed in our laboratory which can accommodate the viewing of most radiologic applications.

12.5.1 Hardware Configuration

The hardware configuration of the workstation was shown in Figure 12.1.

12.5.1.1 Host Computer

The host computer of the workstation is a PC with an Intel Pentium Pro 200 MHz chip, 128 Mbyte of RAM, PCI bus structure, and two 40 Mbit/s Ultra SCSI disks as local storage.

12.5.1.2 Display Devices

Display devices include single or multiple display monitors and video boards. The display monitor can be a 24-in. 1600 × 1280 (or 2.5K × 2K) resolution device in portrait mode (Image Systems Corp., Hopkins, MN). A DOME Md2/PCI (or MD5 for 2K) host adapter (DOME Image Systems, Inc., Waltham, MA) serves as the video board.

12.5.1.3 Network Equipment

In the display workstation, asynchronous transfer mode (ATM) or fast Ethernet can be used as the primary means of communication, with conventional Ethernet as the backup. In the former, the FORE 155 Mbit/s (OC-3) ATM host adapter and the FORE ForeRunner ASX-200BX ATM switch (FORE Systems, Inc. Warrendale, PA) or other manufacturers' products, can be used.

12.5.2 Software System

The software can be developed based on Microsoft Windows NT platform and in the Visual C/C++ programming environment. WinSock communication over TCP/IP, Microsoft Foundation Class (MFC) libraries, DOME Image Processing Library

DICOM-BASED NT/PC DISPLAY WORKSTATION 339

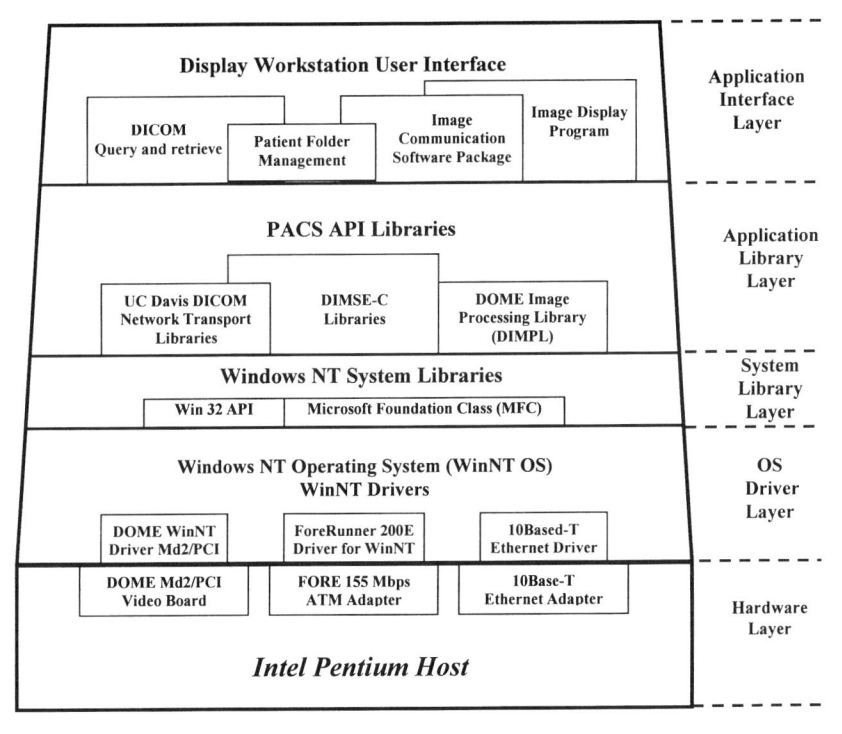

Figure 12.21 Software architecture of the NT/PC-based display workstation. (Courtesy of Lei, Zhang, and Wong.)

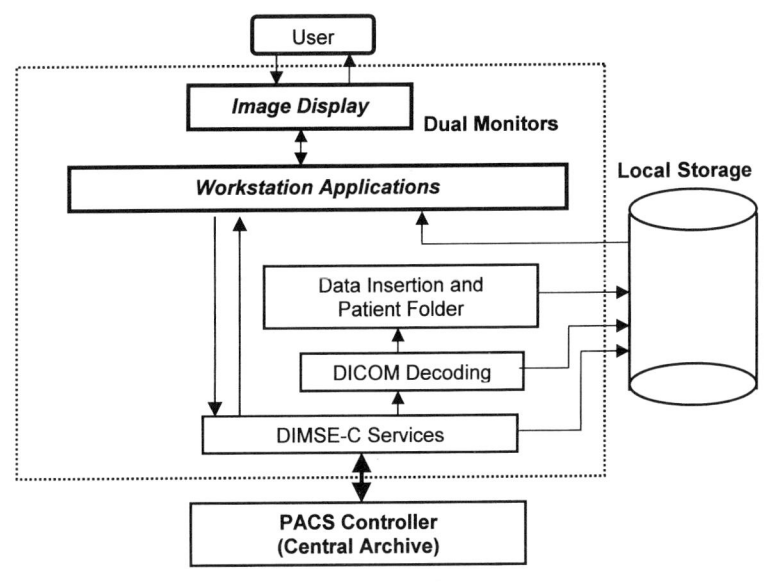

Figure 12.22 Data flow in the DICOM-compliant NT/PC-based display workstation. (Courtesy of Lei, Zhang, and Wong.)

(DIMPL), UC Davis DICOM library, and UCSF Windows NT-based PACS API libraries can be used as development tools. The user interface of the display workstation is icon/menu-driven with user-friendly graphics.

12.5.2.1 Software Architecture

The architecture of the software system is divided into four layers: the application interface layer, the application library layer, the system library layer, and the operating system driver layer, which is over the hardware layer. Figure 12.21 shows the software architecture of the display workstation.

The application interface layer is the top layer of the software system that interfaces with the end user of the display workstation. This layer is composed of four modules: (1) image communication software package, (2) patient folder management, (3) image display program, and (4) DICOM query/retrieve software package. This layer directly supports any application that requires accessing PACS and radiological images.

In the application library layer, the PACS API Libraries provide all library functions to support the four modules in the application interface layer. Here, UC Davis DICOM Network Transport Library and DIMSE-C Library ensure DICOM communication protocols and functions, and DOME Image Processing Library (DIMPL) supplies library functions for image display of the workstation.

The system library layer is responsible for providing Windows NT system library, Win 32 API functions, and Microsoft Foundation Class (MFC) to serve as a developmental platform.

The operating system driver layer provides Windows NT OS and its drivers for connecting with hardware components, which include a DOME Md2/PCI driver for its video board, a ForeRunner 200E driver for FORE 155 Mbit/s ATM adapter, and a 10 BaseT Ethernet driver for 10 BaseT Ethernet adapter.

All data flow between the layers of the software is shown in Figure 12.22.

12.5.2.2 Software Modules in the Application Interface Layer

In the workstation, the user has access only at the application interface layer, which is composed of four modules described in the subsections that follow.

Image Communication The image communication module is responsible for supporting DICOM services with DICOM communication protocols over TCP/IP to perform two DICOM services: Storage service class provider (SCP) and Storage service class user (SCU). The DICOM services include C-ECHO for verification, C-STORE for storage, C-FIND for querying, and C-MOVE for retrieving.

Patient Folder Management The second module manages the local storage with hierarchical, or tree-structure, directories to organize patient folders in the display workstation.

DICOM decoder is used to extract patient demographic data and examination

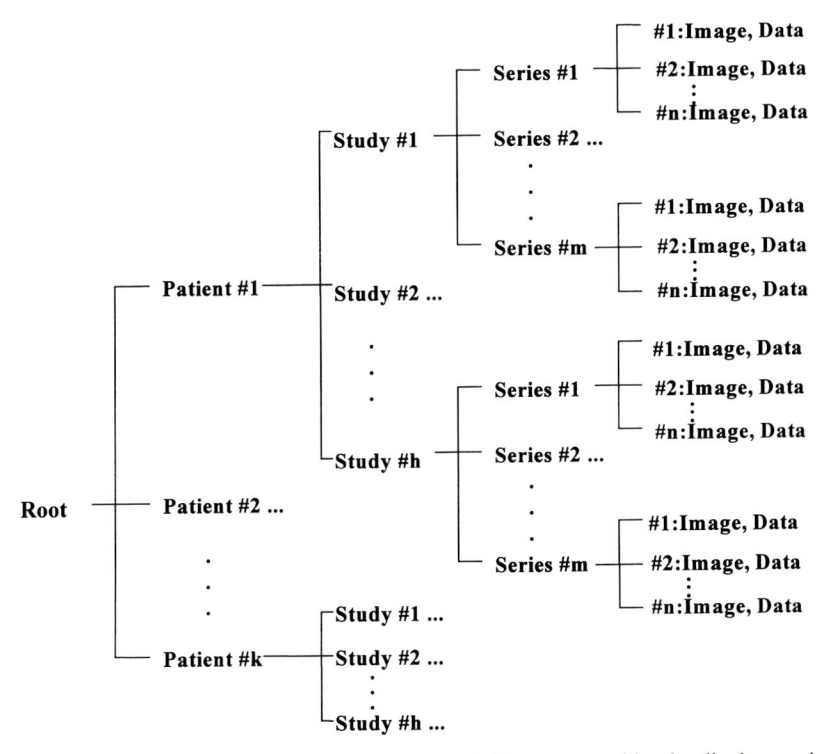

Figure 12.23 Three-level hierarchy of the patient folders managed by the display workstation. (Courtesy of Lei, Zhang, and Wong.)

Figure 12.24 Patient folders in the diagnostic workstation. Each folder contains three hierarchical levels: patient level, study level, and series level. (Courtesy of Lei, Zhang, and Wong.)

records from the header of a DICOM image. The reformatter of the module changes the image from DICOM format to DOME format for display. The extracted data are inserted into an individual patient folder via the DICOM decoder, and the reformatted image by the reformatter. A patient folder contains three hierarchical levels: patient level, study level, and series level. The hierarchy starts with a root directory in the local storage system (i.e., hard disks of the display workstation). Figure 12.23 is a diagram of the patient folder structure.

A patient folder is automatically created in the workstation upon receipt of the first image of the patient. Subsequent images from individual studies and series are inserted into the patient folder accordingly. The patient folder can be automatically deleted from the workstation based on certain aging criteria such as number of days since the folder was created, or the discharge or transfer of the patient. Figure 12.24 presents the interface of three hierarchical levels of patient folders.

Image Display Program   The image display program supports both single and dual 24-inch 1600×1280 (or $2.5K \times 2K$) resolution portrait monitors to display patient information and radiological images in the workstation. Images with the DOME image header format in a patient folder can be displayed via the image display program.

The screen layout of the workstation is user adjustable with one image on one monitor, two on one, four on one, and so on. The display program can support multimodality displays for CT, MR, and CR in the sense that one monitor can display one modality while the second monitor can show images in the other modality.

Image manipulation functions such as zoom, pan, rotation, flip, window and level adjustment, and invert are available. Automatic defaulted window and level preset function is used during imaging loading to minimize the manipulation time. Real-time zoom and contrast adjustment can be easily done by using the mouse.

Query and Retrieve   The application interface layer software module is a DICOM Query/Retrieve service class user (Q/R SCU) to query and retrieve patient studies from the PACS long-term archive or directly from radiological imaging systems. The query and retrieve module supports DICOM C-ECHO, C-STORE, C-FIND, and C-MOVE services. With this module, the workstation has access capability to Query/Retrieve service class poviders, which use the Q/R information models of patient root and study root. The supported Query/Retrieve levels are shown in Table 12.6.

TABLE 12.6 Supported Query/Retrieve Levels in the Display Workstation

Q/R SCP Information Model	
Patient Root	Study Root
Patient Study Series Images	Study Series Images

CHAPTER 13

PACS Data Management, Distribution, and Retrieval

13.1 PACS DATA MANAGEMENT

In Section 10.2 we discussed the PACS system software, for image receiving, stacking, routing, archiving, studies grouping, platter management, and RIS and HIS interfacing. These software functions are needed for optimal image and information management, distribution, and retrieval at the display workstation. This section describes methods and essentials of grouping patients' image and other data effectively based on the patient folder manager concept.

13.1.1 Patient Folder Manager Concept: Preliminary

Folder Manager (FM) is a software package residing in the PACS controller that drives a picture archiving and communication system (PACS) by means of event trigger mechanisms. The concept emphasizes standardization, modularity, and portability.

The primary task of FM is to establish an infrastructure, which includes:

- HIS–RIS–PACS interface
- Image routing
- Image selection
- Online radiology reports
- Patient folder management

The first three functions were described in Sections 11.3.2, 10.2.3, and 10.2.5. We briefly discuss the online reports and folder management here.

13.1.1.1 Online Radiology Reports

The PACS receives radiology reports and impressions from RIS via the RIS-PACS interface and stores these text information files in the PACS database. These reports and impressions can be displayed instantaneously at a PACS display workstation along with the associated images from a given examination. The PACS also supports online queries of reports and impressions from a display workstation.

13.1.1.2 Patient Folder Management

The PACS manages patient studies in folders. Each folder consists of a given patient's demographics, examination descriptions, images from current examinations, selected images from previous examinations, and relevant reports and impressions. A patient's folder will remain online at a specific display workstation during the patient's entire hospital stay or visit. Upon discharge or transfer of the patient, the folder is automatically deleted from the display workstation.

13.1.2 Patient Folder Manager: Modules

Three software modules are in the patient folder manager:

- Archive Management
- Network Management
- Display/Server Management

Table 13.1 describes these three modules and associated submodules and gives their essential level for PACS.

13.1.2.1 Archive Management

The Archive Manager module provides the following functionalities:

- manages distribution of images on multiple storage media
- optimizes archiving and retrieving operations for PACS
- prefetches historical studies to display workstations

TABLE 13.1 Summary of Patient Folder Manager Software Modules

Module	Submodules	Essential Level*
Archive Manager	Image Archive	1
	Image Retrieve	1
	HL7 Message Parsing	2
	Event Trigger	2
	Image Pre-fetch	2
	Platter Management	3
Network Manager	Image Send	1
	Image Receive	1
	Image Routing	1
	Job Prioritizing and Recover Mechanism	1
Display/Server Manager	Image Selection	2
	Image Sequencing	3
	Window/Level Preset	2
	Report/Impression Display	1

*1, minimum requirements to run the PACS; 2, requirements for an efficient PACS; 3, advanced features.

Mechanisms supporting these functions include event triggering, image prefetching, job prioritization, and platter management.

Event Triggering   Event triggering can be achieved by means of the following algorithm and pseudocode.

ALGORITHM NAME: EVENT TRIGGERING
DESCRIPTION
   Events occurring in RIS are sent to the PACS in HL7 format over TCP/IP, which then triggers the PACS controller to carry out specific tasks such as image retrieval and pre-fetching, PACS database update, platter management, and patient folder cleanup. Events sent from RIS include patient admission, discharge, and transfer (ADT), patient arrival, examination scheduling, cancellation, completion, and report approval.
SOFTWARE ALGORITHM
   ESSENTIALS
      HIS/RIS/PACS interface
      HL7 message parsing
      Image prefetching
      PACS database update
      Patient folder management
      Platter management
   PSEUDOCODE
      Wait for HL7 message from the RIS
      receive HL7 message
      parse HL7 message
      case of <message type>:
         patient transfer or discharge:
         group patient images from temporary storage and copy to permanent
            archive
         delete patient image folder form display server
      examination scheduling:
         perform prefetch table lookup
         select previous examinations from PACS database
         schedule retrieval of patient images
         schedule retrieval of patient textual data
      examination cancellation:
         remove scheduled retrieval jobs
      patient arrival:
         check existence of patient images in display server
         retrieve patient's selected images from optical archive
         retrieve patient text data from PACS database
         generate or update patient image folder
      patient demographics, examination description, or radiology reports:
         update PACS database
      loop back

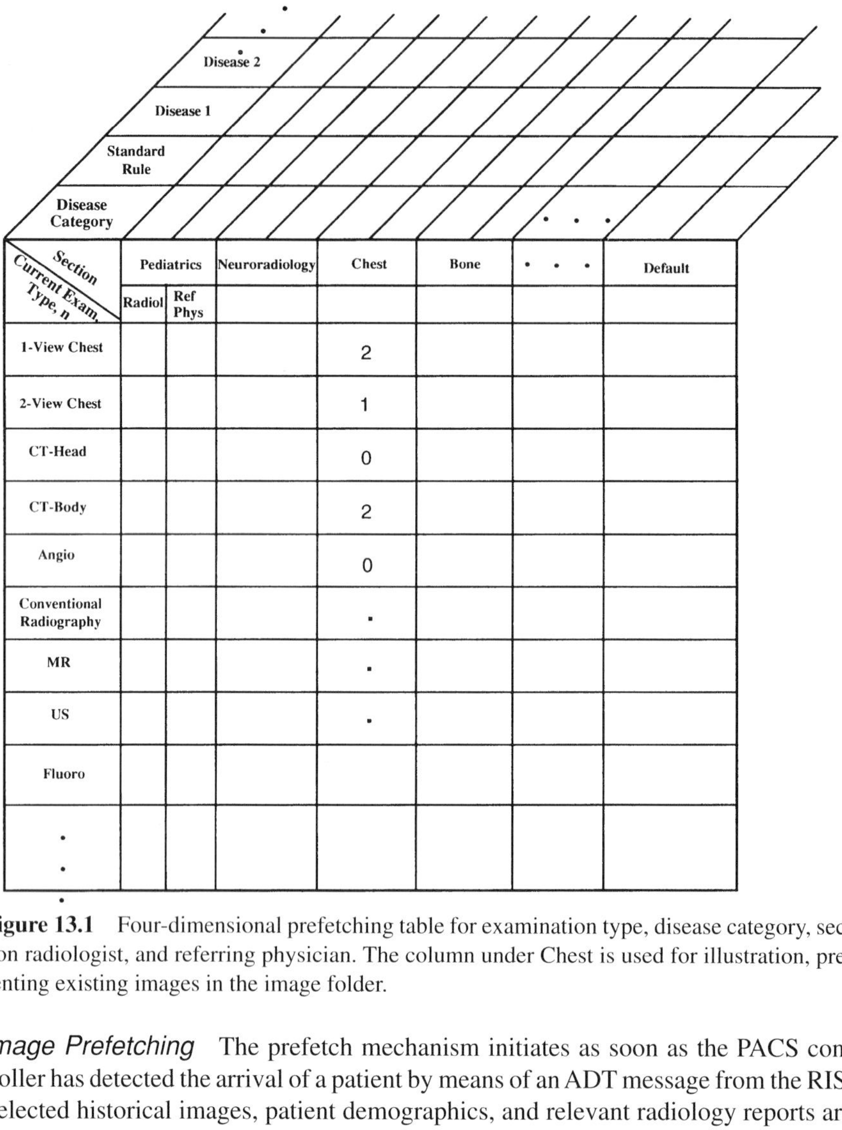

Figure 13.1 Four-dimensional prefetching table for examination type, disease category, section radiologist, and referring physician. The column under Chest is used for illustration, presenting existing images in the image folder.

Image Prefetching The prefetch mechanism initiates as soon as the PACS controller has detected the arrival of a patient by means of an ADT message from the RIS. Selected historical images, patient demographics, and relevant radiology reports are retrieved from the permanent archive and the PACS database. These data are distributed to the destination display workstation(s) before completion of the patient's current examination.

The prefetch algorithm is based on predefined parameters such as examination type, section code, radiologist, referring physician, location of display station, and the number and age of the patient's archived images. These parameters determine which historical images should be retrieved. Figure 13.1 shows a four-dimensional prefetching table that focuses on examination type, disease category, section radiologist, and referring physician. This table determines which historical images should be retrieved from the central archive system. For example, for a patient scheduled for chest examination, the *n*-tuple entries in the chest column (2, 1, 0, 2, 0, . . .) represent an image folder consisting of two single-view chest images, one two-view chest image, no CT head scan, two CT body studies, no angio image, and so on.

In addition to this lookup table, the prefetch mechanism utilizes patient origin, referring physician, location of display station, number of archived images for this patient, and age of these individual archived images in determining the number of images from each examination type to be retrieved.

The Prefetch Algorithm The prefetch mechanism is carried out by several processes within the archive server (see Section 10.2.10). Each process runs independently and communicates simultaneously with other processes utilizing client/server programming, queuing control mechanisms, and job prioritizing mechanisms. The prefetch algorithm can be described in the following algorithm and pseudocode.

ALGORITHM NAME: IMAGE PRE-FETCHING
DESCRIPTION
> The prefetch mechanism is triggered when the examination scheduled, examination canceled, and patient arrived events occur in the RIS. Selected historical images, patient demographics, and relevant radiology reports are retrieved from the optical archive and the PACS database. These data are distributed to the destination display workstation(s) before completion of the patient's current examination.
>
> The prefetch algorithm is based on predefined parameters including examination type, section code, radiologist, referring physician, location of display workstation, and number and age of the patient's archived images.

SOFTWARE ALGORITHM
> *ESSENTIALS*
>> RIS/PACS interface
>> Event triggering
>> Prefetch table lookup
>> Image retrieval
>> Database query
>
> *PSEUDOCODE*
>> Wait for event from the RIS
>> receive event (HL7 message)

case of <event type>
>> examination scheduled:
>>> perform prefetch table lookup
>>> select previous examinations from PACS database
>>> schedule retrieval of historical images
>>> schedule retrieval of patient demographics and radiology reports
>>
>> examination canceled:
>>> remove scheduled retrieval jobs
>>
>> patient arrived:
>>> retrieve patient's selected images from optical archive

348 PACS DATA MANAGEMENT, DISTRIBUTION, AND RETRIEVAL

    retrieve patient demographics and radiology reports from PACS database
    generate or update patient folder
loop back
RULES
    Parameters used in the prefetch table lookup process include:
        Examination type
        Radiologist
        Referring physicians
        Section code
        Display workstation site
        Age of archived image
        Number of historical images in the archive

- Current examination type determines number of images from same type or similar type of previous examinations to be prefetched.
- Radiologists and referring physicians may have individual preferred entries.
- Section code and display station site may alter the maximum number of images to be prefetched by changing the 4-D prefetching table. For example, an ICU station would require fewer historical CR images to be prefetched than a chest station.
- Age and number of a patient's archived images may limit the maximum number of images to be prefetched.

Job Prioritization   The PACS controller manages its processes by prioritizing job control to optimize the archiving and retrieving activities. For example, a request from a display workstation to retrieve an image from the permanent archive will have the highest priority and be processed immediately. And, upon completion of the retrieval, the image will be queued for transmission with a priority higher than other images that have just arrived from the image acquisition nodes and are waiting for transmission. By the same token, an archive process must be compromised if there is any retrieval job executing or pending.

    The use of job prioritizing and compromising between the PACS processes will result in dramatic decreases in delays in servicing radiologists and referring physicians in the clinic.

Platter Management   During a hospital stay or visit, the patient's current images from different examinations are copied to magneto-optical disks (MODs) or other temporary storage device for long-term storage. Upon discharge or transfer of the patient, these images are grouped from the temporary storage and copied contiguously to the permanent storage (see Section 10.2.5).

13.1.2.2 Network Management

The network manager handles the distribution of images and text data from the PACS controller. This module, which controls the image traffic across the entire PACS network, is a routing mechanism based on predefined parameters (see Section 10.2.3). It includes a routing table composed of the predefined parameters and a routing algorithm that is completely driven by the routing table. The routing table should be designed to facilitate updating as needed. Any change of the routing table should be possible without modification of the routing algorithm.

In addition to routing images to their designated display workstations, the network manager performs the following tasks:

- Queues images in the event of network or workstation failure.
- Switches network circuit from the primary network (e.g., ATM) to the secondary network (e.g., conventional Ethernet) when the primary network fails.
- Distributes images based on different priority levels.

The image sending mechanism can be described in the following algorithm and pseudocode. If the DICOM communication standard is used, some pseudocode can be replaced by DICOM DIMSEs.

ALGORITHM NAME : IMAGE SENDING
DESCRIPTION
   The send process catches a ready—to—send signal from the routing manager, establishes a TCP/IP connection to the destination host, and transmits the image data to the destination host.

   Upon successful transmission, the send process dequeues current job and logs a SUCCESS status. Otherwise, it requeues the job for a later retry and logs a RETRY status.

SOFTWARE ALGORITHM
   ESSENTIALS
      TCP connect
      dequeuing
      requeuing
      event logging
   PSEUDOCODE
      Wait for ready_to_send signal from image routing manager
      catch ready_to_send signal
      get next pending job from comm_out queue
      open ATM TCP socket
      if (TCP_OPEN_FAIL)
         open Ethernet TCP socket
         if (TCP_OPEN_FAIL)
            log error
            requeue job
            go to loop back
         else
            go to send_data
      else
         go to send_data

send_data:
  send data to destination host
  wait for acknowledgment
if (NEGATIVE_ACK)
  log error
  requeue job with RETRY status
  go to loop back
else
  dequeue job with SUCCESS status
loop back

13.1.2.3 Display/Server Management

Display/server management includes the following tasks:

- image sequencing
- image selection
- window/level preset
- coordination with reports and impressions

Window/level preset and coordination with reports and impressions were described in Section 12.3.2.2 and 11.3.2, respectively. Image sequencing is one of the most difficult tasks in the display/server management function because it involves users' habits and subjective opinions, but does not supply universal rules to govern these preferences. Algorithm development requires certain artificial intelligence. Current implementation of this model is based on specific applications and requires heavy customization. Image selection can be handled by the display/server management function using basic rules through user interaction by the following algorithm.

ALGORITHM NAME : IMAGE SELECTION
DESCRIPTION
  The image selection process allows a user to select a subset of images from a given image sequence (as in an MR or CT study; see Section 10.2.5) on the display monitor(s). These selected images are then extracted from the original sequence and grouped into a new sequence (e.g., a montage; see Section 12.3.4) for future display.
SOFTWARE ALGORITHM
  ESSENTIALS
    Image display
    Montage function
    PACS database update
  PSEUDOCODE
    Display complete sequence of images
    wait for user to select images through the montage function
    accept selection from user
    while (SELECT_NOT_DONE)
      read index from selected image

group indexes
insert indexes into PACS global database
RULES
- Indexes stored in PACS database are global (i.e., are accessible from any PACS display stations).
- Individual radiologists and referring physicians may select image subsets and save indexes using the montage function in separate index tables under the user's preferred image file names.

13.2 DISTRIBUTED IMAGE FILE SERVER

13.2.1 Concept of Distributed Image File Server

PACS was first developed to meet the need of image management in the radiology department. As the PACS concept evolved, the need increased for applications of PACS to cross borders to other health care disciplines. For this reason, second-generation or hospital-integrated PACS design should include a distributed image file server to provide integrated image and textual data for other departments in the medical center.

The PACS components and data flow diagrammed in Figure 1.1 represent an open architecture design: the display component can accommodate many types of display workstation, as described in Section 12.1.4. When the number of display workstations (e.g., physicians' desktop workstations) increases, each with its own special applications and communication protocols, the numerous queries generated by the more active workstations may affect the performance of the PACS controller (see Section 10.1). Under such circumstances, distributed image file servers linked to the PACS controller should be designed to be incorporated in the PACS infrastructure. Figure 13.2, an extension of Figure 1.1, shows a multiple image server design with a particular one for physicians' desktop Macintosh computers.

13.2.2 Image Retrieval from Physician's Desktop

Consider an example in the radiology department in which an existing departmental Ethernet network is supporting over 100 Macintosh users. In this network, the users have access to a variety of output devices such as laser printers and slide makers, and a QuickMail (CE Software, West Des Moines, IA) server for electronic mail. Based on this working environment, let us design a departmental distributed image file server (DIFS) that will permit these Macintosh users to access images and data from the hospital-integrated PACS via the PACS controller.

13.2.2.1 Distributed Image File Server and Clients

The DIFS consists of a relatively powerful server—for example, a high end Sun SPARC workstation with a large disk capacity for storing images and related data, an ATM connection with Ethernet backup to the PACS controller, and an efficient relational database for client/server queries. In each Macintosh client machine, a C-

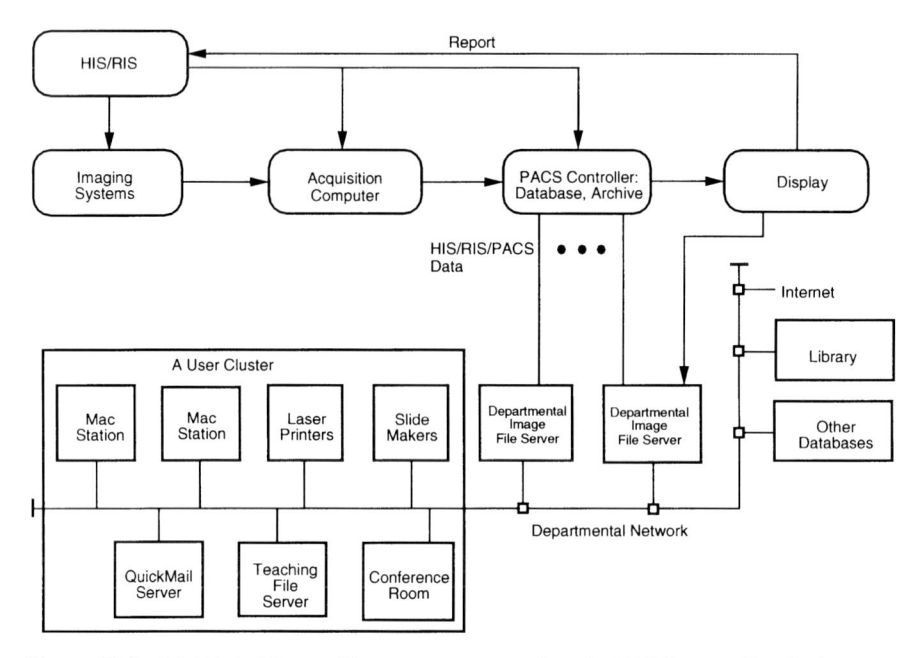

Figure 13.2 Distributed image file servers connected to the PACS controller. Each server provides specific applications for a given cluster of users. The physician's desktop server is used as example for illustration. The concept of Web server is described in Figure 13.6.

language software package (e.g., Radiology Workshop, developed at UCSF, Section 13.2.2.3) enables the computer to establish a network communication link with the PACS controller and other databases connected to the departmental network through the use of a variety of TCP/IP-based messages. Figure 13.3 shows the specifications and the connections between the server and clients.

Let us use the Radiology Workshop software package in the sample client/server queries that follow.

13.2.2.2 Three Types of Query

Text Requests The Macintosh user may request a patient's demographic and examination information and study reports (Figs. 13.4A, 13.5C) based on the patient's name, the patient's ID, or a variety of search parameters (Table 13.2). The DIFS converts these requests into structured query language queries and transmits them to the PACS controller. Any resulting text information is then passed back to the requesting Macintosh.

Thumbnail Image Requests After acquiring the text information concerning a particular study, the user may request a "thumbnail sketch" of the entire study (Fig. 13.4B). The DIFS requests the particular study from the PACS controller in the ACR-NEMA or DICOM format, generates a "thumbnail sketch" consisting of 128×128

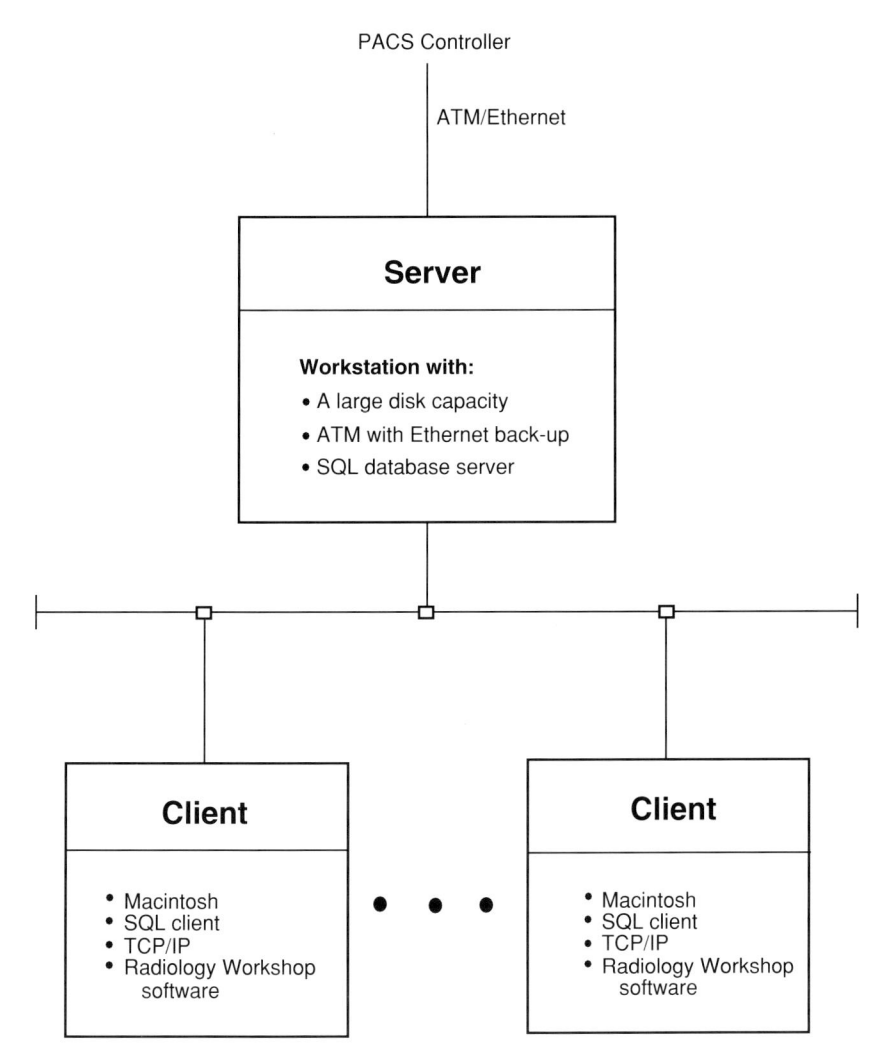

Figure 13.3 The specifications of and the connections between the server and clients in the physician's desktop image file server.

resolution image subsamples, and delivers the entire thumbnail sketch to the requesting Macintosh. After the DIFS has sent this thumbnail sketch to the Macintosh, it discards its own copy. The original ACR-NEMA or DICOM image file, however, can be kept in the DIFS for a certain period of time, perhaps a week, to satisfy any subsequent full-resolution requests. Aside from this temporary storage, no images are archived on the DIFS—it is meant only to act as a gateway into the PACS for radiologists' personal computers. Figures 13.5A and 13.5B show two thumbnail sketches, as well as the screen output of a patient study list, detailed study information, and a diagnostic report.

A. Text Request

```
PACS Controller  ←SQL query──  Departmental Image File Server  ←Text Request──  Macintosh
                 ──Patient Data→                                ──Patient Data→
```

B. Thumbnail Request

```
PACS Archive Controller  ←Study Request──  Departmental Image File Server  ←Thumbnail Request──  Macintosh
                         ──ACR-NEMA/DICOM file→                            ──Thumbnail Sketch 128 X 128→
```

C. Full-Resolution Request

```
Display Workstation  ──Full-Resolution Request→  Departmental Image File Server  ←Full-Resolution Request──  Macintosh
                                                                                 ──PICT or TIFF Image 16 bits/pixel raw data→
```

PACS Network   **Departmental Network**

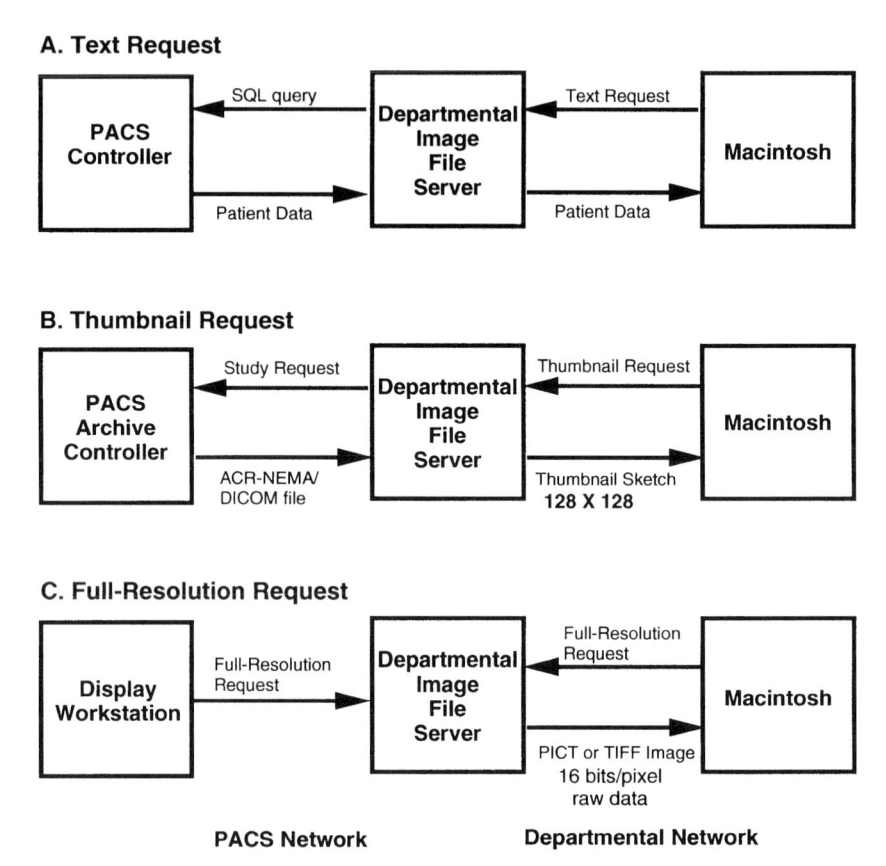

Figure 13.4 Communication between the departmental physician's desktop image file server with the PACS controller, the PACS archive, and the display workstation, respectively, in response to three types of query: (A) text requests, (B) thumbnail image requests, and (C) full-resolution image requests. SQL, structured query language; PICT, Macintosh picture format; TIFF: tagged-image file format.

Full-Resolution Image Requests After viewing a thumbnail sketch, the user may select key images to be retrieved from the DIFS at full resolution using the route outlined in Figure 13.4C (Fig. 13.5D). The DIFS converts these images from the DICOM format to a standard Macintosh format, such as the Macintosh picture (PICT) format or the tagged image file format (TIFF), in full resolution 8 or 12 bits/pixel and transfers them with the user's specific file name(s) to the Macintosh's hard drive, where they may be viewed or manipulated by any standard Macintosh application. Information describing the particular patient and study is inserted into an image header before the image is transferred to the Macintosh. The option of allowing users to create specific file names helps them keep track of their own collections. In addition, interfaces that allow key images to be selected during image interpretation at the display workstation should have been established (see Fig. 13.2: directional arrow from Display box to the image file server). These selected images and related data can be stored

TABLE 13.2 Functionality Provided by the Radiology Workshop

Function	Object
Ability to search for information on the basis of several criteria	Patient's identification number and name
Access to text information	Patient's demographics Examination information Diagnostic reports
Access to image information	Thumbnail images in a study (128×128 or 64×64 resolution)

	Full-resolution images in a study available in three forms:
	    8-bit Macintosh picture format
	    8-bit tagged image file format
	    16-bit raw data file

Ability to receive key full-resolution images selected at remote viewing workstations	Full-resolution images
Access to radiology information system, hospital information system, and library information system through initiation of online session	Related patient data

and tagged with the image file server and later forwarded to the Macintosh by a user's query there.

13.2.2.3 Radiology Workshop Software Package

Radiology Workshop is a C-language software package that allows the user to formulate text, thumbnail, and full-resolution requests to the DIFS and displays any resulting information. Its easy-to-use interface consists of graphic icons and is driven by mouse and keyboard input. The hardware requirements to use this software are minimal—a Macintosh II or better with at least 4 Mbyte of random access memory, a hard drive, and a network connection to the departmental network (either directly or through the Internet). Figure 13.5 shows representative images and patient information retrieved from the PACS through Radiology Workshop. Figure 13.5D shows a subsampled full-resolution CR image displayed by a public domain software package, NIH IMAGE, all within the Radiology Workshop domain.

13.2.3 Some Issues Related to Image and Information Retrieval

The distributed image file server (DIFS) allows users with a minimum desktop computer resource to access a wealth of hospital-integrated PACS data effectively. Since the hospital-integrated PACS is open to every potential user in the medial center com-

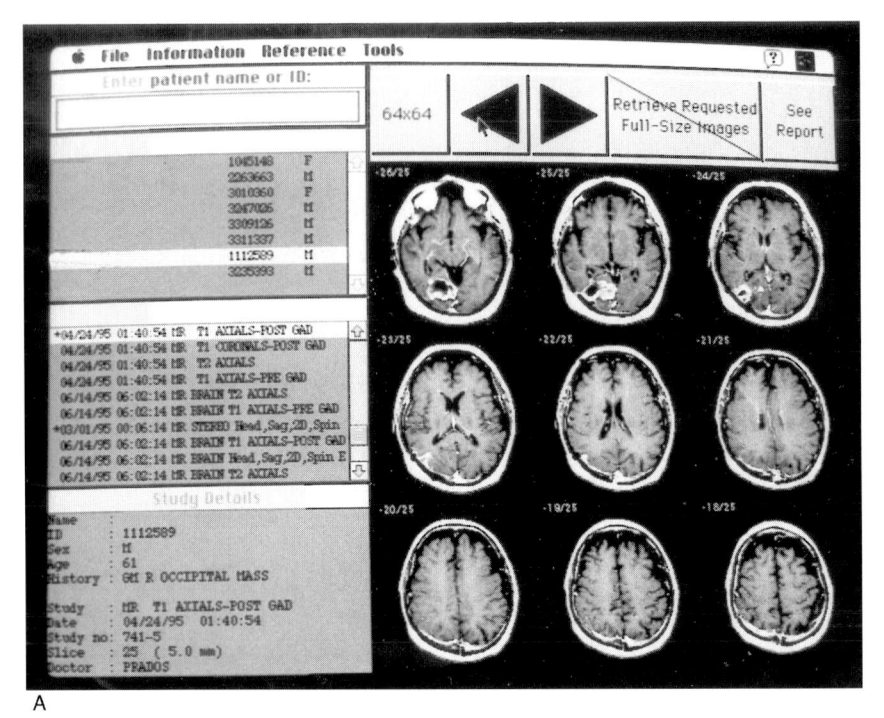

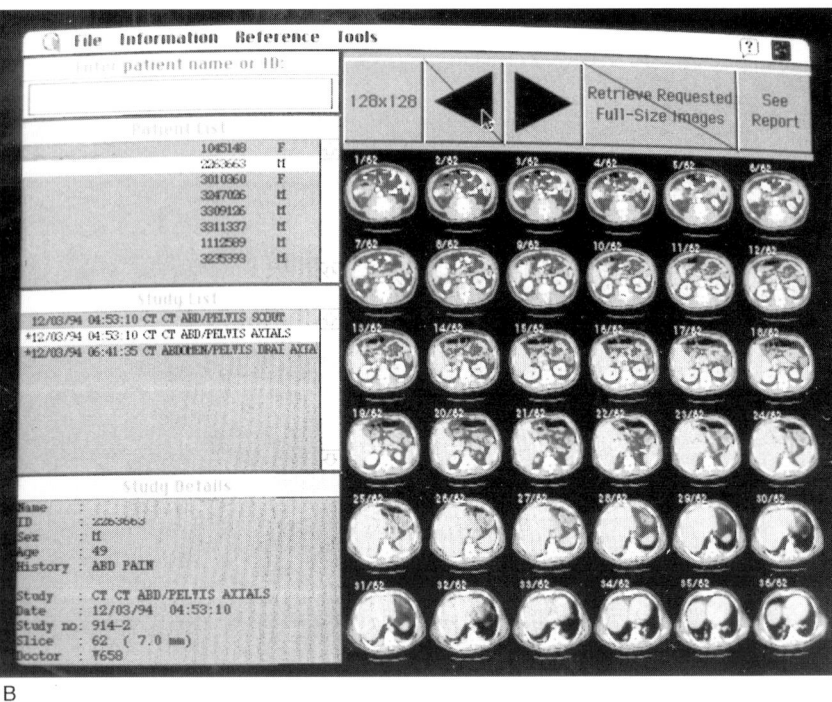

Figure 13.5 (A) Macintosh-based physician's desk workstation used for multimedia display. Upper left, patient list; Middle left, study list; Lower left, patient information; middle and right side, thumbnail screen with a set of MR T1 images subsampled to 128 × 128. (B) Thumbnail screen with a set of CT abdominal images subsampled to 64 × 64.

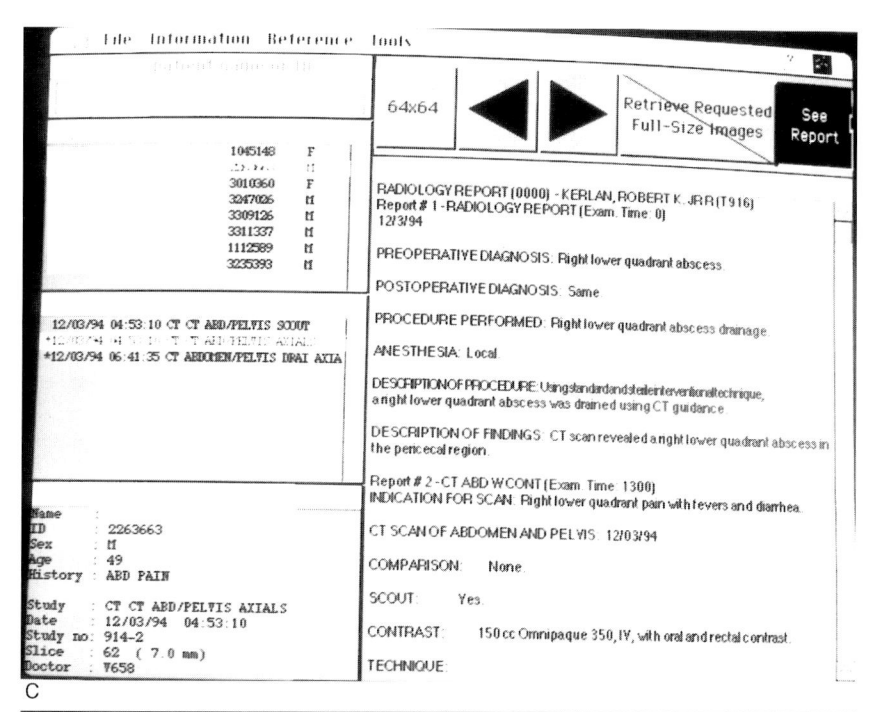

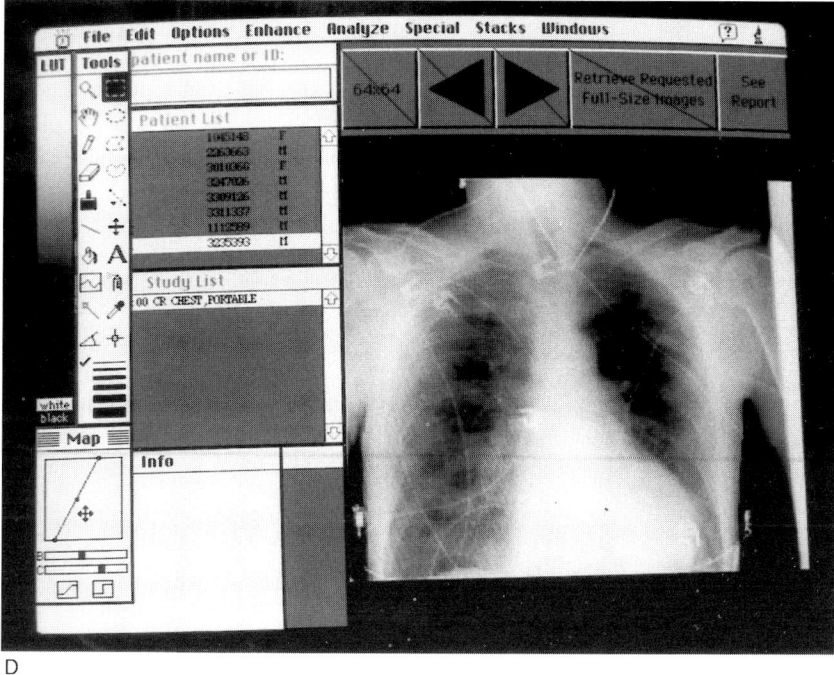

Figure 13.5 (C) Screen showing the diagnostic report describing the images presented in B. (D) Screen with a full-resolution CR image subsampled to 256 × 256 and window and level with the NIH IMAGE software.

munity, several issues arise, related to system usage, system performance, communication bandwidth, access priority, and data security.

13.2.3.1 System Usage

The images and data retrieved from DIFS are best used in two major applications: the acquisition of Macintosh picture images for slide making and the acquisition of raw image data for image processing. Typically, the user has seen an interesting case during readout and wants use the system to transfer a few full-resolution key images to his or her Macintosh for storage in a personal teaching file and for slide production. Because of the large amounts of storage required by these images (in terms of a Macintosh desktop computer), it may be necessary to install other peripheral storage devices, such as the small optical disk drive, to increase the storage capacity for the user. As for slide production, depending on the technique used, the quality of slides varies greatly from user to user, necessitating the identification of a consistent method for producing good quality slides from computer slide printers.

13.2.3.2 System Performance

The system's response to queries of the PACS controller should be timely. For example, queries of text information should be completed within seconds. The time to acquire a thumbnail sketch of a study is quite variable and is generally deemed to be slow, but it depends primarily on the age of the requested study. While a patient is in the hospital, his or her studies are stored in the temporary storage of PACS. After discharge, this study information is moved to a much slower permanent archive. Thumbnail sketches of these recent studies should be ready within one minute, whereas older studies require several minutes (depending on the size of the study). Because 90% of the retrieval time is spent searching and reading the image from the permanent archive, this time is unlikely to be reduced, and the delay must be tolerated by the users. However, users should consider that this image retrieval has a lower priority than the image retrieval from the clinical viewing workstations.

With the PACS and DIFS infrastructure in place, widespread installation of this system for use by students and staff outside the department of radiology will result. However, three fundamental issues must be considered before the PACS administration can provide such unparalleled access to patients' text and image data.

Traffic on the Departmental Network   Although the Macintosh interface is designed for selection of only a few key images from a study, the PACS controller, because of its standard ACR-NEMA or DICOM data format, always delivers an entire image file through the faster PACS network to the DIFS. The DIFS accepts this large image file and extracts only the requested images for delivery to the Macintosh through the slower departmental network. Through a combination of this extraction and the aforementioned data conversion (which typically reduces the number of bytes in an image), the traffic that must be carried on the departmental network is reduced.

This leaves bandwidth available for the other major uses of the network, including electronic mail, printing, file transfer, and Telnet.

Priority of Clinical Activities A priority index must be determined among diagnostic workstations, review workstations, and the DIFS clients. The current thought is that the two former sets of workstations should have higher priority. It is likely that requests from DIFS will have to be handled by the PACS controller at a lower priority than clinical requests.

However, the forwarding of key image requests from the workstations to the DIFS relieves the workstations of the significant amount of work involved in transmitting full-resolution images to the user's Macintosh. Thus, key image selection is allowed to take place with little or no slowing of clinical interpretation. The DIFS also relieves the PACS controller of a significant workload by performing the data format conversion (such as ACR-NEMA or DICOM to PICT) that must precede the transmission of these full-resolution images to a Macintosh.

Data Access Rights and Security Because Radiology Workshop operates through the use of standard TCP/IP protocols, anyone using this software can access the data stored in the PACS archive from anywhere in the world (through the Internet). Therefore, the topic of data security is of paramount importance.

In particular, the issues of data access rights and security give rise to two distinct sets of problems. First of all, data within the PACS must be secure from accidental corruption and tampering, and they must be accessible to authorized users. By limiting access to the PACS to a small number of well-defined read-only requests, the DIFS protects the integrity of the data stored in the PACS. In addition, users wishing to access the DIFS must obtain a password and register their computers with the department. Only requests from authorized machines with valid user passwords should be accepted.

Second, patients' confidentiality must be strictly maintained. One method is the removal of any identifying data from information transmitted to a user's Macintosh. However, without some type of link to this information, valid clinical research would be significantly inhibited. Each institution needs to develop policies based on past experience and clinical requirements, to address these patient confidentiality issues and to establish guidelines specifying who may have access to the data and how the material legitimately may be used.

13.3 WEB SERVER

Section 13.2 describes the concept of the distributed image file server for easy access of PACS images and related data by applications. The physician's desktop Macintosh image server is an example of intrahospital usage. However, this image file server is not ideal for interhospital applications because the design does not include wide area network communication protocols. In this section we present an image file server based on the World Wide Web technology that allows the access of PACS image files and data for both inter- and intrahospital application.

13.3.1 Web Technology

The Internet was developed by the federal government originally for military applications. Through the years, its utilization has been greatly extended. The Internet can be loosely defined as a set of computers, connected together by various wiring methods, that transmit information among each other through TCP/IP network protocols (Section 9.1.2) using a public communication network. An intranet, on the other hand, is a private entity that transmits information through a secured network environment. The World Wide Web is a collection of Internet protocols that provide easy access to many large databases through Internet connections. The Web is based on the hypertext transfer protocol (HTTP), which supports the transmission of hypertext document on all computers accessible through the Internet. The two most popular languages for Web applications that allow for the display of formatted and multimedia documents to be independent of the computers used are HTML (**h**ypertext **m**arkup **l**anguage) and Java language (just another vague acronym) from Sun Microsystems. In Web terminology, there are the Web server and the clients (or sites, or browsers). A Web site can use trigger processes to access information on a Web server through HTTP.

During the past several years, the application of Web technology has been extended to health care information. Some Web sites now support access to textual information from electronic medical record (EMR) systems. These Web-based EMR systems can be categorized according to their characteristics (e.g., completeness and detail of information model, coupling between the Web-based and legacy hospital information systems, machinable quality of data, customization). The use of the Web server as a means to access PACS image data is being considered and implemented by both academic centers and manufacturers. In the next section, we present the design of a Web-based image file server in the PACS environment as a means of accessing PACS images and data for both intra- and interhospital applications.

13.3.2 Concept of Web Server in the PACS Environment

Consider the image file server shown in Figure 13.2. Let us see what properties it needs to be qualified as a Web-based file server. First, the server has to support Web browsers connected to the Internet. Second, the server must interpret queries from the browser written in HTML or Java, and convert the queries to DICOM and HL7 standards. Third, the server must support the DICOM Query/Retrieve SOP to query and retrieve images and related data from the PACS controller. And finally, the server must provide a translator to convert DICOM images and HL7 text to HTTP. Figure 13.6 shows the basic architecture of a Web server allowing Web browsers to query and retrieve PACS image and related data. Figure 13.7 illustrates the eight standard steps involved in a typical query session from the Web browser to the Web server for images and related data stored in the PACS controller.

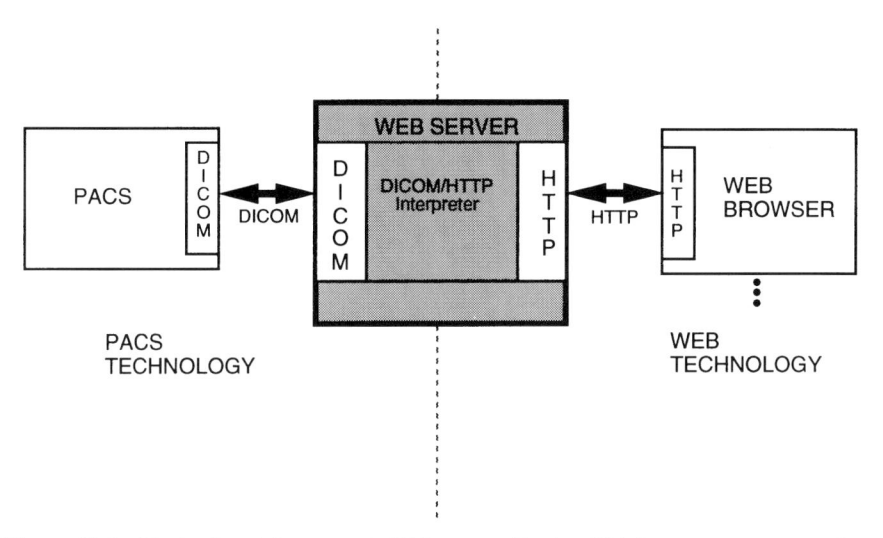

Figure 13.6 The basic architecture of a Web server allowing Web browsers to query and retrieve images and related data from PACS.

The Web server is a nice concept utilizing existing Internet technology available in everyone's desktop computer to access PACS images and related data. There are, however, drawbacks to using the current Internet for image retrieval. First, the response time for image transmission from the Internet is too slow because of the constraints imposed by the WAN speed. As a result, it is feasible to use the Internet for such applications only if the number and the size of images retrieved are small. The proposed next generation Internet (NGI) may alleviate some of these constraints. On the other hand, Web technology is well-suited for intranet applications, especially if the intranet uses a well-designed high speed LAN (e.g., gigabit Ethernet or ATM). Another problem is that Web technology is not designed for high resolution gray-scale image display, especially when real-time lookup table operation is required. In this case, the waiting time for such an operation is intolerably long.

13.4 MEDICAL IMAGE INFORMATICS INFRASTRUCTURE

13.4.1 Concept of MIII

Medical image informatics infrastructure (MIII) is a server designed to take advantage of existing PACS resources and their images and related data for large-scale horizontal and longitudinal clinical, research, and education applications that could not be performed before owing to insufficient data. The MIII is the ultimate goal of the utilization of PACS, in addition to daily clinical service.

13.4.2 MIII Architecture and Components

Medical image informatics infrastructure has the following components: medical images and associated data (including PACS database), image processing, data/knowl-

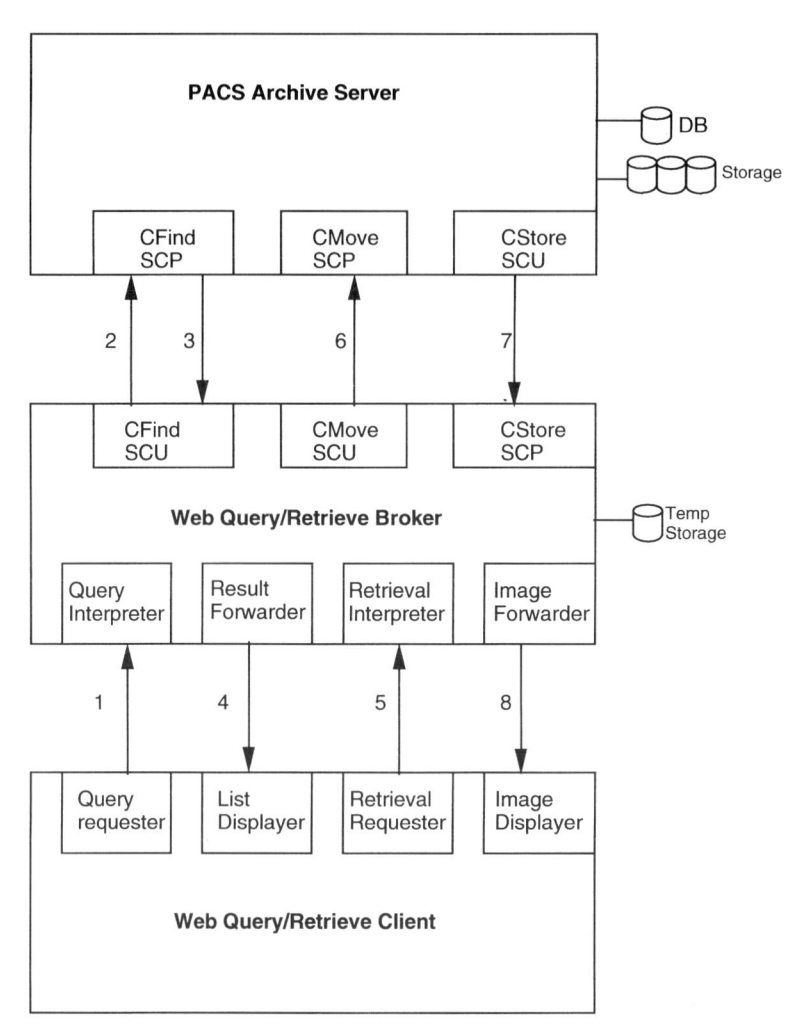

Figure 13.7 A typical query session from the Web browser through the Web server requesting images and related data from the PACS controller. The session requires eight steps involving both Web and PACS technologies. The resources required in the Web server (Fig. 13.6) for such a session are detailed in the Web broker.

edge base management, visualization, graphic user interface, communication networking, and application-oriented software. These components are logically related as shown in Figure 13.8, and their functions are summarized in the subsections that follow.

13.4.2.1 PACS and Related Data

PACS databases and other related health information systems containing patient demographic data, case histories, medical images and corresponding diagnostic reports,

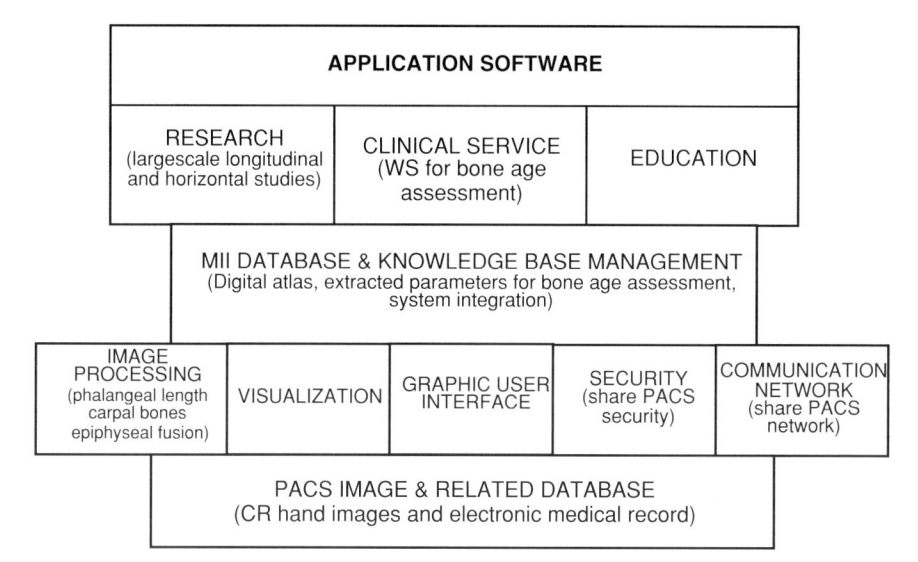

Figure 13.8 Medical image informatics infrastructure (MIII) components and their logical relationship. The bottom layer is image and related data from PACS and other databases. The middle two layers are described in Section 13.4.2. The top-layer software is application specific. Items in parentheses relating to the bone age assessment application are described in Sections 18.1.2.1–18.1.2.4.

and laboratory test results constitute the data source in the MIII. The data are organized and archived by means of standard data formats and protocols, such as DICOM for images and HL7 for text. In addition, a controlled health vocabulary can be based on standards for medical identifiers, codes, and messages proposed by the American Medical Informatics Association.

13.4.2.2 Image Processing

Image processing software allows for setting up the image content indexing and retrieval mechanism. Its functions include segmentation, region of interest determination, texture analysis, content analysis, morphological operations, and image registration. The output from image processing can be a new image or features describing some characteristics of the image. Image processing functions can be performed automatically or interactively on image data from the PACS database by an input server. Data extracted by the image processing functions can be appended to the image data file.

13.4.2.3 Database and Knowledge Base Management

The database and knowledge base management component software has several functions. First, it integrates and organizes PACS images and related data, extracts image features and keywords from image processing, and derives medical heuristics rules and guidelines for incorporation into a coherent multimedia data model. Second, it supports online database management, content-based indexing and retrieval, formatting and distribution for visualization, and manipulation. This component can be developed on top of a commercial database engine with add-on application software.

13.4.2.4 Visualization and Graphic User Interface

Visualization and graphic user interface are output components. Both components are related to workstation design. Visualization includes 3-D rendering, image data fusion, and static and dynamic imaging display. Visualization utilizes extracted data from image processing (i.e., segmentation, enhancement, and shading) for output rendering. Visualization can be performed on a standard workstation (WS) or with high performance graphic engines. For a low performance WS, the final visualization can be precomputed and packaged at the WS; with high performance graphic engines, rendering can be in real time at the WS.

The designers of a graphic user interface (GUI) must consider optimization of workstation design for information retrieval and data visualization with minimal effort from the user. A well-designed GUI is essential for effective real-time visualization and image content retrieval. GUI can also be used for extraction of additional parameters for nonstandard interactive image analysis.

13.4.2.5 Communication Networks

Communication networks include network hardware and communication protocols required to connect MIII components together. The MIII communication networks can have two architectures: a network of its own with a connection to those of the PACS, or it can share the communication networks with the PACS. In the former, the connection between the MIII and the PACS networks should be transparent to the users and should provide the necessary high speed throughput for the MIII to request PACS images and related data and to distribute results to a user's workstation. In the latter, the MIII should have a logical segment, isolated from the PACS networks, to prevent interference with the PACS daily clinical functions.

13.4.2.6 System Integration

System integration includes system interface, and shared data and workspace software. System interface software utilizes existing communication networks and protocols to connect all infrastructure components into an integrated information system. Shared data and workspace software allocates and distributes resources including data, storage space, and workstation to the online users.

13.4.2.7 Security

Security includes data integrity and data access. The former considers image authenticity and the completeness of data. After PACS images have been processed, some validation mechanisms are needed to assure accuracy, completeness, and authenticity. Data access considers who can access what type of data and when.

Once the aforementioned components have been implemented in the MIII, application-oriented software can be designed and developed to integrate necessary components for a specific clinical, research, or education application. This sequence provides rapid prototyping and reduces the development costs of every application. It is in this application layer component that the user encounters the advantages and power of the MIII. We will discuss in Chapter 18 some applications based on the MIII.

CHAPTER 14

Telemedicine and Teleradiology

14.1 INTRODUCTION

Telemedicine and teleradiology have become increasingly important as our country's health care system gradually changes from fee-for-service delivery to managed, capitated care. During the past several years, we have seen the trend of primary care physicians joining health maintenance organizations (HMOs). HMOs purchase smaller hospitals and form hospital groups under the umbrella of the larger business entity. Also, academic institutions form consortia to compete with other local hospitals and HMOs. This consolidation allows the elimination of duplication and the streamlining of health care services among hospitals. As a result, costs are reduced; but at the same time, because of the donwsizing, the number of experts available for service also decreases. Utilization of telemedicine and teleradiology is a method of saving on costs and compensating for the loss of expertise.

One of the most comprehensive reviews in assessing telecommunications in health care was a study reported in 1996 by the Committee on Evaluating Clinical Applications of Telemedicine of the Institute of Medicine. This report, which is an excellent source for future reference, gives detailed discussions of various issues in telemedicine, including technical and human context, policy, and methods of evaluation.

Telemedicine, in terms of applications, can be simply defined as the delivery of health care using telecommunications and computer technologies. The well-established consultation by means of telephone conversation would not alone qualify as telemedicine, since it uses only telecommunications, and not computer technology. There are two models in telemedicine and teleradiology: the referring physician or health care provider can either consult with an individual specialist at various places through a network, or request opinions from a consolidated expert center, where different types of consultation service are provided. In this chapter we concentrate on the expert center model, as this is the trend in the health care delivery system.

In the expert center consultation process, three modes are possible: telediagnosis, teleconsultation, and telemanagement. For telediagnosis, the patient's examination results and imaging studies are done at the referring physician's remote site, and data and images are transmitted to the expert center for diagnosis. The urgency of this service is nominal, and turnaround can take from four hours to all day. For teleconsultation, the patient may be waiting at the examination site, while the referring doctor requests a second opinion or diagnosis from the expert center within half an hour. For telemanagement, the patient may still be on the gantry or in the examination room at the remote site, and the expert is supposed to provide immediate management care to the patient in situ. Because of these three different operational modes, the technology requirements in telemedicine and teleradiology are different.

14.2 TELEMEDICINE

Teleradiology is a subset of telemedicine dealing with the transmission and display of images in addition to other patient-related information between a remote site and an expert center. The technology requirement for teleradiology is more stringent than that of general telemedicine, because the former involves images.

Basically, telemedicine without teleradiology requires only very simple technology: a computer gathers all necessary patient information, examination results, and diagnostic reports, arranges them in proper order at the referring site, and transmits them through telecommunication technology to a second computer at the expert center, where the information is displayed as soft copy on a monitor. In modern hospitals or clinics, the information gathering, and the arrangement of the information in proper order, can be handled by the hospital information system (HIS). In a private practice group or an individual physician's office, these two steps can be contracted out to a computer application vendor. Another requirement of telemedicine is to design communication protocols for sending this prearranged information to the expert center. Special hardware and software components are needed for this task.

Hardware and telecommunication choices vary according to required data throughput. The hardware component includes a pair of communication boards and/or modems connecting the two computers, one at the referring site and the other at the expert center through a telephone line. The type and cost of such hardware depends on which telecommunication service is selected. Depending on the transmission speed required, the line can be a regular telephone line, a DS-0 (digital service, 56 Kbit/s), an ISDN (Integrated Service Digital Network, from 56 Kbit/s to 1.544 Mbit/s), or a DS-1 or private line (T-1), with 1.544 Mbit/s. The costs for these lines are related to the transmission speed, and the distance between sites. For telemedicine applications without images, a regular telephone line, DS-0, or a single ISDN line would be sufficient. In the San Francisco Bay area, a local ISDN line costs between $30 and $40 per month.

The software component includes the information display, and some quality assurance and communication protocol programs. All software programs can be supported either by the HIS department or from a vendor. Efficient information gathering and selecting proper subsets of information for timely transmission are critical to the success of the telesystem. Once diagnostic results are available from the expert center, they can be transmitted back to the referring site with the same communication chain or through a standard fax machine. Figure 14.1 shows a generic telemedicine communication chain.

In teleradiology, since it involves images, the technologies required are more demanding. We turn now to a more detailed discussion of this topic.

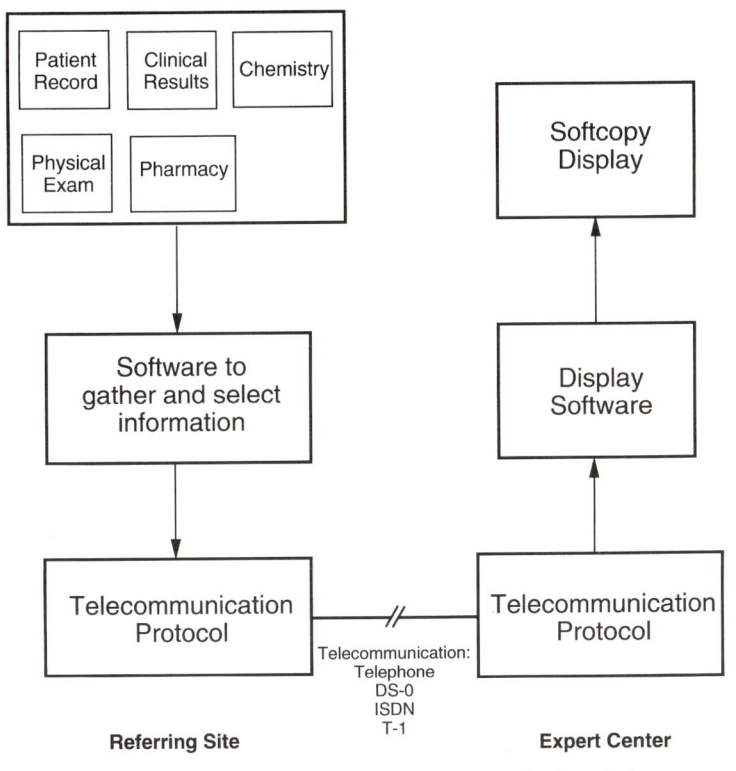

Figure 14.1 A generic telemedicine communication chain.

14.3 TELERADIOLOGY

14.3.1 Background

As discussed in Section 14.1, the trend toward managed, capitated care in the health care industry creates an opportunity to form expert centers in radiology practice. In this model, radiological images and related data are transmitted between examination sites and diagnostic centers through telecommunications. This type of radiology practice is loosely called teleradiology. Figure 14.2 shows an expert center model in teleradiology. In this expert model, rural clinics, community hospitals, and HMOs rely on radiologists at the center for consultation. Figure 14.2 clearly shows that in teleradiology, the turnaround time requirement depends on the mode of service, which in turn determines the technology required and cost involved.

14.3.1.1 Why Do We Need Teleradiology?

The managed care trend in health care delivery is expediting the formation of teleradiology expert centers. However, even without health care reform, teleradiology is still an extremely important component in radiology practice for the following rea-

- Teleradiology -

```
Primary Care Physicians/Patients from
         Rural Clinics,
      Community Hospitals,
              HMOs
                │
                ▼
      Radiological Examinations
                │
                ▼
        Images and information
    Transmitted to the Expert Center
                │
                ▼
      Radiologists Make Diagnosis
```

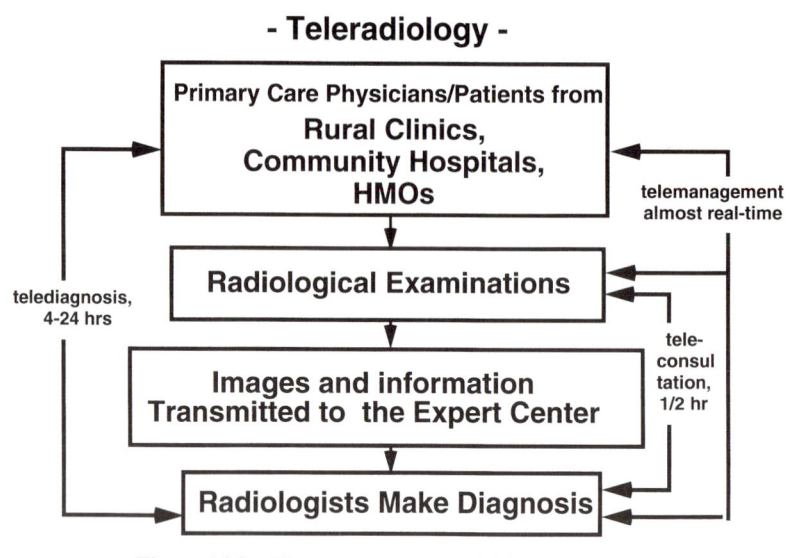

telediagnosis, 4-24 hrs

telemanagement almost real-time

tele-consultation, 1/2 hr

Figure 14.2 The expert center model in teleradiology

sons. First, teleradiology secures images for radiologists to read so that no images will be accidentally lost in transit. Second, teleradiology reduces the reading cycle time from formation of the image to completion of the report. Third, since radiology is subdivided into many subspecialties, even a general radiologist requires an expert's second opinion on occasion. The availability of teleradiology will facilitate the seeking of second opinions. Fourth, teleradiology increases radiologists' income, since no images are accidentally lost, hence not read. Health care reform concerns add two more reasons: (1) health care costs are lowered, since an expert center can serve multiple sites reducing the number of radiologists required, and the efficiency and effectiveness of health care delivery can be improved because turnaround time is faster and there is no loss of images.

14.3.1.2 What Is Teleradiology?

Generally, in teleradiology, an image is sent from the examination site to a remote site, where an expert radiologist will make the diagnosis. The expert's report is sent to the examination site, to a primary physician, who can then prescribe the patient's treatment immediately. Teleradiology can be very simple or extremely complicated. In a simple case, low quality teleradiology equipment and slow speed communication technology might be used to send an image to a radiologist's home, in the evening, for a second opinion. (Many examination sites cannot afford to have a radiologist cover the service at night or on weekends. A resident normally is in charge during these off-hours, and he or she may occasionally require consultation from the staff radiologist, at home.) This type of teleradiology does not require highly sophisticated equip-

TABLE 14.1 Four Models in Teleradiology

Level of Complexity	Historical Images/RIS	Archive
Simple	No	No
Simple to complicated	Yes	No
Complicated	No	Yes
Most complicated	Yes	Yes

ment. It can be handled by a conventional telephone and simple desktop personal computer with modem connection and display software. This type of application originated in early 1970.

The second type of teleradiology is more complicated, with four different models shown in ascending order from simple to complicated in Table 14.1. Complications occur when historical images are required for comparison with the current examination, and when the expert needs information from the radiology information system (RIS) to make a diagnosis. In addition, complications arise when the examination and dictation must be archived and appended to the patient image data file. Teleradiology is relatively simple to operate when no archiving is required. The operation becomes extremely complicated, however, when it is necessary to retrieve archived information on a patient and then return the data to the archive.

14.3.1.3 Teleradiology and PACS

When the teleradiology service requires patient's historical images as well as related information, teleradiology and PACS become very similar. Table 14.2, which compares teleradiology and PACS, shows that the major difference between them is in the methods of image capture. Most current teleradiology still uses a digitizer as the primary method of converting a film image to digital format, although the trend is moving toward the DICOM standard. In PACS, direct digital image capture using DICOM is mostly used. In networking, teleradiology uses slower speed wide area networks (WAN) compared with the higher speed local area network (LAN) used in PACS. In

TABLE 14.2 Differences Between Teleradiology and PACS

Function	Telerad	PACS
Image capture	Digitizer	DICOM
Display technology	Same	Same
Networking	WAN	LAN
Storage	Short	Long
Compression	Yes	Maybe

teleradiology, image storage is mostly short-term, whereas in PACS it is long-term. Teleradiology relies heavily on image compression, whereas PACS may or may not.

Refer back to Table 2.1, which gives sizes of some common medical images. In clinical applications, a single image is not sufficient for diagnostic purposes. In general, a typical examination generates between 10 and 20 Mbyte. The fourth column shows an average size of one typical examination in each of these image modalities. The highest extreme is in digital mammography, which requires 160 Mbyte. To transmit this much information through WAN calls for a very high bandwidth communication technology. One research topic in telemammography entails finding a way to transmit this large file size through WAN with acceptable speed and cost. Telemammography is discussed in more detail in Section 14.4.

14.3.2 Teleradiology Components

Table 14.3 lists the teleradiology components and Figure 14.3 shows a generic schematic of their connections. Among these components, reporting and billing are common knowledge and are not discussed here. Devices generating images in teleradiology applications include film digitizers and the equipment associated with computed tomography (CT), magnetic resonance imaging (MR), computed radiography (CR), ultrasound imaging (US), nuclear medicine (NM), and digital subtraction angiography–digital fluorography (DSA/DF). Images from such acquisition devices are first generated from the examination site and then, if they are already in digital format, sent through the communication network to the expert center. If the images are stored on films, they need to be digitized by a film scanner at the examination site.

14.3.2.1 Image Capture

When the original image data are on film, either a video frame grabber or a laser film digitizer is used to convert them to digital format. A video frame grabber produces lower quality digital images, but it is faster and cheaper. On the other hand, laser film digitizers produce extremely high quality digital data, but compared to the video frame grabber they take longer and cost more. During the past several years, computed radiography has been used extensively in teleradiology. Conventional projec-

TABLE 14.3 Teleradiology Components

- Imaging acquisition device
- Image capture
- Data reformatting
- Transmission
- Storage
- Display
- Reporting
- Billing

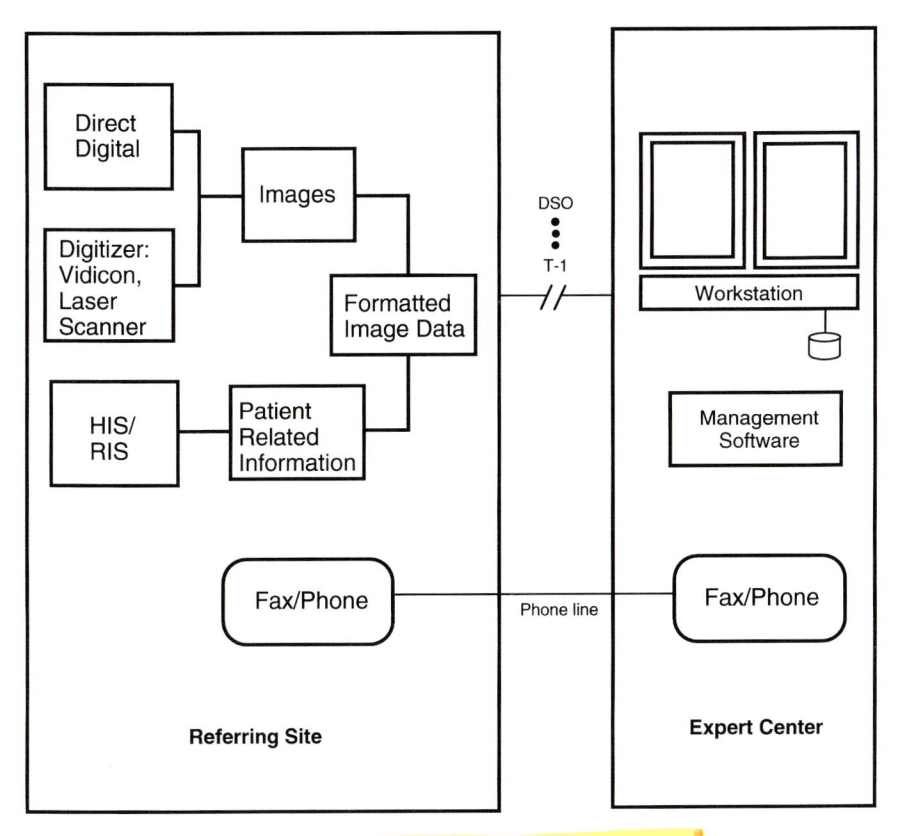

Figure 14.3 A generic teleradiology setup.

tion radiography can be obtained with CR, which produces a direct digital image as the output.

14.3.2.2 Data Reformatting

After images have been captured, it is advantageous to convert them, along with related data, to an industry standard, to allow the use of equipment from multiple vendors in the teleradiology chain. The two common standards used in the imaging industry are the Digital Imaging and Communication in Medicine (DICOM) Standard 3.0 for images and Health Level 7 (HL7) for textual data (see Chapter 7). The DICOM standard includes the image format as well as the communication protocols, whereas HL7 is for textual data only. The communication for textual information generally uses TCP/IP communication protocols.

14.3.2.3 Storage

At the receiving end of the teleradiology chain, a local storage device is needed before the image can be displayed. The capacity of this device can range from several hundred megabytes to 5–10 Gbyte. A long-term archive, such as an optical disk library, is needed at the expert center for teleradiology applications, which must be able to retrieve historical images and radiology information, and for current examination and diagnosis archival. The architecture of the long-term storage device is very similar to that used in PACS, as discussed in Section 10.3.

14.3.2.4 Display Workstation

For an inexpensive teleradiology system, a low cost, 512-line single monitor can be used for displaying images. However, sophisticated multimonitor display workstations are needed for primary diagnosis. The state-of-the-art technology in image workstation design was presented in Chapter 12, and will be revisited in Section 14.3.3.2.

14.3.2.5 Communication Networking

An important component in teleradiology is the communication network used for the transmission of images and related data from the acquisition site to the expert center for diagnosis. Since most teleradiology applications are not confined to the same hospital complex, but are distributed to health care facilities in metropolitan areas or at longer distances, the communication technology involved requires a wide area network. A WAN can be wireless or cabled. In wireless WAN, some technologies available are microwave transmission and communication satellites. Wireless WAN has not been used extensively because of its cost. Table 14.4 shows cable technology available in WAN: it starts from the low communication rate DS-0 with 56 kbit/s, to a very high communication data rate DS-3 with 45 Mbit/s. All these WAN technologies are available through long-distance or local telephone carriers. The cost of using WAN is a function of transmission speed and the distance between sites. Thus, within a fixed distance, for a DS-0 line having a low transmission rate, the cost is fairly low compared to the much faster DS-3. Most of the private lines (e.g., T1 and T3) are point-to-point, and the cost also depends on the distance between connections. Table 14.5 shows the costs of DS-0 and T1 lines between UCSF and Mount Zion Hospital (MZH), two sites about 2 miles apart in the San Francisco Bay area.

Table 14.5 reveals that the initial investment for the DS-0 is $500. The monthly cost is the utility's $30 fixed fee plus the charge per local call. On the other hand, for

TABLE 14.4 Wire Technologies Available for Wide Area Networks

Technology	Speed
DS-0 (digital service)	56 Kbit/s
DS-1 dial up	56 Kbit/s to $24 \times 56 = 1.344$ Mbit/s
DS-1 private line (T1)	1.544 Mbit/s
ISDN (Integrated Service Digital Network)	56 Kbit/s–1.544 Mbit/s
DS-3 private line (T3)	28 DS-1 = 45 Mbit/s

TABLE 14.5 Wide Area Network Cost Using DS-0 (56 Kbit/s) and T1 (1.5 Mbit/s) Between UCSF and MZH: 2 Km Apart

DS-0		T1	
Up-front investment		Up-front investment	
Modems (2)	$400	Modems (2)	$12,000
Installation (2)	$100	Ethernet converters (2)	
	$500	T1 installation	$2,500
			$14,500
Monthly fee $30 + per call		T1 Monthly charge:	$554
(*30 times slower than the T1*)			

the T1 service the up-front investment is $14,500 and the monthly cost is $554, but the user does not have to pay an extra charge per call to use the line. The initial investment for the T1 is much higher than the DS-0, and for longer distances, its monthly charge is expensive. For example, the charge for a T1 line between San Francisco and Washington, D.C., could be as high a $10,000 a month. However, communication using the T1 is about 30 times faster than the DS-0 can deliver. Using T1 for teleradiology is very popular. Some larger companies lease several T1 lines from telephone carriers and sublease portions of them to smaller companies for teleradiology applications.

14.3.2.6 User Friendliness

One aspect of a teleradiology system not listed in Table 14.3 is user friendliness. This quality applied both to the connections of the teleradiology equipment at the examination site and the expert center, and to the display workstation at the expert center, which should not be overly complicated.

To be user friendly, a complete teleradiology operation should be as automatic as possible, requiring only minimal user intervention. For example, a user-friendly image workstation should offer image and related data prefetch, automatic image sequencing at the monitors, and automatic lookup table, image rotation, and unwanted background removal from the image. The first criterion, "image and related data prefetch," means that for the same patient examination, all historical images and related data required for comparison by the radiologist should be prefetched from the patient folder before the image is transmitted and displayed. When the radiologist at the expert center starts to review the case, these prefetched images and related data should be available immediately. "Automatic image sequencing at the display workstation" means that all the images and related data are sequentially arranged so that at the touch of the mouse, properly arranged images and information appear on the monitors. Having prearranged data minimizes the time the radiologist at the expert center must spend to search and organize. This translates to an effective and efficient teleradiology operation. The third factor (automatic lookup table, rotation, and background removal) is necessary because images acquired at the distant site might not

TABLE 14.6 Time Required to Send a 10 MByte X-Ray and 40 MByte CT Study from MZH to UCSF Using T1 and ATM (OC-3): No Compression

System	One X-Ray Exam 2K × 2.5K × 2 byte (10 MByte)		One CT Study (40 MByte)	
	One Image	Two Images	One Study	One Current + One Historical
T1(1.5 Mbits/s) realization 100 Kbits/s	100 seconds (1.6 min)	200 seconds (3.9 min)	400 seconds (6.7 min)	800 seconds (13.4 min)
ATM (155 Mbits/s) realization 60 Mbits/s (7.5 Mbytes/s)	1.3 seconds	2.7 seconds	5.3 seconds	10.7 seconds

have the proper lookup table for optimal visual display, images might not be generated in the proper orientation, and there may be unwanted white background in the image due to radiographic collimation. All these parameters, which were discussed in detail in Chapter 12, affect the quality of a diagnosis based on teleradiology images.

14.3.3 State-of-the-Art Technology

In Section 14.3.2 we discussed the components in a teleradiology operation. In this section, we present the state-of-the-art technology in teleradiology, focusing especially on communication technology, image compression, and image workstations.

14.3.3.1 Wide Area Network: Asynchronous Transfer Mode (ATM) Technology

ATM technology, discussed in Section 9.1.3, is an emerging communication technology both for WAN and LAN. The current commercially available ATM technology is the OC-3, with 155 Mbit/s. Using ATM for data communication between two nodes requires one adapter board at the computer of each node, and an ATM switch connecting both adapters at each node with fiber-optic cables.

In LAN, ATM is being used by many medical centers for image communication, whereas in WAN, ATM still has the obstacle of cost (for expensive long-distance carriers). Table 14.6 compares times needed by the T1 and ATM technologies for the communication of images between Mount Zion Hospital and UCSF. Results demon-

Figure 14.4 (A) FCR 9000, (B) ATM switch, and (C) ISG image workstation (ISG Technologies, Inc. Ontario, Canada). Radiographs generated by a CR system are transmitted through the ATM at UCSF to the ATM main switch at Pacific Bell in Oakland, then to the ATM switch at the SFVA Medical Center, where they are displayed at the 1600-line, two monitor workstation. The completed process takes less than 2 seconds after the generation of images. (Courtesy of Dr. Gretchen Gooding.)

A

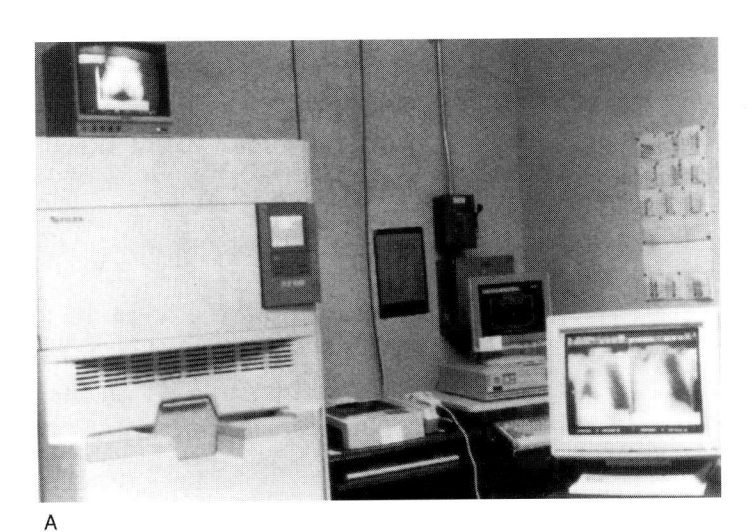

B

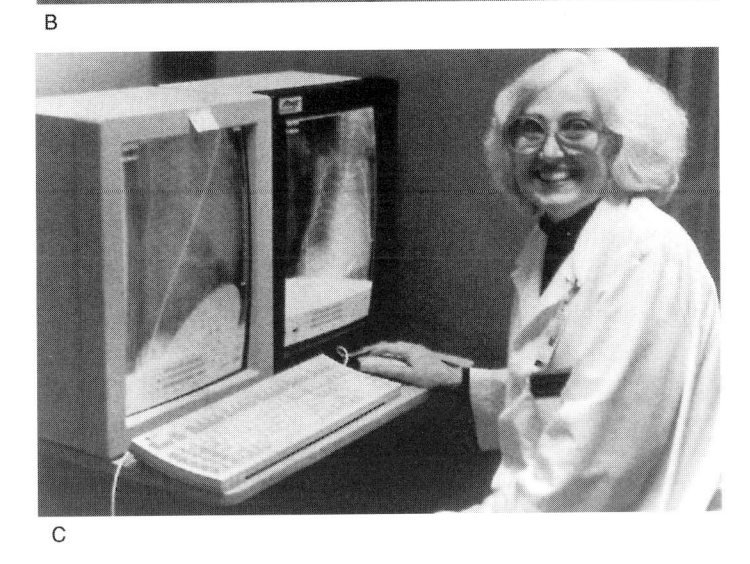

C

377

strate that ATM is almost two orders of magnitude faster than T1. The cost for using ATM technology is still restrictive, not because of the technology, but because of long-distance carrier charges. One way to make the ATM an affordable WAN communication method is to have carriers lower the fiber-optic cable utility cost. Figure 14.4 shows components of a teleradiology testbed between UCSF and SFVA Medical Center using a CR system, a two-monitor display workstation, and the ATM.

14.3.3.2 Display Workstations

Table 14.7 shows the specifications of a 2000-line and a 1600-line workstation used for teleradiology primary readings. These state-of-the-art technology diagnostic units, discussed in Chapter 12, use two monitors with over 2 Gbyte of local storage, displaying images and reports in 1–2 seconds. A 2000-line workstation costs between $50,000 and $60,000, whereas a 1600-line unit costs $30,000 to $40,000. User-friendly software is required for easy and convenient use by the radiologist at the workstation.

14.3.3.3 Image Compression

Teleradiology requires image compression (see Chapter 6) because of the slow speed and high cost of using WAN. For lossless image compression, current technology can achieve between 3:1 to 2:1 compression ratios, whereas in lossy image compression using cosine transform based MPEG and JPEG hardware and software, 20:1 to 10:1 compression ratios can be obtained with acceptable image quality. The latest advance in image compression technology uses the wavelet transform, which offers higher compression ratio and better image quality after decompression than cosine transform. With advances in communications technology, image workstation design, and image compression, teleradiology will move closer to becoming an integrated diagnostic tool in daily radiology practice.

14.3.4 Teleradiology Examples and Models

Teleradiology services started to proliferate around 1996. One of the earliest health care facilities using teleradiology, the Mayo Clinic, has sites in Rochester, Minnesota, Jacksonville, Florida, and Scottsdale, Arizona. To provide service to all three

TABLE 14.7 Specifications of 2000- and 1600- Line Workstations for Teleradiology

- Two monitors
- 1–2 week local storage for current and previous exam
- 1–2 second display of images and reports from local storage
- DICOM conformance
- Simple image processing functions

TABLE 14.8 MGH Operation: Two Regular Grade Voice Lines (9.6 Kbit/s)

- Customer: Saudi Arabia
- 24–48 hour turnaround time
- 4–6 images/case
- Compression: radiograph 20:1, CT 10:1
- Transmission: 3–4 min/image ($7.0)
- Workstations: 2K monitors

sites, a satellite communication method was used. The Mayo Clinic chose IBM at Rochester as the technical partner for the teleradiology service. Another example is the service to Saudi Arabia provided by Massachusetts General Hospital (MGH). In these cases, inexpensive regular voice lines (9.6 Kbit/s) were used. Table 14.8 summarizes the MGH operation. In the following, we generalize two teleradiology models as examples demonstrating the structure of teleradiology and how the service is set up, as well as the operational procedure based on our experience.

14.3.4.1 University Consortium

Telequest is a university consortium formed by the departments of radiology at the following universities: Bowman Graduate School of Medicine, Wake Forest University; the Brigham Radiology Foundation in Boston; Emory University Hospital in Atlanta; the University of California, San Francisco; and the Pennsylvania Medical Center in Philadelphia. A for-profit organization called Telequest was formed to provide a nationwide subspecialty radiology service.

In this model, Telequest provides a turnkey operation for the customer (e.g., an imaging center, an HMO, etc.) and transmits images to the consultation site at one of these five radiology departments. At the customer site, the company provides a turnkey operation, assists the site to interface with the radiology information system and the image acquisition devices, and provides the customer site around-the-clock service coverage. The communication connections is from a third-party vendor, allowing customers to select a desired transmission speed. Customers can also select consultants from any consultation site to read the cases. At the consultation site, high resolution workstations as described in Section 14.3.3.2 are used for the reading, and a rapid turnaround report is guaranteed by the contract. Figures 14.5 and 14.6 show, respectively, the teleradiology operation and data flow in a university radiology department consortium model.

Telequest handles all the marketing, service, communication connections, billing, and management. For example, one customer site, an imaging center located in Ohio, has two image acquisition systems: a General Electric Signa 5x MR scanner and a helical CT scanner. The operational hours are from Monday to Friday, 7:30 A.M. to 10:30 P.M., and Saturday and Sunday from 8:00 A.M. to 2:00 P.M. The image readings are distributed to the various consultation sites at these five universities. The network used is a fractional T1 provided by IBM. Image compression is obtained by means of

380 TELEMEDICINE AND TELERADIOLOGY

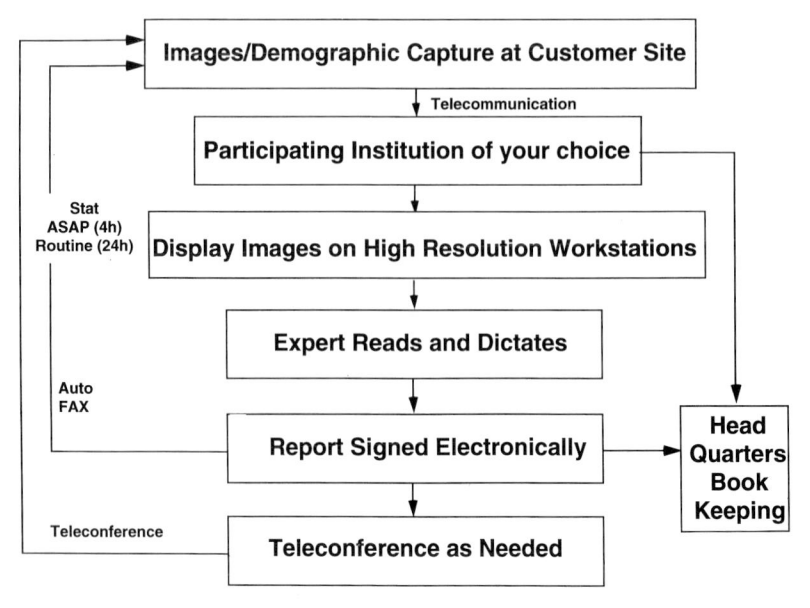

Figure 14.5 Teleradiology operation in a university radiology department consortium model.

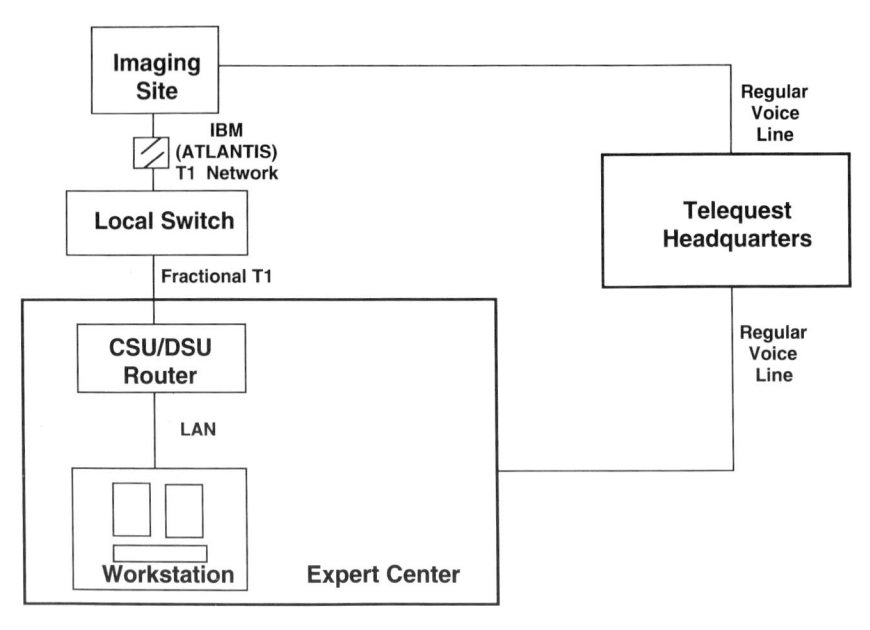

Figure 14.6 Data flow in a university radiology department consortium model.

the 2–3:1 lossless compression method. This teleradiology service model uses the strength of five prestigious radiology departments to attract business from imaging centers and HMOs throughout the nation. The result is that images collected from rural sites, community hospitals, and HMOs are sent to the expert centers, and consultations are distributed geographically to the five universities' radiology departments.

14.3.4.2 Teleradiology Service for Second Opinion

In our final model, a health care insurance company in a foreign country initiates an add-on subscription for its policy holder. For an extra amount of money per year (i.e., on top of the existing health insurance), the holder of an add-on policy has the right to request a second opinion on his or her existing medical diagnosis from a premier medical center in the United States at the subscriber's expense. Table 14.9 shows the operational procedure of this second-opinion teleradiology service.

An example of this model is found in the arrangement between an Israeli health insurance company and the University of California, San Francisco. The current enrollment of this add-on policy is about 800,000 in a country of 5 million people. The physical communication connection between the customer site and the expert site is through international ISDN lines (see Table 14.4), shown in Figure 14.7. The key in this connection is a black box (ASCEND), which provides intelligent software to interpret the number of ISDN lines at the sending site, the number of ISDN lines at the receiving site, and the international ISDN standard conversion. Depending on the speed required, multiple ISDN lines can be used to increase the rate of transmission. At the sending site, a film digitizer is used, and the expert site maintains a 1600-line, two-monitor workstation for interpretation.

This model, like the university consortium of Section 14.3.4.1, indicates the trend in teleradiology service. In the first model, the expert centers expand their capitations in radiology examinations through a consortium. These radiology departments increase their workload and income, which benefits the radiologists as well as the departments. In the second model, second-opinion consultation provides a developing country with easy access to consultations at a premier medical center in the United States. From the customers' point of view, a minimal add-on cost on top of an exist-

TABLE 14.9 Operational Procedure of a Second-Opinion Teleradiology Consultation Service

- Subscriber requests the health insurance company to arrange for a medical second opinion on the radiologic exam
- The insurer arranges for images to be digitized and transmitted from the remote site, possibly a foreign country, to the US consultation site, at the subscriber's expense
- Images are displayed on high resolution workstation and read by experts at the consultation site
- Second opinion is provided to the subscriber via phone, fax, or teleconference with the subscriber's referring physician in the remote location
- Subscriber can schedule follow-up exams at the consultation site at his or her own expense

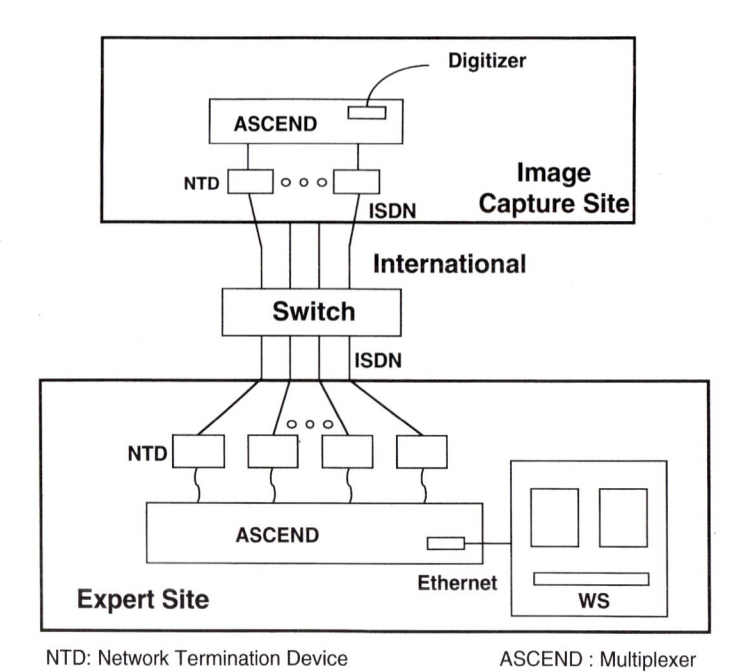

Figure 14.7 The physical communication connection between the customer (image capture site) and the expert site of an international second opinion teleradiology service.

ing health insurance policy is a small amount of pay for peace of mind from a second-opinion consultation if they so desire.

14.3.5 Some Important Issues in Teleradiology

14.3.5.1 Teleradiology Trade-Off Parameters

There are two sets of trade-off parameters in teleradiology. The first set consists of image quality, turnaround time, and cost; and the second set comprises data security, including patient confidentiality, and image authenticity. Table 14.10 shows the teleradiology trade-off parameters between image quality, turnaround time, and cost. These three parameters are affected by four factors: method of image capture, type of workstation used, amount of image compressed, and communication technology selected. The cost in teleradiology is determined by all these four factors.

In terms of data security, we have to consider patient confidentiality as well as image authenticity. Since teleradiology uses a public communication method with no security to transmit images, one must ask what type of protection should be provided to assure patient confidentiality. Moreover, after the image has been created in digital form, can we assure that it has not been altered, either intentionally or unintentionally? Methods such as data encryption and digital signatures, which have been in the domain of defense research for many years, can be used to guarantee image and data authenticity. Some of these techniques may be used to protect the data authen-

TABLE 14.10 Teleradiology Trade-Off Parameters

	Image Capture	Workstation	Compression	Communication Technology
Quality	×	×	×	
Turn around time	×		×	×
Cost	×	×	×	×

ticity as well as patient confidentiality. To impose high security on image data will increase the cost of decryption and decrease ease of access (since there will then be many layers of passwords). The trade-offs between cost and performance, confidentiality and reliability, will become major socioeconomic issues in teleradiology. Figure 14.8 shows a CT image that has been altered digitally by inserting a tumor on the lung (see arrows). Since altering a digital image is not difficult, developing methods to protect the integrity of image data is essential in teleradiology applications. We discuss data integrity and patient confidentiality in more detail in Section 17.6.

14.3.5.2 Medical–Legal Issues

There are four major medical–legal issues in teleradiology: privacy issues, licensure issues, credentialing issues, and malpractice liability issues. The ACR Standard for

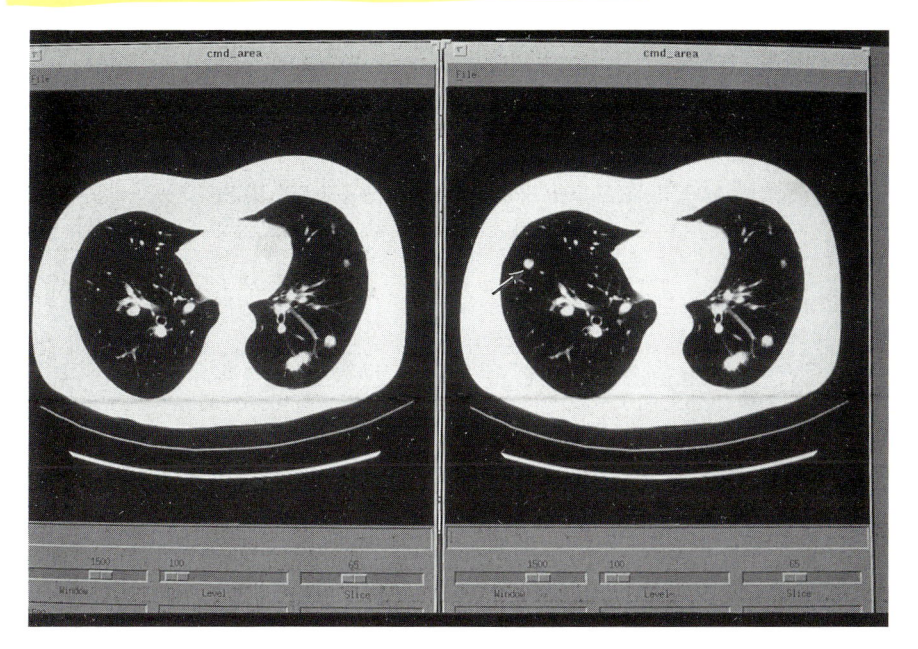

Figure 14.8 *Left:* A CT scan of the chest. *Right:* The same scan with a digitally inserted tumor (arrow). The insertion process requires minimal image processing (Courtesy of Dr. X. Zhu).

Teleradiology adopted in 1994 defines guidelines for "qualifications of both physician and nonphysician personnel, equipment specifications, quality improvement, licensure, staff credentialing, and liability." Although much is uncertain, guidelines to these topics have also been discussed extensively by James, Berger and Cepelewicz, and Kamp. Readers are encouraged to review the ACR standard and these authors' publications for the current status of these issues.

14.4 TELEMAMMOGRAPHY

14.4.1 Why Do We Need Telemammography?

Breast cancer is the fourth most common cause of death among women in the United States. There is no known means of preventing the disease, and available therapy has been unsuccessful in reducing the national mortality rate over the past 60 years. Current attempts to control breast cancer concentrate on early detection by means of mass screening, via periodic mammography and physical examination, because ample evidence indicates that such screening indeed can be effective in lowering the death rate. To perform massive screening, capabilities for digital mammography (Section 4.4.2) and telemammography must be in place. Full-field digital mammography (FFDM) can overcome many inherent problems in the screen/film combination detector and at the same time provide better spatial and density resolutions, and a higher signal-to-noise ratio in the digital mammogram, than are possible from digitized mammograms. Real-time telemammography adds to these advantages the utilization of expert mammographers (rather than general radiologists) as interpreters of the mammography examinations at the expert center. To set up a quality telemammography service requires the FFDM at the examination site, a high speed teleimaging network connecting the examination site with the mammography expert center, and high resolution digital mammogram display workstations for interpretation.

14.4.2 Concept of the Expert Center

Telemammography is built on the concept of an expert center. It allows radiologists with the greatest interpretive expertise to manage and read in real time all mammography examinations, thereby adding to the advantages of the FFDM. Specifically, telemammography increases efficiency, facilitates consultation and second reading, improves patient compliance, facilitates operation, supports computer-aided detection and diagnosis, allows centralized distributive archives, and enhances education through telemonitoring. "Real time" is defined in this context as a very rapid turnaround time between examination and interpretation. In addition, mammography screening in mobile units will be made more efficient, not only by overcoming the need to transport films from the site of examination to the site of interpretation, but also by permitting image interpretation while patients are still available for repeat or additional exposures. Furthermore, telemammography can be used to facilitate second-opinion interpretation, in effect making world-class mammography expertise immediately accessible to radiologists in community practice.

There are three protocols in telemammography: telediagnosis, teleconsultation, and telemanagement.

Telediagnosis uses experts to interpret digital mammograms sent from a remote site. Teleconsultation is used to improve the efficacy on problem cases. Without telemammography, consultations are tedious, time-consuming, and logistically complex. The goal of telemanagement is to replace the on-site general radiologist with remotely located expert mammographers for patient management.

14.4.3 Technical Issues

Telemammography services requires FFDM at the examination site, an image compression algorithm, a high speed tele-imaging WAN connecting the examination site with the mammography expert center, and a high resolution digital mammography display workstation for interpretation.

Present technologies available for telemammography applications include the FFDM with 50 μm spatial resolution with 12 bits/pixel (Section 4.4.2), ATM for both LAN and WAN connections, an optical disk library for long-term archiving, and RAID for rapid image retrieval and display. The telemammograms can be displayed with multiple 2K × 2.5K resolution monitor with 80–100 ft-L brightness. Figure 14.9 depicts schematically two configurations for a telemammography workstation with possible viewing formats and examples of digital mammograms on the 2K display

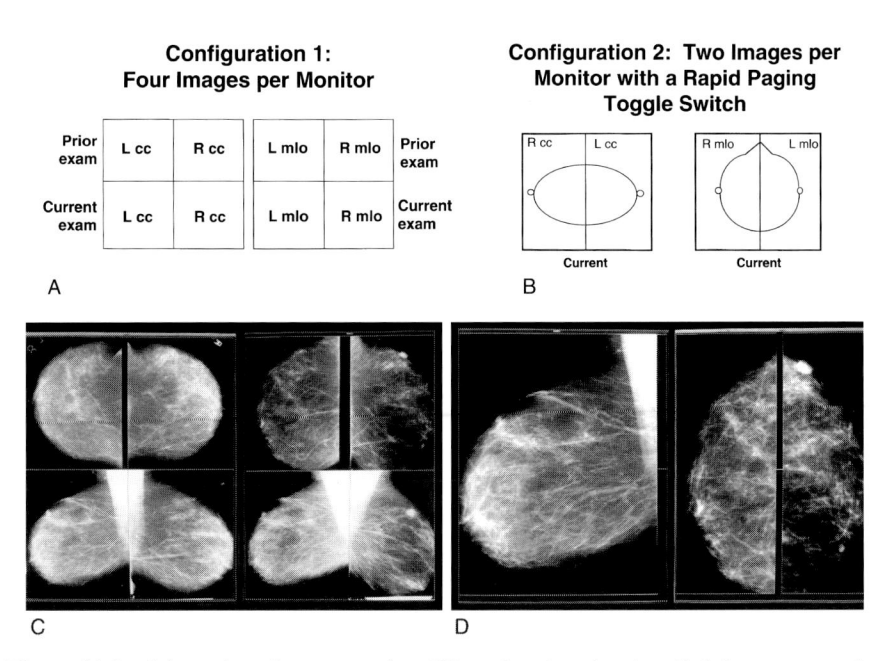

Figure 14.9 Schematics of a two-monitor 2K workstation showing digital mammography display schematic in the four-on-one (A), and two-on-one format (B) formats. Images showing four-on-one (C), two-on-one (D, right) and one-on-one (D, left) on the monitors. (cc: craniocaudal view; mlo: mediolateral oblique view.)

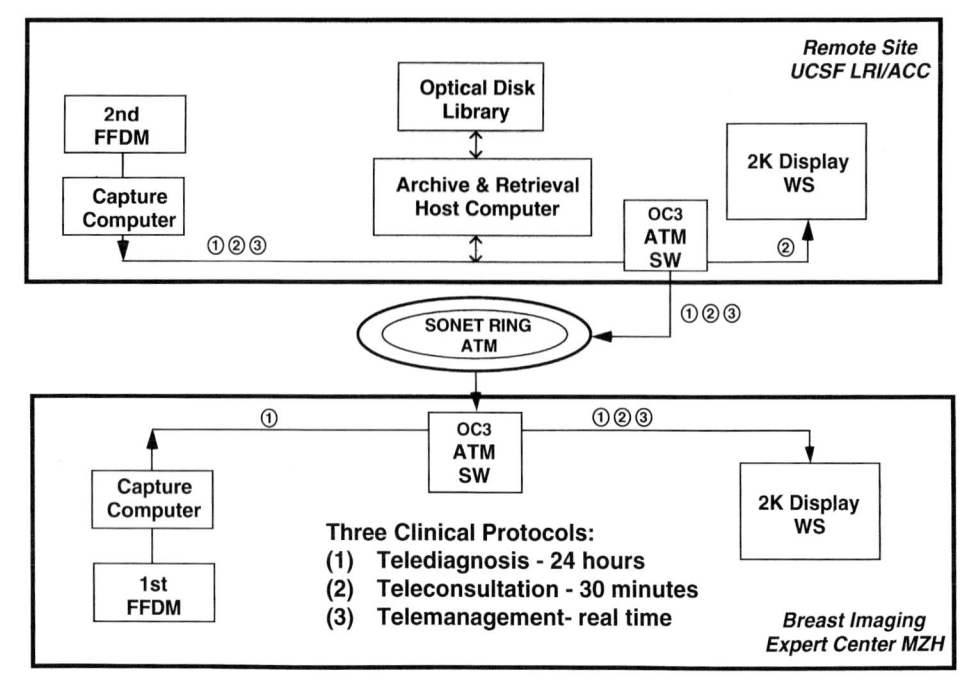

Figure 14.10 Telemammography system being developed for telediagnosis, teleconsultation, and telemanagement. The expert site is located at the breast imaging center, MZH, and the remote site is at the Ambulatory Care Center (ACC), UCSF. (1) *Telediagnosis:* Images sent from FFDM at MZH or ACC to 2K WS at MZH for interpretation. (2) *Teleconsultation:* Images sent from FFDM at ACC to 2K WSs at both MZH and ACC. Referring physician at ACC and expert at MZH use the WSs for consultation. (3) *Telemanagement:* Images sent from FFDM at ACC to 2K WS at MZH. Expert at MZH telemanages the patient, who is still at ACC, based on the reading.

workstation. Figure 14.10 represents a telemammography system being planned for use in telediagnosis, teleconsultation, and telemanagement applications.

Telemammography is still in the experimental stage; issues to be considered are the image quality at the expert's workstation, speed of communication, and the cost of assembling a high quality and efficient digital mammography workstation.

14.5 TELEMICROSCOPY

14.5.1 Telemicroscopy and Teleradiology

Telemicroscopy is the transmission of digital microscopic images (Section 5.7) through a WAN. Under the umbrella of telemedicine applications, telemicroscopy and teleradiology can be combined into one system. Figure 14.11 shows an example of a generic combined telemicroscopy and teleradiology system; its major components and their functions are described as follows:

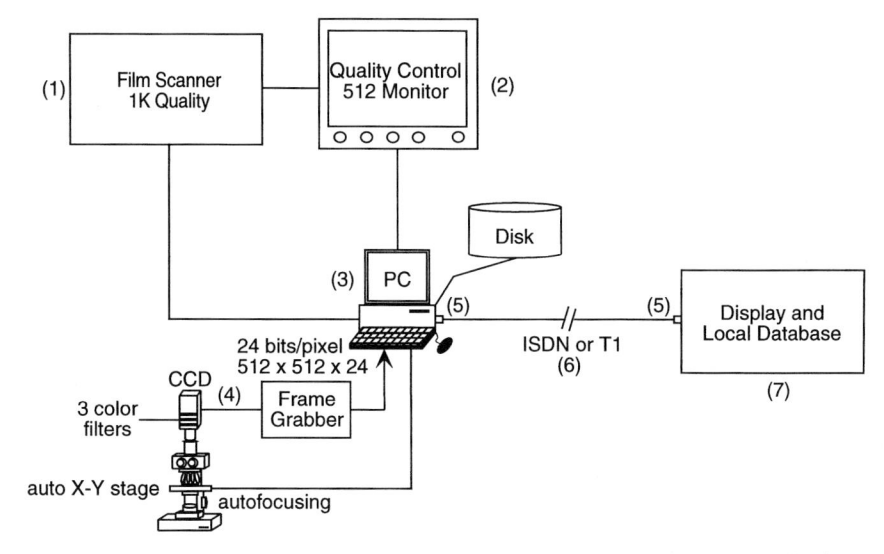

Figure 14.11 A conceptual combined teleradiology and telemicroscopy system for image and textual data transmission (Courtesy of C. Huang).

1. A 1K film scanner for digitization.
2. A 512-line display system for quality control.
3. A personal computer (PC) with four functions:
   (a) For the teleradiology application, software for image acquisition, input patient data, and data communication.
   (b) For the telemicroscopy application, software for automatic focusing, x-y stage motion, color filter switching, and frame grabbing.
   (c) A database for managing images and textual data.
   (d) A standard communication protocol for LAN and WAN.
4. A light microscope with automatic focusing, an x-y stepping motor controlled stage, red, green, and blue color filters, and a CCD camera (see Figure 5.20 (a), (c)).
5. Standard communication hardware for LAN and WAN.
6. Communication carrier (e.g., T1 or ISDN).
7. The display workstation at the expert site should be able to display a 1K × 1K gray level image and 512 color images with standard graphic user interface. It needs a database to manage the local data. The display workstation should be able to control the microscopic stage motion as well as the automatic focusing.

14.5.2 Telemicroscopy Applications

Two major applications of telemicroscopy are in surgical pathology and laboratory medicine. The former deals with samples from surgical specimens at the tissue level, whereas the latter considers samples on the cellular level, from peripheral fluids and biopsy exams. Telemicroscopy requires both static and dynamic images. For this reason, automatic x-y moving stage and focusing are necessary during a teleconsultation process, to permit both the referring physician and the expert to move the microscopic slide during discussion. In Section 5.7 we presented the microscopic image acquisition and display components of a digital microscopic system. The telecommunication component in telemicroscopy uses similar technology in teleradiology except in dynamic images. In this case, because of the rapid transmission requirement in dynamic imaging, it is necessary to rely on high bandwidth WAN and/or image compression. Figure 5.20 showed a telemicroscopy system: in (a) and (c) the left-hand side is the image acquisition component, and the right-hand side is the expert image workstation.

14.6 TRENDS IN TELEMEDICINE AND TELERADIOLOGY

Teleradiology has been used since the 1970s; however, technology was not ready for massive applications until two years ago. This diagnostic modality has become an important topic involving socioeconomic issues because of the role telemedicine will play in health care reform. The trend in telemedicine and teleradiology is to balance the high equipment and utility costs with the advantages in data integrity and image quality, and turnaround time for the service. We see that teleradiology will become a necessity in medical practices of the twenty-first century, and will be an integral component of telemedicine as the future method of health care delivery.

Regarding the use of the Internet or World Wide Web for telemedicine and teleradiology service, it is obvious that the Web could be an excellent tool for telemedicine. However, at the moment, both the Internet and the WWW have problems in teleradiology application: the transmission speed is too slow for imaging; there is no control of data confidentiality; and concerns about security, as well as image authenticity remain to be addressed. Much work is required with respect to these issues before the Internet or the WWW will be suitable for teleradiology applications.

CHAPTER 15
PACS Implementation and System Evaluation

15.1 PLANNING TO INSTALL A PACS

In this chapter we present a methodology of PACS implementation and system evaluation. Our philosophy of PACS design and implementation is that regardless of the scale of a PACS currently being contemplated, the plans should allow for future expansion. Thus, if the intent is to have a large-scale PACS now, the architecture selected should accommodate growth to an even larger scale. On the other hand, if only a PACS module is being planned, its connectivity to future modules or a larger scale PACS is important. Many of the topics introduced in previous chapters, including open architecture, connectivity, standardization, portability, and modularity, should be considered.

15.1.1 Cost Analysis

When is a good time for considering a PACS installation in terms of business investment? Several radiology consulting firms in the nation provide models tailored to the analysis of the operational and cost-benefit situations of individual services. A participating radiology department or health organization inputs its workflow and operating environment, including resources and expenses, and the model predicts the costs of a film-based operation versus digital-based operations. In this section, we present a spreadsheet model developed by the Department of Diagnostic Radiology of the Mayo Clinic and Foundation in Rochester, Minnesota (Langer and Wang, 1996).

The model assumes that the institution being modeled considers only a totally film- or a totally digital-based operation, and that only differential costs including equipment and staff are included. The model tracks events from patient admission to resulting tests, diagnoses, and treatments across departmental boundaries. Through this work flow, staff and equipment requirements are determined, leading to estimates of the total cost of both systems. The model was used to simulate spreadsheets for three hypothetical institutions with 25,000, 50,000, and 105,000 procedures per year. Cost comparisons were drawn between the film-based and the digital-based opera-

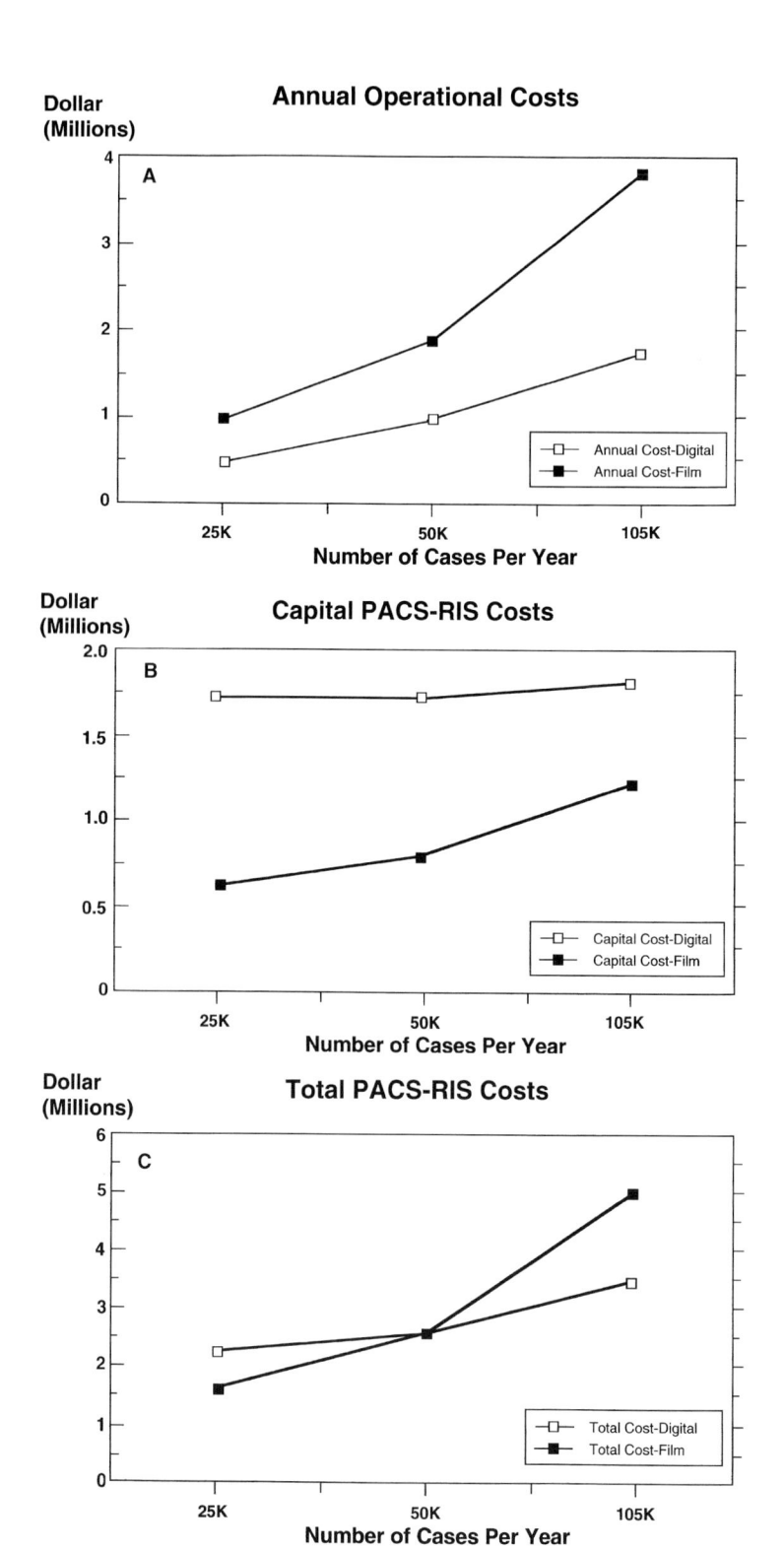

Annual Operational Costs

A

Dollar (Millions) vs Number of Cases Per Year (25K, 50K, 105K)
- Annual Cost-Digital
- Annual Cost-Film

Capital PACS-RIS Costs

B

Dollar (Millions) vs Number of Cases Per Year (25K, 50K, 105K)
- Capital Cost-Digital
- Capital Cost-Film

Total PACS-RIS Costs

C

Dollar (Millions) vs Number of Cases Per Year (25K, 50K, 105K)
- Total Cost-Digital
- Total Cost-Film

tions. Results are shown in Figure 15.1. Figure 15.1A depicts the annual operating expenses, indicating that the film-based operation costs more as the number of procedures increases. On the other hand, Figure 15.1.B demonstrates that capital investment in a digital-based operation is higher when there are fewer procedures, and the gap between the two operations narrows as the number of procedures increases. When the institution performs over 50,000 procedures per year, the total costs for the film-based and the digital-based operations, including capital investment and the annual operating budget (Fig. 15.1C), cross each other in favor of the digital-based operation.

This model allows a first approximation on the cost issue comparing the film-based and digital-based operations. Results from simulation with a mathematical model depend on many assumptions in the model as well as the method of data collection. Care should be exercised in interpreting the results. The spreadsheet file, according to the authors, can be found for both DOS and Macintosh environments, at anonymous FTP sites:

ri-exp.beaumont.edu/pub/diag/Dos/pac-cost.xls
ri-exp,beaumont.edu/pub/diag/Mac/pac-cost.xls

15.1.2 Film-Based Operation

The first step in planning a PACS is to understand the existing film-based operation. In most radiology departments, the film-based operation procedure is run as follows.

Conventional diagnostic images obtained from either X-ray or other energy sources are recorded on films, which are viewed from alternators (light boxes) and archived in the film library. Images obtained from digital acquisition systems (e.g., nuclear medicine, ultrasound, transmission and emission computed tomography, computed radiography, and magnetic resonance imaging) are displayed on the acquisition device's monitor for immediate viewing, then recorded on magnetic tapes or disks for digital archiving. In addition, images are recorded on films for viewing as well as for archival purposes. Since films are convenient to use in a clinical setting, clinicians prefer to view digital images on films even though this method reduces image quality. As a result, most departments still use films as a means for diagnosis and as a storage medium regardless of the image origin. In general, films obtained within 6 months are stored in the departmental film library and older films are stored remote from the hospital. To retrieve older films requires from 0.5 to 2 hours.

Most radiology departments arrange their operations in an organ base, with exceptions in nuclear medicine, ultrasound, and sometimes MRI and CT. Some hospi-

Figure 15.1 Cost comparison between a film- and a digital-based operation derived from a mathematical simulation of three institutions with 25,000, 50,000, and 105,000 procedures per year: (A) annual operating budget, (B) annual capital budget, and (C) capital plus annual operating budget. The crossover is at 50,000 procedures. [From: Langer and Wang, *J. Digital Imaging,* 9:104–112 (1996).]

TABLE 15.1 Record of Number of Procedures, Film Used, and Film Cost

Section (Specialty)	Number of Procedures Year 1, ..., Year N	Film Used (sheets) Year 1, ..., Year N	Film Cost (dollars)* Year 1, ..., Year N
Nuclear medicine			
Ultrasound			
CT/MRI			
Pediatrics			
Genitourinary and gastrointestinal (abdominal)			
Neuroradiology			
Cardiovascular			
Interventional radiology			
General outpatient[†]			
General inpatient[†]			
Mammography			
Emergency radiology			
ICUs[‡]			
Total			

*Film cost is for X-ray film purchase only; film-related costs are not included.
[†]Includes chest and musculoskeletal examinations.
[‡]Includes all portable examinations.

tals group MRI and CT into neurological and body imaging sections. It is advantageous during planning to understand the cost of the film-based operation. The following sample tables are useful for collecting statistics in the planning stage.

Table 15.1, a template for the tabulation of number of procedures, film used, and film cost, will provide an overall view of number of procedures and film usage from each specialty. This information can be used to design the PACS controller routing mechanisms, to determine the number of display workstations required, and to arrive at the local storage capacity needed for each display workstation. The film cost can be used to estimate the film-based operation cost compared with the digital-based or PACS operation cost.

Data recorded in Table 15.1 also can be used to generate estimates of film-based operational costs as suggested by Table 15.2. Direct and indirect film library expenses included under item 1 in Table 15.2 are X-ray film jackets, mailing envelopes, in-

TABLE 15.2 Multiple-Year Estimation of Film and Film-Related Costs

Item	Year 1	...	Year N
1. Film library	$		$
Indirect expenses	$		$
2. Film processor	$		$
Indirect expenses	$		$
3. Personnel:*			
Darkroom	$ (FTE)		$ (FTE)
Film library	$ (FTE)		$ (FTE)
4. Film-related costs			
Total (1 + 2 + 3)	$		$
5. Film cost (from Table 15.1)	$		$
Total costs	$		$

*FTE, Full-time equivalent.

sert envelopes, negative preservers, rental on film storage both inside and outside the department, and fleet services for film delivery; direct (equipment) and indirect (operational) expenses film processor expenses (item 2) include developing solutions, replacement parts, facilities repairs and installations, and other miscellaneous supplies. In a typical film-based operation in a large teaching hospital, 70% of the film-based operation budget is allocated to the film library (item 3). The film cost (item 5) should be derived based on the number of procedures performed and films used per year, as given in Table 15.1. The film operation (not including film viewing) requires a large amount of premium space in the department, which should be translated to overhead cost in the same estimate.

Data from Table 15.2 are necessary in the estimation of the cost of a film-based operation in a radiology department. Using the numbers filled in here and the PACS checklist (Section 15.1.3.2), planners can compare PACS installation and operation costs with those of a film-based operation. Tables 15.1 and 15.2 give the framework for an overview of the film-based operation and its cost. Tables 15.3 and 15.4 provide comparative statistics, as well.

Table 15.3 is an estimated breakdown of the percentage distribution of procedures performed and efforts required in conventional projection X-ray examinations according to body region in a large urban hospital in the northeastern United States. A similar table can be generated for digital sectional images including CT, MR, and US. The effort required is a measure of time and labor required to perform the procedure. Table 15.4 gives estimated annual percentage volumes of procedures from three civilian and three military hospitals. MR head procedures are not entered as an item in either table because there is considerable deviation among hospitals in both number of procedures and number of images generated per procedure. A hospital or a department planning to install a PACS should develop the information needed for such a table to allow comparison with hospitals listed in Tables 15.3 and 15.4, and make judgment accordingly.

TABLE 15.3 Percentage Distribution of Conventional Projection X-Ray Procedures Performed and Effort Required, According to Body Region

Procedure	Percentages* Of Total Departmental Examination	Effort Required
Chest	40	18%
Musculoskeletal	39	25%
Gastrointestinal	9	22%
Genitourinary	1	8%
Neuroradiology	1	9%
Others	7	15%

*For example, the 18% effort required to perform all chest X-ray examinations amounts to 40% of all departmental examinations.

Several commercial two-phase cost analysis models are available to help a hospital to analyze the cost impact of PACS. The first phase is to assess the cost of the present film-based operation. In this phase, the user completes data forms similar to Tables 15.1 and 15.2, and the model will present a detailed costing of the film-based operation. In the second phase, the user evaluates how these costs might differ upon implementation of the PACS. A model like this will allow a hospital to have an overview on the financial impact to the current film-based operation of a PACS implementation.

TABLE 15.4 Estimated Annual Percentage Volume of Procedures: Comparing a Site Planning for PACS with Percentages from Six Other Hospitals

Hospital X, Planning a PACS	Civilian Hospital %(images/procedure)			Military Hospital %(images/procedure)		
	A	B	C	D	E	F
Chest	30 (2)	20 (2)	17 (2)	33 (2)	41 (2)	23 (2)
Extremities	12 (2.5)	10 (2.5)	22 (3)	17 (2.5)	16 (3)	20 (3)
Spine, rib	4 (3)	4 (4)	7 (2)	5 (3)	7 (2)	7 (3)
CT*	4 (12)	8 (20)	7 (12)	5 (/)	4 (/)	6 (/)
Other (MR, US, CT body, etc.)	50	58	47	40	32	44
Total, %	100%	100%	100%	100%	100%	100%
Total Number of Procedures	160,000	98,000	66,000	106,000	79,000	101,000

*Head only.

15.1.3 Digital-Based Operation

15.1.3.1 *Planning a Digital-Based Operation*

Interfacing to Imaging Modalities and Utilization of Display Workstation In a digital-based operation, two components (see Fig. 1.1) are not under the control of the PACS developer/engineer: namely, interfacing to imaging modalities and the use of display workstations. In the former, the PACS installation team must coordinate with imaging modality manufacturers to work out the interface details. When a new piece of equipment is purchased, it is important to negotiate with the manufacturer on the method of interfacing the imaging modality to the PACS controller. It is necessary to include the ACR-NEMA or DICOM standard in the equipment specification for image communication purposes.

With respect to display workstations, however, radiologists and clinicians are the ultimate users to approve the system. Thus, human interface and communication play an important role in planning the installation. In designing the display workstation and its environment, user input is mandatory, and several revisions are necessary to assure user satisfaction.

Cabling We described cabling and the hub room concept in Section 9.2. Now we turn to the overall cable plan. Proper cabling for the transmission of images and patient text information within the department and within the hospital is very crucial for the success of a digital-based operation. The traditional method of cabling for computer terminals is not recommended because as the magnitude of the digital-based operation grows, the web of connecting wires very quickly become unmanageable.

Cabling is much simpler if the entire department is on the same floor. Greater complications ensue when communication cables must traverse the whole hospital, which may occupy many floors or even many building complexes.

The plan of laying out cables to support the digital-based operation should be very carefully thought through. Fiber-optic video broadband communication systems seem to be a good plan, since only two cables (one for backup) will suffice for up to twenty-five 512-line video channels for real-time telemanagement (see Section 9.3.1). When cables become long, signal amplification must be provided at certain strategic points in the network, to sustain the integrity of the signal.

In the case of a digital network, ATM or fast Ethernet with a conventional Ethernet backup is the preferred choice; details were described in Section 9.1.3.

Air Conditioning Most digital equipment in a digital-based operation requires additional air conditioning. If a new radiology department is planned, adequate air conditioning should be supplied to the central computing, server, and image processing facilities. Normally, display workstations do not require special air conditioning, but certain room temperature requirements must be observed.

Because hospitals are always limited in space, it may be difficult to find additional central air conditioning for the large area housing the PACS central facility. Sometimes smaller individual air-conditioning units must be installed. The individual air conditioner can be a stand-alone floor unit or a ceiling-mounted unit.

Each time another air-conditioning unit is installed, additional cool water from the hospital is required. Thus, the hospital's capacity for cooling water should be considered. Also, as noted earlier, additional air-conditioning units create a lot of acoustic noise in the room. To ensure that the room housing the display workstations is suitable for viewing images, adequate soundproofing should be used to insulate these areas from the extra noise created by the air-conditioning and cooling system.

Staffing The hospital or department should allocate special technical staff to support the digital-based operation. In particular, categories in system programming, digital engineering, and quality assurance personnel are necessary to make a digital-based operation run smoothly and efficiently. These new full-time equivalents (FTEs) can be allocated from switching some FTEs in the film-based operation. Even when a manufacturer installs a digital-based operation for a hospital department and provides support and maintenance, the department retains the responsibility for supplying the personnel to oversee the operation. In general, the staff requirements consists of one hardware engineer, one system/software engineer, and a quality assurance technologist, all under the supervision of a PACS manager.

Training The department or hospital should provide four categories of training to the staff.

Continuing Education for the Radiologists/Clinicians. The department should provide adequate training to staff radiologists/clinicians on the concept of a digital-based operation as well as on the use of the display workstations. This training should be periodic, and updates should be offered as new equipment or display workstations are implemented.

Training of Residents. The training for radiology and other specialty residents should be more basic: the four- or three-year residency program should include training in a digital-based operation. A one-month elective in PACS would be advantageous to radiology residents, for example. In this period, one or two residents would rotate through the PACS unit and obtain basic training in computer hardware architecture, software overview, architecture of the image processor, communication protocols, and the concept of the display workstations.

The residents also can learn all the basic image processing functions that are useful for image manipulation, as described in Section 12.3. The training schedule should be in the first or second year of residency, to allow the physicians to understand the concept and the complete procedure involved in a digital-based operation early in their training. This will facilitate future digital-based operation for the department and the health center. In addition, a quick refresher course every year in July, when new staff starts in radiology and other specialties, will minimize the downtime of the display workstations.

Training of Technologists. Some retraining of the technologists in the department must precede the changeover to a digital-based operation. Digitization of images using the laser scanner on X-ray films, and the use of computed radiographic systems with imaging plates, are quite different from the screen/film procedure familiar to technologists. Also, the use of image workstations, computer terminals for patient information in RIS, and image transmission from acquisition devices to PACS gateway computers introduces new concepts that require additional training. The department should provide regular training classes, emphasizing hands-on experience with existing equipment.

Training of Clerical Staff. Experience in training secretarial staff to use word processors rather than a typewriters has proven that the switch to digital operations at the clerical level is not difficult. The training should emphasize efficiency and accuracy. Ultimately, the move to a digital-based operation will reduce the number of FTEs in the department.

15.1.3.2 Checklist for Implementation of a PACS

This section provides a checklist for implementation of a hospital-integrated PACS. The implementation and operational costs can be estimated by multiplying the component price with the number of units and adding the subtotals. The component prices can be obtained from various vendors.

I.	Acquisition gateway computers			
	(one computer for every two acquisition devices)	No. ___		
	Local disk			
	ATM or fast Ethernet connection			
	Interface connections			
II.	PACS controller			
	Database machine	No. ___		
	File server	No. ___		
	Permanent storage	No ___		
	ATM or fast Ethernet connection	No. ___		
III.	Communication networks cabling (contracting)			
	ATM or fast Ethernet switches	No. ___		
	Ethernet hub	No. ___		
	Router	No. ___		
	Bridge	No. ___		
	Video monitoring system	No. ___		
IV.	Display workstations			
	Four-monitor 2K station	No. ___		
	Two-monitor 2K station	No. ___		
	Four-monitor 1K station	No. ___		
	Two-monitor 1K station	No. ___		
	One-monitor 1K station	No. ___		
V.	Interface to other databases			
	HIS	Yes ___	No ___	
	RIS	Yes ___	No ___	
	Other database(s)	Yes ___	No ___	

VI. Software development
   The software development cost is normally about 1–2 times the hardware cost.
VII. Equipment maintenance
   10% of hardware + software cost
VIII. Consumables
   Optical disks, tapes/year   No. ___
IX. Supporting personnel
   FTEs (full-time equivalents)   No. ___

15.2 LARGE-SCALE PACS

PACS has different definitions depending on the user's perspective. It can be as simple as a film digitizer connected to a display workstation with a local database for ICU application, or it can be as complex as a hospital-integrated PACS. As we discussed in Section 1.4.4, commonly accepted criteria for a large-scale PACS are daily clinical use, connection to three or more modalities, with workstations inside and outside of the radiology department, and support to a hospital with over 20,000 examinations per year.

Based on this definition, 13 large-scale PACS systems were identified in 1993, and this list increased to over 20 in 1995. In the early 1998, the number surpassed 40. It is clear that one PACS developmental trend is toward large-scale systems. Generally speaking, when a new hospital or a new radiology department is being planned, the large-scale PACS is included. Whether the plan is eventually carried to the implementation stage very much depends on financial issues rather than on operational or technical conditions. Almost all large-scale PACS plans entail hospital-integrated PACS that interface with other hospital information systems. Implementation of a hospital-integrated PACS is expensive and requires a total commitment from the health center administration. Most earlier plans use the two-team approach; more recent plans favor the partnership arrangement described in Section 1.4.2. Large-scale PACS is a necessary stimulus for the health care community to adopt a digital-based operation.

15.3 PACS MODULES

15.3.1 ICU Module

In the ICU module, the important factor is timeliness in providing radiologic services under critical conditions. Numerous favorable reports on ICUs with teleradiology demonstrate that PACS improves the efficiency as well as the clinical services in these units. There are two possible system designs. The first method is to have only the display component in the ICU; the digital imaging system, including the transmission component, is located in the radiology department. Examinations performed in the unit are brought to the radiology department for processing, either in the film cassettes or with CR imaging plates. In the former case, a film digitizer is used to convert the image on the film to a digital image. A radiologist can perform the wet reading, whereupon the digital image along with the digital voice dictation are transmitted to the ICU referring clinician for immediate service. In the second design, the

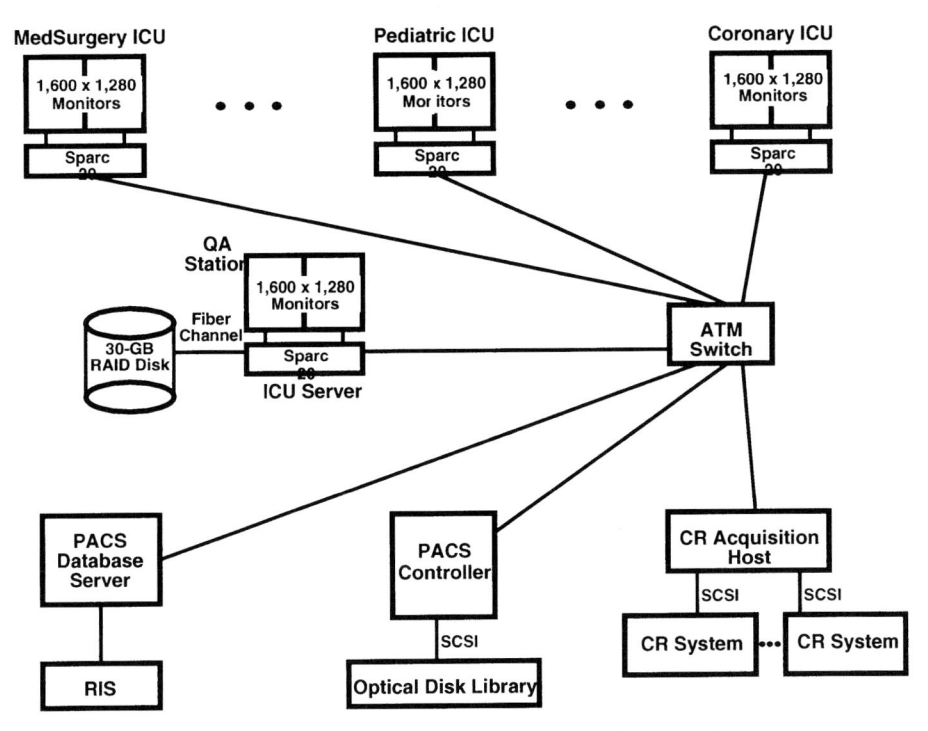

Figure 15.2 Architectural design of an ICU PACS module: only the display component is in the ICU; digital imaging systems, including the transmission component, are located in the radiology department. QA: quality assurance.

imaging system, the transmission component, and the display component are all in the ICU. A high resolution display system is also placed in the radiology department. In this arrangement, the digital image from the radiologic examination is generated at the ICU. Images are also transmitted to the radiology department to be wet-read. Digital voice dictation is transmitted from the radiology department to the ICU and is appended to the image.

Both architectures have advantages and disadvantages. In the first design, the technologist is still required to bring the exposed film cassette or CR plate to the radiology department for processing, which normally takes 30 minutes. In the second design, the hospital must place a CR in the ICU as well as a high resolution display system in the radiology department. Obviously these two additional components increase the cost of a system. Figure 15.2 shows the architectural design of an ICU PACS module serving three ICUs at UCSF.

15.3.2 Emergency Department Module

The emergency room or department module is used to solve the urgent need for images and their interpretation by ER physicians under extremely stressful conditions,

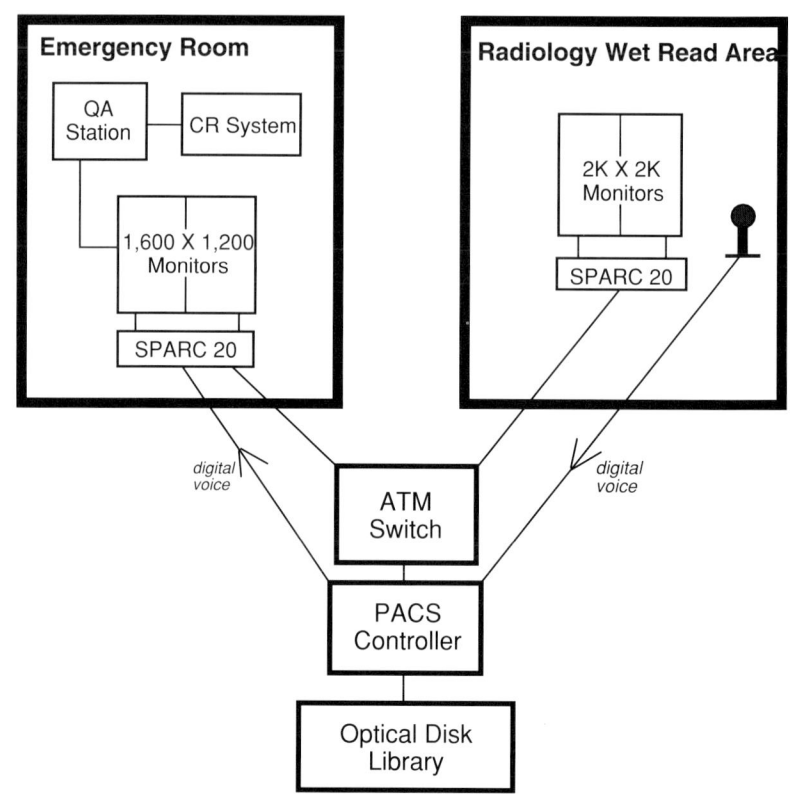

Figure 15.3 Architectural design of an emergency room PACS module: the imaging device, the transmission component, and the display components are all in the ER. A high resolution workstation is also placed in a radiology reading area for wet reading.

where timely arrival of image-related information means life or death to a critical injured patient. For this reason, it is advantageous to have the imaging equipment and display system in the ER. The second design of the ICU module described in Section 15.3.1 fits into this application: that is, the imaging system (CR), the transmission component, and the display component are all in the ER. In addition, a high resolution display system is also placed in the radiology department to facilitate immediate interpretation. During operation, CR images of critical injured patients are taken and processed at the ER. These images are transmitted immediately to both the ER and the radiology department reading area. Voice dictation is transmitted instantaneously to the ER by the radiologist in duty, and this recording is appended to the images by the ER PACS module, ready for the ER physician to use. A well-organized ER PACS operating system can deliver both images and interpretation to the ER reading area less than 5 minutes after the radiographic examination. Figure 15.3 depicts the architectural design of an ER PACS module.

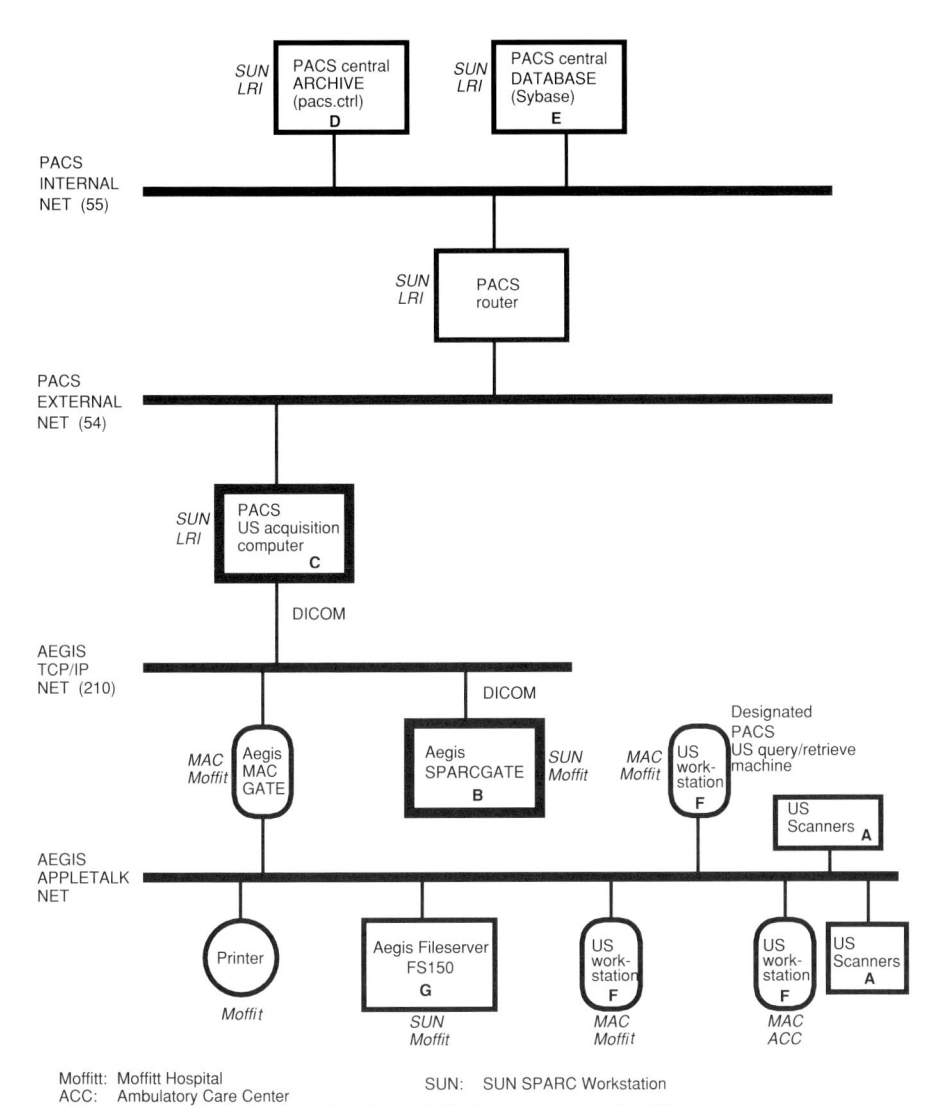

Figure 15.4 An ultrasound PACS module and its connection to the PACS infrastructure. The module (lower right) is connected by the Aegis Appletalk Net. The integration of the module to the PACS is through the Aegis MAC GATE in the module and the US acquisition computer in the PACS infrastructure.

15.3.3 Ultrasound Module

The ultrasound section in a typical radiology department has two distinct characteristics: its operation is very independent, and it uses color and 8 bits/pixel gray scale images for interpretation. The first characteristic makes it easier to go totally digital because a change in operation mode will not impact the entire department operation.

For this reason, the US section is among the first few specialties to change over to digital operation. The second characteristic, however, hinders the US module to be integrated into the PACS infrastructure.

In Chapter 12, we discussed workstation design and functionality, noting that the majority of workstations used in PACS have gray scale displays with 12bits/pixel. For this reason, the workstations used in PACS are not suitable for displaying US images. By the same token, workstations designed for the US scanner cannot be used readily to display other radiologic images without some modifications. The obstacle is in the 24 bits/pixel color and 8 bits/pixel gray scale in US versus the 12 bits/pixel in other modality images. Also, the use of color monitors for US and high resolution gray scale monitors for other services restricts the intermixing of image displays. Thus the display is a major consideration during the system integration of the US module to the PACS infrastructure.

In Section 8.6 we discussed a method to interface a PACS module to the infrastructure. In Figure 8.12 we used the ultrasound (US) module as an example and described the general methodology. In this example, the key component in the US module is the DICOM US PACS gateway, and the corresponding component in the PACS infrastructure is the PACS acquisition gateway. Figure 15.4 illustrates the integration of a US module to the PACS infrastructure. In this case, the US module is located in two buildings, Moffitt Hospital and the Ambulatory Care Center (ACC), UCSF. The module is shown in the lower right connected by the Aegis Appletalk net. The Aegis MAC GATE serves as the connection to the PACS infrastructure through the PACS US acquisition computer (C). This US module with a DICOM gateway is one of the first few US modules in 1994 that could be connected to the outside world. In Section 16.1.2 we present our clinical experience on this system integration.

15.3.4 Nuclear Medicine Module

The nuclear medicine (NM) specialty shares the two characteristics with US. Its operation is very independent, and it uses color for display. The only difference is that its number of bits/pixel is more than 8. Therefore image display should be considered carefully during integration. In addition, NM requires extensive image processing on the acquired images. Its workstation is under the category of analysis workstation, discussed in Section 12.1.4.3.

15.4 INTEGRATION OF PACS MODULES

15.4.1 Background

When a large-scale PACS is implemented, one must consider its longevity, that is, its upgradability to newer technologies when they become available. For example, the large-scale PACS developed for the MDIS project (Section 1.4.1) is very reliable and has operated reasonably well in many institutions. But the system was designed over 10 years ago. Since then PACS-related technologies have advanced tremendously.

The question is, How do we upgrade such a system with current technologies seamlessly, without crippling daily operation? In another example, several institutions developed their own PACS in-house, and those systems have operated for many years. As these systems continue to evolve and become more complex, many institutions are at a disadvantage as a result of the limited manpower and manufacturing skill available to accommodate continuous in-house PACS development. The trend is to seek partnership with manufacturers to sustain the PACS operation and promote its growth.

By the same token, even though a PACS module may be small in scale when installed, it is important to design it from the beginning in a way that allows for efficient integration into future modules.

These three issues—how to upgrade an aging established (or legacy) PACS, how to shift from an in-house PACS to a partnership with manufacturers, and how to ensure a PACS module's connectivity—are important considerations for the PACS system integrator. We consider these questions in Sections 15.4.2 and 15.4.3.

15.4.2 Integration of Existing PACS

15.4.2.1 Upgrading an Aging Established PACS

Assume that an established PACS was designed as a closed system, and has been in operation for several years. As the system continues to acquire data, it may very soon reach the storage capacity and number of workstations limit of the original design. How do we expand its capacity without interrupting its continuous daily clinical operation? One obvious solution, namely, to abandon the original system and transfer its data to a new open architecture, is not feasible because of the logistics of the clinical environment.

Another approach, based on the concept of an incrementally distributive architecture, offers a slow transitional solution to a very difficult problem. In this concept, the functions as well as the data of the aging PACS are gradually relinquished to a new open architecture PACS. First, the workload of the original system is reconfigured. The reconfiguration can be according to body region, patient type, or other criterion depending on the institution's needs. The result of this reconfiguration is a new PACS architecture with multiple clusters, each serving a specific application.

Consider Figure 15.5: in the aging PACS, a new PACS gateway is designed connected to the original central archive. The primary function of the PACS gateway is simply routing. The original PACS continues its archiving function and serves the existing workstations. Based on the new reconfiguration, patient folders belonging to the same category are gradually transferred through the gateway and deposited to the proper cluster. The aging PACS maintains the original patient directory, and a duplicate directory is forwarded to the new PACS. Both directories are continuously updated as new examinations are acquired. The new PACS can start to serve its designated functions, including image viewing at new workstations, whenever the system manager declares that the system is ready. Thus, the demands on the aging PACS gradually diminish, and its functions and data are transferred to the new PACS in-

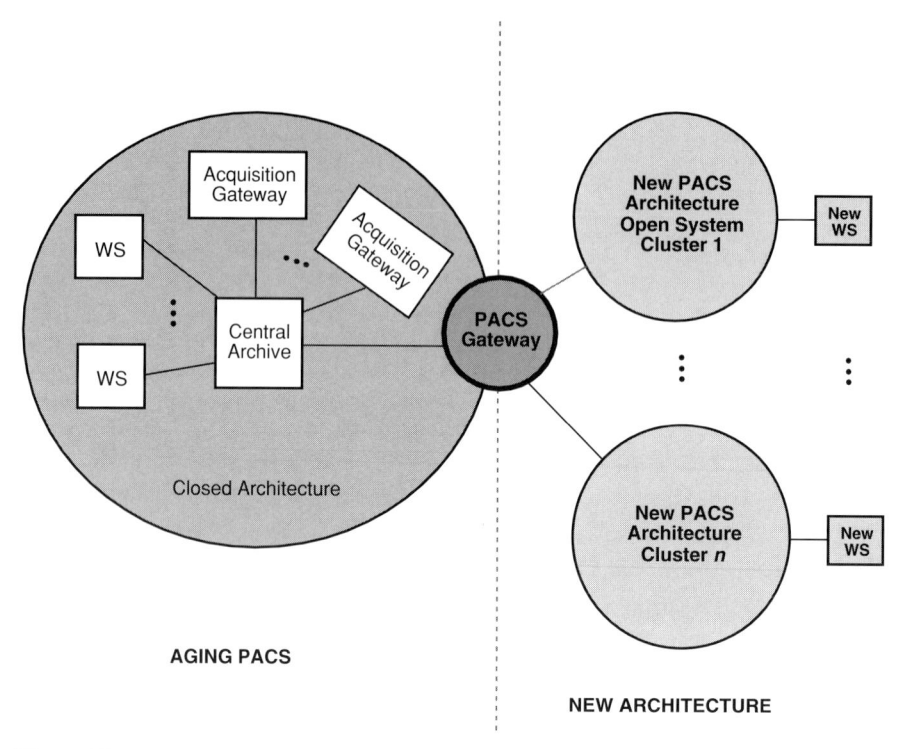

Figure 15.5 Upgrading an aging closed architecture PACS to a new open architecture through a DICOM gateway.

crementally. The aging system can continue its function as an acquisition gateway, or cease its existence when the new PACS is ready to take over the entire operation.

15.4.2.2 Partnership with Manufacturer to Upgrade an In-House PACS

The difference between upgrading an aging PACS and upgrading an in-house PACS is that the latter is not aging because some of its components may use even better technologies than the manufacturer's PACS. The challenge is find a way of combining the two PAC systems by retaining the better components from the in-house PACS while taking advantage of the manufacturer's in-depth resources of service and support. There are many approaches to this problem; we present one method here.

Consider Figure 15.6, in which the state-of-the-art, in-house PACS (left) is in daily operation, and a much larger scale PACS (right) supplied by the manufacturer is being designed. The goal is to continue utilizing the in-house PACS for daily operation until the manufacturer's PACS is ready to be fully functional. Meanwhile the new design takes full advantage of the open architecture of the in-house PACS during the transitional phase. Let us use an example to illustrate the steps involved. Consider the ICU operation, in which CRs are used to acquire images and workstations (WS) are used for display.

INTEGRATION OF PACS MODULES   405

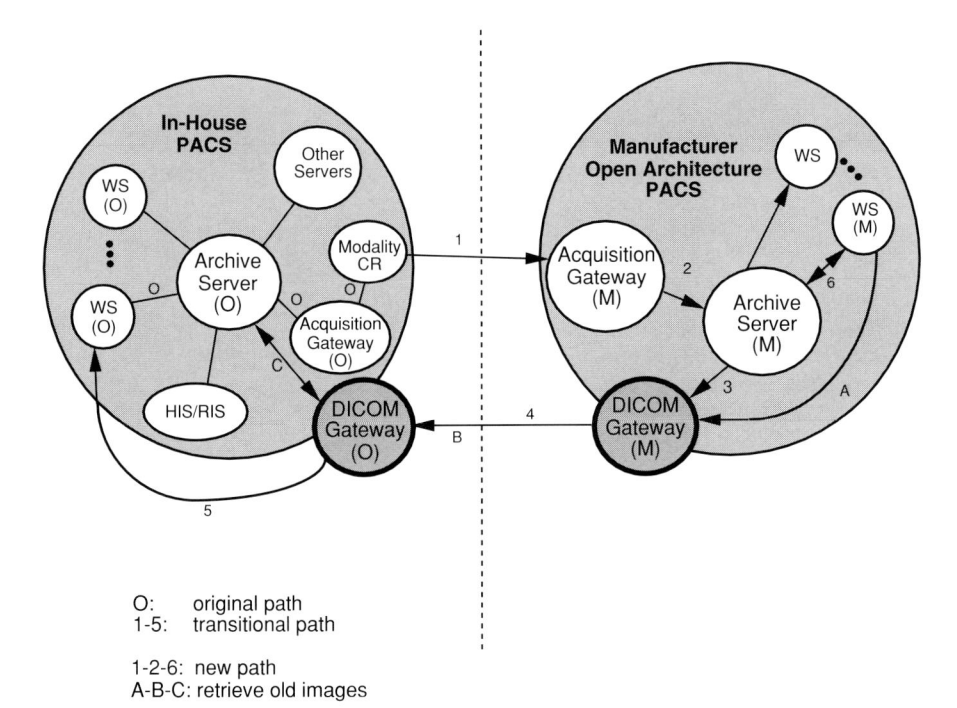

Figure 15.6 Upgrading an in-house PACS through partnership with the manufacturer. Two DICOM gateways, one in the in-house system and the second in the new PACS are used for the integration. Numerals and letters indicate paths of upgrade.

Original steps (O): CR - acquisition gateway (O) - archive server (O) - WS(O). During the transitional phase:

Step I. (1–5 and 6) CR sends a second copy of images to the new acquisition gateway (M)—archive server (M)—DICOM gateway (M)—DICOM gateway (O)—WS (O). Images are also sent to WS (M) from archive server (M) through "6." When this path is completed, and the ICU directory is identical in both archive servers (this can be achieved in about 2 weeks, since the average stay of ICU patients is less than a week), the original path (O) will be disconnected. All CR images are routed to the archive server (M) only, and WS (M) replaces WS (O).

Step II. To retrieve historical images from the original archive server (O) from the new WS (M): (A-B-C); WS (M)—DICOM gateway (M)—DICOM gateway (O)—Archive server (O).

The disadvantage of this method is that the older images of the same patient stored in the original archive server (O) would appear in a separate file. A better way is: WS (M)—archive server (M)—DICOM gateway (M)—DICOM gateway (O)—archive server (O). The latter will require the archive server (M) to integrate the older images to the same patient folder, once it has been retrieved, before sending them to the

WS (M). The integration of old and new images in the archive server (M) is not a trivial task.

Other imaging modalities and workstations can be phased in gradually using a similar approach, although the task may be more complex because of the number of images involved compared with CR. The original archive server (O) can remain as a distributive storage device in the integrated system.

15.4.3 Integration of PACS Modules

Before a PACS module is installed, it is wise to design the long-term PACS architecture of the institution, even though it may be years before a larger scale PACS will be implemented. A DICOM gateway should be included in the module for connectivity during the future expansion. It is sensible to plan an expandable archive system for the PACS module to anticipate other PACS modules in later years. When the future PACS module arrives, either the old or the new module can be treated as an imaging modality, and the integration can be done using techniques similar to those described in Section 8.6.

15.5 MANUFACTURER'S IMPLEMENTATION STRATEGY

15.5.1 System Architecture

A number of PACS manufacturers can install PACS of various scales. For larger manufacturers, the strategy is to install a full PACS for the institution either at one time or incrementally. Smaller vendors tend to want to carve a niche in a market (e.g., teleradiology), which the larger manufacturers do not yet consider financially rewarding. Regardless of the approach, with the advances and the lower costs of the PC computers, high speed networks, and RAID, and the practically free Internet technology, the manufacturer's system architecture design becomes generic, allowing a full or incremental implementation. Figure 15.7 depicts an expandable generic open system architecture.

15.5.2 Implementation Strategy

A generic manufacturer's PACS business unit consists of R&D, service, training, design, implementation, consulting, marketing, and sale components. The marketing and sales components handle the presale phase, with contributions from design and consulting. Information is fed back to R&D for product development. The postsale phase is the responsibility of design and implementation personnel. The operation after implementation is the responsibility of the service and training staffs. It is interesting to see the difference in a manufacturer's point of view according to whether a PACS or an imaging device is being sold (Table 15.5). In PACS, the implementation is 60% versus only 20% in the imaging device. Table 15.6 shows the optimal perception of a manufacturer with respect to manpower allocation in a PACS negotiation and implementation.

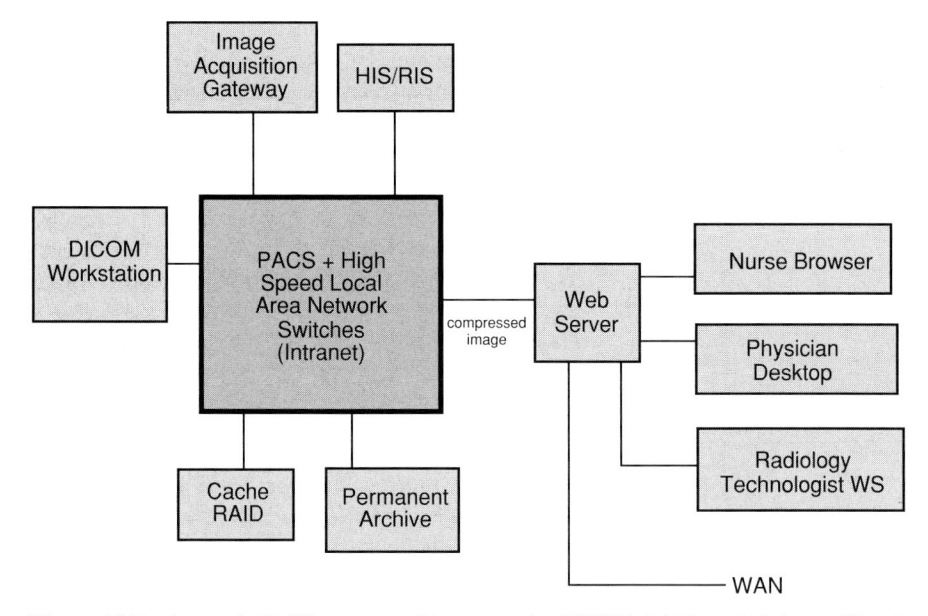

Figure 15.7 A generic PACS system architecture using NT/PC, RAID, and high speed local area network switches.

15.6 TEMPLATE FOR PACS RFP

There are several templates for PACS RFPs (request for proposals) in the public domain. One is entitled A PACS RFP Toolkit (*http://www.xray.hmc.psu.edu/dicom/rfp/RFP.html*) by John Perry, who was with Siemens' Gammasonic Unit and developed the MDIS system. Two others were developed by the military, one for the original Medical Diagnostic Imaging Support project, and the second was the recently released DIN/PACS II. Information on DIN/PACS can be found on the website www.tatrc.org. Another RFP was developed by D.G. Spigos of the American Society of Emergency Radiology's Committee on New Techniques and Teleradiology. These RFPs contain much useful information for those who plan to start the PACS acquisition process.

TABLE 15.5 Comparing Manufacturer's Efforts in Imaging Devices and PACS Sales

	Imaging Device (% Effort)	PACS (% Effort)
Market	40	20
Sale	40	20
Implementation	20	60

TABLE 15.6 Manufacturer's Estimation* on Allocation of Manpower† Required for PACS Implementation

	Presale	Design: 4–6 weeks	Implementation: 6 weeks	Application: 4 weeks	Postimplementation
Institution		2 RT 1 manager	1 manager	2 RT	1 manager, 2 RT + institution staff
Manufacturer	1	2	2	2	1

*The estimation is based on the institution installing the first PACS module with an expandable permanent archive.
†Manpower: person assigned to the task, but not necessarily full time; RT, radiology technologist.

15.7 PACS SYSTEM EVALUATION

In this section, we discuss several methods of PACS system evaluation. The first method is to evaluate subsystem throughputs, which does not involve comparing film-based and digital-based operations. The second is a method of directly comparing the performance of a film-based and digital-based operations. The third method is a standard ROC (receiver operating characteristic) analysis, comparing image quality of hard copy versus soft copy displays. Sections 15.7.1 to 15.7.3 give examples of each method.

15.7.1 Subsystem Throughput Analysis

The overall throughput rate of the PACS is the sum of throughput rates of individual PACS subsystems, including the acquisition, archive, display, and communication network. Figure 15.8 is a diagram of PACS subsystems and image residence times. Table 15.7 defines acquisition, archival, retrieval, distribution, display, and network residence times.

The throughput of a PACS subsystem can be measured in terms of the average residence time of individual images in that subsystem. The residence time of an image in a PACS subsystem is defined as the total time required to process the image in order to accomplish a particular task within that subsystem. The overall throughput of a PACS can then be measured by the total residence time of an image in the various subsystems.

Each of the PACS subsystems may perform several tasks, and each task may be accomplished by several processes. An archive subsystem, for example, performs three major tasks: image archiving, image retrieval, and image routing. To perform the image retrieval task, a server process accepts retrieve requests from the display workstation, a retrieve process retrieves an image file from the permanent archive, and a routing process sends the image file to the destination display workstation. These three processes communicate with each other through a queuing mechanism and run cooperatively to accomplish the same task. The retrieval residence time of an

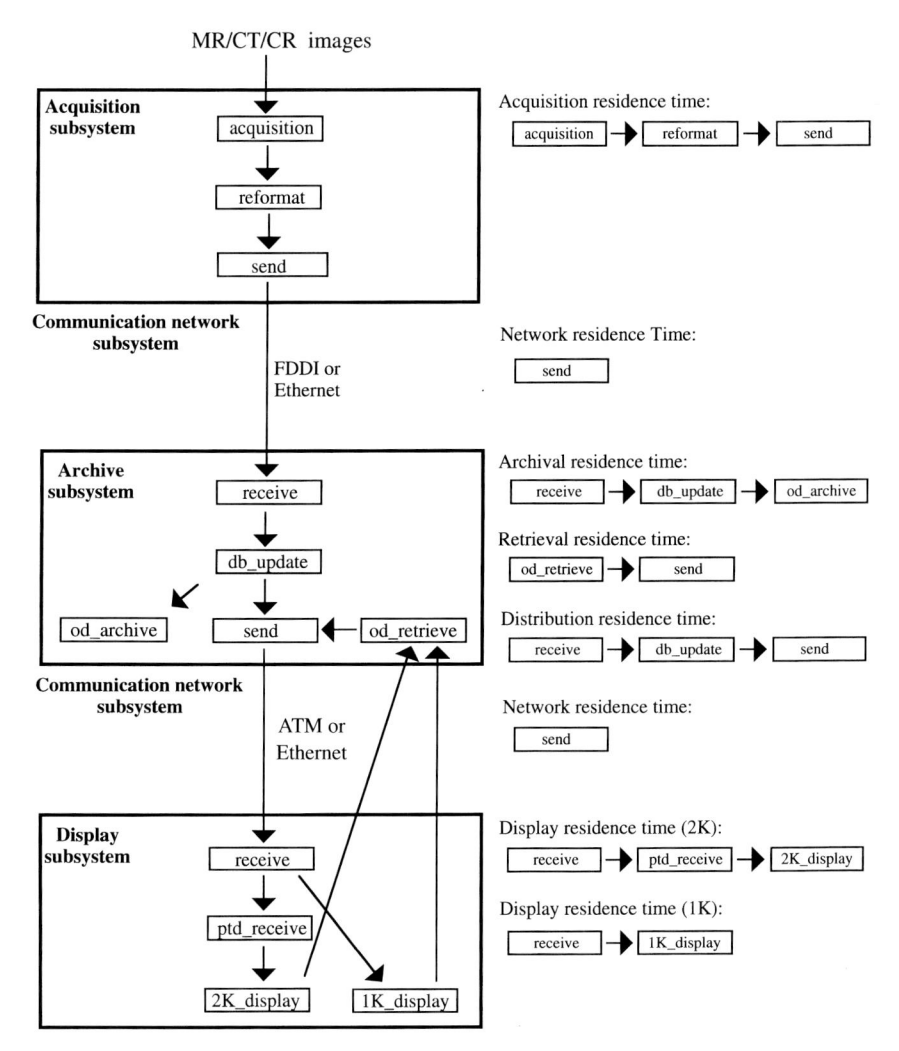

Figure 15.8 PACS subsystems and image residence times: db, database, od, optical disk library, ptd, patient data.

image file in the archive subsystem can be measured by the elapsed time from the moment an archive server receives the retrieve request and retrieves the image file from the permanent archive, to the point at which the server sends the image file to the destination display workstation.

Once these residence times have been broken down into computer processes, a time stamp program can be implemented within each process to automatically log the start and the completion of each process. The sum of all processes defined in each task is the measured residence time.

TABLE 15.7 Definitions: Acquisition, Archival, Retrieval, Distribution, Display, and Network Residence Times

Image Residence Time	Subsystem Where Measurement Performed	Definition
Acquisition	Acquisition	Total time of receiving an image file from a radiologic imaging device, reformatting images, and sending the image file to the PACS controller
Archival	Archive	Total time of receiving an image file from an acquisition computer, updating the PACS database, and archiving the image to the permanent storage
Retrieval	Archive	Total time of retrieving an image file from an optical disk and sending the image file to a display workstation
Distribution	Archive	Total time of receiving an image file from an acquisition computer, updating the PACS database, and sending the image file to a display workstation
Display (2K)	Display	Total time of receiving an image file from the PACS controller, transferring the image file to the disk or RAID, and displaying it on a 2K monitor
Display (1K)	Display	Total time of receiving an image file from a PACS controller and displaying it on a 1K monitor
Network	Network	Total traveling time of an image from one PACS component to another via a network.

15.7.1.1 Residence Time

Image Acquisition Residence Time An acquisition subsystem performs three major tasks: it acquires image data and patient demographic information from radiologic imaging devices, converts image data and patient demographic information to the DICOM format, and sends reformatted image files to the PACS controller. Images from various modalities are acquired via different data interface methods, as described in Sections 8.2, 8.4, and 8.6. The current technology adopted by major manufacturers limits the transfer speed of image data from a radiologic imaging device to its acquisition computer. This constitutes the major factor preventing the achievement of better overall throughput for a PACS.

Archive Residence Time Images in the PACS controllers are archived to permanent storage. However, the archival residence time of an image was found to be significantly affected by the job prioritizing mechanism utilized in the PACS controller. Because of its low priority compared with the retrieve and distribute processes running on the archive subsystem, an archive process always is compromised—that is, it must wait—if there is a retrieve or distribute job executing or pending.

Image Retrieval Residence Time   Images are retrieved from the permanent storage to the PACS controllers. Among the three major processes carried on by the PACS controller, retrieve requests always have the highest priority. Thus images intended for study comparison are always retrieved and sent to the requested display workstation immediately, before archive and distribute processes are initiated.

Distribution Residence Time   All arriving images in the PACS controller are distributed immediately to their destination display workstations before being archived in the permanent storage. These images are sent to the 2K workstations via a high speed network (e.g., the ATM).

Display Residence Time   A display workstation configured with a local disk storage or RAID may need to first receive images from the PACS controller's RAID, and this delays the image display time on the monitor.

Communication Subsystem: Network Residence Time   The residence time of an image in the multiple communication networks can be measured as an overlapped residence time of the image in the acquisition, archive, and display subsystems (see preceding subsections). The ATM or other high speed communication network throughput is limited by the magnetic disk input/output rate.

PACS Overall Throughput: Total Image Residence Time   The overall throughput of the PACS can be determined by the total residence time of an image from its original source (a radiologic imaging device) to its ultimate destination (a display workstation or the permanent archive).

15.7.1.2 *Prioritizing*

The use of job prioritizing control allows urgent requests to be processed immediately. For example, a request from a display workstation to retrieve an image from the permanent archive has priority over any other processes running on the archive subsystem and is processed immediately. On completion of the retrieval, the image is queued for transmission with a priority higher than that assigned to the rest of the images that have just arrived from the acquisition nodes and are waiting for transmission. During the retrieval, the archive process must be compromised until the retrieval is complete. Suppose, for example, that the retrieval of a 20 Mbyte image file from the permanent archive takes 54 seconds; if an attempt is made to retrieve this image file while another large image file is being transmitted to the same archive, increasing the retrieval time for the first image to 96 seconds, the time delay of the retrieval without job prioritizing is 42 seconds.

The bottleneck in PACS performance is the low speed data interface implemented by the major manufacturers in their radiologic imaging and archive devices. For example, current system design of MR and CT scanners has made it difficult for PACS developers to provide prompt clinical service.

15.7.2 System Efficiency Analysis

We can use image delivery performance, system availability, and user acceptance as means of measuring system efficiency.

15.7.2.1 Image Delivery Performance

One method of evaluating PACS system efficiency is to compare image delivery performance from the film management system and from the PACS. For example, consider the neuroradiology PACS component—in particular, the CT and MR images. We can decompose both the film-based and the digital-based operations into four comparable stages. In the case of the film management system, the four stages are as follows:

1. At each CT and MR scanner, technologists create films by windowing images, printing images, and developing films.
2. Film librarians deliver the developed films to the neuroradiology administration office.
3. Neuroradiology clerks retrieve the patient's historical films and combine them with the current examination films.
4. Radiology residents or film library personnel pick up the prepared films and deliver them to a readout area (or neuroradiology reading room).

Similarly, the four stages in the PACS are as follows:

1. The period during which the acquisition gateway computer receives images from the scanner and formats images into the DICOM standard image file.
2. The elapsed time of transferring image files from the acquisition computer to the PACS controller.
3. The processing time for managing and retrieving image files at the PACS server.
4. The time needed to distribute image files from the server to the display workstation.

The time spent in each film management stage can be recorded and estimated by technologists, film clerks, and personnel who have many years of professional experience. Circumstances that should be excluded from the calculation because their performance variances are too large to be valid include retrieving a patient's historical films from a remote film library and the lag time between pickup and delivery of films in the various stages in the film management system described previously. These exclusions apparently make the film-based operation more competitive with that of a PACS module.

The performance of the PACS can be automatically recorded in database files and

TABLE 15.8 Analysis of Image File Delivery Performance of a Neuroradiology PACS Module

Type of File*	Individual Times (min)				Total Time (min)
	Stage 1	Stage 2	Stage 3	Stage 4	
CT file					
Current	40.0	0.50	0.15	1.15	41.80
Previous	0	0	1.25	1.15	2.40
MR file					
Current	7.00	0.15	0.17	0.47	7.79
Previous	0	0	0.57	0.47	1.04

*Current, image file newly acquired from the scanner; previous, image file previously acquired and archived in a permanent storage.

log files by software modules. The data included in these files are date, time, and duration of each modularized process, and size of image file acquired.

The total elapsed time from creation of an image file at a scanner to availability of that file at a display workstation is defined as the image delivery performance of a PACS (which is similar to the residence time defined in Section 15.7.1.1). For example, Table 15.8 shows the results of average image delivery performance for one currently acquired image file from the scanner and one archived image file from the permanent archive in a neuroradiology PACS module. CT and MR image files are quite different in size: on average, the former is approximately five times larger than the latter. Because image file size is one of the fundamental factors affecting the delivery performance, CT and MR image files should be recorded separately.

Table 15.9 compares the image delivery performance of a film management system and a neuroradiology PACS module. Since a consistent comparison baseline is difficult to achieve for both systems, the performance (time to complete tasks in each stage) should be redefined. For example, the images may be based on a patient's film jacket in the film-based management system and on the patient's two examinations in the PACS system. On average, approximately two image files (studies) are created for each CT examination and five image files are generated in an MR examination. The two CT image files are either contrast and noncontrast studies, or one is a scout view image. The five MR files are various pulse sequence studies. Therefore, in a comparison study of a digital-based system, it is reasonable to use two newly acquired and two older CT image files and five newly acquired and five older MR image files. In this particular example, the average image delivery performance of the PACS (88.5 min for CT and 44.2 min for MR) is better than the average performance of the film-based management system (93 min). However, a patient's film jacket can contain many image examinations. If more than two examinations are used to calculate the image delivery performance with the PACS, the comparison study may show

TABLE 15.9 Comparison of Image Delivery Performance Between the Film-Based Operation and the PACS in a Neuroradiology Section

System	Situation	Individual Times (min)				Total Time
		Stage 1	Stage 2	Stage 3	Stage 4	
Film-based	Optimal*	25.0	1.0	2.0	0	28.0
	Regular	50.0	25.0	15.0	3.0	93.0
PACS	CT†	80.0	1.0	2.9	4.6	88.5
	MR‡	35.0	0.75	3.75	4.7	44.2

*The patient, who has no previous radiographs, is scanned with a few images, and the images are reviewed at a film reading room near the scanner and the film administration office.
†Two newly acquired and two previous CT image files are used to calculate the total.
‡Five newly acquired and five previous MR image files are used to calculate the total.

different results. It must be noted that although all historical examinations of a patient are important, the latest previous examination is essential in a clinical comparison study. Most neuroradiologists use the current image examination and the latest previous examination to make the diagnosis, referring to older examinations only if necessary.

In the PACS system, the performance of delivering one MR examination (five image files) is twice as fast as that of delivering one CT examination (two image files). The major difference is at stage 1: capturing and formatting images takes 80 minutes for a CT examination but only 35 minutes for an MR examination. In fact, the performance bottleneck, as we discussed earlier, is not the twin processes of capturing and formatting in the PACS; rather, it is the system design of the CT scanner that causes a lengthy delay. The scanner has no means of indicating to the communication protocol that the last image of a given study in the CT image acquisition process has been sent. Lacking this information, the image capturing program must wait until the first image of the next study has been received before it can close the last image file. Until the system design of the CT scanner is modified, therefore, any improvements in delivering CT examinations will be limited in scope.

15.7.2.2 System Availability

PACS system availability can be examined in terms of the probability that each component will be functional during the period of evaluation. In the neuroradiology example, the components considered to affect the availability of the neuroradiology PACS include (1) the image acquisition subsystem, including all CT and MR scanners and interface devices between the scanners and the acquisition computers, (2) the PACS controller and the optical disk library, (3) the display subsystem, with its display workstation computer and display monitors, and (4) the communication network.

Calculations of the probability that each component will be functional can be based on the 24-hour daily operating time. The probability P that the total system will be functional is the product of each component's uptime probability in the subsystem, defined as follows:

$$P = \prod_{i=1}^{n} P_i \qquad (15.1)$$

where P_i is the uptime probability of each component and n is the total number of components in the subsystem.

15.7.2.3 User Acceptance

The acceptability of the display workstation can be evaluated by surveying users' responses and analyzing data from a subjective image quality questionnaire. Table 15.10 shows a sample item in a user acceptance survey, and Table 15.11 is a typical subjective image quality survey.

15.7.3 Image Quality Evaluation

A major criterion in determining user acceptance of a PACS is image quality in soft copy displays, compared with the quality available from hard copy. In the preceding section, we briefly noted a subjective image quality survey method. In this section, we discuss a more rigorous analysis based on the receiver operating characteristic (ROC) (see Section 6.5.5). Although it is tedious, time-consuming, and expensive to perform, ROC has been accepted in the radiology community as the de facto method for objective image quality evaluation. The ROC analysis consists of the following steps: image collection, observer testing, truth determination, and statistical evaluation. Consider a sample comparison of observer performance in detecting various pediatric chest abnormalities—say, pneumothorax, linear atelectasis, air bronchogram, and interstitial disease—on soft copy (a 2K monitor) versus digital laser-printed film from computed radiography in pediatric radiology. Sections 15.7.3.1 to 15.7.3.5 provide the basic steps of carrying out an ROC analysis.

15.7.3.1 Image Collection

All routine clinical pediatric CR images are sent to the primary 2K workstation and the film printer for initial screening by an independent coordinator, who selects images of acceptable diagnostic quality, subtle findings, disease categories, and matched normal images. To ensure an unbiased test, half the selected images should be determined from the soft copy and half from the hard copy. A reasonably large-scale study should consist of about 350 images to achieve a good statistical power.

The selected images should be screened one more time by a truth committee of at least two experts who have access to all information related to a specific patient, including clinical history and images, obtained by means of other radiologic techniques. During this second screening, some images will be eliminated for various reasons (e.g., poor image technique, signal too obvious, overlying monitoring or vascular

TABLE 15.10 Display Workstation User Survey Form

Attribute	Poor (1)	Fair (2)	Good (3)	Excellent (4)	Average Score
Image quality					
Speed of image display					
Convenience of image layout					
Performance of manipulation functions					
Sufficiency of patient information					
Sufficiency of image parameters					
Ease of use					
Overall impression					

Overall average

lines clouding the image, overabundance of a particular disease type). The remaining images are then entered into the ROC analysis database in both hard copy and soft copy forms.

15.7.3.2 Truth Determination

Truth determination is always the most difficult step in any ROC study. The truth committee usually determines the truth of an image by using the clinical history of each patient, the hard copy digital film image, the soft copy image, all image processing tools available, and biopsy results if they are available.

15.7.3.3 Observer Testing and Viewing Environment

The display workstation should be set up in an environment similar to a viewing room, with ambient room light dimmed and no extraneous disruption. Film images should be viewed in a standard clinical viewing environment.

TABLE 15.11 Subjective Image Quality Survey Form for Comparing the Film/Light Box Setup Versus the Display Workstation

Display System	Ranking Scales (perception of confidence)*					
	1	2	3	4	5	6
Film and lightbox						
Display workstation						

*1, least; 6, most.

```
┌─────────────────────────────────────────────────────────────────┐
│  Case Number_____          Board Number_____        │
│  Patient Name_____     Procedure Date_____Time_____ │
│  Patient I.D._____   Reading Date_____Size_____ │
├─────────────────────────────────────────────────────────────────┤
│                                                                 │
│   Instructions: If abnormality is present, please indicate      │
│                 your level of confidence.                       │
│   Confidence Scale:                                             │
│         0 . . . . 1 . . . . 2 . . . . 3 . . . . 4               │
│      Sure Not Present      50% sure         100% sure           │
│         (default)        It is Present    It is Present         │
│                                                                 │
└─────────────────────────────────────────────────────────────────┘
```

Radiographic Condition	Enter Confidence Ratings					
	Absent	Diffuse	R.U.	R.L.	L.U.	L.L.
1. Pneumothorax						
2. Interstitial Disease						
3. Linear Atelectasis						
4. Air Bronchograms						

Comments:

Figure 15.9 Structured receiver operating characteristic form used in a typical ROC study of chest images. For each disease category, a level of confidence response is required. Chest quadrants assessed were right upper (R.U.), right lower (R.L.), left upper (L.U.), and left lower (L.L.).

Observers are selected for their expertise in interpreting pediatric chest X-rays. Each observer is given a set of sample training images from which to be trained on four steps: (1) learning how to interpret an image with soft copy display, (2) completing an ROC form (see, e.g., Fig. 15.9), (3) viewing the corresponding hard copy film from a light box, and (4) filling out a second ROC form on the hard copy film from a light box.

TABLE 15.12 Order of Interpreting Image Sets Used in the ROC Study

Observer Number	Order of Interpreting Technique Subsets*	
	Round 1	Round 2
1	A1, B1, C2, D2	A2, B2, C1, D1
2	A2, B2, C1, D1	A1, B1, C2, D2
3	C1, D1, A2, B2	C2, D2, A1, B1
4	C2, D2, A1, B1	C1, D1, A2, B2
5	C1, D1, A2, B2	C2, D2, A1, B1

*A, B, C, and D are the four image sets, with equal numbers of images. The numbers 1 and 2 refer to the technique (soft or hard copy). For example, observer 1 views image sets A1, B1, C2, D2 during round 1 and later (>3 months), in round 2, reviews image sets A2, B2, C1, and D1.

15.7.3.4 Observer Viewing Sequences

An experimental design is needed to cancel effects due to the order in which images are interpreted. The image sample from the ROC database can be randomized and divided into four subsets (A, B, C, and D), containing approximately equal numbers of images. Identical subsets are present for both the hard copy and the soft copy viewing. Each observer participates in two rounds of interpretation. A round consists of several sessions (depending on the total number of images). To minimize fatigue, each observer interprets about 30 images during a session. During the first round, the observers interpret all images, half from hard copy and half from soft copy. During the second round, which should be 3 to 5 months later to minimize the learning effect, the observers again interpret all images, but for each image they use the viewing technique not used in round 1. The viewing sequence is shown in Table 15.12.

15.7.3.5 Statistical Analysis

The two ROC forms filled out for each image modality by each observer are entered in the database. Results are used to perform the statistical analysis. A standard ROC analysis program—for example, CORROC2, developed by Charles Metz of the University of Chicago—can be used to calculate the area under the ROC curve (see Fig. 6.22), along with its standard deviation for a given observer's results for the hard copy and soft copy viewing methods. The ROC area can be compared by the disease category with the paired t test. The results will provide a statistical comparison of the effectiveness of using soft copy and hard copy on these sets of images in diagnosing the four disease categories. This statistical analysis forms the basis of an objective evaluation of image quality of the hard copy and soft copy displays derived from this image set.

CHAPTER 16

PACS Clinical Experience, Pitfalls, and Bottlenecks

16.1 CLINICAL EXPERIENCE WITH PACS MODULES

In Sections 16.1 and 16.2, we describe some clinical experience based on the PACS at the University of California, San Francisco (UCSF), which was developed in-house and has been operating since 1994. In January 1997 the in-house PACS was expanded in partnership with a manufacturer to promote continued growth and operation. The clinical experience presented here is as of November 1996.

UCSF is a health sciences campus in the San Francisco Bay area. Its two medical centers, the UCSF Medical Center and the Mount Zion Medical Center (MZH) are 2 km apart. Table 16.1 shows some statistics for the two campuses. In addition, the main campus, UCSF, affiliates with the San Francisco Veterans Administration Medical Center (SFVAMC) and the San Francisco General Hospital. The HI-PACS (hospital-integrated PACS) at UCSF was designed to connect all four medical centers. The infrastructure provides intrahospital as well as interhospital digital image communication and management. For interhospital communication between UCSF and MZH, a two-tier communication network is used with the 155 Mbit/s ATM as the primary network and a T1 line as the secondary. Figure 16.1 shows the UCSF PACS infrastructure as of January 1997. Section 16.1 covers three areas of applications: ICU workstation utilization, physician desktop image and report access, and connection of a US PACS module to the infrastructure. Section 16.2 is devoted to neuroradiology workstations for teleradiology applications.

16.1.1 ICU PACS MODULE

16.1.1.1 ICU Server

Not shown in Figure 16.1 is an ICU server connected to the PACS central node. The ICU server presented in Figure 15.2 serves three units: pediatric (16 beds), medical/surgical (16 beds), and cardiac care (14 beds). Three workstations, one at each ICU, were installed sequentially in a period of one month in 1995. The ICU server, containing a 30 Gbyte RAID, can be easily expanded as needed. Instead of configuring a large global database, which could bring all three ICU applications to a halt if the global database were to become inoperative, the ICU server maintains a separate

TABLE 16.1 The University of California at San Francisco Medical Center Statistics: Annual*

Parnassus Campus	Mount Zion Campus
560 beds with 76% occupancy	230 beds with 61% occupancy
22,200 admissions	6,800 admissions
7.1-day average length of stay	7.9-day average length of stay
289,000 patient visits	29,500 patient visits
23,000 emergency room visits	17,500 emergency room visits

*From 1993 survey.

database for each ICU workstation. In other words, images are stored centrally, and yet, in a distributed database environment.

Local directories containing all the current patients of the respective ICUs are maintained. A user can request images of a patient by first selecting the patient ID from the patient directory. On receiving the request, the ICU server routes the patient's images and demographic data back to the ICU workstation through an ATM network. Images are transferred in their original sizes to the workstation's memory cache, but are interpolated to 1600×1200 for the two display monitors. While one monitor maintains the most current image, the other monitor can be used to review the set of remaining images.

To manipulate images, many user-friendly, easy-to-use functions are available.

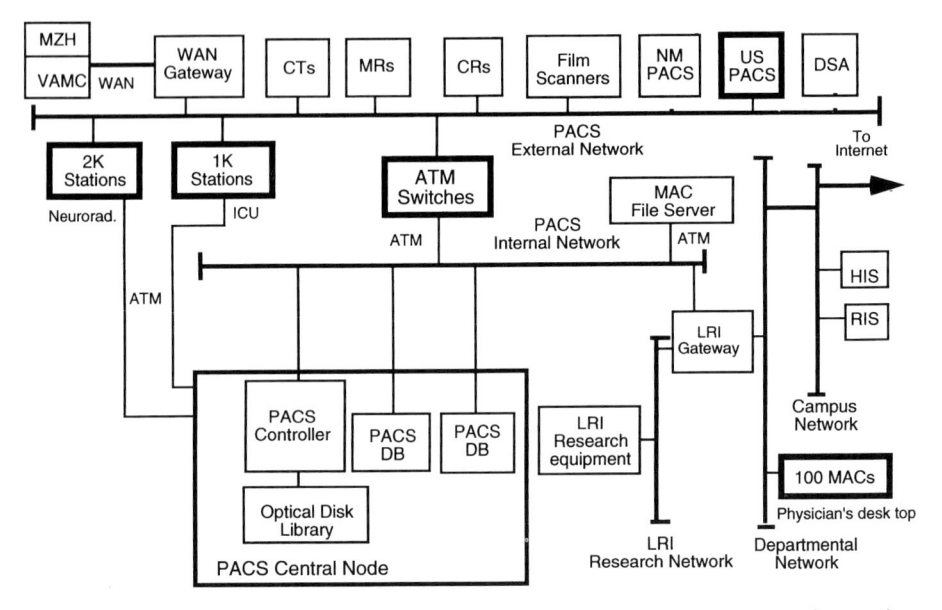

Figure 16.1 UCSF PACS network architecture as of January 1997: bold rectangles are the components used to describe our clinical experience.

Some of the most frequently used features include window and level, zoom, rotation, and image layouts. Through a popup window, a patient's demographic data and study information can be obtained. Real-time access to historical images and diagnostic reports also is available. The image retrieval icon allows a user to retrieve from the PACS archive images that are not in the ICU server. The report icon allows instantaneous access to the PACS database, which stores all the diagnostic reports obtained from the RIS. When a report request is initiated, a report window will open, and a user can browse through the directory of all available reports. Because of direct access, historical images and diagnostic reports can be forwarded from the PACS to an ICU workstation without severely affecting the performance of the ICU server.

The image acquisition process is through an FCR-9000 and an FCR AC-II CR system. The technologist enters a two-letter code designating a particular ICU when the CR reads the imaging plate. During the acquisition process, the CR image is first converted to DICOM 3.0 format. It then validates the patient ID, runs a special utility to remove any white background (Section 4.1.6), and sends the image to the PACS. On receiving the CR image, the PACS archives it into permanent storage, updates the mirrored PACS databases, and routes a copy of the image to the ICU server. An acknowledgment is also sent back to the acquisition gateway computer so that the local image in the host computer can be purged.

16.1.1.2 Clinical Experience

The ICU workstation performance has been excellent with minimum interruption from hardware, software, or ATM network failure. Physicians, on the average, are able to request and review the first image within 1.5 to 2.0 seconds. A typical 24-hour CR image acquisition and viewing activity distribution in an ICU workstation is shown in Figure 16.2. The workstation was accessed at almost every hour of the day, with two peaks at early morning and midafternoon. Clinical experience with these three ICU workstations yielded the following conclusions in the areas of robustness and physicians' reactions.

1. *Robustness.* There was no downtime in these three workstations from February to July 1997. This is probably due to robustness in hardware components and software design. In terms of hardware, all components are off the shelf and therefore, maintenance and service requirements are minimal. The software was developed jointly by ISG Technologies, Inc. (Toronto, Canada) and the Laboratory for Radiological Informatics at UCSF. It went through three revisions with input from clinicians before the workstations were installed. The software is user friendly and easy to use.

2. *Physicians' reaction.* The physicians at the ICUs accepted the system the first day it was installed. It has become an integral part of their daily clinical operation. The viewing time of a patient's image is usually less than one minute. The three workstations differ with respect to location in the ICUs. In the medical/surgical unit (MICU), the workstation is side by side with other patient monitoring systems at the nurses' station. The workstation in the cardiac ICU is located in the conference area with a large window, and because of the ambient light, the image quality on the mon-

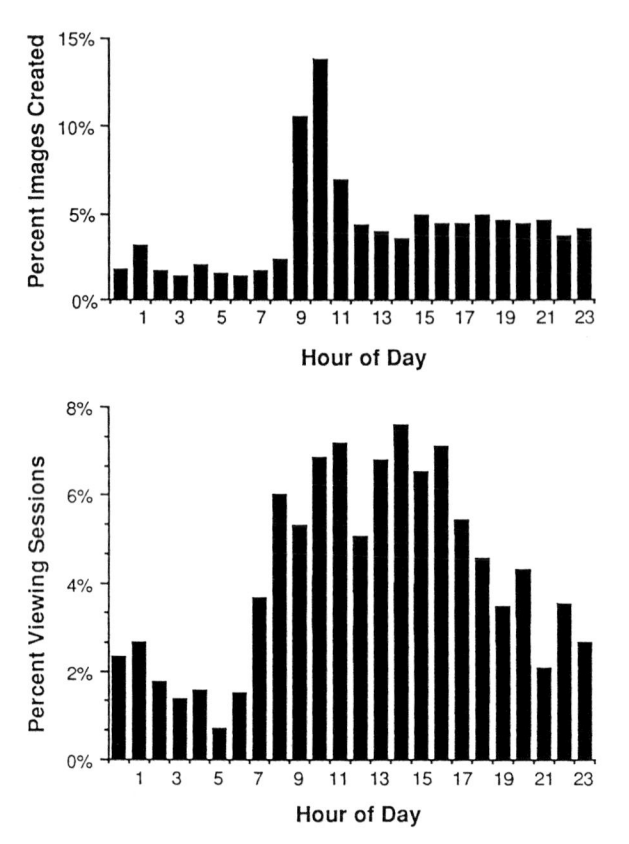

Figure 16.2 Typical image acquisition and viewing activity distribution of an ICU workstation over a 24-hour period. (Courtesy of Dr. P. Cho.)

itors is suboptimal. In the pediatric ICU, the workstation is at the entrance of the unit. As for the workstation usage, although reports from RIS are usually available within 6 to 12 hours, they are seldom requested. The clinicians say they can interpret easy cases themselves; for difficult cases, they would have consulted with the radiologist already. In either situation, a report delayed 6 hours adds little value if any.

Two requests from the users at these ICUs are worth mention. In the pediatric ICU, since the workstation is at the entrance of the unit, the users requested a very short screensaver duration that causes images to disappear from the screen if no action is taken for one minute. The rationale behind this request was that the physicians did not want relatives or visitors of ICU patients to see the images when they walk into the unit, whereas in the MICU and cardiac ICU, no such precaution was necessary. Originally, each workstation had a patient image retrieval icon, and any images from the PACS archive could be retrieved through a request. A couple of months after the workstations were installed, MICU requested that the retrieval button be removed, since house staff rotating through other ICUs that lacked workstations had learned to retrieve their patients' images from the MICU workstation. The MICU physicians felt that such requests interfered with their daily clinical work progress and also accumulated patients in the local database directory who did not belong to MICU.

16.1.2 Ultrasound PACS Module

In 1994 UCSF acquired an ultrasound PACS (Aegis) from Acuson (Mountain View, CA). This PACS module links seven Acuson ultrasound scanners (Figure 15.4A) in two buildings. This ultrasound PACS module features a network server with 1.5 Gbyte disk storage used for short-term archiving, with images stored in a compressed format (DICOM compatible). Refer again to Figure 15.4, which shows the connectivity between the ultrasound module and the UCSF PACS infrastructure through Ethernet protocol. The connectivity is provided by the ultrasound module Aegis SPARC GATE (B) and the PACS ultrasound Sun SPARC acquisition gateway (C) in the infrastructure through a DICOM interface.

16.1.2.1 Data Flow

Because this ultrasound PACS module is the first such system developed by the manufacturer, which lacked PACS experience, the data flow from the module to the PACS infrastructure was cumbersome, requiring four routes. The first route transmits DICOM-formatted compressed ultrasound images from the SPARC GATE (Fig. 15.4B) to the ultrasound acquisition gateway (Fig. 15.4C) and to the PACS central archive (Fig. 15.4D) for long-term storage. In the PACS database (Fig. 15.4E), either a new patient folder is opened or the images are appended to an existing folder with historical ultrasound or other type images. The second route allows the retrieval of ultrasound images from the long-term archive through a request from any ultrasound workstation (Fig. 15.4F). The third route is the same as the second route except that, in addition, other modality images belonging to the same patient can be retrieved from this patient's image folder. The fourth route allows other workstations in the PACS to retrieve ultrasound images along with other modality images. Both routes 1 and 2 were completed, but the data transmission rate was very slow—in the neighborhood of 180 Kbyte/s. Great difficulties were encountered during the implementation of routes 3 and 4, and they were never completed.

16.1.2.2 Clinical Experience

The ultrasound section now is filmless in that it acquires and stores images digitally, and radiologists and clinicians read from soft copy. The ultrasound section prints several selected images from each study on films and inserts them in the patient's record. Currently, the ultrasound section keeps its own erasable optical disks.

The design of this ultrasound PACS module was very crude. During each transfer, the image file had to go through at least the ultrasound internal networks (Appletalk and Aegis TCP/IP net) four times before it went to the PACS infrastructure's acquisition computer. The handshaking between computers (especially Apple computers) during the transfer became tedious and created some network bottleneck problems.

The original plan was to complete routes 1 and 2 in-house in 3 months; the job ended up taking over a year, during which time complications were introduced because both the manufacturer and the laboratory had personnel changes. Fortunately, both parties were committed to the project, and eventually routes 1 and 2 were completed. The manufacturer was very cooperative during this venture.

During the implementation of routes 3 and 4, two difficulties were encountered. First, in the third route, after a US workstation successfully received a patient image folder from the PACS long-term archive, it did not have the capability of displaying modalities other than US images, even though these non-US images were in DICOM format. The US workstation was a Macintosh-based Quadra computer (Apple Computer, Cupertino, CA), and an attempt to obtain such a display would cause the workstation to crash. This was a fundamental problem that could only be resolved by the manufacturer. Second, in route 4, when an existing PACS workstation retrieved a patient folder that had ultrasound images, the workstation could not display the compressed ultrasound color images because it lacked both a decoder to decompress the images and a color monitor. The decoder part of the problem could be resolved easily, since the compression algorithm used was in the public domain. To add the color capability for displaying Doppler ultrasound images, however, required extensive hardware and software modifications in existing gray scale monitors. An easy, but not desirable solution was to just display colors in gray scales. The lesson we learned from this integration of a PACS module with an existing infrastructure is that the manufacturer of the module must be knowledgeable about PACS; otherwise, the module will end up being a closed component in the PACS environment.

16.1.3 Physician Desktop Access to PACS Images

16.1.3.1 *System Usage*

In Section 13.2.1 we introduced the concept of a distributed image file server to access PACS images from a physician's desktop workstation. Since July 1994, over 100 Macintosh computers have been connected to the server, but only 10–15 are active. Most clinicians use the workstation to access selected CT or MR images from cases of interest to them (Fig. 13.4). Several radiology specialty sections trained their administrative assistants to retrieve cases for research projects or teaching material. The availability of full-resolution images at the desktop is a quantum leap from the traditional method of getting images from tapes or disks in the CT or MR scanner rooms.

16.1.3.2 *System Performance and Reliability*

The connection of the Macintosh computer to the server is through conventional Ethernet. The response time to retrieve demographic and historical text data from the PACS database through the Macintosh, using the patient ID as the search key, ranges from less than 2 seconds to 5 seconds (Fig. 13.4A). However, when the patient name is used as the search key, the response time can vary between 4 and 15 seconds, since this is a nonindexed search.

Response to thumbnail sketch requests also varies and depends on the size of the study (Fig. 13.4B). In general, a successful retrieval takes between 5 and 45 seconds. The performance is significantly better in the evening than during the peak hours of the day because there is less contention for network access.

Once a thumbnail sketch has been received, the response time to requests for full-resolution images is very fast, because the server retains a copy of the original full-size images after the thumbnail set has been sent to the desktop (Fig. 13.4C). Requesting full-resolution images can bypass the PACS central archive and the database, resulting in a very impressive response time. The average time to receive a single CT slice is less than 2 seconds; multiple-slice requests may take slightly longer. However, performance can be degraded tremendously during peak traffic hours because of the large file size of such images.

System availability is considered satisfactory. It operates 24 hours/day, 7 days/week. The server has been running without interruption since its release, except during periodic preventive maintenance. The system requires little operator intervention and maintenance other than a system administration routine to maintain users' log-in accounts and the Internet addresses of the client machines.

16.1.3.3 Users' Feedback

Users, in general, are happy that the PACS allows them access to both images and text at the desktop with minimal effort. However, several criticisms should be considered before the next revision is undertaken.

In the infrastructure design, accessing PACS information from a physician's desktop has low priority compared with accessing from clinical workstations. For this reason, the PACS allocates the server a maximum of 3 minutes for each request. After 3 minutes, if the retrieval is not completed, the server aborts the request automatically and does not requeue it. Since the communication from the Macintosh to the server is through Ethernet, the retrieval of a large image file like a CT body examination may not be completed within the 3-minute limit during peak hours. Users are usually frustrated under this circumstance. Although we tried to extend the 3-minute limit, this measure did not help much because of the characteristics of Ethernet protocol. Once network transmission has slowed down, retrying normally creates more network collisions. A fundamental change in design, for example, would be to put the request in a dormant state whenever the system senses a slowdown in transmission, notify the user, and retry during off-hours. This scheme can also be used in the Web server described in Section 13.3.2.

Because of the limited storage capacity in the server (Sun SPARC 10 with 8 Gbytes of disk storage), the retrieval program allows a maximum of 32 most recent sequences (or studies) per patient. In the case of CT retrieval, this does not pose a problem, since a patient would seldom have more than 32 studies. However, in the case of MR, a patient can have many studies and each study can have many sequences, with the result that the person's older MR studies cannot be retrieved. This situation is specially acute in a longitudinal research protocol, when researchers need to go back several months to retrieve data from the same patient. Future designs can have larger capacity disks, but as the PACS database grows with time and has to support more users throughout the health center, similar situations will arise again. It is a classical cost versus capacity trade-off problem.

Note that the retrieval problem at the level of the physician's desktop is different from the PACS central archival requirement problem. The PACS archival requirement is predictable in the sense that the number of images archived can be estimated once the health center/radiology department operation environment is known. In desktop retrieval, user demand is variable because it depends on the number of users, the research topics, each user's preference, and retrieval characteristics.

16.2 NEURORADIOLOGY

16.2.1 Neuroradiogy Image Acquisition

Five MR and five CT scanners (CT: 3 GE Spiral, Milwaukee, WI; 1 GE 9800 Quick; 1 Imatron, South San Francisco, CA; MR: 4 GE Signa 5x, 1 Siemens Vision, Erlangen, Germany), located in different buildings of UCSF and MZH for neuroradiology and other types of examination, are connected to the PACS infrastructure. Images acquired from the scanners are converted to either ACR-NEMA 2.0 or DICOM 3.0 format at the acquisition gateway computers. In addition, data from the hospital information system (HIS) and the radiology information system (RIS) are available in the PACS network. The PACS controller organizes images from CT and MR neuro examination with related data from HIS and RIS and creates a new patient folder or inserts the images into an existing folder. The folder is transmitted to designated workstations for review. On average, the folder is available at the workstations within half an hour of completion of the examination.

Beginning in May 1995, two 2K-line, two monitor workstations were placed in the inpatient and outpatient neuroradiology reading areas at two separate buildings in UCSF. The 2K workstation is based on a Sun SPARC server 470 computer, two 2500-line monitors (UHR-4820P MegaScan display system, AVP, Littleton, MA) for images, and a text monitor for patient and study directories . Each workstation has a local 5.2 Gbyte RAID, which can display a page (twenty 512-line CT or MR) of images in 1.5 seconds (Storage Concepts, Irvine, CA). All software programs, developed in-house, were written in C programming language for the UNIX operating system and X-Windows user interface. Current inpatient and outpatient folders are available in the local RAID. The workstations have identical image databases, each with a capacity of storing over a week's worth of current neuro CT/MR examinations, and some with historical images. The workstation is also equipped with easy-to-use, real-time simple image processing functions such as cine mode, tile mode, window/level, preset lookup table, zoom/scroll, and region of interest measurement (see Fig. 12.4). Neuroradiologists can use either workstation (i.e., in the inpatient or the outpatient reading area) or both at the same time to review or discuss cases. The neuroradiology section currently still uses a dual display system with both films and soft copy. Neuroradiologists are free to use either display mode or both for their daily clinical practice.

16.2.2 Neuroradiology Examinations

Figure 16.3 shows a 19-month summary from September 1994 to March 1996 of total neuro CT/MR procedures performed in both UCSF and MZH as well as the soft copy reading statistics. At the workstation, the user first scans the patient directory monitor, which shows all current examinations by patient name and ID in the local RAID. The user scrolls through the directory and finds the desired patient by clicking the mouse to activate the Patient Select function. If the patient has more than two image sets, clicking Image Select1 and Image Select2 will display the two proper sets on monitors 1 and 2, respectively. The next step is to scroll to the selected patient and click the mouse constituting one Patient Select request (Fig. 16.3). After a patient has been selected, if some older images required for comparison are not in the local disk, clicking the Lib Search (library research, Fig. 16.4) button allows the user to search for older images from the global database in the permanent storage.

After the patient has been selected, the images will be displayed on the 2K monitor in about 1–1.5 seconds if they are in the local disk; if they are in the permanent storage, there will be a wait of about 45 seconds. For example, in August 1995 (Fig. 16.3), about 59% of all neuro examinations were read with the soft copy method, permitting the assumption that each patient was only read once, from the workstation. Also, in August, coincidentally, about 59% of the time, the user wanted to see whether a selected patient had previous examinations. Having such data allows the derivation of a workstation utilization index to measure the utility of workstations, as described in Section 16.2.4.3.

One unique feature in the neuroradiology PACS application is that all CT/MR images from MZH are transmitted directly to UCSF through the ATM network. For these images, although a neuroradiology fellow may be at MZH interpreting them with films, all readings are verified at UCSF through the two 2K workstations.

16.2.3 Users' Reading Habits

The neuroradiology section at UCSF manages and supervises all neuroradiology cases at UCSF and MZH. We describe the similarity and differences of the inpatient and outpatient neuro workstation utilization. Figure 16.5 shows the inpatient and outpatient workstation (WS) usage by hour in August 1995. The inpatient workstation was used almost hourly, with a bimodal distribution showing two peaks at 8–10 A.M. and 4–5 P.M. The outpatient workstation usage was different. It was used from 8 A.M. to 6 P.M. with two peaks at 10 A.M. and 12 P.M. Figure 16.6 shows the duration of workstation use after a patient selection. Both workstations exhibit similar trends, with duration from 0 to 4 minutes. More than 20 minutes' duration means there were no other activities at the workstation during the next 20 minutes after the last usage. For inpatient and outpatient workstation usage by function, refer back to Table 12.4. As described in Section 12.3.5, the most common functions used were Patient Select, Library Search, Image Select, Cine Mode, Window Level, and Find Patient. Image Select is used when an examination has more than one study (sequence). The surprise from Table 12.4 is that even though reports were available at the workstation through

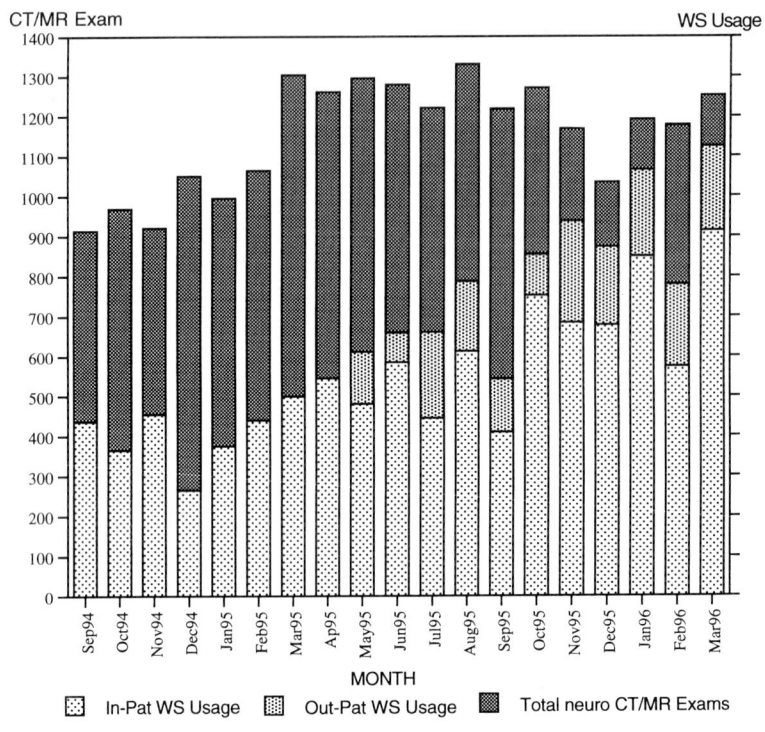

428 PACS CLINICAL EXPERIENCE, PITFALLS, AND BOTTLENECKS

Figure 16.3 Total neuro CT/MR examinations and inpatient and outpatient workstation (WS) utilization. The WS utilization index given in Figure. 16.7 is derived by (inpatient WS + outpatient WS) / (total neuro CT/MR exams).

an RIS interface with instant retrieval, the (REPORT__SELECT) usage was almost negligible. The last function, WS__MAIN__STARTUP, means that during the month, the inpatient workstation crashed for various reasons and rebooted itself eight times. Similar trends in workstation usage were found during other months.

16.2.4 Neuroradiology PACS Workstation System Utilization

In Sections 16.2.1 to 16.2.3 we discussed some clinical experience with neuroradiology workstations, and Section 15.7 presented methods of PACS system evaluation. Now we develop a workstation utilization index as a measure of the workstation utility. The two neuroradiology workstations are used as examples. Although workstation viewing can have various impacts on the operation in a radiology department, the objectives of studying the neuroradiology workstation utilization are to focus on two questions:

1. Do the two workstations placed in the neuroradiology inpatient and outpatient reading areas facilitate interhospital reading?

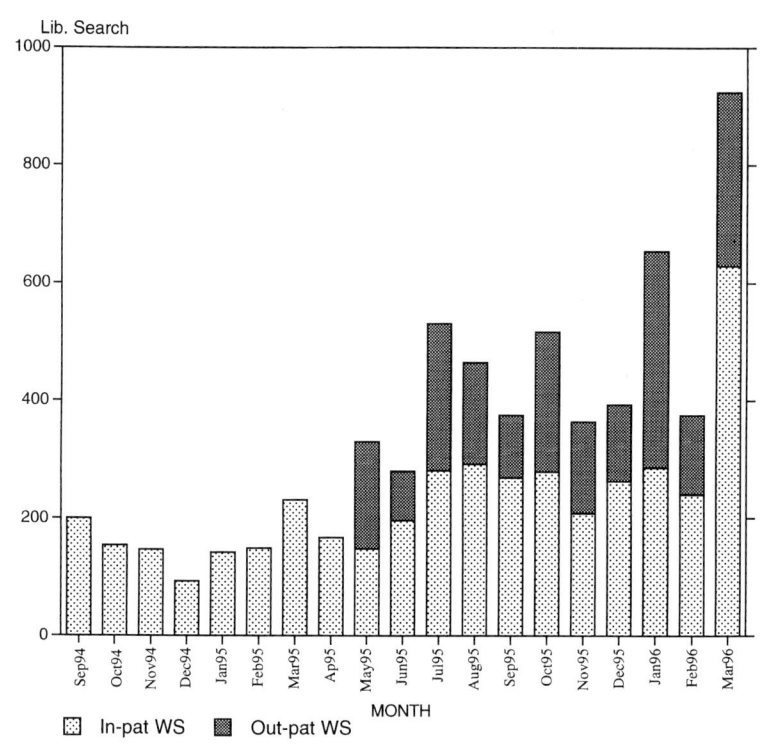

Figure 16.4 Total number of library searches for historical images of the patient being reviewed.

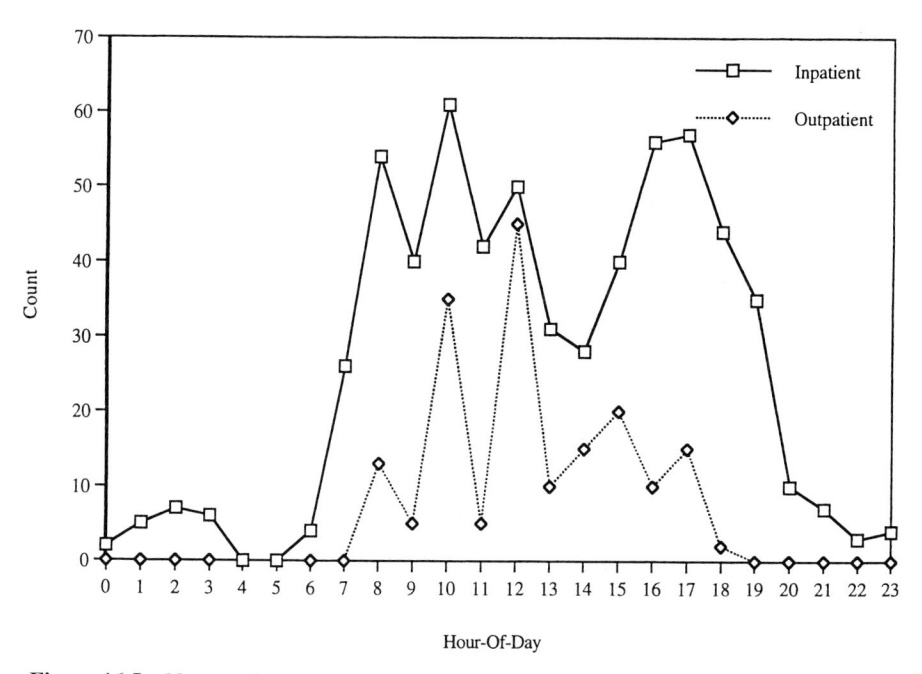

Figure 16.5 Neuroradiology workstation image usage by hours of the day (August 1995).

429

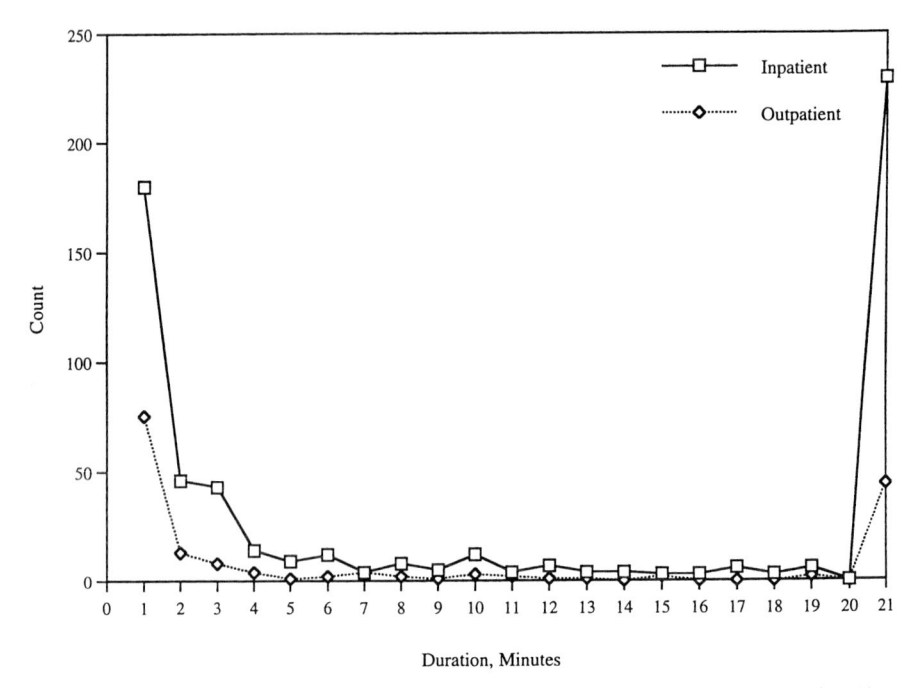

Figure 16.6 Duration of the neuroradiology workstation in use after a patient selection (August 1995).

2. Does the interhospital reading of images performed at MZH from UCSF save operational costs?

16.2.4.1 Neuroradiology Clinical Services

The neuroradiology section, with five neuroradiologists and five fellows, provides clinical service for the radiology departments at both UCSF and MZH. At MZH, there is an active neuroradiology service performing from 15 to 20 CT/MR cases per day and 1 to 4 CT scans per night from the emergency department request. A neuroradiology fellow and an attending physician provide coverage during the day until approximately 6:00 P.M. During this time, all examinations are also transmitted to UCSF and read by other experts in the neuroradiology section. Members of the neuroradiology faculty from UCSF rotate to MZH daily, either by shuttle or by personal automobile.

Emergency call at MZH is provided on a first-line basis by the UCSF resident on call, who is physically at UCSF. Before the workstations were installed, films were made after the scan and were delivered to UCSF by the technologist (courier service) for the on-call resident to read. Now that the workstations have been installed, the resident reviews emergency cases with the two workstations, and a verbal and a written report are transmitted to the referring physician at MZH.

16.2.4.2 Operational Environment

During the time of collecting data for this study, the operational environment in the neuroradiology section can be summarized as follows:

1. All neuro images from 10 CT and MR scanners from UCSF and MZH were transmitted to the PACS. The PACS distributed **all** neuro images, regardless of inpatient or outpatient status, to both workstations. Both workstations had similar equipment, the same database, and identical images. There was no distinction as to which workstation was the source and which the destination.
2. We placed one workstation in the neuro inpatient reading room and the other in the outpatient reading room, both at UCSF. We put the workstations in two different rooms not to separate inpatient and outpatient images, but because neuroradiologists rotated to these two different areas to perform their duties. Having workstations at both sites would allow them to review both in and outpatient images at either site. The outpatient room was open only from 8 A.M. to 6 P.M., whereas the inpatient reading room was open 24 hours. The workstation in the inpatient room was used more often, not because of the number difference in inpatient and outpatient examinations, but because of the availability of access.
3. Neuroradiologists could read both inpatient and outpatient images from either workstations or films, and they had no preference as to where to read them.
4. MZH had no workstation. All images obtained there, either from inpatient or outpatient examinations, were transmitted to the two workstations at UCSF. All MZH neuro images could be read at both workstations. During regular working hours, an attending staff from UCSF was always stationed at MZH, where films were used as the primary means for reading. The attending consulted with a subspecialist at UCSF, who could use either the inpatient or the outpatient area workstation. All off-hour cases were read from UCSF with the two workstations.
5. There was no modality difference in the two workstations. In the database, there was a patient folder for each patient containing **all** modality images either CT or MR, in- or outpatient exam, performed at MZH or at UCSF, or both.

16.2.4.3 Two Parameters

Answers to question 1 in Section 16.2.4 can be complex because the word "facilitate" can be interpreted differently. For this reason, we choose two parameters as a measure of "facilitation." The first parameter, T is "time required before images become available for viewing after the examination." This parameter can be used to predict when images will become available for film and workstation readings.

The second parameter, **workstation utilization index,** is defined as the percentage of neuro examinations performed that are read via the workstation. To measure this parameter, we select a passive approach that allows neuroradiologists to choose either the film or the workstation they prefer to read a case. If the workstation is used, relevant data needed to compute this index are recorded automatically and will count as one entry, even though films of the same patient may also be used at a certain time during the diagnostic process. Since both the film and the workstation reading are available, and the neuroradiologists are free to select the reading method for their convenience, a steady increase of workstation usage through time means that neuroradiologists find the workstation useful and are using them more frequently. This upward trend can be interpreted as a "facilitation" of the neuroradiology section operation.

In doing this analysis, some by-products of workstation utilization can also be generated. These include user habits, workstation functions utilization frequency (Section 12.3.5), and a **library search index,** defined as the total number of times the user looks for a patient's historical images while current images are being reviewed from the workstation. This index can be computed by dividing the total number of Library Search functions requested by the total number of instances of workstation usage. This index can also be used as a measure of "facilitation" of the neuroradiology operation.

The parameter T is also used to compute the costs required to prepare images obtained from MZH for interpretation by neuroradiologists at UCSF as a means to answer the second question. Note that we are not attempting to compute the cost effectiveness, which is a very difficult parameter to measure. Instead, we try to estimate whether preparing for the workstation reading actually costs less than the film reading, assuming both the systems are in place. In doing so, we focus on the weekend and evening examinations, since these periods are most problematic in the radiology operation owing to the shortage of personnel.

16.2.4.4 Data Collection

We collected data of two types as a means of analyzing the workstation utilization and the operational cost of preparing the film and workstation readings. First, all CT/MR monthly procedures performed at UCSF and MZH from September 1994 to March 1996 were extracted through the RIS. The data, tabulated as monthly neuro CT/MR examinations (see Fig. 16.3), served as a baseline for computing the workstation utilization index. We implemented a user log program in each workstation to automatically record the workstation utilization by functions, and user's habit. Data for computing the workstation utilization index were collected from September 1994 to March 1996 for the inpatient workstation, and from May 1995 to March 1996 for the outpatient workstation.

Even though we selected a passive approach, we still would like to be able to track whether the workstation was used for a particular case, how often films were used in conjunction with the workstation, and why any users chose not to use the workstation. Such data were very difficult to obtain online and could be collected only retrospectively. Thus a survey form was distributed in July 1996. Results demonstrate that in 85% of the cases performed at MZH during evenings and weekends, the radiologists did not read the films again. Examinations performed in daytime, during the

TABLE 16.2 Definitions of Time Periods for Image Delivery for the Film and the Workstation Reading

T = from T_0 to T_2	Film	Workstation
T_0	Start of neuro scan at MZH	Start of neuro scan at MZH
T_1	All images are windowed and printed onto films and ready for delivery to UCSF	All images are ready to be sent to PACS
T_2	Film are delivered by courier service to UCSF neuro reading room and ready to be viewed	Images are transmitted to UCSF via the wide area network and ready to be displayed on the workstation at the neuro reading rooms

week, were reread about 50% of the time. The mode of the choice depended on which was available first. For most MR studies performed at UCSF that required more than 100 images, films were first, followed by the workstation with the cine mode.

Data of the second type are helpful for cost analysis. Since we wanted to compare the costs of preparing the film reading and the workstation reading, we had to record relevant data pertinent to a period of time when both methods were in use. For this reason, we recorded all neuro CT procedures performed at MZH from February 1 to October 31, 1994, and computed the T for both preparation times. After October 1994, film reading was used sparsely. Only neuro CT examinations were collected because almost all evening and weekend emergency cases at MZH were CT examinations. Table 16.2 shows how T was computed for preparing the film and the workstation reading, and Table 16.3 tabulates the time required for each time period within T. For each time period within T, we can associate a value based on the cost estimate. The result is the operational costs of preparing images for the film and the workstation reading.

We selected afterhours and weekend cases at MZH for the cost analysis for several reasons. First, this time duration was most suitable for comparing the difference in costs between film reading and soft copy readings because both readings were done at UCSF, but the images generated were outside UCSF. Before the installation of the workstations, all readings were from film, whereas after the installation, all readings were from workstations. This environment is very similar to two controlled periods, which enforced the method of reading for each period. Second, daytime cases at MZH were read by an attending staff member at MZH (using film) and consulted by staff

TABLE 16.3 Time Required (min) Before Images Become Available for Reading After an Examination

	T_0-T_1	T_1-T_2	T
Film	6–8	23	29–31
Workstation	10–15	13–19	23–34

at UCSF (using workstations). Third, for all UCSF cases, both films and workstations were available. In the two latter situations, the conditions were too random to render significant results. Moreover, there was no need for courier service and thus the computation would have omitted this communication component.

16.2.4.5 System Utilization

Figure 16.3 shows the total number of monthly neuroradiological examinations performed at both UCSF and MZH as well as the total number of patients reviewed via the two workstations from September 1994 to March 1996. The data demonstrate that the inpatient workstation usage is much higher than that of the outpatient workstation: the inpatient reading room is inside the hospital and open 24 hours a day, whereas the outpatient area is closed from 6 P.M. to 8 A.M. Figure 16.4 shows the Library Search usage from the two workstations while a patient's images are being reviewed. Figure 16.7 depicts the workstation utilization index and the library search index: the former shows that the usage of the workstations moves up steadily from 40% to over 80% (slope estimate 2.7 ± 0.53, $p < .001$). That is, almost 80% of the neuro cases are reviewed from the two workstations. The chi-square test for linear trend is significant at $p < .0001$, demonstrating a definite increase of workstation utilization. We interpret this upward trend as indicating facilitation of the neuroradiology operation. The library search index shows that about 50% of the time the neuroradiologist also looks for images from older examinations while current images are being reviewed. The chi-square test for linear trend is significant at $p < .0001$, demonstrating a definite increase linear trend to over 50% (slope estimate 1.6 ± 0.56, $p < .001$).

One purpose of this study was to see whether the workstations facilitate the neuroradiology operation. The library search index is a parameter to measure whether neuroradiologists used the workstations to search for historical exams. An increased linear trend means that neuroradiologists relied more on the workstations for image retrieval, an indication that the workstations contributed to a facilitation of neuroradiology operation.

Table 16.4 compares the operational costs of preparing images for the film and workstation readings. In generating Table 16.4, we assumed that all the film-based and workstation equipment was already in place. Thus, the amounts represent the operational cost per case. We estimated the costs for examination done during weekends and evenings only, since a neuroradiologist/fellow is always on site at MZH and no courier service is required during normal operation hours. The courier is normally the technologist who performed the examination, then delivers the films to UCSF from MZH and charges for the extra time. Although the cost for the T1 line lease is for the entire month, we made the assumption that it was installed as if for weekend and evening use only, which inflates the rate for the workstation preparation cost. For the storage cost estimation, we computed only the costs of producing the films and storing the images on the optical disk as a long-term archive. Other possible costs were ignored. Results from Table 16.4 demonstrate that the cost for preparing images for weekend and evening workstation reading is substantially less than that for the film reading.

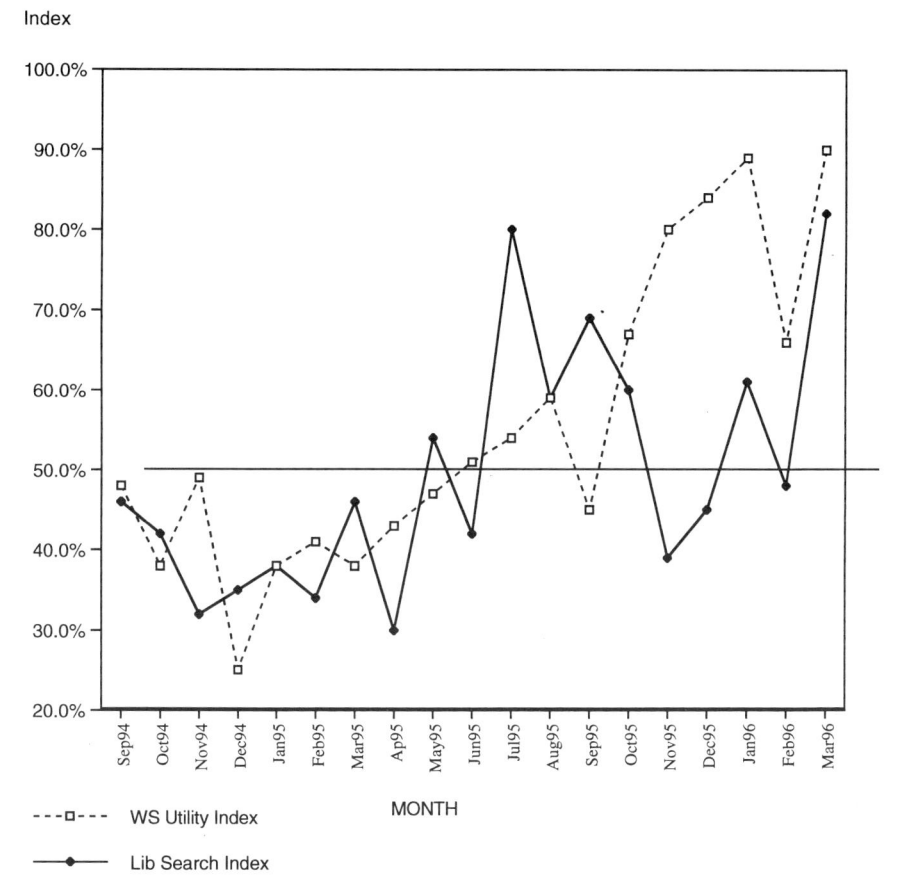

Figure 16.7 WS utilization index derived from Figure 16.3 and Library search index derived from Figures 16.3 and 16.4: (total Lib Search)/(total WS utilization).

Other results derived from this study include the workstation utilization hours, workstation functions used, and the time duration of each workstation session (Figs. 16.3–16.6). Of the 29 available functions in the workstations (Table 12.4), the following: Patient Select, Image Select, Zoom and Scroll, Cine Mode, Window/Level, Library Search, and Sort Patient were used most often. Statistics collected in August 1995 indicates that for the inpatient and the outpatient workstations, these functions were used 95, and 91%, respectively. Again, as in the ICU workstations, Select Report was very seldom activated, even though it can be used to retrieve previous diagnostic reports of the patient from the RIS instantaneously.

Pitfalls and bottlenecks are two major obstacles hindering a smooth PACS operation after its installation. Sections 16.3 and 16.4 identify most of these problems based on clinical experience. Methods are also suggested to circumvent these pitfalls and minimize the occurrence of bottlenecks.

TABLE 16.4 Image Preparation Costs ($/case) for the Film and Workstation Readings

	Film	Workstation
Image delivery	12.50*	13.50†
Storage	10.00‡	1.00§
Total	22.50	14.50

*Weekend and evening rate for Courier Service: $22/h × 1.5; delivery time was computed as the difference between $T_2 - T_1$ in Table 16.2: $22/h × 1.5 × 23/60 h = $12.50.
†Image transmission T1 line lease from phone company, $540/month; 40 cases in evenings and weekends/month, $540/40 cases = $13.50/case.
‡Film cost average 30 images/case on 2–4 sheets: $10/case.
§Digital storage optical disk (2600 Mbyte)/$100 = 26 Mbyte/$1. One CT study averages 20 Mbyte or less than $1.

16.3 PACS PITFALLS

PACS pitfalls are mostly created from human error, whereas bottlenecks are due to imperfect design in either the PACS or image acquisition devices. These drawbacks can be recognized only through accumulated clinical experience.

Pitfalls due to human error are often initiated at imaging acquisition devices and at workstations. Three major errors at the acquisition devices are entering wrong input parameters, stopping an image transmission process improperly, and incorrect patient positioning. The error occurring most often at the workstation is due to users entering too many keystrokes or clicking the mouse too often before the workstation can respond. Pitfalls at the workstation unrelated to human error are missing location markers in a CT or MR scout view, images displayed with unsuitable lookup tables, and white borders in CR images due to X-ray collimation. Pitfalls created due to human intervention can be minimized by instituting a better quality assurance program, scheduling periodic in-service training, and interfacing image acquisition devices directly to the HIS/RIS.

16.3.1 During Image Acquisition

16.3.1.1 Human Errors at Imaging Acquisition Devices

The two most common errors at CR acquisition are using the wrong imaging plate ID card at the reader (Fig. 16.8, left) and entering the wrong patient's ID, name, accession number, or birthdate, and invalid characters at the scanner's operator console (Fig. 16.8, right). These errors can result in loss of images, assignment of images to a wrong patient, a patient image folder that contains other patients' images, orphaned images, and crashing the acquisition process due to illegal characters. Routine quality assurance (QA) procedures checking the CR operator log book or the radiology

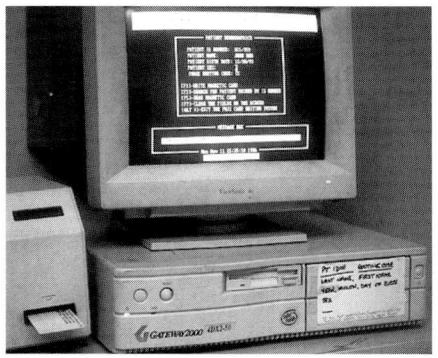

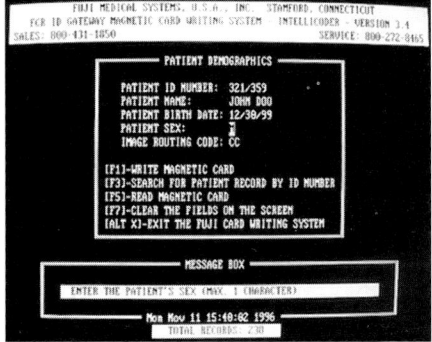

Figure 16.8 *Left:* ID card of the last patient was used at the card reader (lower left). *Right:* At the CR terminal: enter wrong patient's name: "Doo", wrong ID character: "/", wrong birthdate: "1999".

information system examination records against the PACS patient folder normally will disclose these errors. If a discrepancy is detected early enough (i.e., before images are sent to the workstation and the long-term archive), the PACS manager can perform the damage control by manually editing the PACS database to:

1. Correct for patient's name, ID, etc., and other typographical errors.
2. Delete images not belonging to the patient.
3. Append orphaned images to the proper patient image folder.

Lost images in a patient's folder can usually be found in the orphaned image directory. If images were sent to the workstation before the PACS manager had a chance to do the damage control described earlier, the PACS coordinator should alert the users immediately. If, however, these images had already been archived in the long-term storage before the damage control was performed, recovery of the errors will be more complicated. In this case, the PACS controller should have a mechanism allowing the PACS manager to correct the error at the PACS database.

16.3.1.2 Procedural Errors at Imaging Acquisition Devices

Procedural errors can be categorized in CT/MR and in CR during image acquisition separately. In CT/MR, the three most common errors are as follows:

terminating a scan while images are being transmitted
manually interrupting an image transmission process
realigning the patient during scanning

These errors can result in CT/MR image files that are missing images, images out of order in the sequence, and crashing the scanner due to the interruption of the image transmission.

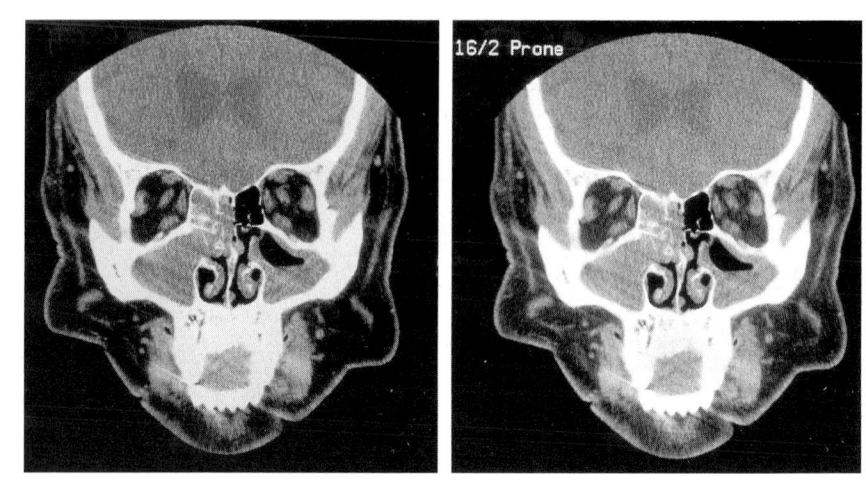

Figure 16.9 *Left:* Coronal view of a CT scan without a "left" or "right" indicator. *Right:* Label "16/2 Prone" can be generated by means of DICOM header information.

Another pitfall during CT acquisition that does not stem from human error lies in the coronal head scan protocol. Images appearing on the CT display monitor according to this protocol, have the left and right directions reversed. If film output is used, the technologist manually inputs the orientation as annotation on the screen, which is then printed on the film with the image. Such an interactive step in the PACS is not possible because graphics on the CT display console are not included in the DICOM image header. A method for circumventing this shortcoming is to detect the scanning protocol from the DICOM image header and automatically annotate the orientation on the image during its display on the PACS workstation (Fig. 16.9).

In CR, the most common error occurs when the technologist places the imaging plate under the patient in the wrong direction during a portable examination (Fig. 16.10). The result is the wrong image orientation during the display.

Errors due to manually interrupting the transmission procedure can be alleviated by using the DICOM communication protocol for automatic image verification and recovery during the transmission. Images archived out of order in the sequence can be manually edited during the QA procedure. Wrong CR orientation during display can be detected by an algorithm with automatic rotation (Fig. 16.11), or manual rotation can be instituted during the QA procedure.

Pitfalls due to human error can be minimized by scheduling regular in-service training and continued education for technologists. However, the most effective method is to use a direct HIS/RIS interface between the image acquisition device and the PACS components, which in essence eliminates the human interaction for inputting patient-related data (Fig. 16.12). Currently, it is possible to interface CR to RIS for direct patient data input. However, direct interface from RIS to CT/MR is still not available.

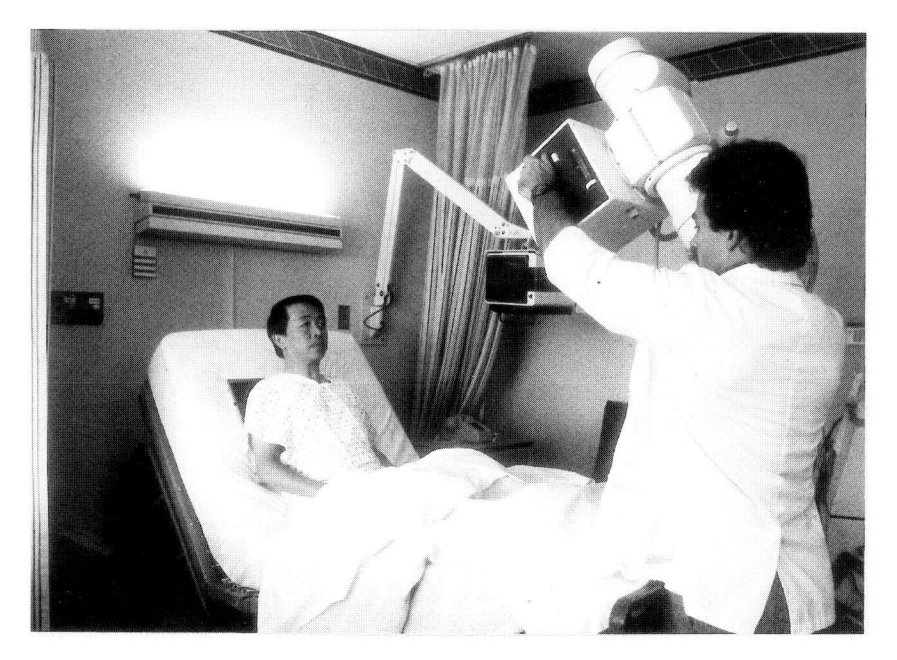

Figure 16.10 IP behind the patient is in the wrong orientation.

16.3.2 At the Workstation

16.3.2.1 Human Error

Two human errors occur often at the workstation. First, the user enters too many keystrokes or clicks the mouse too often before the workstation can respond to the last request. As a result, the workstation does not respond properly or the display program crashes. When the workstation response is slow, the impatient user may enter the next few commands while the workstation is still executing the last request, causing the display program either to crash unexpectedly or to hang up. Another possible result is that the workstation continues executing the next few commands by the user after the current one is completed. Since the user may have forgotten what commands he or she had entered, the display appearing on the screen may be unexpected, hence confusing. The second error occurs when the user forgets to close the window of a previous operation. In this case, the workstation may not respond to the next command. If the user panics and enters other commands, errors similar to those described in the first case may occur.

Two remedies can be used. The workstation can provide a big visible timer on the screen, to let the user know that the last command or request is being processed. This measure will minimize the impatient user's tendency to enter commands prematurely. A better solution is to have an improved workstation design that will tolerate such human errors.

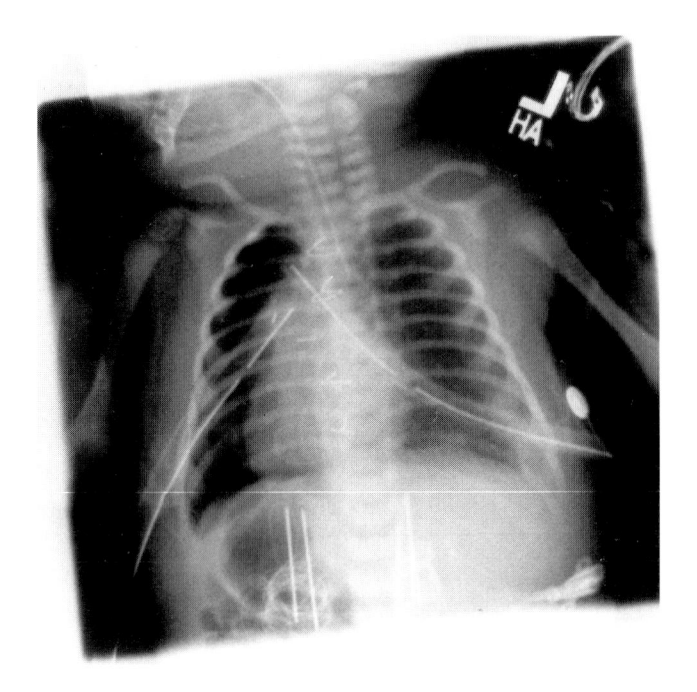

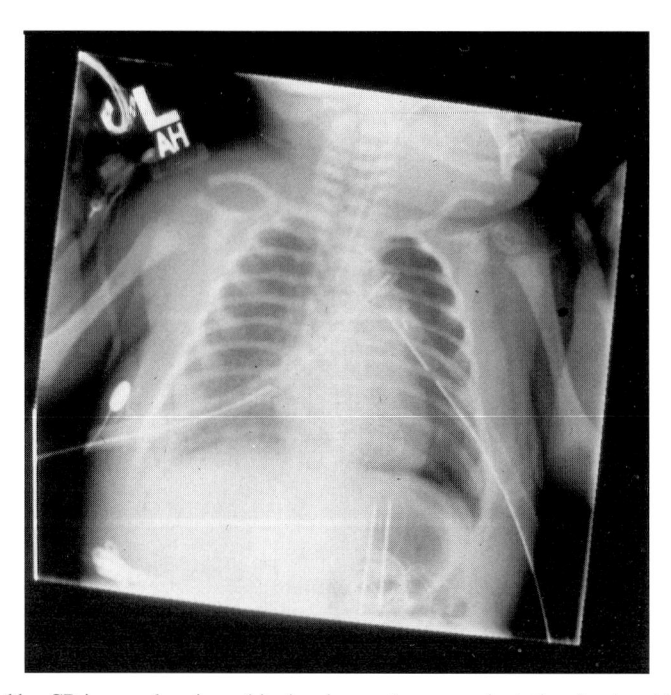

Figure 16.11 CR image showing white borders and wrong orientation (top) and background removal and automatic rotation to correct for the orientation (bottom).

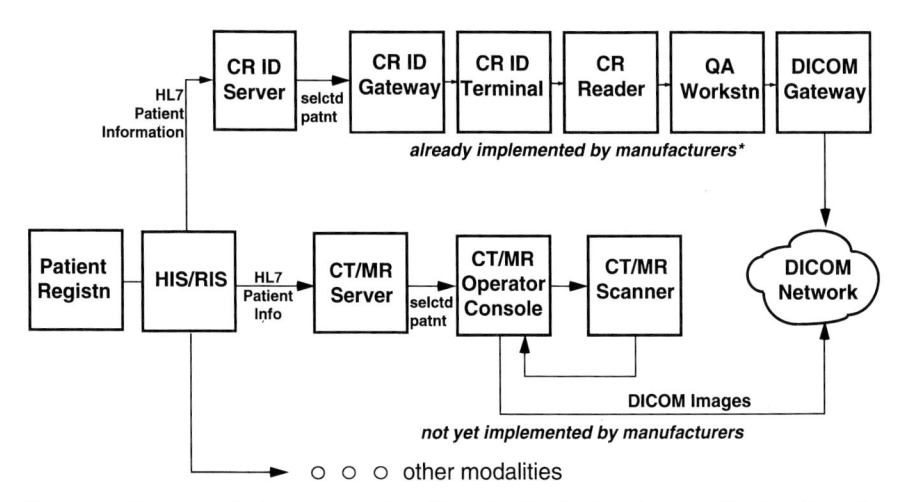

Figure 16.12 Method of connecting the RIS to the CR. Patient demographic data from the RIS can be transmitted directly to the CR in lieu of typing at the ID terminal, a feature that minimizes typographic errors.

16.3.2.2 System Deficiency

Four system deficiencies at the workstation are no localization markers on a CT/MR scout view (Fig. 16.13), incorrect lookup table for CT/MR display (Fig 16.14), orientation of the CT head image in the coronal scan protocol discussed earlier (Fig. 16.9), and white borders in CR due to X-ray collimation. No localization markers on a CT/MR scout view can be remedied by creating the localization lines using the information from the DICOM image header (See Figure 16.13). The use of an incorrect lookup table for a CT/MR display is case dependent. Correct lookup tables for CT can be generated by means of the histogram technique. There are still some difficulties in obtaining a uniform correct lookup table for all images in a head MR sequence. Sometimes it is necessary to use the histogram method to investigate every image individually (see Fig. 16.14). The correction for the CT head coronal scan has been discussed previously (Fig. 16.9). White borders in CR due to X-ray collimation can be corrected using an automatic background removal technique (Section 4.1.6, Fig. 16.11).

16.4 PACS BOTTLENECKS

Bottlenecks affecting the PACS operation include contention among networks, CR, CT, and MR images stacked up at acquisition devices, slow responses from workstations, and long delays for image retrieval from the long-term archive. Bottlenecks can be alleviated by improving the system architecture, reconfiguring the networks, and streamlining operational procedures as a result of coming to understand the clinical environment.

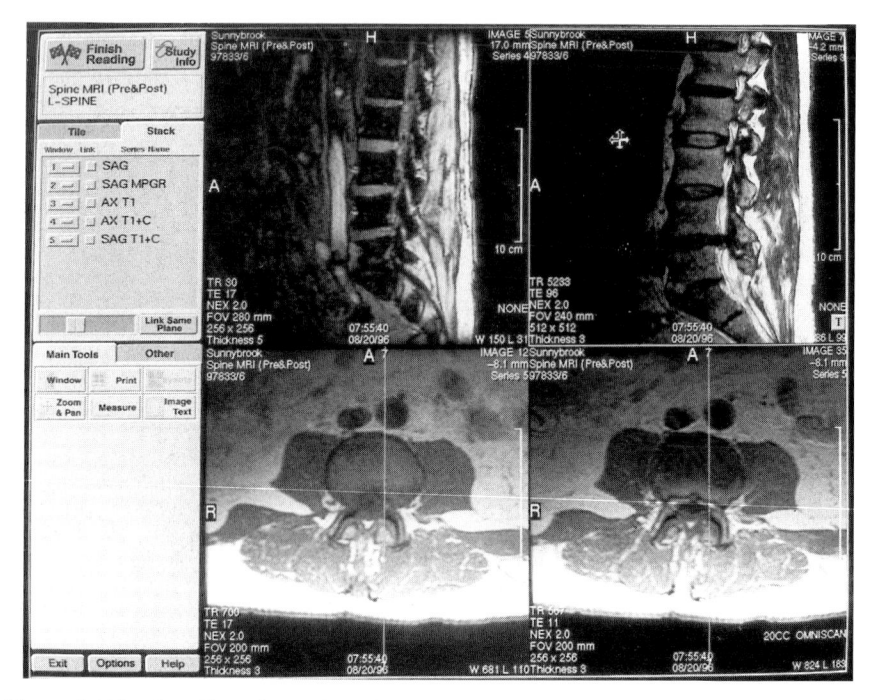

Figure 16.13 Scan lines (bottom) can be generated from the DICOM header information to correlate scans between planes: Sagittal, top; transverse, bottom.

16.4.1 Network Contention

Network contention will cause many bottlenecks. First, CR/CT/MR images may stack up at the image acquisition computers, causing the computer disks to overflow and eventually lose some images. Or, the PACS controller may take longer to collect a complete sequence of images from one MR or CT examination, delaying the transmission of the sequence file to the workstation for review. Network contention can also cause long delays for image retrieval from the long-term archive, especially when the retrieved image file is large.

Methods of correction can be divided into general and specific. The general category includes redesigning the network architecture, using a faster network, and modifying the communication protocols. To redesign the network architecture, for example, one might separate the network into segments and subnets and redistribute the heavy traffic routes to different subnets, perhaps by dividing CT/MR acquisition and CR acquisition into two subnets. Assigning priorities to different subnets based on the use and time of day is one way to address the user's immediate needs.

Using a faster network can speed up the image transfer rate. If the current network is conventional Ethernet, consider changing to Ethernet hub or fast Ethernet. If optical fibers are available, consider upgrading the network to asynchronous transfer mode (ATM, Fig. 9.7) or gigabit Ethernet technology (Fig. 9.11). Conventional network protocols often use default parameters that are suitable only for small file trans-

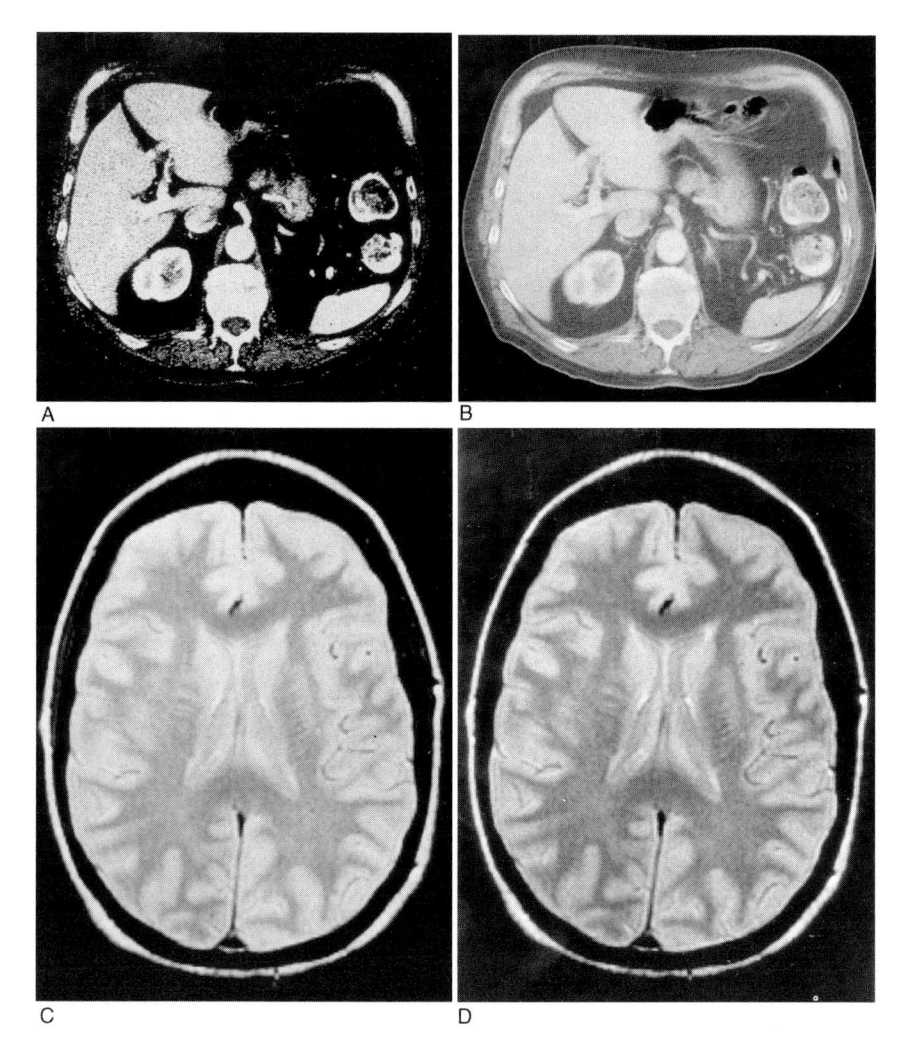

Figure 16.14 Body CT and MR head scan: *Left:* wrong LUT, *right:* correct LUT.

fer. Changing some parameters in the protocol (e.g., enlarging the TCP window and the image buffer size) may speed up the transfer rate.

In the specific category, the modification depends on the operational environment. Methods of correction may involve changing the operational procedure in the radiology department. Consider two examples: CR images stacked up at the CR readers, and CT/MR images stacked up at the scanners. Most CR applications are for portable examinations, and they tend to be performed in the early morning. One obvious method of correction is to rearrange the portable examination schedule on the wards. CT/MR images stacked up at the scanners may indicate a design fault in the communication protocol at the scanners. There are two methods of correction. First, use DICOM autotransfer mode to "push" images out from the scanner as soon the image

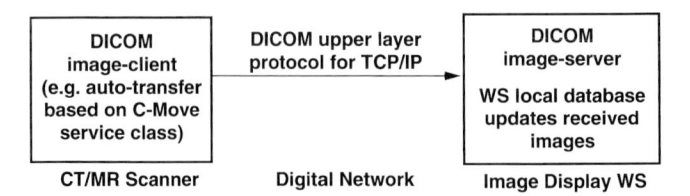

```
┌─────────────────┐                          ┌─────────────────┐
│     DICOM       │  DICOM upper layer       │     DICOM       │
│  image-client   │  protocol for TCP/IP     │  image-server   │
│ (e.g. auto-transfer ├────────────────────► │                 │
│  based on C-Move│                          │ WS local database│
│  service class) │                          │ updates received│
│                 │                          │     images      │
└─────────────────┘                          └─────────────────┘
   CT/MR Scanner         Digital Network       Image Display WS
```

Note: The auto-transfer software at the scanner automatically "pushes" an image whenever ready. The image server receives an image one at a time at the workstation.

Figure 16.15 A push operation at the scanner to transmit an image out of the scanner as soon as it is generated.

is ready to be sent to the acquisition gateway or the workstation (Section 7.6.4.1; Fig. 16.15). Second, from the acquisition gateway or the workstation, use DICOM to "pull" images from the scanner periodically (Section 7.6.4.2; Fig. 16.16).

16.4.2 Slow Response at the Workstation

A slow response at the workstation is generally due to bad local database design and insufficient image memory in the workstation. An example of a poorly designed workstation database is one that uses a large file in the local disk for image storage. During the initial configuration of the workstation software, this storage space is contiguous. As the workstation starts to accumulate and delete images during use, the space becomes fragmented. Fragmented space causes an inefficient I/O transfer rate, rendering a slow response in bringing images from the disk to the display. Periodic cleanup is necessary to retain contiguous space in the disk. Insufficient image memory in the workstation, which requires continuous disk–memory swap, slows down the image display speed (Fig. 12.2). This is especially problematic when the image file is large.

Several methods for correcting a slow response at the workstation are possible. First, one can increase the image memory size to accommodate a complete image file, which will minimize the requirement for memory–disk swap. The use of RAID tech-

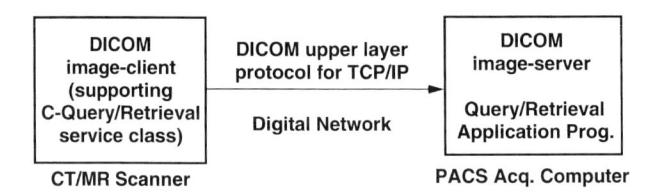

```
┌─────────────────┐                          ┌─────────────────┐
│     DICOM       │  DICOM upper layer       │     DICOM       │
│  image-client   │  protocol for TCP/IP     │  image-server   │
│  (supporting   ├────────────────────►     │                 │
│ C-Query/Retrieval│                         │ Query/Retrieval │
│  service class) │   Digital Network        │ Application Prog.│
└─────────────────┘                          └─────────────────┘
   CT/MR Scanner                              PACS Acq. Computer
```

Note: The query/retrieval program "pulls" images by sending query/retrieval requests to the scanner for a complete study.

Figure 16.16 A pull operation at the acquisition gateway or the WS to receive an image from the scanner as soon as it is generated.

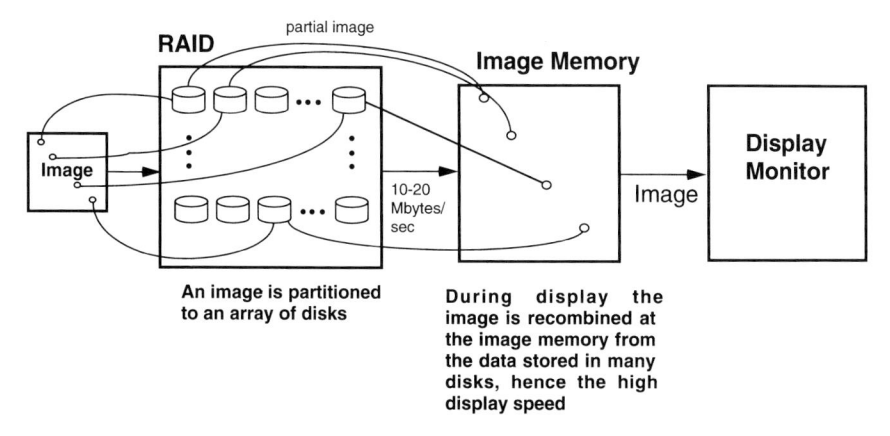

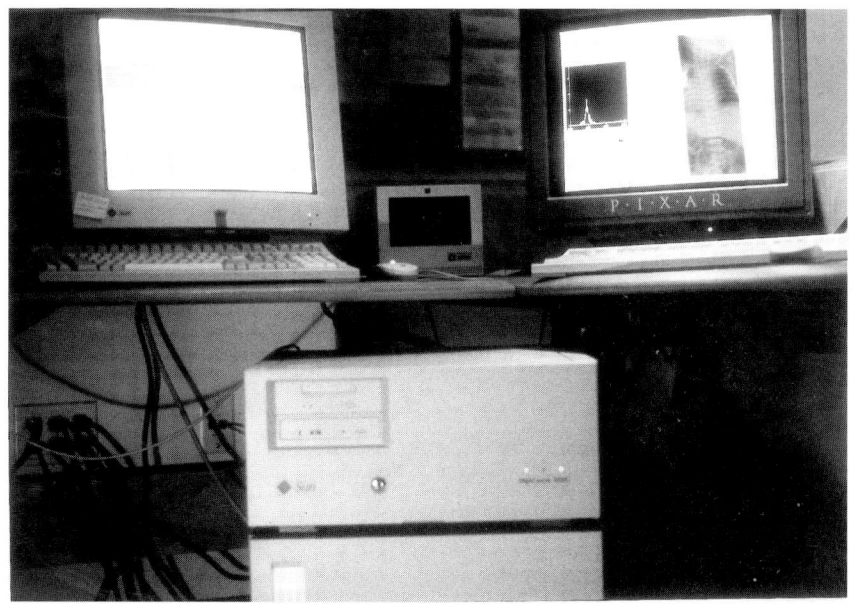

Figure 16.17 RAID Technology: scheme of concept and 30 Gbyte RAID in a WS.

nology is another way to speed up the disk I/O for faster image display. Better local database design and image search algorithm, along with RAID at the workstation, can speed up the image seeking and transfer time (Fig. 16.17).

16.4.3 Slow Response from the Archive Server

A slow response from the long-term archive can be caused by slow optical disk search and read/write operations, patient images scattering in different optical disk platters, and many simultaneous requests. A normal optical disk read/write data rate is about 400–500 Kbyte/s. When many large image files have images scattered in many plat-

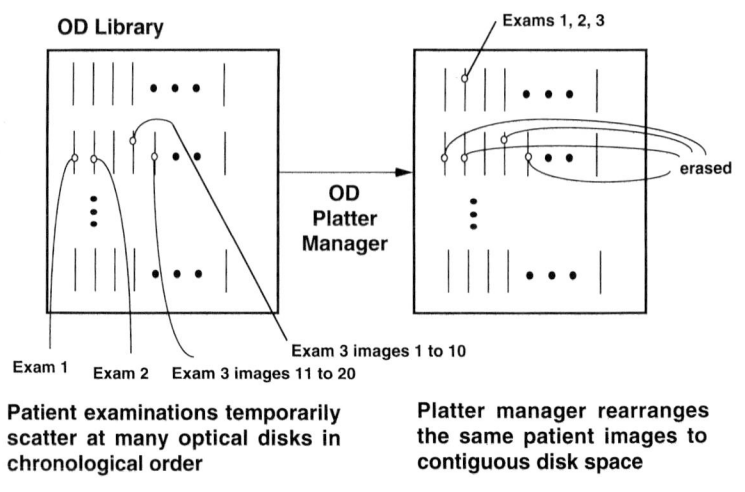

446 PACS CLINICAL EXPERIENCE, PITFALLS, AND BOTTLENECKS

Figure 16.18 Concept of the platter manager.

ters, the seek time and disk I/O will be slow. This will delay retrieval of these files from the long-term archive.

There are three possible methods of improvement. First, an image platter manager software can be used to rewrite scattered images to contiguous optical disk platters (Section 10.2.6; Fig. 16.18). This mechanism will minimize the future retrieval time for images. However, this method works only if optical disks used are erasable. Another method is to use the image prefetch mechanism (Section 10.2.10; Fig. 16.19), which anticipates what images the clinician will need for a particular patient. A combination of both mechanisms will speed up the response time from the long-term archive. In addition to these two mechanisms, a permanent storage upgrade (e.g., to optical disk library with multiple optical drives) can also improve the overall throughput of the retrieval operations, provided the library unit is capable of supporting a multidrive configuration.

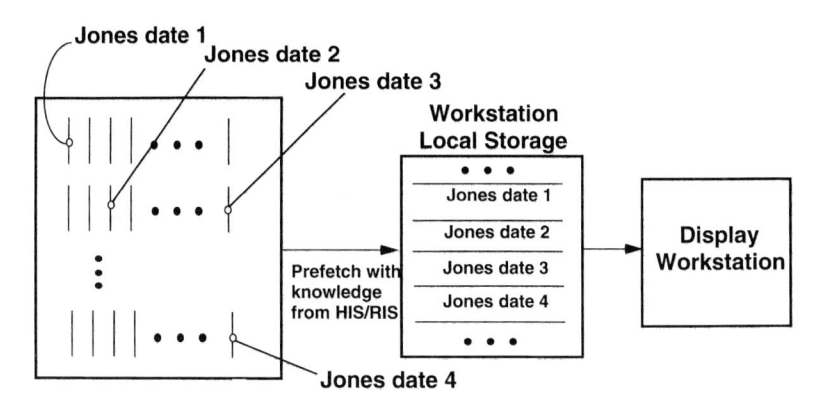

Figure 16.19 Concept of image prefetch.

16.5 PITFALLS IN DICOM CONFORMANCE

16.5.1 Incompatibility in a DICOM Conformance Statement

During the integration of multivendor PACS components, even though each vendor's component may come with a DICOM conformance statement, there may still be incompatibility. We have identified some representative pitfalls.

1. *Missing image(s) from a sequence during an acquisition process:* when a CT or MR scanner (Storage SCU) transmits individual images from a sequence to an image acquisition gateway (Storage SCP), the scanner initiates the transfer with a push operation. The reliability of transmission is dependent on the transfer mechanism implemented by the scanner.
2. *Incorrect data encoding in image header:* examples include missing type 1 data elements, which are mandatory attributes in the DICOM standard, incorrect value representation (VR) of data elements, and encoded data in data elements exceeding their maximum length.
3. *SOP service class not fully supported by the SCP vendor:* this happens when an SCU vendor and an SCP vendor implement a SOP service class with different operation supports. For example, a C-GET request initiated from a display workstation is rejected by an archive server because the latter accepts only C-MOVE requests, even though both C-GET and C-MOVE are DICOM standard DIMSE-C operations that support the Q/R service class.
4. *DICOM conformance mismatching between the individual vendors:* when an SCU vendor and an SCP vendor implement the Q/R service class in different information models or with different support levels, a C-FIND request in patient level initiated from a display workstation is rejected by a CT scanner because the latter supports only the Q/R study root model, which does not accept query requests in the patient level.
5. *Shadow group conflict between the individual vendors:* when both vendor A and vendor B store proprietary data in the same shadow group, data previously stored in the shadow group by vendor A are overwritten by vendor B's data.

16.5.2 Methods of Remedy

The pitfalls outlined above can be minimized through the implementation of two DICOM-based mechanisms, one in the image acquisition gateway (IAG), and the second in the PACS controller, to provide better connectivity solutions for multivendor imaging equipment in a large-scale PACS environment, the details of which were discussed in Sections 10.5.3.2 and 10.5.4.2.

CHAPTER 17
PACS Current Development Trends and Future Research Directions

17.1 INTRODUCTION

PACS originated as an image management system for improving the efficiency of radiology practice. It is evolved into a hospital-integrated system dealing with information media in many forms, including voice, text, medical records, images, and video recordings. To integrate these various types of information requires the technology of multimedia: hardware platforms, information systems and databases, communication protocols, display technology, and system interfacing and integration. We have discussed most of these topics in earlier chapters. As a PACS grows, so does the content of its database. The richness of information within the PACS provides an opportunity for a completely new approach in medical research and practice via the discipline of medical informatics. Our last two chapters touch on some new research frontiers and applications in PACS.

17.2 MEDICAL IMAGE INFORMATICS INFRASTRUCTURE IN A PACS ENVIRONMENT

In Section 13.4 we presented the medical image informatics infrastructure (MIII) as a server designed to utilize existing PACS resources including images and related data for large-scale research and clinical studies. In this section, we describe the MIII developed in our laboratory based on an existing hospital-integrated PACS.

17.2.1 Hospital-Integrated (HI) PACS at UCSF

The HI-PACS at UCSF is an integrated hospital imaging system, the details of which are described in Section 9.5.3. As of January 1997, the system consisted of a 2.6 Tbyte optical disk library as the long-term archive, and a two-tier communication network with asynchronous transfer mode (ATM) technology as the primary network and the Ethernet as the secondary. The PACS interfaces the hospital information system (HIS) and the radiology information system (RIS) with TCP/IP communication protocols and HL7 data format. Workstations of various types are distributed in both the radiol-

TABLE 17.1 Major Image Acquisition Devices and Databases Connected to the UCSF HI-PACS

- 5 CTs (4 GE, 1 Imatron)
- 5 MRs (4 GE 1.5T, 1 Siemens)
- 1 US PACS (Acuson)
- 2 CRs (Fuji AC-II, FCR-9000)
- 2 Film digitizers (Konica, Lumisys)
- HIS (IBM mainframe)
- RIS (IDXRAD)
- Digital Voice (Dictaphone DX7000)
- MEDLINE and LocalTalk

ogy department and intensive care units. Figure 16.1 showed the architecture, and Table 17.1 lists the image acquisition devices and databases connected to the HI-PACS.

17.2.2 MIII Based on the HI-PACS

The MIII based on the UCSF HI-PACS includes the components given in Section 13.4, as well as some additional special features described in the subsections that follow.

17.2.2.1 Communication Networking

The communication of the HI-PACS consists of a two-tier, wide area network (WAN) and local area network (LAN). The WAN connects UCSF, the San Francisco VA Medical Center, the San Francisco General Hospital, and Mount Zion Hospital, all in the Bay area, with a 155 Mbit/s ATM as the primary and a 1.5 Mbit/s T1 as the secondary network. The LAN (see Fig. 16.1) consists of a 155 Mbit/s ATM as the primary and a 10 Mbit/s Ethernet as the secondary network. The MIII shares these communication networks with the PACS for clinical images and data, thus guaranteeing high bandwidth image delivery for clinical service, education, and research requirements. In addition, an independent research ATM network is built in parallel with the PACS network (Fig. 17.1). The former is used for certain high speed communication requirements in research so that it does not interfere with the daily clinical service. Telemammography research, which requires large image files to be transmitted instantaneously (Section 14.4), is an example.

17.2.2.2 Content-Based Image Indexing

PACS database is designed to retrieve information by artificial keys, such as patient name and hospital ID. This mode of operation is sufficient for traditional radiology operations, but not adequate for image data storage of large-scale research and clinical applications. Therefore, in the MIII we develop a separate database containing

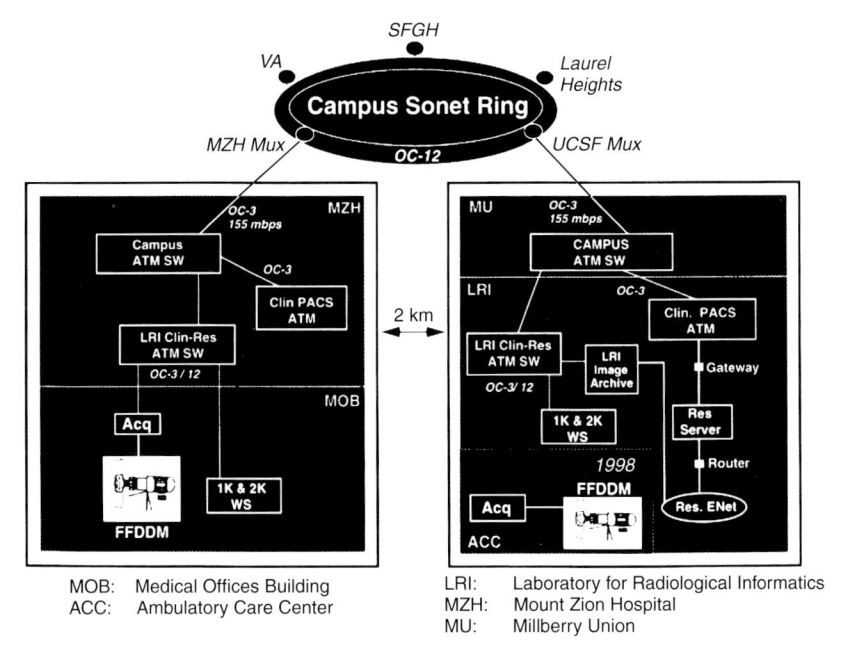

Figure 17.1 Dual ATM OC-3 networks supporting the MIII. The campus ATM OC-12 SONET ring (top) is supported by Pacific Bell. An OC-3 connection is available at each campus to the SONET ring through the campus ATM switch. Each campus switch is connected to two other ATM switches: one supports the PACS daily research and clinical service; the second, dedicated research projects.
FFDM: full-field digital mammography (Section 4.4.2); SW, switch; WS, workstation. (Courtesy of D. Hoogstrate.)

keywords of diagnostic reports, patient history, and imaging sequences, as well as certain features of images for content-based indexing of underlying MR/CT/CR images in the PACS database. The content-based image indexing, which is discussed in more detail in Section 17.4, allows for efficient image storage and retrieval and is used in the applications described in Section 17.2.3.

17.2.2.3 Volumetric Visualization of 3-D Images

A volumetric visualization node is for use as a MIII computing resource. The user at a workstation in a satellite site wishing to view fusion volumetric images from different imaging modalities (e.g., MRI and CT) in the PACS database can use the visualization node. Figure 17.2 shows the steps to accomplish this task through the central visualization node consisting of a high end graphic computer:

1. From the image workstation, the request is sent to either the PACS database or the MIII server to retrieve the volumetric image sets.

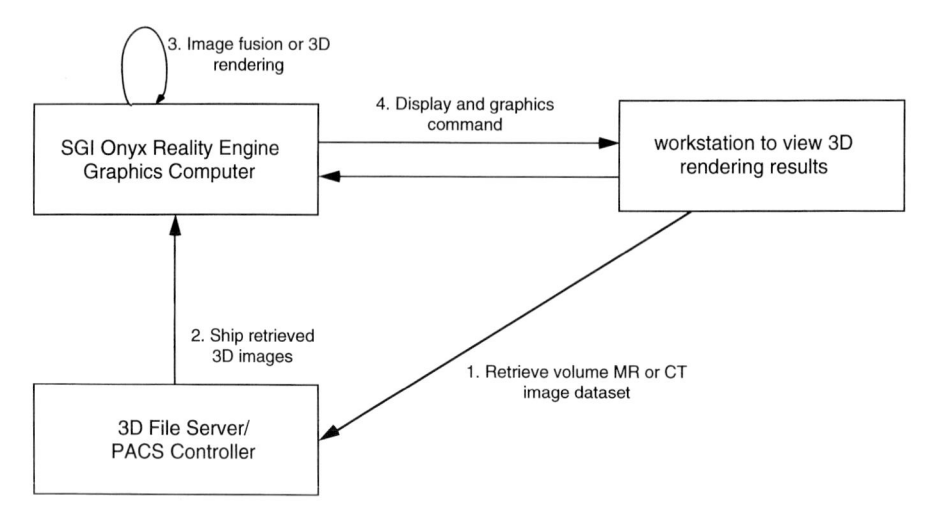

Figure 17.2 Visualization of volumetric images using the client/server visualization node for high speed image processing with an SGI Onyx Reality Engine Graphic Computer. The node is a major component in the MIII.

2. The image set is sent to the visualization node (Onyx, Silicon Graphics, Inc., Mountain View, CA).
3. The visualization node performs the necessary 3-D computation and rendering functions.
4. Results are sent back to the workstation for viewing after the task is completed.

In step 4, the user can also communicate with the visualization node directly for further instructions or manipulation.

17.2.3 Some Research Using the MIII

We turn briefly to a discussion of four ongoing projects in our laboratory based on the concept of the MIII. In each of these projects, we describe the utilization, the hypothesis, the conventional method and its drawback, and the MIII approach. We also mention components required in the MIII and their utilization. In Sections 18.1, 18.2.5, and 18.4, we elaborate on topics of bone age assessment, temporal image database, and teleconsultation.

17.2.3.1 Bone Age Assessment with a Digital Hand Atlas

Utilization: Research and clinical service.

Hypothesis: Bone age of children can be assessed automatically by comparing a left hand and wrist digital X-ray image with a comprehensive hand digital atlas.

Conventional method: Compares a hand X-ray film with an atlas developed in the 1930s from a limited number of films. Thus, the conventional method is inaccurate and has bias because of the limited data available for comparison.

MIII approach: Uses computed radiography (CR) images and related data from the PACS database to generate a digital atlas. Image processing software is used to extract parameters from CR images for bone age assessment. A visualization engine is used to match the image with extracted parameters with those from the digital atlas. Specific application software based on the match can be developed for bone age assessment.

17.2.3.2 Temporal Image Database as a Means to Evaluate the Effectiveness of Therapy Treatment Planning

Utilization: Research and clinical service.

Hypothesis: Progression of lung nodules over time can be tracked and analyzed using spiral CT scans. The results can be used to determine the effectiveness of a treatment plan.

Conventional method: There is no conventional method to quantitatively evaluate the effectiveness of a treatment planning for a disease. Without the PACS database, it is tedious to track down temporal CT images along with patient's records through time. It is difficult, as well, to append the extracted nodule data with the images to perform longitudinal comparison.

MIII approach: Quantitative nodule attributes from spiral CT images with relevant patient records can be obtained from the PACS database. Image processing can be used to extract sizes and shapes of lung nodules from longitudinal sequential CT images. MIII database, knowledge base, and special application software organize the extracted data with therapeutic treatment planning results to determine the effectiveness of the therapeutic plan.

17.2.3.3 Collaborative Consultation with High Resolution Images

Utilization: Clinical service.

Hypothesis: Communication and visualization tools can be integrated with the PACS database to enable collaborative consultation among radiologists and referring physicians at various sites, resulting in a better health care delivery system.

Conventional method: Referring physicians use telephones or walk to the radiology department for consultation or review of images.

MIII approach: Utilizes PACS database, communication protocols, graphic user interface, visualization engines, and specific application software for interactive collaborative consultation with high resolution images from PACS as needed.

17.2.3.4 Noninvasive Surgical Planning Using Multimodal Neuroimages

Utilization: Research and clinical service.

Hypothesis: Multimodality neuro images can be fused to aid noninvasive planning of epilepsy surgery.

Conventional method: It is tedious to assemble the necessary neuro images and related data from various modalities to locate the epileptic site and to determine its extensiveness in the patient. To perform image fusion requires offline computing and online visualization from noninterconnected computing resources.

MIII approach: Use the MIII input server to acquire neuro images from the PACS database, the image processing software for segmentation and registration, and the visualization engine for 3-D rendering. Special application software can be developed to aid noninvasive planning of epilepsy surgery based on the derived results.

17.3 COMPUTATION AND THREE-DIMENSIONAL RENDERING NODE

PACS is designed as a data management system; it lacks the computational power for image content analysis at the image workstation or at the PACS controller. To facilitate the effectiveness of the medical image database server, it will be necessary to append a computation and 3-D rendering node in the PACS network, to perform high power computations requested by image workstations. On the completion of a given computation, the results are distributed with visualization capability to other image workstations through the high speed PACS network. The architecture of a computation and 3-D rendering node in a PACS environment at UCSF is shown in Figure 17.3: the PACS integrated database is at the left; the computation and 3-D rendering node is on the top, connected to the HI-PACS networks, with ATM and with 10 BaseT as the backup. The Mac server provides a connection of the PACS with the Mac users, and the image workstations are for clinical use. Let us consider two scenarios.

Scenario 1: Volumetric Visualization of Clinical Images. Suppose that the user wishes to view fusion volumetric images from different imaging modalities (e.g., MRI and PET) in the PACS database, either from the image workstation or from a Macintosh computer through the Mac server. Current PACS controller and image workstation design does not support such a capability. Figure 17.2 and Section 17.2.2.3 illustrated the steps that would be needed to accomplish this task through the computation node. In this scenario, we assume that the image workstation has the capability to view 2-D and 3-D images with graphics. Figure 17.4 shows the mapping of 2-D brain function (PET, color) to anatomy (MRI, black and white).

Scenario 2: Video/Image Conferencing with Image Database Query Support. Now suppose that the referring physician at a workstation requests a video conference with a radiologist who is located elsewhere. Figure 17.5 shows the data flow. In this case,

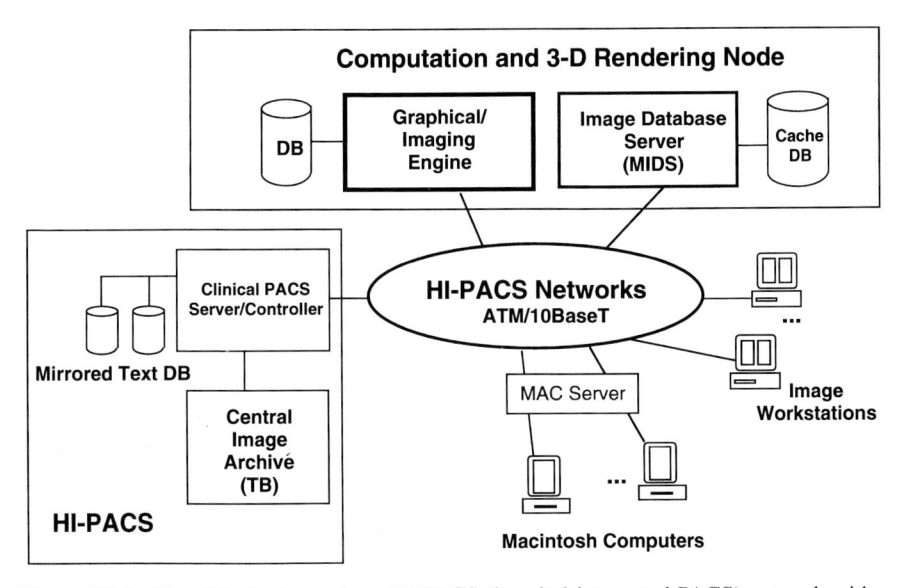

Figure 17.3 Simplified scheme for a HI-PACS (hospital-integrated PACS) network with a computation and 3-D rendering Node at UCSF: MIDS, medical image database server; DB, database.

we demonstrate how to utilize the medical image database server and the computation node to accomplish the task. The data flow starts with establishment of a video conference between two image workstations (1); then the referring physician requests the case from the PACS database and sends necessary queries to the MIDS, the medical image database server (2). The PACS database transmits data (3), and the MIDS sends synthesized query instructions to the computation node. The computation node performs necessary computation and 3-D rendering and sends results back almost in real time to both image workstations (4), and the results (5) allow a real-time video conference with the 3-D high resolution image set and related data at both workstations. Note that to accomplish this scenario, three components are necessary in addition to the PACS database: the MIDS, the computation node, and the high speed ATM network. Figure 17.6 shows such a video/image conferencing. Note that video/image conferencing does not allow the manipulation of images by either site. Simultaneous and instantaneous image manipulation of images requires other resources, and we define this operation as teleconsultation (see below: Section 18.4).

17.4 IMAGE CONTENT INDEXING

Current image retrieval is through artificial indexing using a patient's name, ID, age group, disease category, and so on. With the combination of the MIDS and the computation node, it is possible to explore image content indexing. In one-dimensional

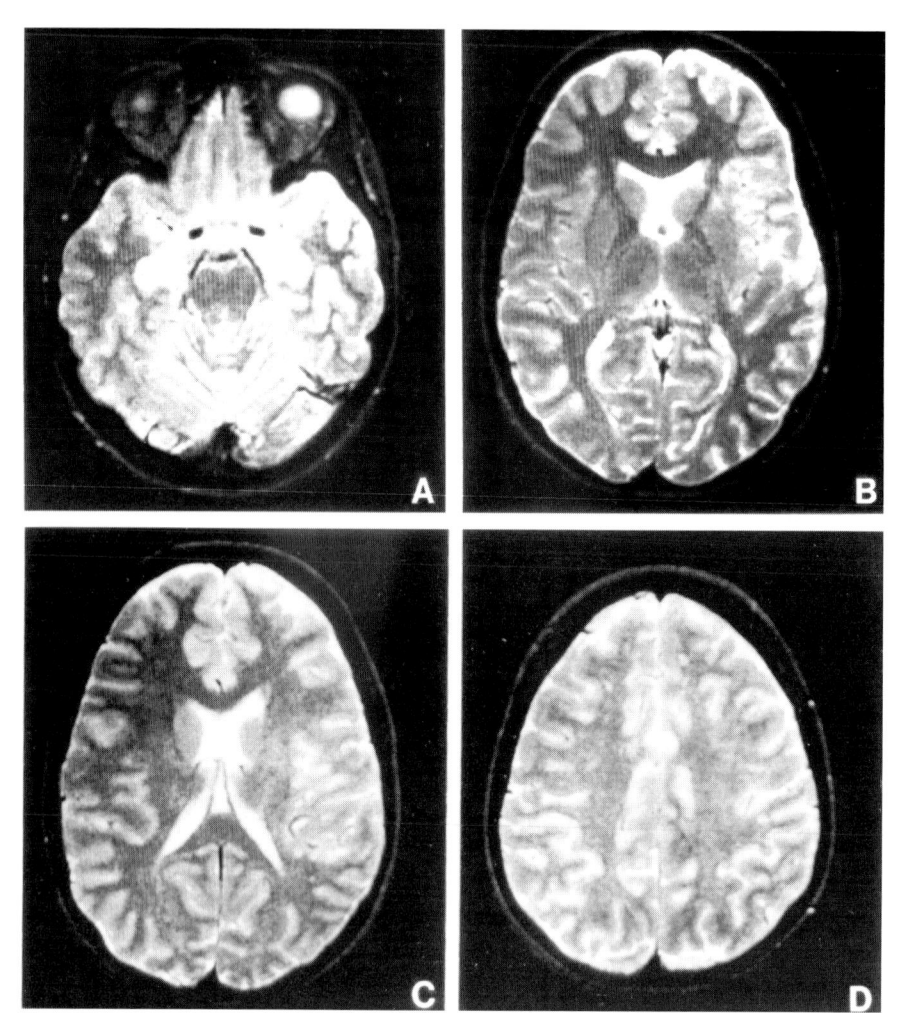

Figure 17.4 Mapping of 2-D brain function (PET, color) to anatomy (MRI, gray scale). Areas of high activity are colored red and orange, whereas lower activity are green and blue: (A) midbrain, (B) striatum, (C) head of the caudate, and (D) anterior pole of the cortex. (See color plate.) (Courtesy of D. Valentino.)

data, indexing can be through keywords, which is a fairly simple procedure. On the other hand, indexing through image content is complicated because the computation node and the MIDS first must understand the image content, which can include abstract terms (e.g., objects of interest) derived quantitative data (e.g., area and volume of the object of interest), and texture information (e.g., interstitial disease). Figure 17.7 shows some preliminary results acquired using indexing via image content in brain myelination disorder research. Indexing via image content is a frontier research topic in image processing, and the PACS-rich database will allow the validation of new theories and algorithms. As an example, refer to Figure 12.6, which shows the

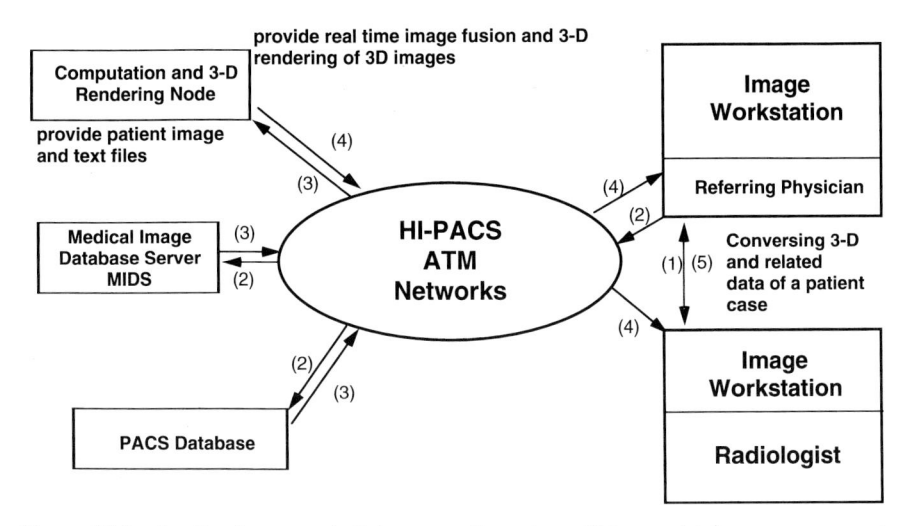

Figure 17.5 Application scenario 2: image conferencing with image database query support. Refer to text for numerals.

mapping of the 3-D-rendered brain function (PET, red) to anatomy (MRI, black and white) based on image content matching.

17.5 DISTRIBUTED COMPUTING

17.5.1 Concept of Distributed Computing

The basic idea of distributed computing is that if several computers are networked together, the workload can be divided into smaller pieces for each computer to work on. In principle, when n computers are networked, the total processing time can be reduced down to $1/n$ of the processing time of a single computer. It should be noted that this theoretical limit is unlikely to be achieved because of the unavoidability of various overheads, most likely due to data communication latency.

Two important factors affect the design of a distributed computing algorithm. Processor speed variations in different computers make it important to implement the mechanism to balance the workload in distributed computing in a way that allows faster computers to be given more work to do. Otherwise, the speed of the processing is essentially dictated by the capabilities of the slowest computers in the network. Data communication speed is another factor to consider. If workstations are connected by conventional Ethernet, with a maximum data transfer rate of 10 Mbit/s, the slow data transfer rate will limit the application of the distributed computing to CPU-intensive problems and areas where data communication is sparse. Increased implementation of the ATM and gigabit Ethernet technologies will widen the parameter regime in which distributed computing is applicable.

The minimum requirement for distributed computing is a networked computer sys-

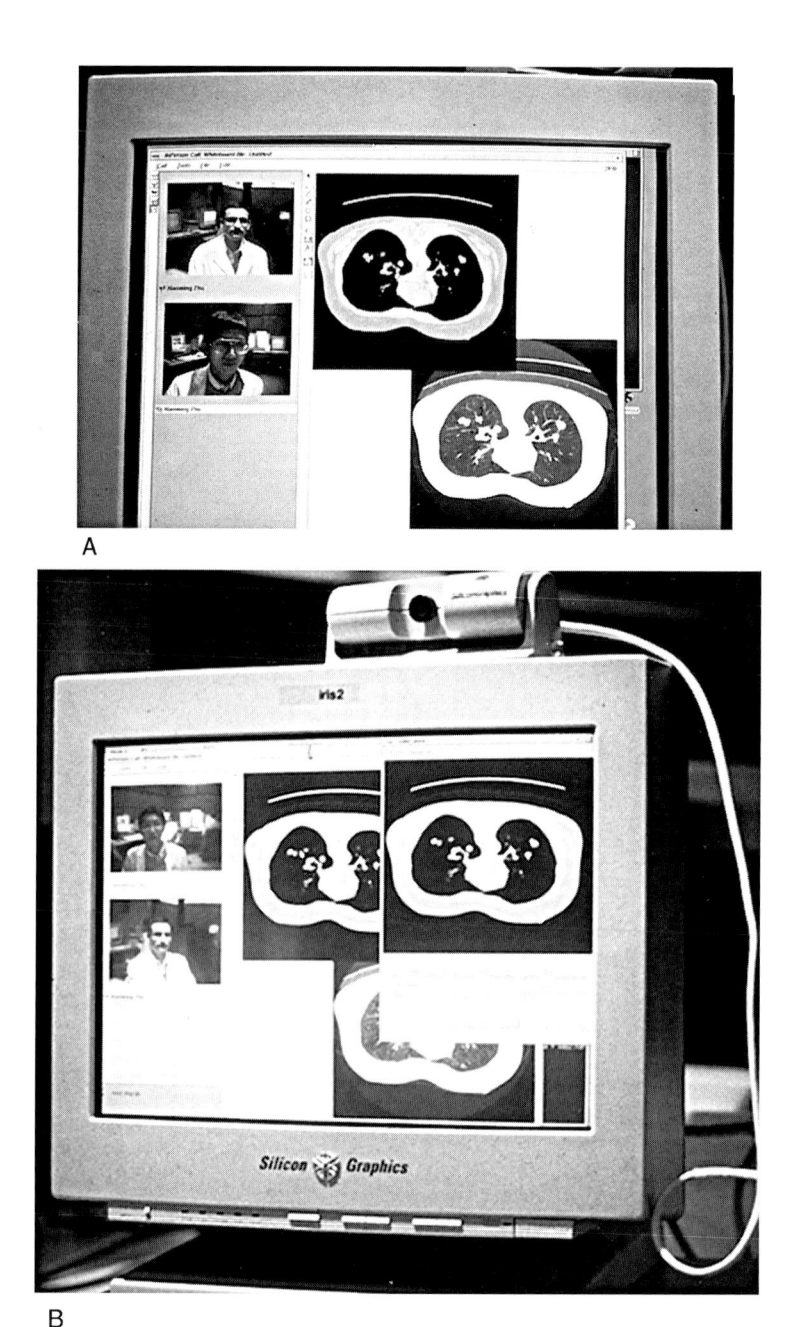

Figure 17.6 Video/image conferencing with PACS images at two workstations. (A) A video/image conferencing workstation with the left window showing two participants; right window shows two CT chest images with one active (controlled by this workstation) and one passive (controlled by the other workstation) arrows pointing to two lesions. CT images are shown with 8 bits/pixel without LUT capability. (B) The workstation at the other site with the participants in reverse positions. The two arrows are also in reversed positions. A third CT image has been requested by this workstation but it has not appeared in the first workstation yet. (Courtesy of Xiaoming Zhu.) (See color plate.)

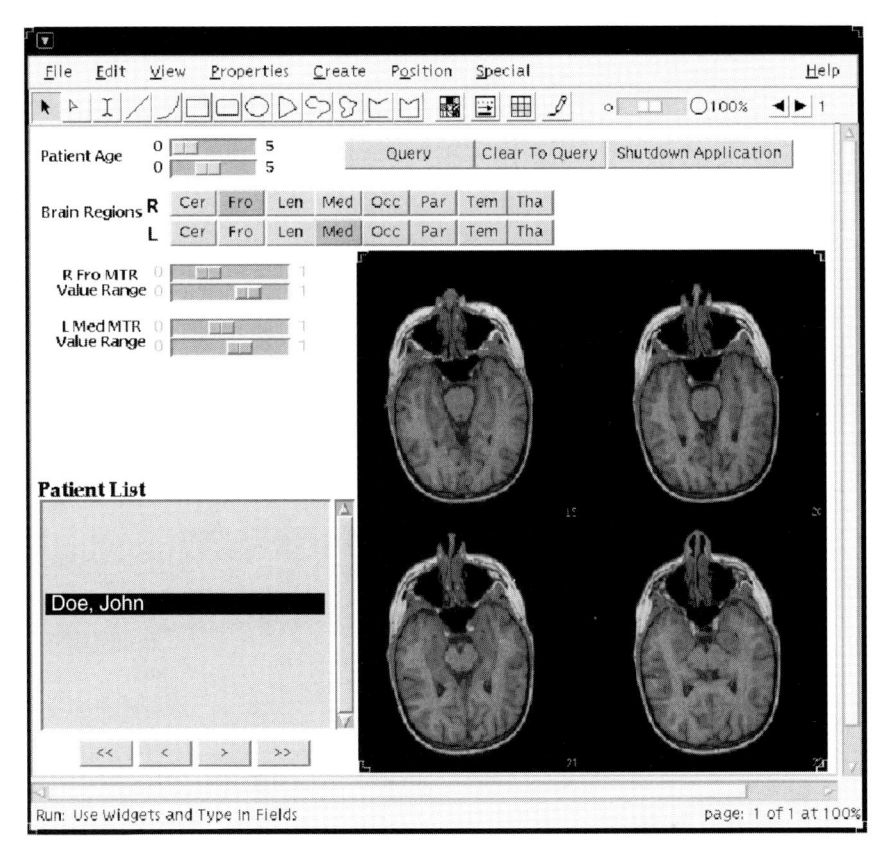

Figure 17.7 Image query by content and features in brain myelination disorders: R (L) FRO MTR, right (left) front magnetization transfer ratio. Easy-to-use graphic user interface allows image query by image content. (Courtesy of Steven Wong.)

tem with software that can coordinate the computers in the system to work coherently to solve a problem. There are several software implementations available for distributed computing; an example is the parallel virtual machine (PVM) system developed jointly by Oak Ridge National Laboratory, the University of Tennessee, and Emory University. PVM supports a variety of computer systems, including workstations by Sun Microsystems, Silicon Graphics, Hewlett-Packard, DEC/Alpha, and IBM-compatible personal computers running on a LINUX operating system.

After the PVM system has been installed in all computer systems, one can start the PVM task from any computer. Other computers can be added to or deleted from the PVM task interactively or by a software call to reconfigure the virtual machine. For computers under the same PVM task, any computer can start new PVM processes in others. Intercomputer communication is realized by passing messages back and forth, thus allowing the exchange of data among the computers in the virtual machine.

The parameter regimes for applicability of distributed computing are both problem and computer dependent. For distributed computing to be profitable, t_1, the time

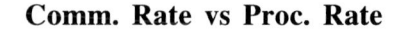

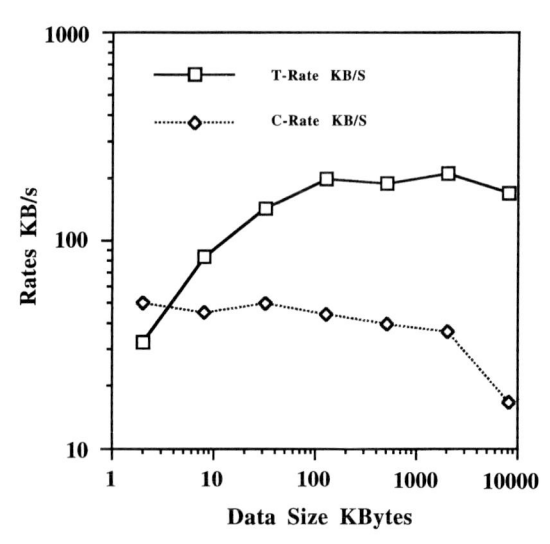

Figure 17.8 Distributed computing in a PACS environment. The solid curve represents computer-to-computer transmission rate (T-rate) under PVM and TCP/IP Ethernet connection, as a function of data size. The dotted curve represents data processing rate (C-rate) required to perform a 2-D FFT in a Sun SPARC-LX computer. The squares and diamonds represent the measured data points. Distributed computing is applicable only when the solid curve exceeds the dotted curve. (Courtesy of Xiaoming Zhu.)

interval required to send a given amount of data between two computers across the network, should be much shorter than t_2, the time needed to process them in a host computer. In other words, the network data communication rate (proportional to $1/t_1$) should be much higher than the data processing rate (proportional to $1/t_2$). The smaller the ratio of t_1 to t_2 or the higher the ratio of the two rates, the more advantages for distributed computing. If the ratio of the two rates is equal to or less than 1, there is no reason to use distributed computing, since too much time would be spent waiting for the results to be sent across the network back to the host computer. Thus, for $t_1 \leq t_2$, it is faster to use a single computer to do the calculation.

While the data communication rate can be estimated based on the network type and the communication protocol, the data processing rate depends both on the computer and on the nature of the problem. For a given workstation, more complex calculations lower the data processing rate. Since the computer system and the network are usually fixed within a given environment, the data processing rate depends more on the nature of the problem. Therefore, whenever a problem is given, one can estimate the ratio of the two rates and determine whether distributed computing is worthwhile. Figure 17.8 depicts the concept of distributed computing based on the data communication rate and processing rate. The graphics were obtained using the Sun SPARC LX computers and the Ethernet communication protocol. With the advances of ATM and gigabit Ethernet technologies in desktop computers, communication rates will render distributed computing attractive. Distributive computing is applicable only when the communication rate is above the computation rate. Immediate applications using distributed computing are image compression, unsharp masking, and enhancement, as well as computer-aided diagnosis, as discussed in Chapter 6 and Section 12.3.

17.5.2 Distributed Computing in a PACS Environment

Each image workstation in a PACS, when it is not in active use, consumes only a minimum of its capacity for running the background processes. As the number of image workstations grows, this excessive computational power can be exploited to perform value-added image processing functions for PACS images. Image processing is used extensively in the preprocessing stage, as in unsharp masking in CR, but it has not been popular in postprocessing (see Sections 4.1.6 and 12.3). One reason is that preprocessing can be done quickly through manufacturer's imaging modality hardware, which is application specific, and the execution time is fast. On the other hand, postprocessing depends on the image workstation which, in general, does not provide hardware image processing functions beyond such simple functions as lookup table, zoom, and scroll. For this reason, at the image workstation, the user very seldom uses time-consuming image processing functions, even though some, like unsharp masking, are effective. The multi-image workstation PACS environment allows the investigation of distributed computing for image processing by taking advantage of the excessive computational power available from the workstations. Conceptually, distributed computing will allow the acceleration of time-consuming image processing functions, with the result that the user will demand image postprocessing tools that can improve medical service by providing near-real-time performance at the image workstation.

In distributed computing, several networked image workstations can be used for computationally intensive image processing functions by distributing the workload to these workstations. Thus, the image processing time can be reduced at a rate inversely proportional to the number of workstations used. Distributed computing requires several workstations linked together by means of a high speed network, but these conditions are within the realm of a PACS in its number of workstations and the ATM and gigabit Ethernet technologies. Figure 17.9 depicts the concept of distributed computing in a PACS network environment using a three-dimensional data set as an example.

17.6 AUTHENTICITY FOR PACS IMAGES AND RECORDS

17.6.1 Background

A digital radiology environment supported by picture archiving and communication systems raises a new issue: how to establish trust in multimedia medical data that exist only in the easily altered memory of the computer. Trust is characterized in terms of integrity and privacy of digital data. Two major self-enforcing techniques can be used to assure the authenticity of electronic images and text—key-based cryptography and digital time stamping.

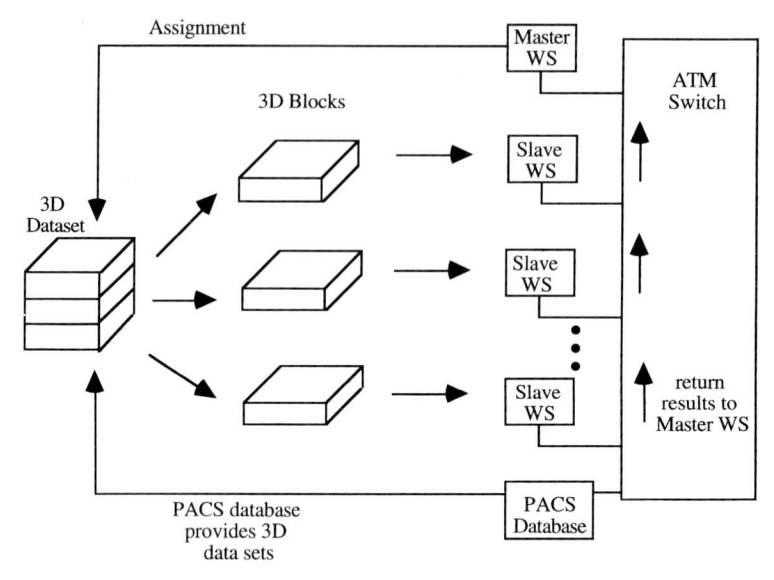

Figure 17.9 Procedure in distributed computing: master workstation requests 3-D data from the PACS database and assigns 3-D blocks to each slave workstation (WS) for the computation task. Each slave WS returns results to the master workstation, which compiles all results. (Courtesy of Jun Wang.)

Key-based cryptography associates the content of an image with the originator, using one or two distinct keys, and prevents alteration of the document by anyone other than the originator (Schneier, 1993). It can be further classified into algorithms of three general types. First, in secret key algorithms, the encryption key and the decryption key are the same. Second, in public key algorithms, the public encryption key is different from the private decryption key. Third, in digital signatures, image data are encrypted with the private key and decrypted with the public key. On the other hand, a digital time-stamping algorithm does not involve keys. It generates a characteristic "digital fingerprint" for an image when it is first generated, using a mathematical hash function, and checks that it has not been modified since then by anyone. The digital notary concept involving a third party further refines the time-stamping method by blending several sequential time stamp requests into a chain or tree structure (Cipra, 1993).

17.6.2 Key-Based Cryptographic Algorithms

The three general forms of key-based cryptographic algorithms are classified according to the nature of the encryption and decryption keys. This section reviews their principles briefly and provides an example. Secret or private key algorithms use an encryption key that can be calculated from the decryption key and vice versa. In many such cryptosystems, the encryption and the decryption key are the same. These algorithms require the sender and the receiver to agree on a key before they pass messages back and forth. This key must be kept secret, and therefore the security of such symmetric algorithms rests in the key.

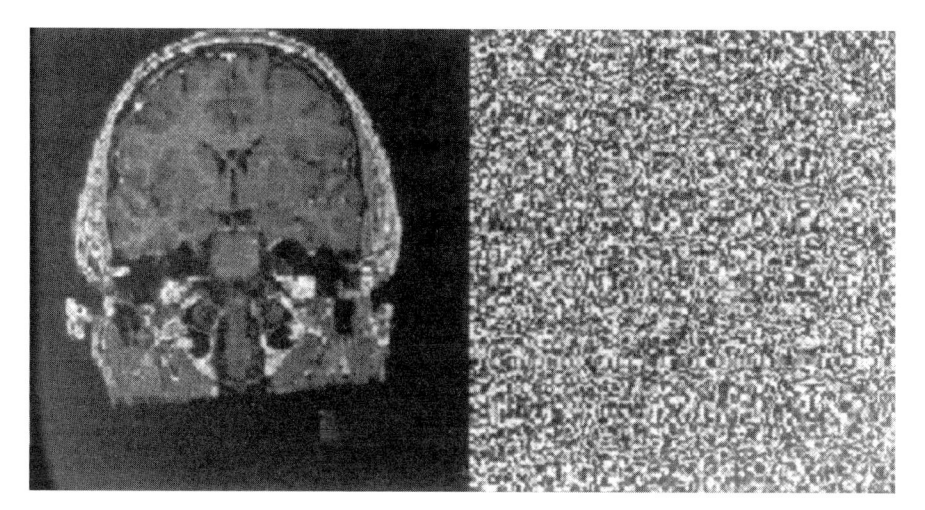

Figure 17.10 An MR image (L) and its encrypted form (R) using the IDEA PGP package. (Courtesy of Steven Wong.)

Figure 17.10 presents an example of software implementation of a secret key cipher on an 8-bit magnetic resonance image, where the left-hand side is the original, and the right-hand side is the encrypted image. The cipher used is the IDEA (International Data Encryption Algorithm) implementation from Phil Zimmermann's PGP (Pretty Good Privacy) package (Davies and Price, 1980). The secret key length is 128 bits and it would require 2^{128} (or 10^{38}) encryptions to recover the key. Figure 17.11 is the corresponding histogram of the encrypted image. Note that the gray level frequencies are very evenly distributed over all gray levels. The main drawback to a private key algorithm is that anyone with the key can both encode and decode messages

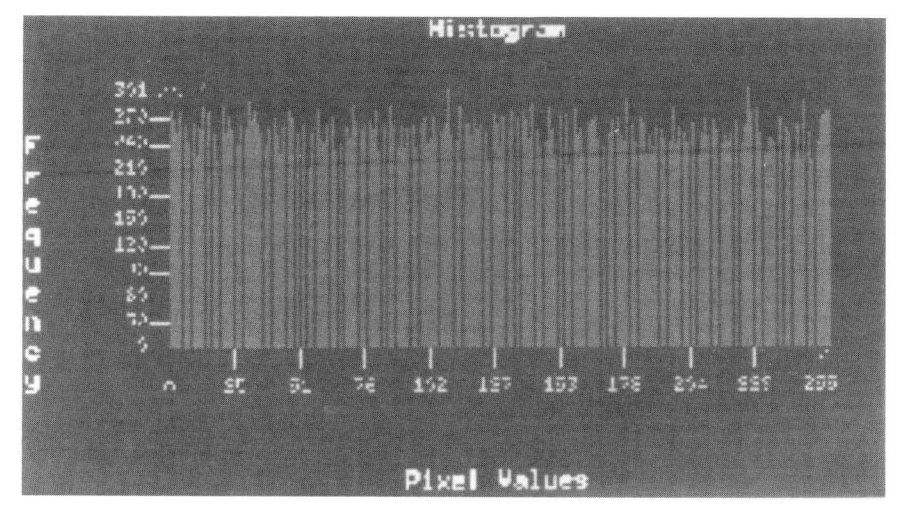

Figure 17.11 Histogram distribution of the encrypted image shown in Figure 17.10 (R). (Courtesy of Steven Wong.)

TABLE 17.2 Three General Types of Key-Based Cryptography

Type of Cryptography	Status of Keys*	
	Same or Different	Public or Private
Secret Key	e = d	e and d are private
Public-key	e ≠ d	e public, d private
Digital Signature	e ≠ d	e private, d public

*e, encryption key; d, decryption key.

and images. If the key is intercepted, any message can be compromised. Also, the management of keys involved in a cryptographic protocol creates a problem, since the total number of keys increases rapidly as the number of users increases.

The key management problem of secret key ciphers can be alleviated by the public key cryptography. In this case, two different keys are used: one public and one private. Information is encoded by the sender with the recipient's public key but can be decoded only by the designated recipient, who possesses the private key. Moreover, the public key contains no hint as to the nature of the private key. Anyone with the public key (which, presumably, is made public by the owner) can encrypt a message but not decrypt it. Only the person with the private key can decrypt the message. The disadvantage of the public key encryption algorithm is that it is much slower than conventional single key encryption, and therefore is impractical for implementation.

Digital signatures can be accomplished in some public key algorithms by encoding images with the sender's private key and deciphering them with the sender's public key. Encrypting a medical image using the physician's private key generates a secure digital signature. Often, digital signatures include time stamps. The date and time of the signature are attached to the image and signed along with the rest of the images. The PACS can store this time stamp in its image archive, which can be used for future reference. In practical implementation, public key algorithms are often too inefficient to use in the encryption of large documents such as medical images. Table 17.2 summarizes the three general types of key-based cryptography.

Key-based encryption techniques, along with digital time stamp methods, form the foundation for investigating the authenticity of PACS images. However, as of today, no dedicated research is being carried out in the medical imaging field. Image authenticity will become a major social issue as more PACS are gradually integrated into daily clinical practice. A concentrated effort by the medical imaging community is needed to resolve this important issue.

17.7 INTEGRATION OF MULTIPLE PACS

When health care centers with large-scale or small-scale PACS are merging for managed care or other financial and operational reasons, the need to integrate multiple PACS as a single operational unit must be addressed. The U.S. military establishment also faces similar problems when images and related data must be transmitted through

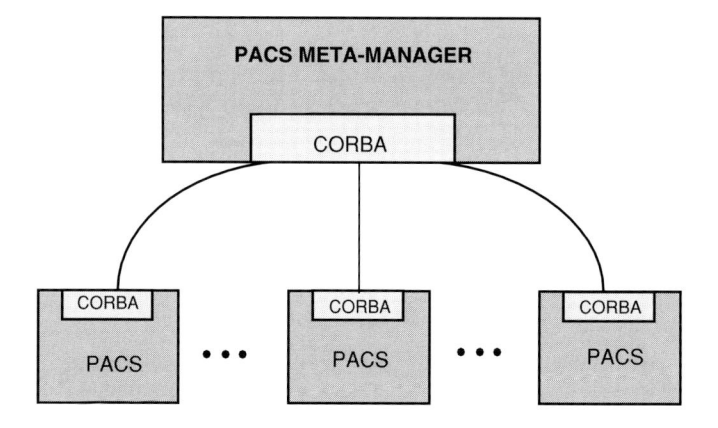

Figure 17.12 Concept of using a meta-manager for the integration of multiple PACS.

CORBA: Common Object Request Broker Architecture

different army medical centers, regional medical commands, and medical treatment facilities. This question is not unique in PACS, for other information systems face similar challenges when they have to be merged. The difference between PACS and other information systems is that the former contains many large image files, which the traditional information systems do not have. Therefore, the integration of multiple PACS calls for consideration of the archiving, transmission, retrieval, and display of image files, and their integration. Merging these files created from different imaging modalities and various PACS, with technology ranging from very primitive to advanced, results in a nontrivial instance of system integration.

The current thought in this area of research and development is to create a virtue radiology environment (VRE) based on a metamanager. The result is a hyper-PACS. Figure 17.12 illustrates such a concept, where the connection between a PACS and the metamanager is through current software technology like CORBA (**c**ommon **o**bject request broker architecture) and Java (Section 13.3.1), and communication networks like the ATM. The U.S. military has defined such a project, called USAVRE (U.S. Army Virtual Radiology Environment), and is planning such an integration for all existing and future MDIS sites (Section 1.4.1).

17.8 CAD IN A PACS ENVIRONMENT

17.8.1 Computer-Aided Detection or Diagnosis

Computer-aided detection or diagnosis (CAD) is traditionally performed off-line in the sense that the data is acquired from an imaging modality either through a peripheral device or a network connection, from which image processing is performed to

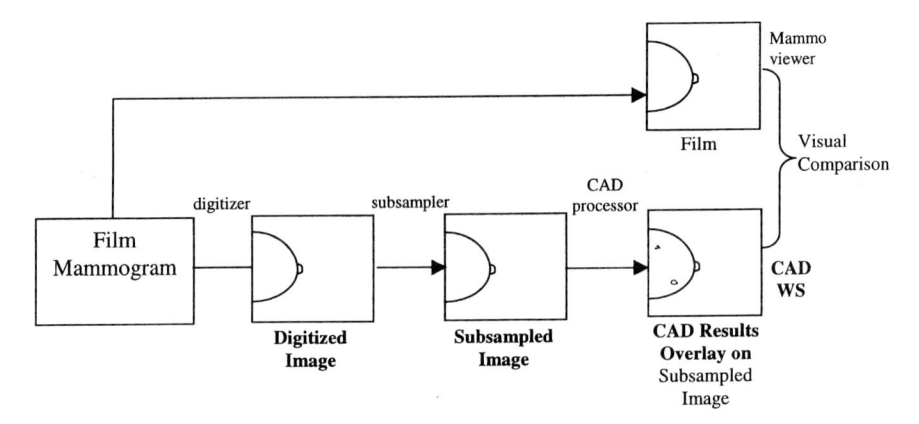

Figure 17.13 Dataflow in current method of CAD mammography.

extract relevant parameters. These parameters are used to alert the physician to pay more attention to certain regions in the image for potential ailment. This approach does not take advantage of PACS infrastructure. An example is CAD in mammography.

The current method of CAD in mammography uses film-based mammogram as input. The film is first digitized, subsampled, and then fed into a processor containing CAD algorithms for detection of microcalcification and masses. Results from the CAD are superimposed on the subsampled mammogram and displayed on a CAD workstation with a low resolution monitor(s). A standard light box is used to display the mammogram so that a visual comparison between the film and the subsampled image overlayed with CAD-detected lesions can be performed. This off-line method is a two-step process requiring special hardware to accomplish the CAD task. Hardware components in such a system consist of a film digitizer, a workstation, a CAD processor, and a light box. Figure 17.13 depicts the hardware configuration and the operation procedure.

CAD can be integrated in a PACS environment by taking advantage of the resources already available in PACS: image storage, retrieval mechanism, communication network, and display workstation. The bone age assessment described in Sections 17.2.3.1 and 18.1 is an example of integrating CAD in a PACS environment. In Section 17.8.3, we will discuss methods of integrating CAD in PACS from a system point of view.

TABLE 17.3 CAD Without PACS and with or Without Digital Input

- Collect films or digital images based on patient's record
- Digitize films or develop interface programs to read digital images
- Input images to the CAD workstation (WS)
- CAD algorithm
- Return results to CAD workstation WS

17.8.2 CAD without PACS

CAD without PACS can use either direct digital input or film with a digitizer. In either case, CAD is a totally isolated system. Table 17.3 lists the procedure of performing CAD in such a system. The current CAD system for mammography is an example.

17.8.3 Methods of integrating CAD in A PACS Environment with DICOM

There are four alternative approaches for the integration of CAD with DICOM PACS.

17.8.3.1 PACS WS Query/Retrieve (Q/R), CAD WS Detect

In the first approach the PACS workstation (WS) queries images from the PACS database, which are sent to the CAD WS where CAD is performed. Table 17.4 and Figure 17.14 illustrate the steps for the CAD. This method involves the PACS server, the

TABLE 17.4 CAD with DICOM PACS: First Approach (for PACS WS Q/R, and CAD WS Detect)

At the PACS server
- Connect CAD WS to PACS
- Register CAD WS (IP address, port number, application entity (AE)) title to receive images

At the PACS WS
- Use DICOM Query/Retrieve to select Patient/Studies/Images
- Use C-GET to select images from server to CAD WS

At the CAD WS
- Develop DICOM storage class provider to accept images
- CAD
- Develop database to archive results

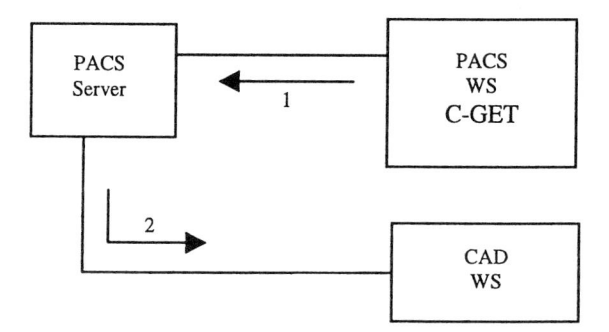

Figure 17.14 PACS WS Q/R, CAD WS Detect.

PACS WS, and the CAD WS. A DICOM Storage Service Class has to be installed in the CAD WS.

17.8.3.2 CAD WS Q/R and Detect

It is also possible for the CAD WS to query and retrieve the images, and then perform the CAD. This method involves only the PACS server and the CAD WS. The function of the PACS server is identical to that of the last method. The difference is that the last method uses the PACS WS to query, whereas in this method the CAD WS queries. Because of this, DICOM Q/R and Storage Service Class must be installed in the CAD WS. Table 17.5 and Figure 17.15 describe the steps.

17.8.3.3 CAD Server

In another method, a CAD server, developed to be connected to the PACS server, is used to serve all CAD workstations. Figure 17.16 shows the schematic of how the architecture of the CAD server is connected to the PACS. This concept is similar to the

TABLE 17.5 CAD With DICOM PACS: Second Approach (for CAD WS Q/R, and Detect)

At the PACS server
- Connect CAD WS to PACS
- Register CAD WS (IP address, port number, AE title) at PACS

From the CAD WS
- Develop DICOM Q/R Client and Storage Class to select/accept Patient/Study/Images
- CAD
- Develop database to archive results

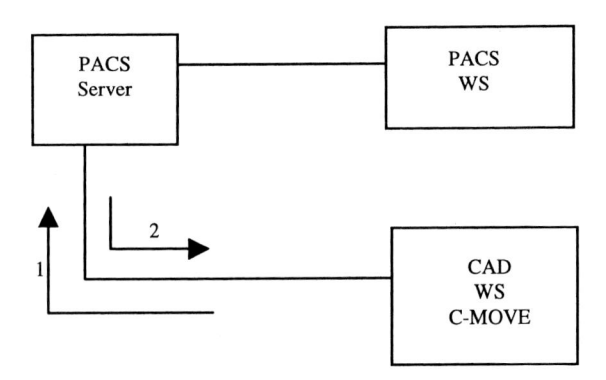

Figure 17.15 CAD WS Q/R and Detect.

TABLE 17.6 CAD with DICOM PACS: Third Approach (for CAD Server)

- Connect CAD server to PACS
- Server performs Q/R Patient/Study/Images from PACS
- Archive
- DICOM format decoder
- Distribute images to CAD WS

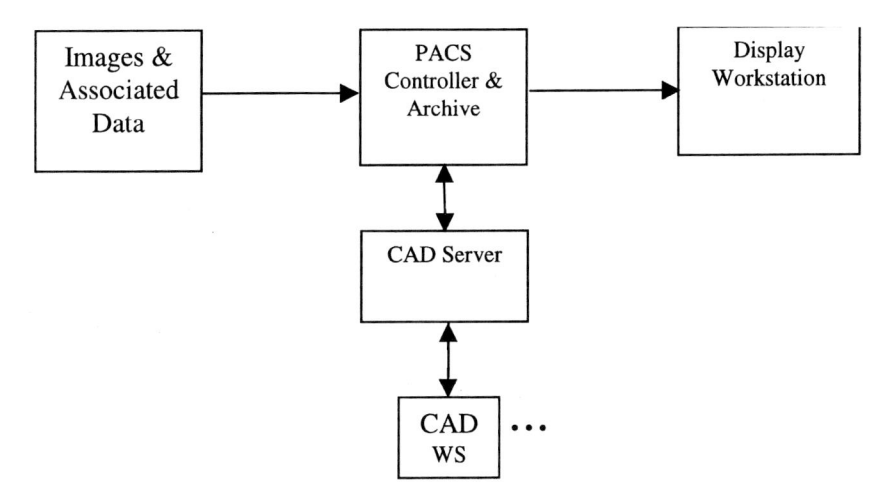

Figure 17.16 Integration of the CAD server in PACS.

distributed and Web servers described in Sections 13.2 and 13.3. Table 17.6 and Figure 17.16 describe the steps involved.

17.8.3.4 PACS WS with CAD Algorithm

The last approach is to install the CAD software in the PACS WS. This will eliminate all components in the CAD system and its connection to the PACS. Table 17.7 shows the steps involved.

TABLE 17.7 CAD with DICOM PACS: Fourth Approach (for PACS WS with CAD Software)

- Install CAD software at PACS WSs
- PACS WSs Q/R Patient/Study/Images
- Establish linkage for CAD software to access DICOM images
- Develop DICOM format decoder to CAD format
- CAD at PACS WS
- Develop CAD database to archive results

CHAPTER 18

PACS Applications

In Chapter 17, we presented PACS current development trends and future research. We emphasized the importance of developing the medical image informatics infrastructure (MIII) based on the resources from PACS as a vehicle for large-scale horizontal and longitudinal research and clinical services. In this chapter we discuss four applications based on the MIII. These applications are either in the developmental stage or in clinical use.

18.1 BONE AGE ASSESSMENT WITH A DIGITAL HAND ATLAS

18.1.1 Background

Bone age assessment based on a radiological examination of a left hand and wrist is a procedure frequently performed to evaluate the growth of pediatric patients. It is universally used because of the multiple advantages of simplicity, minimum of radiation exposure, and availability of multiple ossification centers for evaluation of maturity. The main clinical uses of this examination include (1) evaluation of growth disorders due to endocrine abnormalities in the thyroid, pituitary, or gonads; (2) determination of growth potential in children with abnormal stature and in children with various bone dysplasias, syndromes, and nutritional abnormalities; (3) monitoring of therapy effects, such as administration of growth or sex hormones; and (4) determination of the best time for intervention to correct scoliosis or limb length discrepancies.

Atlas matching methods currently used in radiological diagnosis compare the diagnosed image with a set of atlas patterns that in most cases includes one hand image pattern per year of age. A reference set of data, developed in the 1930s and published in the Greulich and Pyle atlas (1959), is not fully applicable to children of today. It does not reflect the standard development, particularly in black girls and white boys. The discrepancy in these two groups can range from 0.4 to 0.9 year.

To increase the accuracy of the bone age assessment, an upgraded set of reference radiographs must be collected. For each age group, various images should be available. Moreover, the diagnosis ought to be based on quantitative features extracted from the diagnosed images and their comparison with the corresponding values of an upgraded reference set. The goal of the digital atlas is to collect a large standard set of normal hand and wrist radiographs associated with automatically extracted measures, to form a basis for computer-assisted bone age assessment. This application is based on three hypotheses:

1. A reference set of clinically normal radiographs can serve as a digital atlas for use in clinical diagnosis, teaching, and research.
2. Computer-assisted assessment of skeletal development can extract radiological findings from a patient image and allow for comparison with corresponding values extracted from the digital atlas.
3. The database system can archive image data and radiological findings and allow them to be accessed from clinical workstations for automatic comparison.

18.1.2 Methodology

18.1.2.1 Selection of Reference Images for the Digital Atlas

MIII can access images and related data from the PACS database. The first step in this application is to select normally developed hand and wrist computed radiography (CR) or digitized film images from children by searching the PACS database. This collection of hand images and related data formulate the digital atlas.

18.1.2.2 Image Processing and Bone Age Assessment

Image processing functions are used to extract from hand images attributes that are related to bone age. These extracted attributes, obtained from three regions of interest (phalangeal, carpal, and epiphyseal), include phalangeal length and diameter, number and size of carpal bones, and degree of epiphyseal fusion. Based on these extracted attributes, derived parameters can be computed to compare with those extracted from images of known chronological age. From these comparisons, heuristic rules can be derived to assess the bone age of a patient from a CR hand image.

18.1.2.3 Database and Knowledge Base Management

The database is the digital hand atlas. The atlas is comprised of two types of data obtained from PACS: CR or digitized film hand images and related data from male and female subjects of various ethnic origins, and ages, and extracted attributes and derived parameters from these images. The knowledge base consists of heuristic rules for bone age assessment. These rules are derived by correlating the patient chronological age from PACS-related data with extracted parameters from the hand images. Software integration permits the digital atlas to associate with the knowledge base to allow for bone age assessment.

18.1.2.4 User Graphic Interface and Workstation

The graphic user interface and interactive communication software is located at the hand atlas workstation. Its major function is to assist the user to perform an automat-

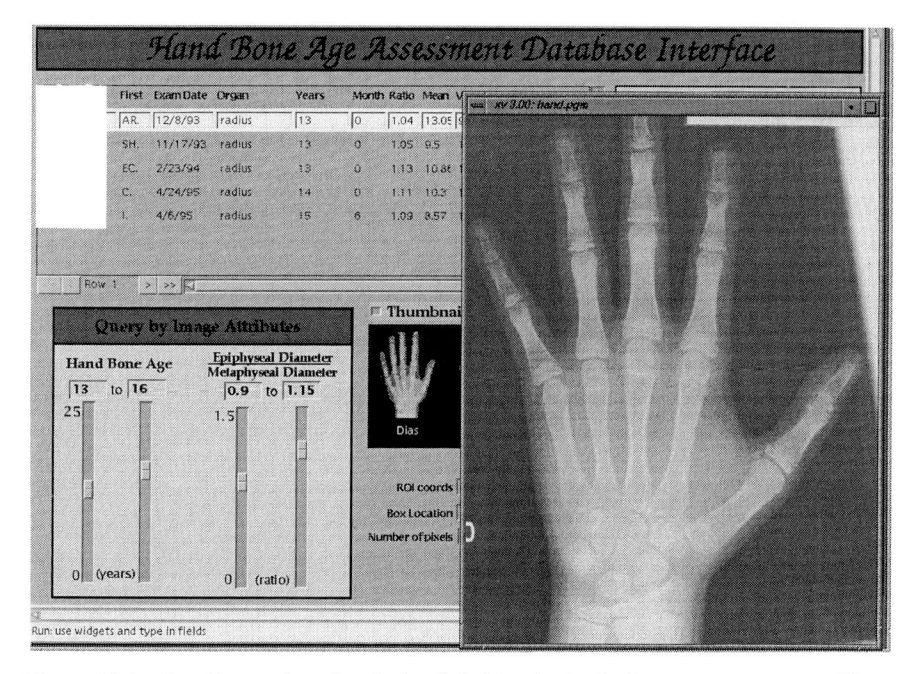

Figure 18.1 Graphic user interface in the digital hand atlas for bone age assessment. (Courtesy of K. Soo Hoo.)

ic bone assessment of a CR image from a patient based on the digital atlas. Other functions include requests from the database and the knowledge base to retrieve, compare, manipulate, analyze, and update related information concerning the patient under consideration. Figure 18.1 shows a page of the graphic user interface in a Sun SPARC workstation. A user-friendly environment allowing additional findings to be extracted interactively is the key to success of such a workstation. The connection of the input and workstation of the digital hand atlas for bone age assessment is depicted is Figure 18.2.

18.1.3 Operational Procedure

When a bone age assessment is required, the first step is to obtain a hand/wrist CR image from the patient. The physician retrieves this image from the PACS database and requests the digital atlas for an automatic bone assessment from the workstation. The system returns the bone age and the physician can request comparisons among patients with similar symptoms and age group. If the user is satisfied with the result, both the image and extracted data will be automatically appended in the atlas to increase its statistical power. If the result is doubtful, different queries can be invoked to elicit other alternatives from the atlas. Figure 18.3 shows the use of the digital atlas to assess bone age.

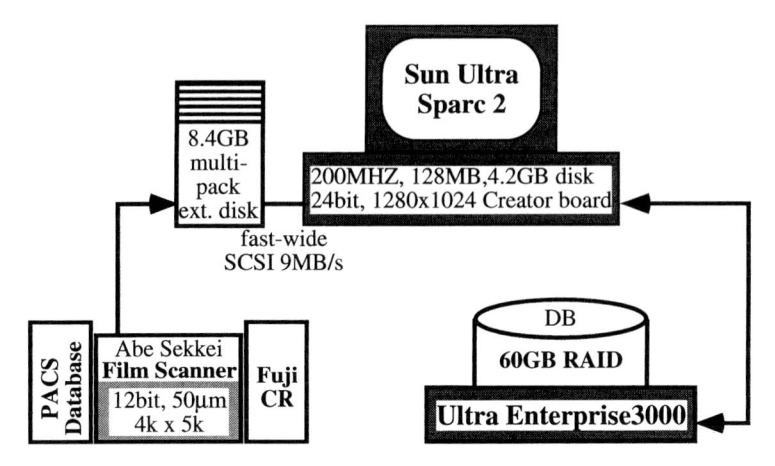

Figure 18.2 Digital hand atlas system configuration and the workstation.

18.1.4 Clinical Evaluation

A digital atlas approach for bone age assessment permits the diagnosis to be standardized and to become more objective and reproducible. All findings (radiological and clinical) can be stored to enrich the atlas for future reference. An advantage of using the MIII approach for large-scale longitudinal and horizontal clinical studies and applications is the ease of developing evaluation criteria and improving the performance of the digital atlas. The accuracy of each assessment can be automatically logged and scored. The results can be used to improve the performance of the atlas.

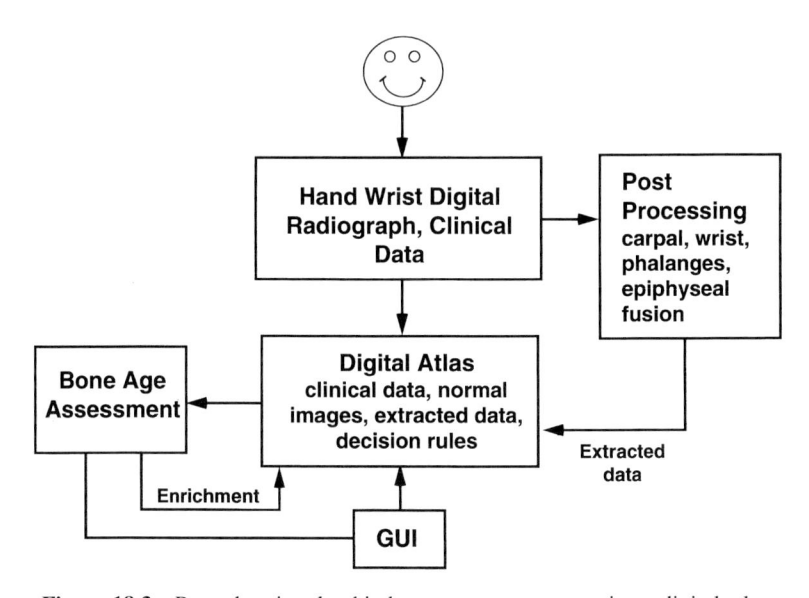

Figure 18.3 Procedure involved in bone age assessment using a digital atlas.

The current status of this application is in data collection and knowledge base development.

18.2 OUTCOME ANALYSIS OF A LUNG NODULE WITH TEMPORAL CT IMAGE DATABASE

18.2.1 Background

Although the progression of lung nodules over time can be monitored qualitatively by means of spiral CT scans, a qualitative result alone is not sufficient for assessing the effectiveness of ongoing therapeutic treatment. Outcome analysis using CT requires an application-specific temporal image database management system connected to the PACS server, and necessary image processing tools to extract the tumor volume from longitudinal CT scans. Without these tools, the quantitative description of the effectiveness of a treatment plan to control the disease is a formidable task. However, to perform a longitudinal quantitative analysis requires access to temporal CT images with related patient records through time using the PACS database, and derivation of quantitative measures from the lesions. These requirements fall into the domain of the MIII.

18.2.2 System Architecture

The design of the temporal medical image database is based on a three-tiered client/server architecture (Fig. 18.4). The image database (DB) server is a centrally located core of application programs for accessing, processing, and managing chest CT images and associated textual reports from the RIS and HIS. The server consists

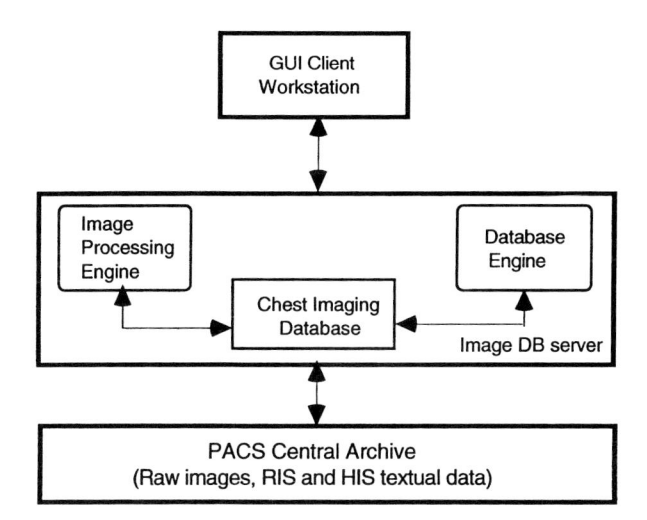

Figure 18.4 The three-tiered client/server architecture of the temporal chest imaging database system.

476 PACS APPLICATIONS

of three components: a chest imaging database to store CT images and processed multimedia chest data, a relational database engine, and an image processing engine.

Medical images and text are retrieved from the PACS archive server through the DICOM interface. The image processing engine consists of necessary segmentation and user interface tools for interactive editing of the outline of the segmented tumor. It also has functions for various quantitative measurements related to tumor size and shape. The CT images, the extracted tumors, and their measurements are stored in the chest image database. The relational database engine is used for the tabulation of data from the chest image database for outcome analysis. Since the image processing functions are standard tools available in the public domain, they are not elaborated here. Instead, we discuss the graphic user interface at the workstation.

18.2.3 Graphic User Interface

Figure 18.5A shows the layout of the graphic user interface. When a particular patient is selected, the image of a predetermined spiral CT slice is displayed in the left window.

When a nodule is identified visually, the user initiates the image processing tools by moving the mouse pointer anywhere within the nodule and then clicking the mouse button to activate a series of image processing steps to segment out the nodule and to calculate 3-D information of the nodule automatically. When the calculation is complete, a popup window will appear to allow the user to inspect the result of automatic segmentation, as shown in the right bottom window in Figure 18.5A. If the result is satisfactory, the 3-D nodule information will be stored in the chest imaging database. Otherwise, the user can interactively correct any segmentation errors as follows. A second popup window magnifies the image, with all pixels segmented as the nodule marked by a plus "+" sign. The user can easily include or exclude one pixel by clicking the mouse at the pixel position. The corrected nodule is then stored. The top row in the upper window in the Figure 18.5A shows the segmented nodules from different CT slices.

To ensure that a nodule is not calculated twice, the processed nodules will turn red on the display (Fig. 18.5B). This feature is found to be helpful for metastatic applications, since a patient with lung metastases usually has many nodules and it is difficult to keep track of which ones have been processed.

18.2.4 An Example

18.2.4.1 Case History

We illustrate a case of a woman with lung metastases to demonstrate the usefulness of the temporal database system. In 1989 the patient, who had a family history of breast cancer, complained of a small lump in her breast, which was found to be benign after aspiration. Two years later (1991), she complained of two small masses, one in each breast. Excisional biopsy and pathology showed that the right one was a breast carcinoma. The patient was treated with radiation therapy and chemotherapy. In 1993 multiple small lung nodules were detected in chest radiographs. Biopsy of

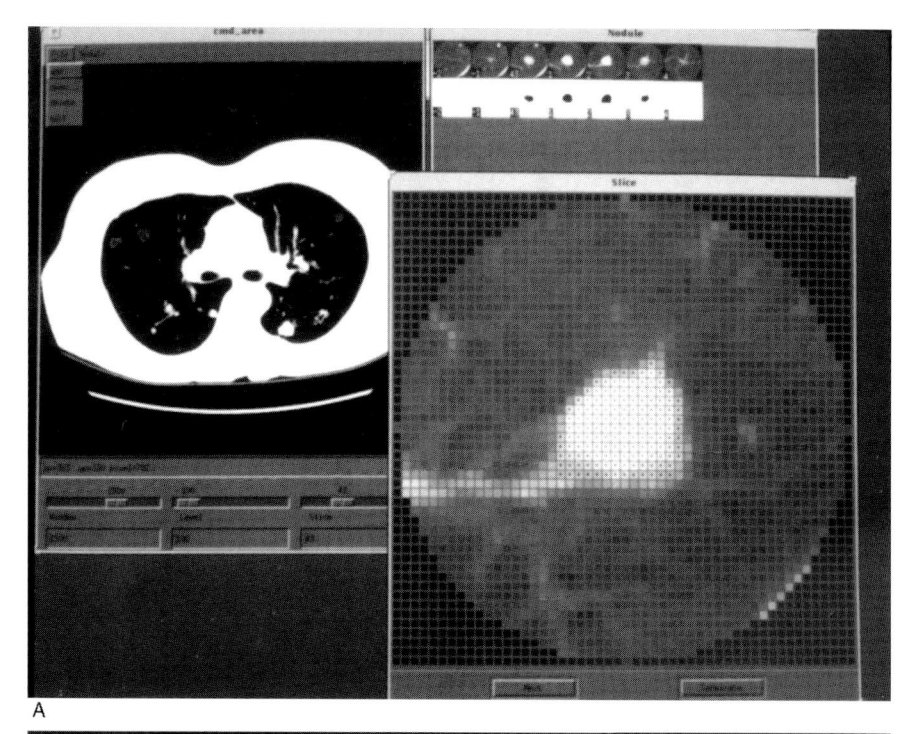

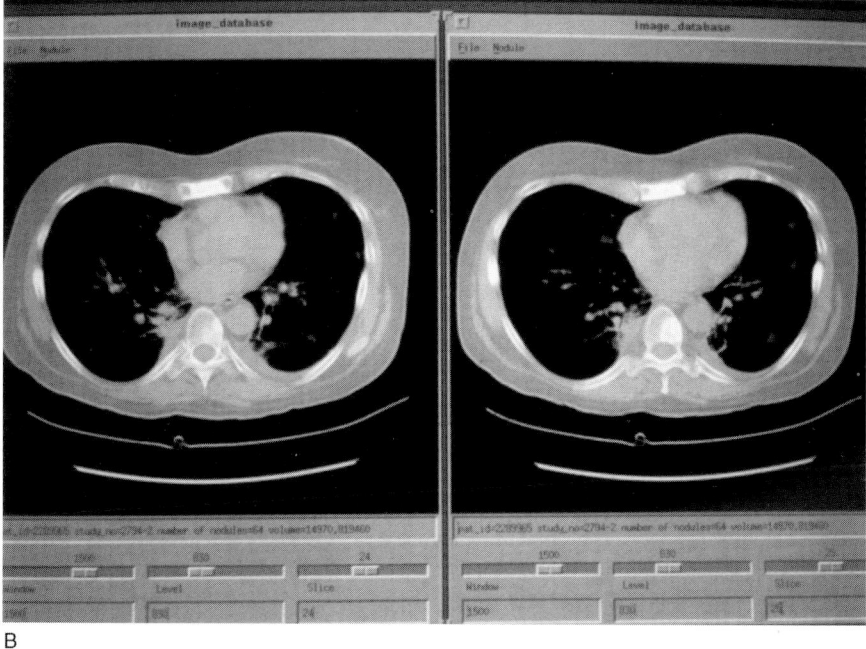

Figure 18.5 (A) Three windows in the graphic user interface. *Left:* a CT image. *Lower right:* an enlarged segmented nodule; + signs are the lesion pixels. *Upper right:* segmented nodules from CT scans stored in the chest image database. (B) Processed nodules in a CT image is turned "red" color to ensure that a nodule is not processed twice. Two consecutive sections are shown. (See color plate.)

the nodules revealed adenocarcinomas. The patient was given various chemotherapeutic agents. Between September 1994 and March 1995, the patient was given several experimental agents. In March 1995, marked progression of the lung metastatic nodules was found on a chest CT examination. Diffuse bone metastasis were also noted. After March 1995, the patient received Taxol treatment (chemotherapy) and in June radiation therapy (4500 cGy) to her thoracic spine. After radiation therapy, adriamycin (chemotherapy) was administered. The problem posed is how to assess the effectiveness of the treatment plan quantitatively.

18.2.4.2 Temporal Assessment

From the PACS archive server, a total of five spiral CT studies of the patient were retrieved and deposited in the temporal image database management system. The first was in August 1994, while the most recent one was in November 1995. The first two studies were scanned at 5 mm collimation, and the images were reconstructed with 3 mm slice thickness. The last three studies, which were performed by a different radiologist, were scanned at 7 mm collimation and reconstructed with 7 mm slice spacing. Nodule segmentation and volume estimates were performed by a radiologist aided with the software tools. The total volume and the mass center of each nodule were saved into the database. After all nodules in five studies had been segmented, the progression of the lung disease was tabulated by means of the relational database engine and could be graphically displayed as in Figure 18.6. The horizontal axis plots time. The vertical axes plots number of nodules (scale at left) and total volume of the nodules in each study (scale at right). The volume is measured in cubic millimeters. Below the horizontal axis, two lines denote the intervals during which the patient was under different treatment plans. In the first interval, the patient was taking an experimental medication. Unfortunately both nodule volume and nodule number grew with time. Total nodule volume tripled during this experimental period. After March 1995, the patient was under a combination of chemotherapy and radiation therapy, which effectively in controlled tumor volume. We can note that the total volume of the cancer reduces by a factor of 5 from its peak value in March 1995.

18.2.5 Temporal Image Database and the MIII

The temporal image database relies on extensive searching of the PACS archive server for relevant CT examinations. This search is simple, quick, and reliable. Without the PACS search, this type of outcome analysis using longitudinal images is extremely difficult to perform owing to the logistics of data collection. The image processing engine contains standard image processing functions for segmentation and interactive editing. The chest image database is designed such that the original, segmented nodules, as well as the processed data, are organized to permit the relational database to analyze the treatment outcome. The three major components in the temporal image database are subcomponents in the MIII infrastructure shown in Figure 13.8 and described in Section 13.4. Once the MIII has been established, the majority building blocks of the temporal image database are always readily available.

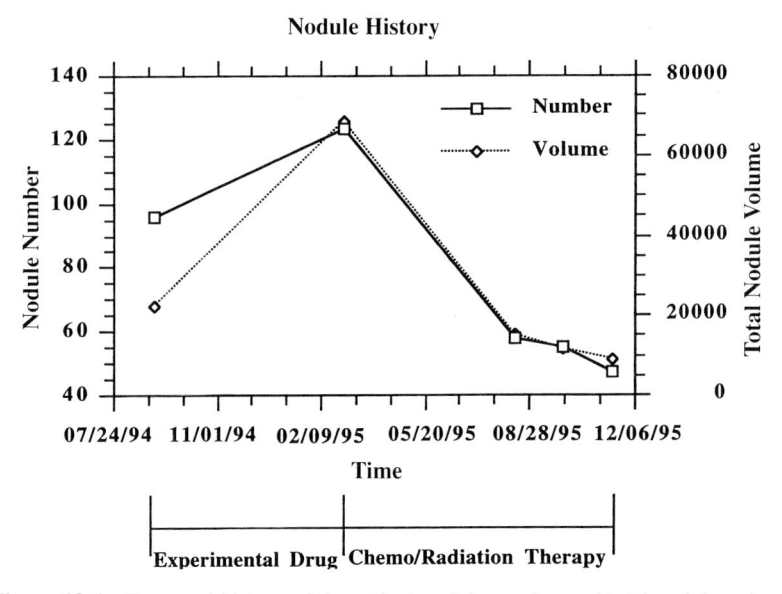

Figure 18.6 Temporal history of the patient nodule number and total nodule volume.

18.3 INTERACTIVE DIGITAL BREAST IMAGING TEACHING FILE

18.3.1 Background

Routine screening with periodic mammography has proven to be effective for the early detection of breast cancer and in lowering its death rate. Because of limited resources and facilities that provide hands-on instruction in breast imaging interpretation, there is a need to develop an alternate method to supplement or replace the current film-based teaching file method of training. A digital-based system could alleviate this shortage, since a digital teaching file can be duplicated easily with preservation of quality. Copies so created can be disseminated widely, for simultaneous use by many individuals at different sites providing continuing medical education. This approach promises to improve the quality of breast imaging interpretation, and thereby facilitate mass screening with mammography and the problem-solving imaging evaluation of screening-detected abnormalities.

Currently there is no digital mammography teaching file fully adequate for clinical use. This is due in part to the relatively low resolution of currently affordable display monitors and to the relatively slow speed required to manipulate large digital mammogram images (20–40 Mbyte for each image). The basic requirement for the general use of a mammography display workstation is the ability to show an entire breast with such fine detail that tiny structures are readily visible (Figs. 12.7, 12.8).

There has been only limited success in applying computer-aided instruction (CAI) to mammography teaching files, in part because of difficulties in handling high resolution images and in simulating an interactive teaching session. Furthermore, previous CAI models have not required the user to identify abnormalities by marking displayed images, a substantial deficiency because this practice represents one of the key elements in breast imaging interpretation. In addition, CAI models should be designed to allow the user to follow more than one suitable approach to working up a specific breast imaging problem for cases in which several such approaches are valid. These features all should be incorporated into a successful, clinically relevant CAI model. To serve as a useful instructional tool, an interactive digital teaching file should also contain large sets of cases selected and prepared by expert mammographers. These images can be retrieved from the PACS database.

This application is to develop an interactive digital breast imaging teaching file as a training tool for educational purposes using some existing components in the MIII. The CAI model was developed based on a digital mammography workstation described in Figures 12.7 and 12.8 (this workstation has since been upgraded to the Sun UltraSPARC II and DOME imaging display boards).

18.3.2 Computer-Aided Instruction Model

The interactive teaching file is based on a computer-aided instruction model, which specifies the sequence of questions, image display, instructions, and explanations of cases dynamically, based on user responses during an interactive teaching session. CAI permits image visualization, allows the user to detect imaging abnormalities by pointing and clicking on the 2K monitors, provides questions, displays both correct and incorrect answers, and leads the user through the analysis and management of each case in a clinically relevant sequence. Follow-up questions are included in most cases, once the user has determined the correct diagnosis and management.

The CAI is best explained by using the general work flow of this model shown in Figures 18.7 and 18.8. Figure 18.7 shows the workup sequence of a question with a simple true/false or multiple-choice answer, whereas Figure 18.8 involves follow-up questions based on the choice of the first answer. At the start of a case, the system gives a brief description of the case history and then presents to the user a set of digital mammograms on a two monitor 2K workstation (left-most box, Exam Images, Fig. 18.7). After examining those images, the user is asked to use a mouse pointer to identify on the monitors any mammographic abnormalities, as shown in Figure 18.7. The user's selection is compared with prerecorded region of interest (ROI) data. A user who succeeds in identifying the ROI will proceed to a multiple-choice or true/false question that is relevant to these findings; otherwise, he or she must try again. If a user has not marked the abnormality after three tries, the system will display the ROI on the monitor, accompanied by an explanation; the user then proceeds to the next question.

Based on user response, the computer system presents different workup sequences, defined in the CAI model as illustrated in Figure 18.7. The system provides instructions, explanations, and answers to the question, guiding the user toward the next question. During this process, additional images are displayed when appropriate. This work flow serves, in a structural way, to aid the user in navigating through the medical knowledge embedded in the teaching file cases. Note that a user cannot proceed beyond a multiple-choice question until the question has been answered correctly.

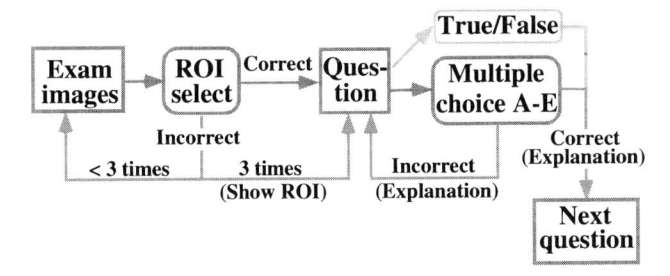

Figure 18.7 General algorithm for the CAI model and basic workup sequences.

The immediate repetition of an incorrectly answered question serves as a powerful educational device to reinforce correct answers.

There is often more than one suitable approach to working up a specific breast imaging problem. The questions and instruction sequences built into the CAI support this by accepting more than one choice as correct and by providing different pathways using tailored follow-up questions. Figure 18.8 shows, as an example, how the system can call up different workup sequences and follow-up questions in responding to user choices. Marking the abnormality, multiple-choice, and true/false questions are the three basic building blocks of the interactive teaching file. They are nested together to create an effective teaching tool.

18.3.3 The Teaching File Script and Data Collection

The teaching file consists of over 1000 pathologically proven cases, each of which begins with a mammography examination no more than 7 years old. The case material demonstrates the various problem-solving imaging approaches available in reaching accurate imaging diagnoses. Mammograms, as well as breast sonograms, CT images, and MR images (if they are included in the case), are collected from screening

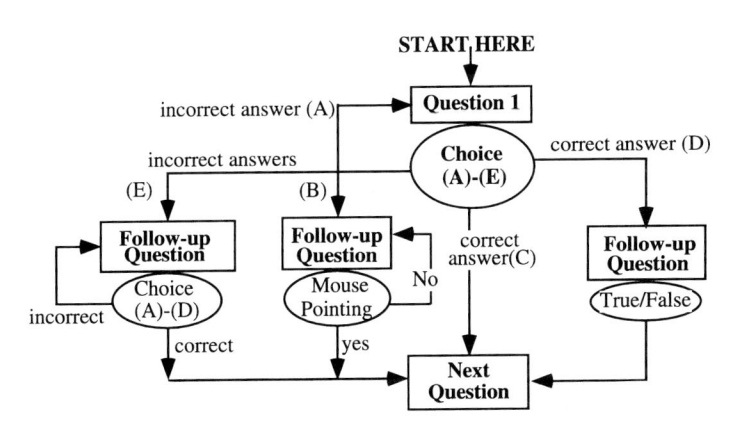

Figure 18.8 Example of nested building blocks and different workup sequences based on five possible choices, (A)–(E), for a hypothetical Question 1.

mammography examinations, digitized with the high resolution film scanner (2K × 2.5K × 12) if they are not already in digital format. Related medical information and image description textual data from PACS and RIS are inserted into the header record of the image files. The digitized images are currently formatted to the ACR-NEMA 2.0 standard.

To prepare a case for the teaching file, a radiologist uses the CAI interface to mark the appropriate regions of interest on the digital images, and uses the teaching file script (TFS) language to write the accompanying interactive teaching text. The TFS language is similar to but much simpler than the Hypertext Markup Language (HTML) used in home pages on the World Wide Web. It is simply an ordinary text file together with tags that tell the computer how to identify each element in the teaching file, how to query and display images, and how to respond to a teaching file user's actions.

After a case has been prepared, a navigational browser in the CAI package can be used to read and navigate through the TFS file, producing an interactive response-driven teaching session.

18.3.4 Graphic User Interface

An easy-to-use graphical user interface was designed for the interactive teaching file. It responds dynamically with detailed instructions to every action of the user. Combined with online help, the GUI makes it easy for the user to manipulate digital mammograms and navigate through the teaching session.

A user first types in his or her name on the login screen. The login process then captures the user name and starts the interactive teaching file program. User performance scores are time-stamped and recorded in a log file. Users also can click the Comments button to get a popup text editor window in which they can write comments and suggestions on how to improve the teaching file. Figure 18.9 shows the main control screen of the interactive teaching file.

Following Figure 18.9, the teaching session begins when the user selects the Start here button on the top-left corner, which presents the choice of starting a new session, resuming the preceding session, or starting at a specific case. At the left, the left-bottom, and the middle bottom of the screen, there is an array of image tools that allow the user to do window/level adjustments, image magnification, measurement, and image scrolling (up/down and left/right). At the right-bottom corner, there is a depiction of a mouse with three selections for manipulating individual images on the two 2K monitors. The online description of mouse button function is displayed dynamically during the session. The information window at the mid-right portion of the screen displays the case and question number, the number of correct and wrong answers, as well as the total elapsed time. The user navigation buttons are located at the middle of the screen. The user must click on these buttons to make choices, answer questions, and initiate the pointer for marking abnormalities on the 2K monitors. Teaching file text (questions and answers) and system navigation instructions are shown dynamically in the large upper central text window, according to the user's actions.

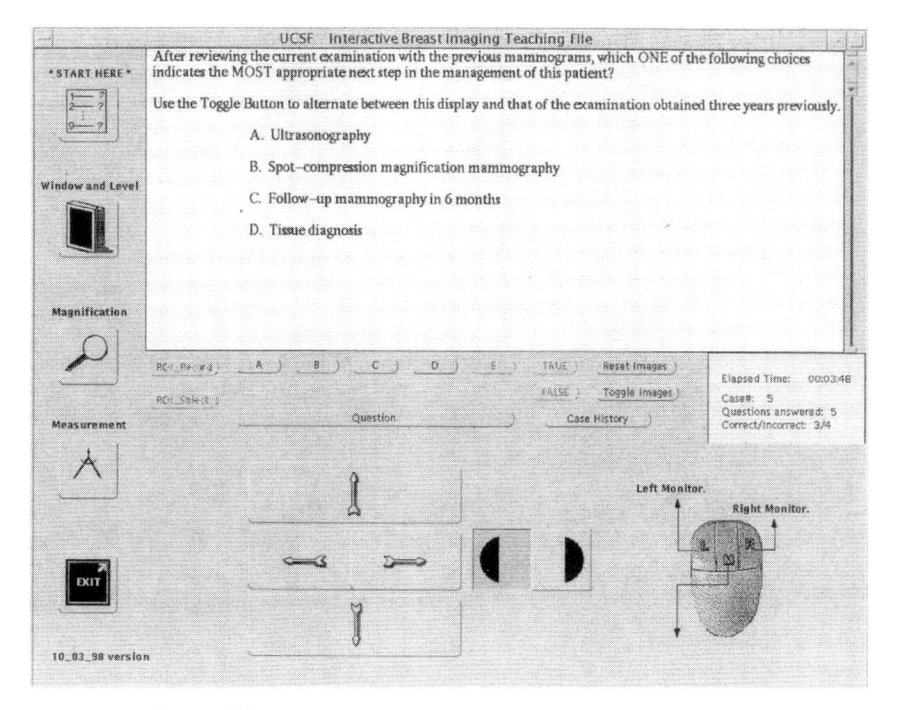

Figure 18.9 Main control screen of the interactive teaching file.

18.3.5 Interactive Teaching File as a Training Tool

The digital teaching file is available to all radiology residents, fellows, staff radiologists, and visiting radiologists for continuing medical education at UCSF. All radiology residents are now required to complete a set of 25 cases in the digital teaching file during each 4-week breast imaging rotation at UCSF. We also have incorporated the digital teaching file into several of the San Francisco–based postgraduate breast imaging courses given at UCSF. As of August, 1998, over 1,000 residents and fellows have been trained with this interactive teaching file in breast imaging.

The digital teaching file currently maintains 50 active cases, with approximately 500 digital mammograms and approximately 800 questions. It takes about 10 hours for an average user to complete a 50-case set. By means of the teaching file script and the image management tool described in Section 18.3.3, the breast imaging section constantly adds new cases, thereby replenishing the teaching file with new material. Mammograms of 1000 carefully selected cases are maintained in digital format in the PACS database, from which active case sets are updated periodically.

A comprehensive user log mechanism is used to record user activities. This system documents user progress and performance by time-stamping the user activity and recording the user's correct/wrong answers. The user is allowed to log off at any time in the middle of a session. The system automatically saves an unfinished session so that the user can resume from the point of logging off. The user log provides performance evaluation feedback for users and can be used to test the effectiveness of the digital teaching file compared with traditional film-based methods of teaching file instruction.

A mammography display must be able to portray the entire breast with such fine detail that tiny structures are readily visible. This display must be done at near real-time speed. The quality of digital mammograms is highly dependent on the original digital image, the film digitizer, and the display system; while the speed of image display and the on-screen image manipulation are determined by system hardware architecture and image processing software. All these components are included in the MIII. With hardware consisting of a two-monitor 2K display workstation and a high resolution film digitizer, the image quality of digitized and displayed mammograms has been found to be adequate and acceptable for interactive clinical teaching. The images from the new full-field direct digital mammography systems (Section 4.4.2) provide better quality mammograms, which are DICOM conformant for easier input to the interactive teaching file.

18.4 REAL-TIME TELECONSULTATION WITH HIGH RESOLUTION AND LARGE-VOLUME MEDICAL IMAGES

18.4.1 Background

The managed care trend in health care delivery systems is expediting the formation of teleradiology expert centers. In the expert center model of teleradiology (Section 14.3.1, Fig. 14.2), medical images are sent from the examination site to a remote site, where an expert radiologist makes the diagnosis. The report is sent to the examination site, where a primary physician can then prescribe the patient's treatment immediately. If the teleradiology procedure does not require manipulation of images by both sites, we call the arrangement telediagnosis or teleconferencing (Section 17.3, Fig. 17.6). If, on the other hand, interactive manipulation of images by both sites is required during teleradiology, the term "real-time teleconsultation" is applied. In real-time consultation, both sites need to synchronously manipulate and interpret high resolution digital radiographic images (16 MByte/exam) and/or large-volume MR/CT sequential images (8–20 MByte/exam). This application presents a teleconsultation system with bidirectional remote control using high resolution and large-volume medical images in a limited-bandwidth network environment.

The teleconsultation system meets the following requirements:

1. Provides real-time teleconsultation services with high resolution and large-volume medical images (MR, CT, CR, US, digital mammography).
2. Synchronously manipulates images on both local and remote sites, including remote cursor, window/level, zoom, cine mode, overlay, and measurement.
3. Supports multimedia, including audio and video (option) communications.
4. Interfaces to PACS database for image retrieval through the DICOM standard.
5. Allows the use of intranet (LAN) and Internet (WAN) environments with TCP/IP protocol.

6. Provides scalable network connections including ATM, Ethernet, and modem.
7. Uses low cost NT/PC-based hardware and software platform.

18.4.2 System Design

Teleconsultation involves a referring site and an expert site. Between these sites three kinds of data communication are necessary: images transferred from the referring physician or general radiologist site to the expert site; remote control messages between the two sites; and voice/video communication between the referring physician and the expert. Among these three types of data, image transmission requires a very high bandwidth network, but normally (i.e., in nonemergency cases), the images can be preloaded before the consultation session. Image preloading can be done with various kinds of network (e.g., ATM, T1 line, Ethernet, or telephone line through nonpeak hours, evenings, or weekends, dependent on the turnaround time requirement). Remote control message routing and voice communication are real-time, online procedures but with a low bandwidth requirement. Video communication requires ISDN with compression. Figure 18.10 shows a schematic of a teleconsultation system.

The hardware configuration of the teleconsultation system at each site includes the following:

1. One or more Pentium II NT workstations, each with 128 MB SDRAM, and 4 GByte hard disk, as well as Ethernet, ATM and modem connections.
2. One DOME Md2/PCI high resolution display board that can be configured to support a single monitor or dual monitors.
3. Two high resolution gray scale monitors.
4. One telephone or teleconference connection for audio or video communication.

The software package in the teleconsultation system consists of the following:

1. Image display graphic user interface for teleconsultation.
2. Event interpreter for local and remote message dispatching.
3. Remote control manager for routing messages between local and remote sites.
4. View and memory manager for view controlling and image data memory management.
5. Graphic manager for image rendering and display.
6. DICOM communication services for DICOM image receiving and sending between the teleconsultation workstations, scanners, and PACS server.
7. Image database for medical image display and teleconsultation authoring.

The data flow and network connection of the teleconsultation system in a clinical environment entail three sites: the general physician or radiologist site, the PACS archive server, and the expert site (Fig. 18.11).

486   PACS APPLICATIONS

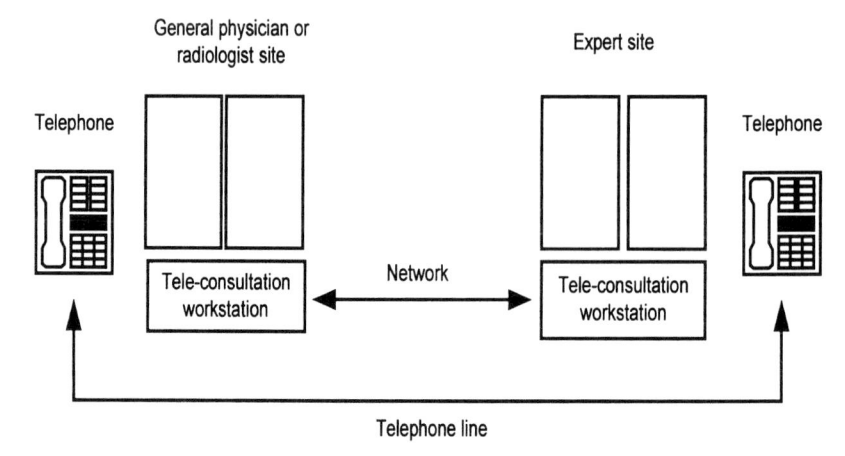

Figure 18.10   Schematic of the teleconsultation system.

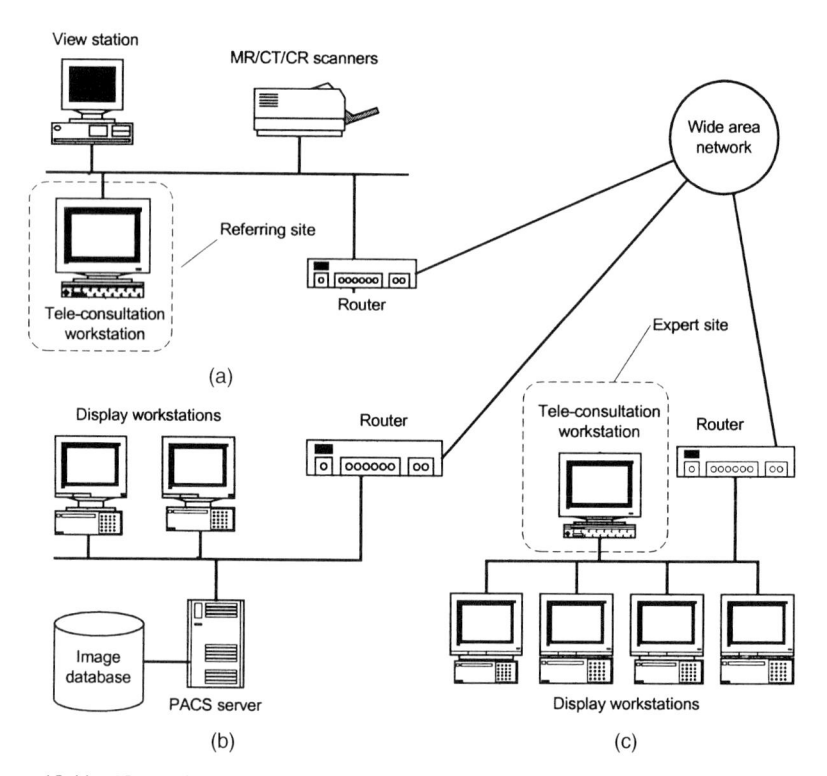

Figure 18.11   Network connection of teleconsultation system in clinical environment: (a) general physician or radiologist site, (b) PACS central server, and (c) expert site.

18.4.3 Teleconsultation Procedure and Protocol

The teleconsultation protocol consists of three steps: data formatting, data authoring, and data presentation.

18.4.3.1 Data Formatting

A teleconsultation session proceeds as follows. When cases need to be consulted, a general physician or radiologist collects the images from the scanners, display workstations, or PACS image database, and pushes them to the teleconsultation workstation located at the local reading site. If the data are not already in DICOM format, they must be converted to DICOM.

18.4.3.2 Data Authoring

The authoring procedure serves to authorize data for teleconsultation. The authoring function module is an integrated component in the software package. At the teleconsultation workstation, the referring physician inspects the data supplied by the teleconsultation system and sends them to the teleconsultation workstation located at the expert site, either through the local area network (if it is within the same building or campus) or through the wide area network (if distant). This large-volume data transfer can take place in off-hours or in a lower priority queue if there is no emergency. Later, either the general physician or an expert can call the other site to start the consultation session. There are three steps in data authoring, as shown in Figure 18.12:

1. The general physician or radiologist uses the software program to create an object called the virtual envelope, which includes information of the selected patient, studies, and series, as well as the host name of the expert site, and the name of the consultant from the teleconsultation local database. Note that the virtual envelope does not contain images. The virtual envelope is sent to the expert site through a network with DICOM communication services.

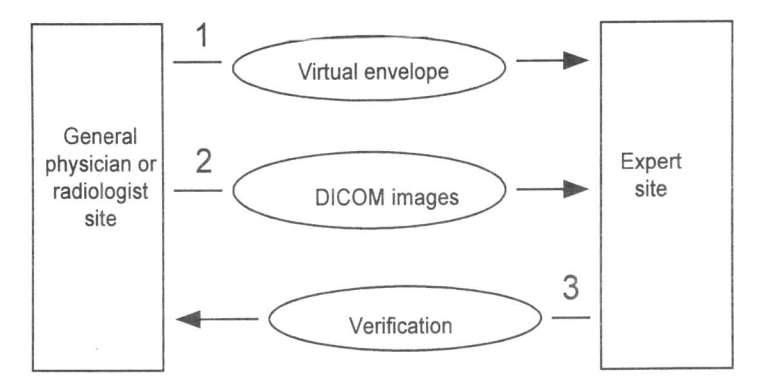

Figure 18.12 Data authoring steps in teleconsultation.

2. After the expert site has received the envelope, the general physician site sends the DICOM image objects related to the patient as dictated by the virtual envelope to the expert site.
3. After sending the images, the general physician site automatically performs a DICOM query to the expert site, and the expert site verifies the receipt of the virtual envelope and image objects from the general physician site. The consultation session can start once the data have been verified.

18.4.3.3 Data Presentation

Before the data presentation, both the expert site and the general physician site have the virtual envelope and image data. Either site can operate the teleconsultation software package to display and manipulate images and related information. The software synchronizes the operation of image display and manipulation at both sites. The teleconsultation operation procedure in either site proceeds as follows (using the numerals in Fig. 18.13).

1. Either the expert site or the general physician site can start the consultation procedure by selecting a session and loading image objects from the site's local database to the memory and displaying them at both sites.

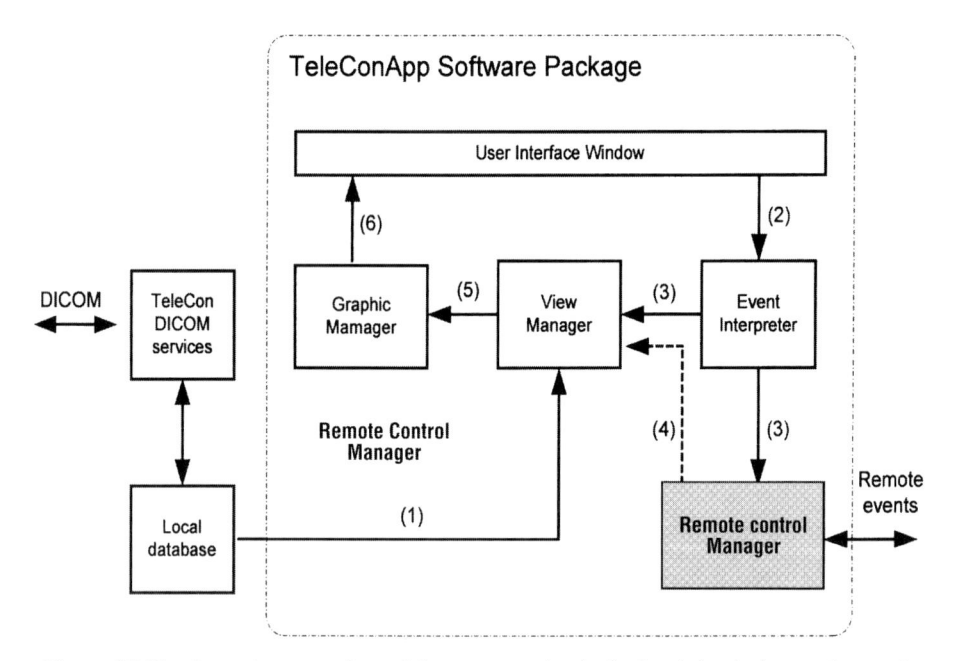

Figure 18.13 Operation procedure of data presentation in the local site during a teleconsultation session. Identical procedure also happens at the remote site. Shaded area and dashed line represent events happened at the remote site related to the local procedure. Numerals represent the data flow.

2. Either site can manipulate the displayed images at the user interface window to create events, which are received by event interpreter. The site that starts an event is called the local, whereas the other is the remote.
3. Event interpreter sends the events to the local view manager and remote control manager.
4. Remote control manager encodes events and sends them to the remote site. (*Note:* If the general physician site starts the event, it is the local and the expert is the remote. On the other hand, if the expert site starts the event, it is the local and the physician site is the remote.) At the remote site, events are received and decoded by remote control manager and sent to view manager (shaded (4) and dotted line).
5. View manager handles both local and remote events, processes images according to the event types, and sends processed image data to the graphic manager.
6. Upon receiving processed image data, the graphic manager renders them to display windows, which are managed by user interface window.

18.4.4 Clinical Evaluation

The teleconsultation is under clinical evaluation through LAN and WAN with Ethernet and modem connections, respectively. During consultation, both sites manipulated images, performed ROI, and talked via telephone. There were no crashes, no data lost, and no delays at either site in a 2-month test in the laboratory setting. The system is now under clinical evaluation in neuroradiology between MZH and UCSF (see Figures 9.8, 17.1, 17.6). This system, based on low cost NT/PC technology connecting to the PACS archive server through DICOM, provides data authoring, and also synchronizes image display and manipulation at both the general physician/radiologist site and the expert site during consultation through remote cursors. This system allows real-time collaborative consultation on serious or difficult cases with high resolution and large-volume medical images in a limited-bandwidth network environment.

References

Aberle, D., Gleeson, F.V., Sayre, J.W., Brown, P., Batra, P., Young, D., Stewart, B.K., Ho, B.K.T., and Huang, H.K. The Effect of Irreversible Image Compression on Diagnostic Accuracy in Thoracic Imaging. *Invest. Radiol.,* Vol. 28, 1993, pp. 398–403.

Aberle, D.R., Hansell, D., and Huang, H.K. Current Status of Digital Projection Radiography of the Chest. *J. Thorac. Imaging,* Vol. 5, 1990, pp. 10–20.

ACR/NEMA Digital Imaging and Communication Standard Committee. *Digital Imaging and Communications ACR-NEMA* 300–1988. Washington, DC: National Electrical Manufacturers Association, 1989.

Agresti, A. *An Introduction to Categorical Data Analysis.* New York: Wiley, 1996, pp. 34–35.

Allen, P.S. Nuclear Magnetic Resonance Imaging. *In Imaging with Non-ionizing Radiations,* D.F. Jackson, Ed. Glasgow: Surrey University Press, 1983.

Alvarez, R.E., and Macovski, A. Energy-Selective Reconstructions in X-ray Computerized Tomography. *Phys. Med. Biol.* Vol. 21, No. 5, 1976, pp. 733–744.

AMASS: Storage management systems (version 4.0). Greenwood Village, CO: Advanced Archival Products, Inc., 1993.

American College of Radiology, National Electrical Manufacturers Association. Digital Imaging and Communications in Medicine (DICOM): Network Communication Support for Message Exchange. Washington, DC: NEMA. Publication PS 3.8–1992, 1992.

American College of Radiology, National Electrical Manufacturers Association. Digital Imaging and Communications in Medicine (DICOM): Point-to-Point Communication Support for Message Exchange. Washington, DC: NEMA. Publication PS 3.9–1993, 1993.

American College of Radiology, ACR Standard for Teleradiology, Reston, VA: American College of Radiology, 1996.

Andriole, K.P., Gooding, C.A., Gould, R.G., and Huang, H.K. Analysis of a High-Resolution Computed Radiography Imaging Plate Versus Conventional Screen-Film Radiography for Neonatal Intensive Care Unit Applications. *SPIE,* Vol. 2163, 1994, pp. 89–97.

Arenson, R.L., Seshadri, S., Kundel, H.L., et al. Clinical Evaluation of a Medical Image Management System for Chest Images. *Am. J. Roentgenol.,* Vol. 150, 1988, pp. 55–59.

Arenson, R.L., Chakraborty, D.P., Seshadri, S.B., and Kundel, H.L. The Digital Imaging Workstation. *Radiology* Vol. 176, 1990, pp. 303–315.

Arenson, R.L., Avrin, D.E., Wong, A., Gould, R.G., and Huang, H.K. *Second Generation Folder Manager for PACS,* SCAR, 1994.

ATM Forum. ATM User–Network Interface Specification, version 3.0. Englewood Cliffs, NJ: Prentice-Hall, 1993.

Barnes, G.T. Radiographic Mottle: A Comprehensive Theory. *Med. Phys.,* Vol. 9, 1982, pp. 656–667.

Barnes, G.T. Noise Analysis of Radiographic Imaging. In *Recent Developments in Digital Imaging,* D. Doi, L. Lanzi, and P.P. Lin, Eds. New York: American Institute of Physics, 1985, pp. 16–38.

Barnes, G.T. Digital X-Ray Image Capture with Image Intensifier and Storage Phosphor Plates: Imaging Principles, Performance and Limitations. *Proc. AAPM Summer School, "Specifications, Acceptance, Testing, and Quality Control of Diagnostic X-ray Imaging Equipment,"* Vol. II, July 12–19, 1991.

Barnes, G.T., et al. Digital Chest Radiography: Performance Evaluation of a Prototype Unit. *Radiology,* Vol. 154, 1985, pp. 801–806.

Barnes, G.T., Morin, R.L., and Staab, E.V. Teleradiology: Fundamental Considerations and Clinical Applications. Syllabus: A Special Course in Computers for Clinical Practice and Education in Radiology, *Radiological Society of North America,* 1992, pp. 139–146.

Barrett, H.H., and Swindell, W. *Radiological Imaging: The Theory of Image Formation, Detection, and Processing.* New York: Academic Press, 1981.

Bauman, R.A. Large Picture Archiving and Communication Systems (PACS). *Proc. Computer Assisted Radiology 95,* 1995, pp. 537–541.

Bauman, R.A., Gell, G., and Dwyer, S.J. III. Large Picture Archiving and Communication Systems of the World—Part 1. *J. Digital Imaging,* Vol. 9, No. 3, 1996, pp. 99–103.

Bauman, R.A., Gell, G., and Dwyer, S.J. III. Large Picture Archiving and Communication Systems of the World—Part 2, *J. Digital Imaging,* Vol. 9, No. 4, 1996, pp. 172–177.

Benedetto, A.R., Huang, H.K., and Ragan, D.P., Eds. *Computers in Medical Physics.* New York: American Institute of Physics, 1990.

Bennett, B., and McIntyre, J. Understanding DICOM 3.0. Dallas, TX: Kodak Health Imaging Systems. 1993.

Berger, S.B., and Cepelewicz, B.B. Medical-Legal Issues in Teleradiology, *Am. J. Roentgenol.,* Vol. 166, 1996, pp. 505–510.

Berlin, L. Malpractice Issues in Radiology-Teleradiology. *Am. J. Roentgenol.,* Vol. 170, 1998, pp. 1417–1422.

Bertram, S. On the Derivation of the Fast Fourier Transform. *IEEE Trans. Audio Electroacoust.,* Vol. AU-18, March 1970, pp. 55–58.

Bidgood, W.D., and Horii, S.C. Introduction to the ACR-NEMA DICOM Standard. Syllabus: A Special Course in Computers for Clinical Practice and Education in Radiology, Radiological Society of North America, 1992, pp. 37–45.

Bidgood, W.D. Jr., and Horii, S.C. Modular Extension of the ACR-NEMA DICOM Standard to Support New Diagnostic Imaging Modalities and Services. *J. Digital Imaging,* Vol. 9, 1996, pp. 67–77.

Bjorkholm, P.J., et al. Digital Radiography. *SPIE,* Vol. 233, 1980, pp. 137–144.

Blume, H., Roehrig, H., Browne, M., and Ji, T.-L. Comparison of the Physical Performance of High Resolution CRT Displays and Films Recorded by Laser Image Printers and Displayed on Light Boxes and the Need for a Display Standard. *Proc. SPIE,* Vol. 1232, 1990, pp. 97–114.

Boag, J.W. Xeroradiography. *Phys. Med. Biol.,* Vol. 18, 1973, pp. 3–37.

Board of Directors, American Medical Informatics Association. Standards for Medical Identifiers, Codes, and Messages Needed to Create an Efficient Computer-Stored Medical Record. *J. Am. Med. Informat. Assoc.* Vol. 1, 1994, pp. 1–7.

Boring, C.T., et al. Cancer Statistics. *Chem. Abstr.,* Vol. 42, 1992, pp. 19–38.

Boyd, D., Herrnannsfeldt, W.B., Quinn, J.R., and Sparks, R.A. X-ray Transmission Scanning System and Method and Electron Beam X-Ray Scan Tube for Use Therewith. U.S. Patent 4,352,021 (Sept. 28, 1982).

Bracewell, R. *The Fourier Transform and Its Applications.* New York: McGraw-Hill, 1965.

Bracewell, R.N. Strip Integration in Radio Astronomy. *Aust. J. Phys.,* Vol. 9, 1956, pp. 198–217.

Bramble, J.M., Huang, H.K., and Murphy, M.D. Image Data Compression. *Invest. Radiol.,* Vol. 23, 1988, pp. 707–712.

Breant, C.M., Taira, R.K., and Huang, H.K. Integration of a Voice Processor Machine in a PACS. *J. Comput. Med. Imaging Graphics,* Vol. 17, 1993, pp. 13–19.

Breant, C.M., Taira, R.K., and Huang, H.K. Interfacing Aspects Between the PACS, RIS, and HIS. *J. Digital Imaging,* Vol. 6, 1993, pp. 88–94.

Brigham, E.O. *The Fast Fourier Transform.* Englewood Cliffs, NJ: Prentice-Hall, 1974, pp. 148–183.

Brody, W.R. *Digital Radiography.* New York: Raven Press, 1984.

Brooks, R.A., and Chiro, G.D. Principles of Computer Assisted Tomography (CAT) in Radiographic and Radioisotopic Imaging. *Phys. Med. Biol.,* Vol. 21, No. 5, 1976, pp. 689–732.

Budginer, T.F. Physical Attributes of Single-Photon Tomography. *J. Nucl. Med.,* Vol. 21, No. 6, 1980, pp. 579–592.

Budinger, T.F., et al. "Emission Computer Assisted Tomography with Single-Photon and Positron Annihilation Photon Emitters. *J. Comput. Assist. Tomogra.* Vol. 1, No. 1, 1977, pp. 131–145.

Cao, F., Sickles, E.A., and Huang, H.K. An Interactive Digital Breast Imaging Teaching File. *RSNA EJ* 1:26 pars. Available Online: http://ej.rsna.org//EJ_0_96/0037-97.fin/mammo.html. 18 July 1997.

Carlson, C.R., Cohen, R.W., and Gorog, I. Visual Processing of Simple Two-Dimensional Sine Wave Luminance Grating. *Vision Res.,* Vol. 17, 1977, pp. 351–358.

Castleman, K.R. *Digital Image Processing.* Englewood Cliffs, NJ: Prentice-Hall, 1979.

Chacko, A., and Griffin, B.G.G. The Vision and Benefit of a Virtual Teleradiology Environment for the DoD. *Proc. SPIE Med. Imaging,* Vol. 3339-23, 1998, p. 389.

Chan, H., Doi, K., Vyborny, C., et al., Improvement in Radiologists' Detection of Clustered Microcalcifications on Mammograms. *Invest. Radiol.,* Vol. 25, 1990, pp. 1102–1110.

Chan, K.K., Lou, S.-L., and Huang, H.K. Full-Frame Transform Compression of CT and MR Image. *Radiology,* Vol. 171, 1989, pp. 847–851.

Chan, K.K., Lou, S.L., and Huang, H.K. Radiological Image Compression Using Full-Frame Cosine Transform with Adaptive Bit-Allocation. *Comput. Med. Imaging Graphics,* Vol. 13, No. 2, 1989, pp. 153–159.

Chang, L.T. A Method for Attenuation Correction in Radionuclide, Computed Tomography. *IEEE Trans. Nucl. Sci.,* Vol. NS-25, No. 1, 1978, pp. 638–643.

Chimiak, W.J., Wolfman, N.T., and Boehme, J.M. Results of a Clinical Test of an ATM Tele-Ultrasound System. *Proc. SPIE Med. Imaging,* Vol. 2711, 1996, pp. 180–184.

Chipman, K., Holzworth, P., Loop, J., et al. Medical Applications in a B-ISDN Field Trial. *IEEE J. Sel. Areas Commun.* Vol. 10, No. 7, 1992, pp. 1173–1182.

Cho, P.A., and Huang, H.K. Architecture and Ergonomics of Imaging Workstations. In *The Perception of Visual Information,* 2nd ed., W.R. Hendee and P.N.T., Wells, Eds. New York: Springer, pp. 343–358.

Cho, P.S. Design and Implementation of a Remote Viewing System for a Coronary Care Unit. Ph.D. dissertation, UCLA, 1989.

Cho, P.S., Huang, H.K., Tillisch, J., and Kangarloo, H. Clinical Evaluation of a Radiologic Picture Archiving and Communication System for a Coronary Care Unit. *Am. J. Roentgenol.*, Vol. 151, 1988, pp. 823–827.

Choplin, R.H., Boehme, J.M., and Maynard, C.D. Picture Archiving and Communication Systems: An Overview. Syllabus: A Special Course in Computers for Clinical Practice and Education in Radiology, Radiological Society of North America, 1992, pp. 33–35.

Chotas, H.G., Dobbins, J.T., Floyd, C.E., and Ravin, C.E. Single-Exposure Conventional and Computed Radiography Image Acquisition. *Invest. Radiol.*, Vol. 26, 1991, pp. 428–445.

Cipra, B. Electronic Time-Stamping: The Notary Public Goes Digital. *Science.* Vol. 261, 9 1993, pp. 162–163.

Cochran, W.T., et al. What Is the Fast Fourier Transform? *IEEE Trans. Audio Electroacoust.*, Vol. AU-15, June 1967, pp. 45–55.

Cohen, M.D., Katz, B.P., Kalasinski, L.A., White, S.J., Smith, J.A., and Long, B. Digital Imaging with a Photostimulable Phosphor in the Chest of Newborns. *Radiology,* Vol. 181, 1991, pp. 829–832.

Cook, J., and Chimiak, W. Multimedia Architecture for Teleradiology in the US Army Virtual Radiology Environment. *Proc. SPIE Med. Imaging,* Vol. 3339-23, 1998, p. 390.

Cowart, R.W. Realtime Radiation Exposure Monitor and Control Apparatus. U.S. Patent 4,268,750 (May 19, 1981).

Creasy, J.L., Thompson, B.G., Johnston, R.E., and Parrish, D. PACS Development at UNC: Evaluation of the Neuroradiology Service Concept. *Proc. SPIE,* Vol. 767, 1987, pp. 808–811.

Curry, T.S., et al. *Cristensen's Introduction to the Physics of Diagnostic Radiology,* 3rd ed. Philadelphia: Lea & Febiger, 1984.

Curry, T.S. III, Dowdey, J.E., and Murry, R.C. Jr. *Introduction to the Physics of Diagnostic Radiology,* 4th ed. Philadelphia: Lea & Febiger, 1987.

Curtis, D.J., et al. Teleradiology: Results of a Field Trial. *Radiology,* Vol. 149, 1983, pp. 415–418.

Cushman, W.H. Illumination. In: Salvendy G., Ed. Handbook of Human Factors. New York: Wiley, 1987, pp. 670–695.

Dainty, J.C., and Shaw, R. *Image Science.* New York: Academic Press, 1974, Chap. 5.

Das, M., and Burgett, S. Lossless Compression of Medical Images Using Two-Dimensional Multiplicative Autoregressive Models. *IEEE Trans. Med. Imaging,* Vol. MI-12, No. 4, 1993, pp. 721–726, Dec. 1993.

Daubechies, I. Orthonormal Bases of Compactly Supported Wavelets." *Commun. Pure Appl. Math.,* Vol. 41, 1988, pp. 909–996.

Davies, D., and Dance, D. Automatic Computer Detection of Clustered Calcifications in Digital Mammograms. *Phys. Med. Biol.,* Vol. 35, 1990, pp. 1111–1118.

Davies, D.W., and Price, W.L. The Application of Digital Signatures based on Public-Key Cryptosystems. Proc. Fifth International Computer Communication Conference, Oct. 1980, pp. 525–530.

de Groot, P.M. Image Intensifier Design and Specifications. In *Specification, Acceptance Testing and Quality Control of Diagnostic X-ray Imaging Equipment, Proc. AAPM Summer School,* J.A. Seibert, G.T. Barnes, and R.G. Gould, Eds. Vol. I, 1991, pp. 477–510.

de Prycker, M. *Asynchronous Transfer Mode—Solution for Broadband ISDN.* New York, Ellis Horwood, 1993.

De Valk, J.P.J. *Integrated Diagnostic Imaging—Digital PACS in Medicine.* New York: Elsevier, 1992.

Dick, C.E., and Motz, J.W. Image Information Transfer Properties X-Ray Fluorescent Screens. *Med. Phys.,* Vol. 8, 1981, pp. 337–346.

Digital Imaging and Communications in Medicine (DICOM). National Electrical Manufacturers' Association. Rosslyn, VA: NEMA, 1966; PS 3.1-1966-3. 13-1966.

Donovan, J.L. X-Ray Sensitivity of Selenium. *J. Appl. Phys.,* Vol. 50, 1979, pp. 6500–6504.

Dorenfest, S. Creating a "Top 100" HIS Firm: The Lessons of History. *Healthcare Inf.,* Vol. 11, No. 6, 1994, pp. 49–72.

Duerinckx, A., Ed. Picture Archiving and Communications Systems (PACS) for Medical Applications. First International Conference and Workshop. *Proceedings SPIE—International Society for Optical Engineering,* Vol. 318, 1982.

Duerinckx, A.J., Hayrapetian, A.S., Valentino, D.J., et al. Assessment of Asynchronous Transfer Mode (ATM) Networks for Regional Teleradiology. *Proc. SPIE Med. Imaging,* Vol. 2711, 1996, pp. 61–70.

Dunn, J.F. Cathode Ray Tube (CRT) Film Recording of Video Based Medical Images. *Society of Photo-Optical Instrumentation Engineers, Picture Archiving and Communication Systems for Medical Applications,* Vol. 318, 1982.

Dwyer, S.J. III, Ed. Picture Archiving and Communication Systems (PACS) for Medical Applications. Second International Conference Workshop for Picture Archiving and Communication Systems (PACS) for Medical Applications. *Proceedings SPIE—International Society for Optical Engineering,* Bellingham, WA, Vol. 418, 1983.

Dwyer, S.J. III, Stewart, B.K., Sayre, J.W., Aberle, D.R., Boechat, M.I., Honeyman, J.C., Boehme, J.M., Roehrig, H., Ji, T.-L., and Blaine, G.J. Performance Characteristics and Image Fidelity of Gray-Scale Monitors. Syllabus: A Special Course in Computers for Clinical Practice and Education in Radiology. Radiological Society of North America, 1992, pp. 107–124.

Emmel, P.M. System Design Consideration for Laser Scanning. *Laser Scanning and Recording for Advanced Image and Data Handling, SPIE,* Vol. 222, 1980.

Fairchild, Semiconductor Co., CCD Device Catalog, 1983–1984.

Fajardo, L, Yoshino, M., Seeley, G., et al., Detection of Breast Abnormalities on Teleradiology Transmitted Mammograms. *Invest Radiol.,* Vol. 25, 1990, pp. 1111–1115.

Feig, S. Decreased Breast Cancer Mortality Through Mammographic Screening: Results of Clinical Trials. *Radiology,* Vol. 167, 1988, pp. 659–665.

Field, M.J. *Telemedicine—A Guide to Assessing Telecommunications in Health Care.* Washington DC: National Academy of Sciences Press, 1996, p. 271.

Frost, M.M., Honeyman, J.C., and Staab, E.V. Image Archival Technologies. Syllabus: A Special Course in Computers for Clinical Practice and Education in Radiology. *Radiological Society of North America,* 1992, pp. 69–72.

Fuji Photo Film Co., Ltd., Digital image processing, *Fuji Computed Radiography Technical Review,* Vol. 1, p. 8, 1993.

Fujita, H., Doi, K., Giger, M.L., and Chan, H.P. Investigation of Basic Imaging Properties in Digital Radiography. V. Characteristic Curves of II-TV Digital Systems. *Med. Phys.,* Vol. 13, 1986, pp. 13–18.

Fukushima, E., and Roeder, S.B.W. *Experimental Pulse NMR: A Nuts and Bolts Approach.* Reading, MA: Addison-Wesley, 1981.

Fullerton, G.D., et al. Electronic Imaging in Medicine. *Med. Phys. Monogr.* No. 11. New York: American Institute of Physics, 1984.

Georinger, F. Medical Diagnostic Imaging Support Systems for Military Medicine in Picture Archiving and Communication Systems (PACS). In NATO ASI Series F, Vol. 74, H.K. Huang et al., Eds. Springer-Verlag, Berlin: Springer-Verlag, 1991, pp. 213–230.

Getty, D., Pickett, R., D'Oris, C., and Swets, J. Enhanced Interpretation of Diagnostic Images, *Invest. Radiol.,* Vol. 23, 1987, pp. 240–252.

Giger, M., and Doi, K. Investigation of Basic Imaging Properties in Digital Radiography. I. Modulation Transfer Function. *Med. Phys.,* Vol. 11, 1984, pp. 287–295.

Giger, M., Doi, K., and Metz, C.E. Investigation of Basic Imaging Properties in Digital Radiography. II. Noise Weiner Spectrum, *Med. Phys.,* Vol. 11, 1984, pp. 797–805.

Giger, M.L., Doi, K., and MacMahon, H. Automatic Detection on Nodules in Peripheral Radiography, *Med. Phys.* Vol. 15, 1988, pp. 158–166.

Glass, H.I., and Slark, N.A. PACS and Related Research in the United Kingdom in Picture Archiving and Communication Systems (PACS). In NATO ASI Series F, Vol. 74, H.K. Huang et al., Eds. Berlin: Springer-Verlag, 1991, pp. 319–324.

Golomb, S.W. Run Length Encodings. *IEEE Trans. Inf. Theory,* Vol. IT-12, 1966, pp. 399–401.

Gonzalez, C.R., and Wintz, P. *Digital Image Processing.* Reading, MA: Addison-Wesley, 2nd Ed. pp. 13–60.

Gonzalez, R.C., and R.E. Woods, *Digital Image Processing.* New York: Addison-Wesley, 1993, p. 27.

Goodman, J.W. *Introduction to Fourier Optics.* New York: McGraw-Hill, 1968, pp. 21–25.

Graham, L.S. Clinical Applicable Modifications of Auger Camera Technology, *Nuclear Medicine Annual,* L.M. Freeman and H.S.S. Weissman, Eds. New York: Raven Press, 1983.

Greulich, W.W., and Pyle, S.I. *Radiographic Atlas of Skeletal Development of Hand/Wrist.* Stanford CA: Stanford University Press, 1959.

Gullberg, G.T. The Attenuated Radon Transform: Theory and Application in Medicine and Biology. Ph.D. thesis, University of California, Berkeley, 1979. Lawrence Berkeley Laboratory, LBL-7486.

Gur, D. Requirements for PACS: Users' Perspective. Syllabus: A Special Course in Computers for Clinical Practice and Education in Radiology. Radiological Society of North America, 1992, pp. 65–68.

Haff, A.V., Shaio, S. and Starbuck, O. *Hooked on Java.* Reading, MA: Addison-Wesley, 1996.

Halsall, F. *Data Communications, Computer Networks and Open Systems.* New York: Addison-Wesley, 1992, Chaps. 7 and 8.

Han, B.K. Large Scale PACS and Its Challenges. *Proc. PACS-Restructuring Tools Toward Year 2000,* IMAC'97 Seoul, Korea; October 1997, p. 44.

Hayrapetian, A., Aberle, D.R., Huang, H.K., Morioka, C.R., Valentino, D., and Boechat, M.I. Comparison of 2048 Matrix Digital Display Formats: An ROC Study. *Am. J. Roentgenol.,* Vol. 152, 1989, pp. 1113–1118.

Health Level Seven (HL7). *An Application Protocol for Electronic Data Exchange in Health Care Environments Version 2.1.* Ann Arbor, MI: Health Level Seven, Inc., 1991

Heiken, J.P., Brink, J.A., and Vannier, M.W. Spiral (Helical) CT. *Radiology,* Vol. 189, 1993, pp. 647–656.

Helsall, F. *Data Communications, Computer Network, and Open Systems,* 3rd ed. Wokingham, England: Addison-Wesley, 1992.

Hendee, W.R., et al. *Radiologic Physics, Equipment and Quality Control.* Chicago: Year Book Medical Publishers, 1977.

Hendee, W.R., and Wells, P.N.T., Eds. *The Perception of Visual Information,* 2nd Ed. New York: Springer, 1997.

Henschke, C.L., and Moreau, J.F. Interactive Telecommunication and Internet Use for Radiology Education. *Radiology,* Vol. 197, 1995, p. 42.

Hersh, W.R. The Electronic Medical Record: Promises and Problems. *J. Amer. Soc. Inf. Sci.,* Vol. 46, No. 10, 1995, pp. 772–776.

Hillen, W., Schiebel, U., and Zaengel, T. Imaging Performance of a Digital Storage Phosphor System. Med. Phys., Vol. 14, 1987, pp. 744–751.

Hindel, R., Ed. *Implementation of the DICOM 3.0 Standard.* Oak Brook, IL: Radiological Society of North America, 1994.

Hisatoyo, K. Photostimulable Phosphor Radiography Design Considerations, *Proc. AAPM Summer School: Specification, Acceptance Testing and Quality Control of Digital X-ray Imaging Equipment,* Vol. 2, 1991.

Ho, B.K.T. Automatic Acquisition Interfaces for Computed Radiography, CT, MR, US, and Laser Scanner. *Comput. Med. Imaging Graphics,* Vol. 15, 1991, pp. 135–145.

Ho, B.K.T., and Huang, H.K. Specialized Module for Full-Frame Radiological Image Compression. *Opt. Eng.,* Vol. 30, 1991.

Ho, B.K.T., Chao, J., Wu, C.S., and Huang, H.K. Full-Frame Cosine Transform Image Compression for Medical and Industrial Application. *Machine Vision Appl.,* Vol. 3, 1991, pp. 89–96.

Ho, B.K.T., Chao, J., Zhu, P., and Huang, H.K. Design and Implementation of Full-Frame Bit-Allocation Image-Compression Hardware Module. *Radiology,* Vol. 179, 1991, pp. 563–567.

Hoffman, E.J., et al. ECAT III—Basic Design Considerations. *IEEE Trans. Nucl. Sci.,* Vol. NS-30, No. 1, 1983, pp. 729–733.

Hoffman, J.G. Reliability Requirements in a Digital Imaging Environment. *Proc. SPIE,* Vol. 767, 1987, pp. 834–838.

Honeyman, J.C., Messinger, J.M., Frost, M.M., and Staab, E.V. Evaluation of Requirements and Planning for Picture Archiving and Communication Systems. Syllabus: A Special Course in Computers for Clinical Practice and Education in Radiology, Radiological Society of North America, 1992, pp. 55–64.

Horii, S.C. Electronic Imaging Workstations: Ergonomic Issues and the User Interface. Syllabus: A Special Course in Computers for Clinical Practice and Education in Radiology, Radiological Society of North America, 1992, pp. 125–134.

Horii, S.C. A Nontechnical Introduction to DICOM. *RadioGraphics,* Vol. 17, 1997, pp. 1297–1309.

Horii, S.C., and Bidgood, W.D., Jr. Network and ACR-NEMA Protocols. Syllabus: A Special Course in Computers for Clinical Practice and Education in Radiology. Radiological Society of North America, 1992, pp. 97–106.

Hounsfield, G.N. A Method and Apparatus for Examination of a Body by Radiation Such as X- or Gamma Radiation. British Patent No. 1,283,915. (1972).

Huang, H.K. Recent Development in Medical Digital Radiography, *Transactions of the American Nuclear Society,* Vol. 45, Oct.–Nov., 1983, pp. 249–251.

Huang, H.K. *Elements of Digital Radiology,* Chapter 3, Prentice-Hall, 1987.

Huang, H.K. Image Storage, Transmission, and Manipulation. *J. Minimally Invasive Therapy,* Vol. 1, 1991, pp. 85–92.

Huang, H.K. PACS-A Review and Perspective in *Integrated Diagnostic Imaging: Digital PACS in Medicine.* Ed. J. deValk J.-P., Elsevier, Amsterdam, The Netherlands, Chapter 3, 1992, pp. 39–58.

Huang, H.K. Three Methods of PACS Research, Development, and Implementation. *Radiographics.,* Vol. 12, 1992, pp. 131–139.

Huang, H.K. Medical Imaging. In *Encyclopedia of Computer Science and Engineering,* 3rd ed. Ed. A. Ralston and E.D. Reilly. Van Nostrand Reinhold, 1993, pp. 842–847.

Huang, H.K. Ultrasonic Picture Archiving and Communication Systems in Wells PNT Ed. *Advances in Ultrasound Technologies and Instrumentation. Ch. 11.* Churchill Livingstone, NY, NY. 1993, pp. 141–150.

Huang, H.K. 1996. PACS and Teleradiology Revisited. *Advance Adm. Radiolgy & Rad. Oncol.,* Vol. 6, No. 8, pp. 28–36.

Huang, H.K. PACS in Academic Medical Centers. In Siegel E.L. *Filmless Radiology.* Springer-Verlag: NY., Chap. 21 (in press) 1998.

Huang, H.K. PACS-Picture Archiving and Communication Systems in Biomedical Imaging. New York: VCH/Wiley, 1996.

Huang, H.K. Some Aspects of Medical Imaging. In *Principles of Medical Biology,* Vol 4., E.E. Bittar and N. Bittar, Eds. Greenwich, CT: 1996, pp. 211–239.

Huang, H.K. Telemedicine and Teleradiology. *San Francisco Medicine,* Vol. 69, No. 7, 1996, pp. 22–23.

Huang, H.K. Teleradiology Technologies and Some Service Models. *Computerized Med. Imaging and Graphics,* Vol. 20, 1996, pp. 59–68.

Huang, H.K. Towards The Digital Radiology Department. Editorial. *European J. Radiology,* Vol. 22, 1996, p. 165.

Huang, H.K. Multimedia Applications in Health Care. Editorial, *IEEE Multimedia,* Special Issue: *Multimedia in Medicine* Vol. 4, No. 2, 1997, p. 23.

Huang, H.K. Telemedicine and Teleradiology Technologies and Applications. *Min. Invasive Ther.,* Vol. 6., 1997, pp. 387–392.

Huang, H.K., Aberle, D., Lufkin, R., Grant, E., and Hanafee, W. Advances in Medical Imaging. UCLA Conference. *Annals of Internal Medicine,* Vol. 112, 1990, pp. 157–240.

Huang, H.K., Andriole, K., Bazzill, T., Lou, A.S.L., and Wong, A.W.K. Design and Implementation of PACS—The Second Time. *J. Digital Imag.,* Vol. 9, No. 2, 1996, pp. 47–59.

Huang, H.K., Arenson, R.L., Dillon, W.P., et al. Asynchronous Transfer Mode (ATM) Technology for Radiologic Communication. *Am. J. Roentgenol.,* Vol. 164, 1995, pp. 1533–1536.

Huang, H.K., Arenson, R.L., Lou, S.L., et al. Multimedia in the Radiology Environment: Current Concept. *Comput. Med. Imaging Graphics,* Vol. 18, 1994, pp. 1–10.

Huang, H.K., Bassett, L.W., Mankovich, N.J., Cho, P., Kangarloo, H., and Seeger, L. Instruction in Image Processing for Residents in Diagnostic Radiology, *Am. J. Roentgenol.,* Vol. 149, 1987, pp. 435–437.

Huang, H.K., and Cho, P.S. Architecture and Ergonomics of Imaging Workstations. In *The Perception of Visual Information,* Ed. W.H. Hendee and P.N.T. Wells. Springer-Verlag, Ch. 11, 1993, pp. 316–334.

Huang, H.K., Cho, P.S., Ratib, O., et al. Personal Digital Image Filming System. *Radiology* 173, 1989, pp. 292.

Huang, H.K., Cho, P.S., Taira R., et al. Picture Archiving and Communication Systems in Japan: 3 Years Later. *Am. J. Roentgenol.,* 154, 1990, pp. 415–417.

Huang, H.K., Gould, R.G., Callen, P.W., Filly, R.A., et al. Initial Clinical Experience with Ultrasound PACS. *SPIE,* Vol. 2435, 1995, pp. 246–251.

Huang, H.K., Kangarloo, H., Cho, P.S., et al: Planning a total digital radiology department, *Am. J. Roentgenol.,* Vol. 154, 1990, pp. 635–639.

Huang, H.K., and Ledley, R.S. Scanning Methods and Reconstruction Algorithms for Computerized Tomograph. In *Medical Imaging Techniques,* K. Preston, et al., Eds. Plenum Press, 1979, pp. 313–327.

Huang, H.K., Lo, S.-C., Ho, B.K., and Lou, S.L. Radiological Image Compression Using Error-Free and Irreversible Two-dimensional Direct-Cosine-Transform Coding Techniques. *J. Optical Society of America A.,* Vol. 4, 1987, pp. 984–992.

Huang, H.K., Lou, S.L., Cho, P.S., et al. Radiologic image communication methods. *Am.J. Roentgenol.,* Vol. 155, 1990, pp. 183–186.

Huang, H.K., Lou, S.L., and Dillon, W.P. Neuroradiology Workstation Reading in an Inter-Hospital Environment: A Nineteen Month Study. *J. Comp. Med. Imag. & Graphics* 21, 5, 1997, pp. 309–317.

Huang, H.K., Lou, S.L., and Wong, W.K. PACS pitfalls and bottlenecks, *SPIE Proceedings,* Vol. 3035, 1997, pp. 1–5.

Huang, H.K., Mankovich, N.J., Taira, R.K., Cho, P., Stewart, B., Ho, B., Cho, K., and Ishimitsu, Y. PACS for Radiological Images: State of the Art. *CRC Critical Review in Diagnostic Imaging,* Vol. 28, 1988, pp. 383–427.

Huang, H.K., Ratib, O., Bakker, A., and Witte, G. *Picture Archiving and Communication Systems.* NATO ASI Series F, Vol. 74. Springer-Verlag: Germany, 1991.

Huang, H.K., and Taira, R.K. Infrastructure Design of a Picture Archiving and Communication System. *Am. J. Roentgenol.,* Vol. 158, 1992, pp. 743–749.

Huang, H.K., Taira, R.K., Lou, S.L., Wong, W.K., et al. Implementation of a Large Scale Picture Archiving and Communication System. *J. Comp. Med. Imaging and Graphics.,* Vol. 17, 1993, pp. 1–11.

Huang, H.K., Tecotsky, R.H., and Bazzill, T. A Fiber-Optic Broadband CT/MR Video Communication System. *J. Digital Imaging.* Vol. 5, 1992, pp. 22–25.

Huang, H.K., Wong, A.W.K., Bazzill, T.M., Andriole, K.P., Lee, J.K., and Zhang, J.G. Asynchronous Transfer Mode-Distributed PACS Server for Intensive Care Unit Applications. *Radiology,* Vol. 197, No. P, 1995, pp. 247.

Huang, H.K., Wong, A.W.K., and Lou, S.L. Architecture of a Comprehensive Radiologic Imaging Network. *IEEE J. Sel. Areas in Communications,* Vol. 10, No. 7, 1992, pp. 1188—1196.

Huang, H.K., Wong, A.W.K., Lou, S.L., Bazzill, T.M., et al. Clinical Experience with a Second Generation PACS. *J Digital Imag.* Vol. 9, No. 4, 1996, pp. 151–166.

Huang, H.K., Wong, A.W.K., and Zhu, X. Performance of Asynchronous Transfer Mode (ATM) Local Area and Wide Area Networks for Medical Imaging Transmission in Clinical Environment. *Comp. Med. Imaging and Graphics,* Vol. 21, No. 3, 1997, pp. 165–173.

Huang, H.K., and Wong, C.K. Dual-Potential Imaging in Digital Radiography, *IEEE Proc. Intern. Workshop on Physics of Medical Images,* 1982, pp. 122–129.

Huang, H.K., Wong, S.T.C., and Pietka E. Medical Image Informatics Infrastructure Design and Applications. *Medical Informatics,* Vol. 22, No. 4, 1997, pp. 279–289.

Huffman, D.A. A Method for the Construction of Minimum-Redundancy Codes. *Proc. IRE V,* Vol. 40, 1952, pp. 1098–1101.

Irie, G. Clinical Experience—16 Months of Hu-PACS in Picture Archiving and Communication Systems (PACS). In NATO ASI Series F, Vol. 74, H.K. Huang et al., Eds. Berlin: Springer-Verlag, 1991, pp. 183–188.

Ishida, M., Kato, H., Doi, K., and Frank, P.H. Development of a New Digital Radiographic Image Processing System. *SPIE,* Vol. 347, 1982, pp. 42–48.

Ishida, M., Frank, P.H., Doi, K., and Lehr, J.L. High Quality Digital Radiographic Images: Improved Detection of Low-Contrast Objects and Preliminary Clinical Studies. *Radiographics,* Vol. 3, 1983, pp. 325–338.

Ishida, M., et al. Digital Image Processing: Effect on Detectability of Simulated Low-Contrast Radiographic Patterns. *Radiology,* Vol. 150, 1984, pp. 569–575.

Ishimitsu, Y., Arai, K., Taira, R.K., and Huang, H.K. Radiological Laser Film Scanner Sampling Artifact, *Comput. Med. Imaging Graphics,* Vol. 14, 1990, pp. 25–33.

Jain, A.K. Image Data Compression: A Review, Proc. *IEEE,* Vol. 69, March 1981, pp. 349–389.

James, A.E. Jr., James, E. III, Johnson, B., and James, J. Legal Considerations of Medical Imaging. *Leg. Med.* 1993, pp. 87–113.

Ji, T.-L., Roehrig, H., Blume, H., Seeley, G., and Browne, M. Physical and Psychological Evaluation of CRT Noise Performance. Proc. *SPIE,* Vol. 1444, 1991, pp. 136–150.

Johns, H.E., and Cunningham, J.R. *The Physics of Radiology,* 4th ed. Springfield, IL: Charles C. Thomas, 1983.

Kalender, W.A., Sissler, W., Klotz, E., and Vock, P. Spiral Volumetric CT with Single-Breath-Hold Technique, Continuous Transport, and Continuous Scanner Rotation. *Radiology,* Vol. 176, 1993, pp. 181–183.

Kamp, G.H. Medical-Legal Issues in Teleradiology: A Commentary. *Am. J. Roentgenol.,* Vol. 166, 1996, pp. 511–512.

Kangarloo, H., Boechat, M.I., Barbaric, Z., Taira, R.K., Cho, P.S., Mankovich, N.J., Ho, B.K.T., Eldredge, S.L., and Huang, H.K. Two-Year Clinical Experience with a Computed Radiography System. *Am. J. Roentgenol.,* Vol. 151, 1988, pp. 605–608.

Karssemeijer, N. A Stochastic Model for Automated Detection of Calcifications in Digital Mammograms. *Image Vision Comput.,* Vol. 10, 1992, pp. 369–375.

Kato, H. Photostimulable Phosphor Radiography Design Considerations. In *Specification, Acceptance Testing and Quality Control of Diagnostic X-Ray Imaging Equipment: Proceedings of the 1991 AAPM Summer School,* Vol. II, J.A. Seibert, G.T. Barnes, R.G. Gould, Eds. pp. 860–898.

Kaufman, L., et al. *Nuclear Magnetic Imaging in Medicine.* New York: Igaku-Shoin, 1982.

Keller, P.A. Cathode-Ray Tube Displays for Medical Imaging. *J. Digital Imaging,* Vol. 3, 1990, pp. 15–25.

Kim, J.H., Yeon, K.M., Han, M.C., Lee, D.H., and Cho, H.I. Development of Hospital-Integrated Large Scale PACS in Seoul National University Hospital. *SPIE,* Vol. 3035, 1997, pp. 248–255.

Kohane, I.S. Exploring the Functions of World Wide Web-Based Electronic Medical Record Systems. *M.D. Comput.,* Vol. 13, No. 4, 1996, pp. 339–346.

Koo, J.I., Lee, H.S., and Kim, Y. Applications of 2-D and 3-D Compression Algorithms to Ultrasound Images. *SPIE Image Capture, Formatting, Display,* Vol. 1653, 1992, pp. 434–439.

Korn, D.M., et al. A Method of Electronic Readout Electrophotographic and Electroradiographic Images. *J. App. Photogr. Eng.,* Vol. 4, 1978, pp. 178–182.

Kotsas, P., Piraino, D.W., Recht, M.P., and Richmond, B.J. Comparison of Adaptive Wavelet-Based and Discrete Cosine Transform Algorithm in Image Compression. *Radiology,* Vol. 93(P), 1994, Suppl., p. 331.

Krestel, E. *Imaging Systems for Medical Diagnostics.* Berlin: Siemens Aktiengesellschaft, 1990, p. 334.

Krongauz, V.G., and Parfianovich, I.A. Photostimulated Luminescence of Phosphors. *J. Lumin.,* Vol. 9, 1974, pp. 61–70.

Kruger, R.A., Mistretta, C.A., Houk, T.L., et al. Computerized Fluoroscopy in Real Time for Noninvasive Visualization of the Cardio-Vascular System. Preliminary Studies. *Radiology,* Vol. 130, 1979, pp. 49–57.

Kuhl, D.E., and Edwards, R.Q. Image Separation Radioisotope Scanning. *Radiology,* Vol. 80, No. 4, 1963, pp. 653–661.

Kundel, H.L. Visual Perception and Image Display Terminals. *Radiol. Clin. North Am.,* Vol. 24, 1986, pp. 69–78.

Kundel, H.L., Seshadri, S.B., Langlotz, C.P., et al. A Prospective Study of a PACS: Information Flow and Clinical Action in a Medical Intensive Care Unit. *Radiology* 1997.

Langer, S., and Wang J. A Goal-Based Cost-Benefit Analysis for Film Versus Filmless Radiology Departments. *J. Digital Imaging,* Vol. 9, No. 3, 1996, pp. 104–112.

Langer, S., and Wang, J. An Evaluation of Ten Digital Image Review Workstations. *J. Digital Imaging,* Vol. 10, No. 2, 1997, pp. 65–78.

Langlotz, C.P., Even-Shoshan, O., Seshadri, S.B., et al. A Methodology for the Economic Assessment of PACS. *SPIE Med. Imaging,* Vol. 2165, 1994, pp. 584–592.

Lee, H., Kim, Y., Rowberg, A.H., and Riskin, E.A. Statistical Distributions of DCT Coefficients and Their Application to an Interframe Compression Algorithm for 3D Medical Images. *IEEE Trans. Med. Imaging,* Vol. 12, No. 3, 1993, pp. 478–485.

Lee, J.K., Wong, A.W.K., Ramaswamy, M., Yin, L., and Huang, H.K. Access to Multimedia PACS Information from a Mac-based workstation. *SPIE,* Vol. 2435, 1995, pp. 33–42.

Lee, J.K., Wong, A.W.K., Huang, H.K., et al. ATM Distributed PACS Server for ICU Application. *Proc. SPIE Med. Imaging,* Vol. 2711, 1996, pp. 14–21.

Lei, G.P., Zhang, H., and Wong, A. PC/NT- Based PACS Display Workstation with ATM and DICOM Connectivity. *Proc. SPIE Med. Imaging,* 3339–16, 1998.

Lemke, H.U. The Berlin Communication System (BERKOM). In *Picture Archiving and Communication Systems (PACS) in Medicine,* NATO ASI Series F, Vol. 74. H.K. Huang et al., Eds. Berlin: Springer-Verlag, 1989, pp. 275—281.

Leverenz, H.W. *An Introduction to Luminescence of Solids.* New York: Dover, 1962, p. 150.

Lo, S.C. Radiological Image Compression, Ph.D. thesis, University of California, Los Angeles, December 1985.

Lo, S.C., and Huang, H.K. Error-Free and Irreversible Radiographic Image Compression, *Society of Photo-Optical Instrumentation Engineers Picture Archiving and Communication Systems (PACS III) for Medical Application,* 536, Newport Beach, CA, February 1985, pp. 170–177.

Lo, S.C., and Huang, H.K. Radiological Image Compression: Full-Frame Bit-Allocation Technique. *Radiology,* Vol. 155, No. 3, 1985, pp. 811–817.

Lo, S.-C., and Huang, H.K. Compression of Radiological Images with 512, 1024, and 2048 Matrices. *Radiology,* Vol. 161, No. 2, 1986, pp. 519–525.

Lo, S.C., Taira, R.K., Mankovich, N.J., Huang, H.K., and Takeuchi, H. Performance Characteristics of a Laser Scanner and Laser Printer System for Radiological Imaging. *Comput. Radiol.,* Vol. 10, 1986, pp. 227–237.

Lo, S.-C., Mun, S.K., and Chen, J. A Method for Splitting Digital Value in Radiological Image Compression. *Med. Phys.,* Vol. 18, No. 5, 1991, pp. 939–946.

Lou, S.L. The Design and Implementation of a CT/MR Picture Archiving and Communication System Applied to Neuroradiology. *Dissertation,* University of California, Los Angeles, 1991.

Lou, S.L., Huang, H.K., Mankovich, N.J., et al. A CT/MR/US Picture Archiving and Communication System. *Proc SPIE,* Vol. 1093, 1989, pp. 31–36.

Lou, S.L., Lufkin, R.B., Valentino, D.J., et al. A Neuroradiology Viewing Station. *Proc SPIE,* Vol. 1232, 1990, pp. 238–245.

Lou, S.L., Loloyan, M., Weinberg, W., et al. Image Delivery Performance of a CT/MR PACS Module Applied in Neuroradiology. *Proc SPIE,* Vol. 1446, 1991, pp. 302–311.

Lou, S.L., and Huang, H.K. Assessment of a Neuroradiology PACS in the Clinical Environment. *Am. J. Roentgenol.,* Vol. 159, 1992, pp. 1321–1327.

Lou, S.L., Huang, H.K., Taira R., et al. A 2K Radiological Image Display Station. *Proc. SPIE, Med. Imaging,* Vol. 1899, 1993, pp. 95–102.

Lou, S., Sickles, E., Wang, J., and Huang, H. A High Resolution Display System for Mammograms. *Radiology,* Vol. 193P, 1994, p. 474.

Lou, S.L., Huang, H.K., Bazzill, T., Gould, R.G., Dillon, W.P., and Schomer, B.G. Inter-hospital Image Communication: T-1 line Versus Courier Service. *Proc. SPIE Med. Imaging,* Vol. 2435, 1995, pp. 188–194.

Lou, S.L., Wang, J., Moskowitz, M., et al. Methods of Automatically Acquiring Images From Digital Medical Systems. *Comput. Med. Imaging Graphics,* Vol. 19, No. 4, 1995, pp. 369–376.

Lou, S.L., Huang, H.K., and Arenson, R.L. Workstation Design—Image Manipulation, Image Set Handling, and Display Issues. *Radiol. Clin. North Am.,* Vol. 34, No. 3, 1996, pp. 525–544

Lou, S.L., Hoogstrate, D.R., Huang, H.K. An Automated PACS Image Acquisition and Recovery Scheme for Image Integrity Based on the DICOM Standard. *J. Comput. Med. Imaging Graphics,* Vol. 21, No. 4, 1997, pp. 209–218.

Lou, S.L., Sickles, E., Huang, H.K., Cao, F., Hoogstrate, D., and Jahangiri, M. Digital Mammography—Preliminary. *Proc. SPIE Med. Imaging,* Vol. 3035, 1997, pp. 369–79.

Lou, S.L., Sickles E.A., Huang, H.K., et al. Full Field Direct Digital Telemammography: Technical Components, Study Protocols, and Preliminary Results. *IEEE Trans. Inf. Technol. Biomed.,* Vol. ITB-1, No. 4, 1997, pp. 270–278.

Lowe, H.J., Loma, E.C., and Poonkey, S.E. The World Wide Web: Review of an Emerging Internet-Based Technology for the Distribution of Biomedical Information. *J. Am. Med. Inf. Assoc.,* Vol. 3, 1996, pp. 1–4.

Lubinsky, A.R., Owen, J.F., and Korn, D.M. Storage Phosphor System for Computed Radiography: Screen Optics. *SPIE,* Vol. 626, 1986, pp. 120–132.

Lubinksy, A.R., Whiting, B.R., and Owen, J.F. Storage Phosphor System for Computed Radiography: Optical Effects and Detective Quantum Efficiency (DQE). *SPIE,* Vol. 767, 1987, pp. 167–177.

Maekawa, M., Oldehoeft, A.E., and Oldehoeft, R.R. *Operating Systems—Advanced Concepts.* New York: Benjamin/Cummings Publishing Company, 1987.

Mallat, S.G. A Theory for Multiresolution Signal Decomposition: The Wavelet Representation. *IEEE Trans. Pattern Anal. Machine Intell.,* Vol. PAMI-11, No. 1, 1989, pp. 674–693.

Mankovich, N.J., Taira, R.K., Cho, P.S., and Huang, H.K. An Operational Radiological Image Archive and Digital Optical Disks. *Radiology,* Vol. 167, 1988, pp. 139–142.

Mansfield, P., and Morris, P.G. *NMR Imaging in Biomedicine.* New York: Academic Press, 1982.

Masahiro, Ito. Ed. *Nuclear Medicine in Japan.* Instrumentation in Nuclear Medicine. Takeshi A. Iinuma, International Medical Foundation of Japan, 1975.

Mason, R.O. Ethics to Information Technology Issues. *Commun. ACM,* Vol 38, 1995, pp. 55–57.

Masser, H., Mandl, A., Urban, M., et al. The Vienna Project SMZθ in Picture Archiving and Communication Systems (PACS). In NATO ASI Series F, Vol. 74, H.K. Huang et al., Eds. Berlin: Springer-Verlag, 1991, pp. 247–250.

McDonald, C.L. The Barriers to Electronic Medical Record Systems and How to Overcome Them. *J. Am. Inf. Assoc.,* Vol. 4, 1997, pp. 213–221.

McDysan, D.E., and Spohn, D.L. *ATM—Theory and Application.* New York: McGraw-Hill: 1994, Chaps. 7 and 10.

McNitt-Gray, M.F., Pieka, E., and Huang, H.K. Image Preprocessing for a Picture Archiving and Communication System. *Invest. Radiol.,* Vol. 27, 1992, pp. 525–535.

McNitt-Gray, M.F., Huang, H.K., and Sayre, J.W. Feature Selection in the Pattern Classification Problem of Digital Chest Radiograph Segmentation. *IEEE Trans. Med. Imaging,* Vol. MI-14, 1994, pp. 537–547.

Medical Imaging Technology. *The Fifth MIT and the Third PACS/PHD Symposia,* Vol. 4, No. 2, 1986.

Mengers, P. Low Contrast Imaging, *Electro-Opt. Syst. Design,* October, 1978, pp. 1–5.

Merritt, C.R.B., et al. Clinical Application of Digital Radiography. *Radiographics,* Vol. 5, No. 3, May 1985.

Merritt, C.R.B, Matthews, C.C., Scheinhorn, D., and Balter, S. Digital Imaging of the Chest. *J. Thorac. Imaging,* Vol. 1, 1985, pp. 1–13.

Miller, E.R., McCury, E.M., and Hruska, B.B. Immediate Hospital Wide Access to X-Ray Film Images. *Radiology,* Vol. 192, 1969, pp. 13–16.

Mitchell, W. When Is Seeing Believing? *Sci. Am.,* Vol. 270, 1994, pp. 68–73.

MITRE Corporation. Installation Site for Digital Network and Picture Archiving and Communication Systems (DIN/PACS). *RFP B52-1545,* 1985.

Miyahara, J., and Kato, H. Computed Radiography. *Oyo Buturi* (Japanese), Vol. 53, 1984, pp. 884–890.

Moore, S.M. Observation on DICOM Demonstration at the RSNA Annual Meetings. *Proc. SPIE, Med. Imaging,* Vol. 2711, 1996, pp. 89–97.

Moskowitz, M., Gould, R.G., Huang, H.K., et al. Initial Clinical Experience with Ultrasound PACS. *Proc. SPIE Med. Imaging,* Vol. 2435, 1995, pp. 246–251.

Moskowitz, M.J., Wang, J., Allen, J.D., Huang, H.K., Sickles, E.A., Allen, J., and Giles, A. High-Resolution Display System for Mammograms. *Proc. SPIE Med. Imaging,* Vol 2431, 1995, pp. 447–454.

Mosser, H.M., Partan, G., and Hruby, W. Clinical Routine Operation of a Filmless Radiology Department: Three Year Experience. *SPIE Med. Imaging,* Vol. 2435, 1995, pp. 321–327.

Multiple Viewing Station for Diagnostic Radiology *RO1 CA 39063 National Cancer Institute.* Washington, DC: Department of Health and Human Services, 1985.

Murphey, M.D., Huang, H.K., Siegel, E.L., and Hillman, B.J. Clinical Experience in the Use of Photostimulable Phosphor Radiographic Systems. *Invest. Radiol.,* Vol. 26, 1991, pp. 590–597.

Nahmias, C.D.B., Kenyon, L.T., and Coblentz, C.L. Design and Implementation of an Integrated PACS Workstation in the ICU. *SPIE,* Vol. 3035, 1997, pp. 268–275.

Nakamori, A., Doi, K., Sabeti, V., and MacMahon, H. Automated Analysis of Sizes of Heart and Lung in Digital Chest Images. *Med. Phys.,* Vol. 17, 1990, pp. 342–350.

Nakazawa, M., et al. Effect of Protective Layer on Resolution Properties of Photostimulable Phosphor Detector for Digital Radiographic System. *SPIE,* Vol. 1231, Medical Imaging IV: Image Formation, 1990, pp. 350–363.

National Electrical Manufacturers Association. *Digital Imaging and Communications in Medicine (DICOM).* Rosslyn, VA: NEMA Standards Publication PS 3.3, 1993.

National Electrical Manufacturers Association. *Digital Imaging and Communication in Medicine (DICOM).* Rosslyn, VA: NEMA Standards Publication PS 3, 1994.

National Electrical Manufacturers' Association. *Digital Imaging and Communications in Medicine (DICOM).* Rosslyn, VA: NEMA, 1996; PS 3.1–1996–3.13–1996.

Nelson, M. *Data Compression Book,* San Mateo, CA: M&T Publishing, Inc., 1992.

Nelson, M. 1995. A Clinician's View of Digital Mammography. In *Proc. 4th Int. Conf. Imaging Manage. and Commun.,* 1995.

Noriaki, O., and Koichi, Y. Improved Detection Rate of Early Breast Cancer in Mass Screening Combined with Mammography. *Jap. J. Cancer Res.,* Vol. 84, No. 7, 1993, pp. 807–812.

Oishi, I. *Frequency Characteristics of the Mosaic Type Display System.* Television Society of Japan, 1970 (in Japanese).

Olendorf, W.H. Isolated Flying Spot Detection of Radiodensity Discontinuities—Displaying the Internal Structural Pattern of a Complex Object. *IEEE Trans. Biomed. Electron.,* Vol. BME-8, No. 1, 1961, pp. 68–72.

Ophir, J., and Maklad, N. Digital Scan Converters in Diagnostic Ultrasound Imaging. *Proc. IEEE,* Vol. 67, No. 4, April 1979.

Osteaux, M. *A Second Generation PACS Concept.* Berlin: Springer-Verlag, 1992.

Ottes, F.P., Bakker, A.R., and VanGennip, C. Overall System Design of a PACS for Nuclear Medicine Images. *SPIE Med. Imaging,* Vol. 2711, 1996, pp. 553–559.

Papin, P.J. A Prototype Amorphous Selenium Imaging Plate System for Digital Radiography. Ph.D. Dissertation, University of California, Los Angeles, 1985.

Papin, P.J., et al. Sensitivity Characteristics of a Prototype Selenium Detection System for Digital Radiographic Imaging. *Soc. Photo-Opt. Instrum. Eng.,* Vol. 535, 1985, pp. 222–227.

Partain, C.C.L., et al. *Nuclear Magnetic Resonance Imaging.* Philadelphia: Saunders, 1983.

Pietka, E., McNitt-Gray, M.F., and Huang, H.K. Computer-Assisted Phalangeal Analysis in Skeletal Age Assessment. *IEEE Trans. Med. Imaging,* Vol. MI-10, 1991, pp. 616–620.

Pietka, E., and Huang, H.K. Orientation Correction for Chest Images, *J. Digital. Imaging,* Vol. 5, 1992, pp. 185–189.

Pietka, E., Kaabi, L., Kuo, M.L., and Huang, H.K. Feature Extraction in Carpal-Bone Analysis. *IEEE Trans. Med. Imaging,* Vol. MI-12, 1993, pp. 44–49.

Pietka, E., Kaabi, L., Kuo, M.L., and Huang, H.K. Feature Extraction in Carpal Bone Analysis. *IEEE Trans. Med. Imaging,* Vol. MI-12, 1993, pp. 44–49.

Pietka, E., and Huang, H.K. Epiphyseal Fusion Assessment Based on Wavelet Decomposition Analysis. *J. Comput. Med. Imaging & Graphics* Vol. 19, No 6, 1996, pp. 465–472.

Pietka, E. and Huang, H.K. Image Processing Techniques in Bone Age Assessment. In *Medical Imaging Techniques and Applications,* C.T., Leondes, Ed. Philadelphia: Gordon & Breach, 1997, Chap. 5, pp. 221–272.

Prior, F.W. Specifying DICOM Compliance for Modality Interface. *Radiographics,* Vol. 13; 1993, pp. 1381–1388.

Protopapas, Z., Siegel, E.L., Reiner, B.I., et al. PACS Training for Physicians: Lessons Learned at the Baltimore VA Medical Center. *J. Digital Imaging,* Vol. 9, No. 3, 1996, pp. 131–136.

Queisser, H.J. Luminescence, Review and Survey. *J. Lumin.* Vol. 24/25, 1981, pp. 3–10.

Ramachandran, G.N., and Lakshminarayanan, A.V. Three-Dimension Reconstruction from Radiographs and Electron Micrographs: Applications of Convolutions Instead of Fourier Transforms. *Proc. Natl. Acad. of Sci.,* Vol. 68, No. 9, 1971, pp. 2236–2240.

Ramaswamy, M.R., Wong, A.W.K., Lee, J.K., and Huang, H.K. Accessing a PACS' Text and Image Information Through Personal Computers. *Am J. Roentgenol.,* Vol. 163, 1994, pp. 1239–1243.

Razavi, M., Sayre, J.W., Taira, R.K., et al. A ROC Study of Pediatric Chest Radiolographs Comparing Digital Hardcopy Film and 2K × 2K Softcopy Images. *Am. J. Roentgenol.,* Vol. 158, 1992, pp. 443–448.

Reeve, H.C. III, and Lim, J.S. Reduction of Blocking Effects in Image Coding. *Opt. Eng.,* 1984, pp. 34–37.

Richardson, M.L., and Gillespy, T. An Inexpensive Computer-Based Digital Imaging Teaching File. *Am. J. Roentgenol.,* Vol. 160, 1993; pp. 1299–1301.

Riederer, S.J. The Application of Matched Filtering to X-Ray Exposure Reduction in Digital Subtraction Angiography: Clinical Results. *Radiology,* Vol. 146, 1983, pp. 349–354.

Riederer, S.J,. and Kruger, R.A. Intravenous Digital Subtraction: A Summary of Recent Development in Radiology. *Radiology,* Vol. 147, 1983, pp. 633–638.

Riskin, E.A., Lookabaugh, T., Chou, P.A., and Gray, R.M. Variable Rate Vector Quantization for Medical Image Compression. *IEEE Trans. Med. Imaging,* Vol. MI-9, 1990, pp. 290–298.

Robb, R.A. *Three-Dimensional Biomedical Imaging.* New York: VCH/Wiley, 1995.

Roehrig, H., Blume, H., Ji, T.-L., and Browne, M. Performance Tests and Quality Control of Cathode Ray Tube Displays. *J. Digital Imaging,* Vol. 3, 1990, pp. 134–145.

Roos, P., and Viergever, M.A. Reversible Interframe Compression of Medical Images: A Comparison of Decorrelation Methods. *IEEE Trans. Med. Imaging,* Vol. MI-10, No. 4, 1991, pp. 538–547.

Roos, P., and Viergever, M.A. Reversible 3-D Decorrelation of Medical Images. *IEEE Trans. Med. Imaging,* Vol. MI-12, No. 3, 1993, pp. 413–420.

Rosenfeld, A., and Kak, A.C. *Digital Picture Processing.* New York: Academic Press, 1976.

Rossman, K. Image Quality. *Radiol. Clin. North Am.,* Vol. VII, No. 3, 1969.

Roth, K. *NMR—Tomography and Spectroscopy in Medicine.* Berlin: Springer-Verlag, 1984.

Rowberg, A.H., and Williamson, B., Jr. SCAR 97: PACS in Practice. *J. Digital Imaging,* Vol. 10, No. 3, Suppl. 1, 1997, pp 1–231.

Rowlands, J.A., and Taylor, K.W. Absorption and Noise in Cesium Iodide X-Ray Image Intensifiers. *Med. Phys.,* Vol. 10, 1983, pp. 786–795.

Rowlands, J.A., and Taylor, K.W. Detective Quantum Efficiency of X-Ray Image Intensifiers: Comparison of Scintillation Spectrum and rms Methods. *Med. Phys.,* Vol. 11, 1984, pp. 597–601.

Sanada, S., Doi, K., Su, X.W., Yin, F.F., Giger, M.L., and MacMahon, H. Comparison of Imaging Properties of a Computed Radiography System and Screen-Film Systems. *Med. Phys.,* Vol. 18, 1991, pp. 414–420.

Sanders, J.N., Cattell, C.L., Bender, N.E., and Tesic, M.M. Design Consideration of a Laser Based Multiformat Camera for Medical Imaging, *Appl. Opt. Instrum. Med. XII, SPIE,* Vol. 454, 1984.

Sayre, J.W., Ho, B.K.T., Boechat, M.I., Hall, T.R., and Huang, H.K. The Effect of Full-Frame Image Compression on Diagnostic Accuracy in Hand Radiographs with Subperiosteal Resorption. *Radiology,* Vol. 185, 1992, pp. 559–603.

Schaetzing, R., Whiting, B.R., Lubinksy, A.R., et al. Digital Radiography Using Storage Phosphors. In *Digital Imaging in Diagnostic Radiology,* J.D. Newell Jr. and C.A. Kelsey, Eds. New York: Churchill Livingstone, 1990, pp. 107–138.

Schaffert, R.M. The Nature and Behavior of Electrostatic Images. *Photogr. Sci. Eng.,* Vol. 6, 1962, pp. 197–215.

Scheffer, P.A., and Stone, A.H. A Case Study of SREM. *Computer,* Vol.18, 1985, pp. 47–54.

Schneider, R.H., Dwyer, S.J. III, and Jost, R.G., Ed., Medical Imaging III. *Proc. SPIE,* Vols. 1090, 1091, 1092, and 1093, 1989.

Schneier, B. Applied Cryptography: *Protocols, Algorithms, and Source Code in C.* New York: John Wiley & Sons. 1993.

Seshadri, S.B. Software Suite for Image Archiving and Retrieval. Syllabus: A Special Course in Computers for Clinical Practice and Education in Radiology. Radiological Society of North America, 1992, pp. 73–78.

Sezan, M.I.A, Tekalp, M., and Schaetzing, R. Automatic Anatomically Selective Image Enhancement in Digital Chest Radiography. *IEEE Trans. Med. Imaging,* Vol. MI-8, 1989, pp. 154–162.

Shade, O.H. *Image Quality: A Comparison of Photographic and Television Systems.* Princeton, NJ: RCA, 1975, p. 2.

Shaprio, S.W. Venet, P.S., et al., Selection, Follow-Up, and Analysis of the Health Insurance Plan Study: A Randomized Trial with Breast Cancer Screening. *J. Natl. Cancer Inst. Monogr.,* Vol. 67, 1985, pp. 65–74.

Sheep, L.A., and Logan, B.F. The Fourier Reconstruction of a Head Section. *IEEE Trans. Nucl. Sci.*, Vol. NS-21, No. 3, 1974, pp. 21–43.

Sherrier, R.H. and Johnson, G.A. Regionally Adaptive Histogram Equalization of the Chest. *IEEE Trans. Med. Imaging,* Vol. MI-6, 1987, pp. 1–7.

Sickles, E. Quality Assurance: How to Audit Your Own Mammography Practice. *Radiol. Clin. North Am.,* Vol. 30, 1992, pp. 265–275.

Sickles, E. Current Status of Digital Mammography. In *Proceedings of the 7th International Congress on Senology* (Excerpta Medica International Congress Series). Amsterdam: Elsevier, 1993.

Sickles, E., Ominsky, S., Sollitto, R., Galvin, H., and Monticciolo, D. Medical Audit of a Rapid-throughput Mammography Screening Practice: Methodology and Results of 27,114 Examinations. *Radiology,* Vol. 175, 1990, pp. 323–327.

Siegel, E.L. Assessment of Filmless Hospital. *Proc. PACS-Restructuring Tools Toward Year 2000,* IMAC'97 Seoul, Korea, October 1997, p. 51.

Sinha, S., Sinha, U., Kangarloo, H., and Huang, H.K. A PACS-Interactive Teaching Module for Radiological Sciences. *Am. J. Roentgenol.,* Vol. 159, 1992, pp. 199–205.

Smathers, R., Bush, E., and Drace, J., et al., Mammographic Microcalcifications: Detection with Xerography, Screen–Film and Digitized Film Display. *Radiology,* Vol. 159, 1986, pp. 673–677.

Smith, D.V., Smith, S., Bender, G.N., et al. Evaluation of the Medical Diagnostic Imaging Support System Based on 2 Years of Clinical Experience. *J. Digital Imaging,* Vol. 8, No. 2, 1995, pp. 75–87.

Sones, R.A., and Barnes, G.T. A Method to Measure the MTF of Digital X-Ray Systems. *Med. Phys.,* Vol. 11, 1984, pp. 166–171.

Sonoda, M., et al. Computed Radiography Utilizing Scanning Laser Stimulated Luminescence. *Radiology,* September 1983, pp. 833–838.

Sorenson, J.A. and Phelps, M.E. *Physics in Nuclear Medicine,* 2nd ed. New York: Grune &Stratton, 1986.

Sprawls, P. *The Physics and Instrumentation of Nuclear Medicine.* Baltimore: University Park Press, 1981.

Steckel, R.J. Daily X-Ray Rounds in a Large Teaching Hospital Using High-Resolution Closed-Circuit Television. *Radiology,* Vol. 105, 1972, pp. 319–321.

Stevels, A.L.N., and Pingault, F. BaCl:Eu^{2+} A New Phosphor for X-Ray Intensifying Screen. *Philips Res. Rep.,* Vol. 30, 1975, pp. 277–290.

Stewart, B.K., and Huang, H.K. Single-Exposure Dual-Energy Computed Radiography. *Med. Phys.,* Vol. 17, 1990, pp. 866–875.

Stewart, B.K. Three-Tiered Network Architecture for PACS Cluster in Picture Archiving and Communication Systems (PACS). In NATO ASI Series F, Vol. 74, H.K. Huang et al., Eds. Berlin: Springer-Verlag, 1991, pp. 113–118.

Stewart, B.K. Local Area Network Topologies, Media, and Routing. Syllabus: A Special Course in Computers for Clinical Practice and Education in Radiology. Radiological Society of North America, 1992, pp. 79–95.

Stewart, B.K., Lou, S.L., Wong, A., and Huang, H.K. An Ultrafast Network for Communication of Radiologic Images. *Am. J. Roentgenol.,* Vol. 156, 1991, pp. 835–839.

Strickland, N.H. Hammersmith PACS: Some Lessons Learned in Implementing a Filmless Hospital. *Proc. 14th Int. EuroPACS Meeting,* October 3–5, 1996, Crete, pp. 12–17.

Strickland, N.H. Implications of a Filmless Hospital for a Radiologicsl Service. *Proc. PACS—Restructuring Tools Toward Year 2000,* IMAC'97 Seoul, Korea, October 1997, p. 45.

Sun, H.F., and Goldberg, M. Radiographic Image Sequence Coding Using Two-Stage Adaptive Vector Quantization. *IEEE Transactions on Medical Imaging,* Vol. 7, No. 2, June 1988, pp. 118–126.

Swank, R.K. Absorption and Noise in X-Ray Phosphors. *J. Appl. Phys.,* Vol. 44, 1973, pp. 4199–4203.

Swank, R.K., et al. The Development of a Self-Contained Instant-Display Erasable Electrophoretic X-Ray Imager, *J. Appl. Phys.,* Vol. 50, 1979, p. 6534.

Tabar, L., Faberberg G., Duffy, W., Day, N., Gad, A., and Grontoft, O. Update of the Swedish Two-County Program of Mammographic Screening for Breast Cancer. *Radiol. Clin. North Am.,* Vol. 30, 1992, pp. 187–210.

Taira, R.K., Mankovich, N.J., Boechat, M.I., Kangarloo, H., and Huang, H.K. Design and Implementation of a Picture Archiving and Communication System (PACS) for Pediatric Radiology. *Am. J. Roentgenol.,* Vol. 150, 1988, pp. 1117–1121.

Taira, R.K., and Huang, H.K. A Picture and Communication System Module for Radiology. *Comput. Methods Programs Biomed.* Vol. 30, 1989, pp. 229–237.

Takahashi, K., et al. Mechanism of Photostimulated Luminescence in BaFX:Eu^{2+} (X = Cl, Br) Phosphors. *J. Lumin.,* Vol. 31/32, 1984, pp. 266–268.

Takano, T.L. Ed. *Computed Radiography.* Berlin: Springer-Verlag, 1987, pp. 1–6.

Takeuchi, H., et al. Preliminary Experience with a Laser Scanner and Printer System for Radiological Imaging. *Society of Photo-Optical Instrumentation Engineers 536: Picture Archiving and Communications Systems (PACS III) for Medical Applications.* Newport Beach, CA, February 1985, pp. 65–71.

Tanenbaum, A.S. *Computer Networks,* 2nd ed. Englewood Cliffs, NJ: Prentice-Hall, 1989, pp. 373–375.

Tasto, M., and Wintz, P.A. Image Coding by Adaptive Block Quantization. *IEEE Trans. Commun. Technol.,* Vol. CT-19, 1971, pp. 957–971.

Tecotsky, R. FCR ID gateway: Theory of operation. Private communication, 1996.

Tesic, M., and Piccaro, M. *Digital Mammography Scanner: Performance Characteristics and Preliminary Clinical Results.* IEEE Colloquium Digital Mammography, London, 1996, pp. 3/1–3/7.

Thiel, A., and Bernarding, J. Distributed Medical Services Within the ATM-Based Berlin Regional Test Bed. *Proc. SPIE Med. Imaging,* Vol. 2711, 1996, pp. 32–43, 1996.

Toker, E., and Piccaro, M. Design and Development of a Fiber Optic TDI CCD-Based Slot-Scan Digital Mammography System. *SPIE Proc., Med. Imaging,* Vol. 2009, 1993.

Tsai, M., Ho, B.K., Villasenor, J., and Saipetch, P. Full-Frame Wavelet Video Compression with Incorporation of Block Classification. *Radiology,* Vol. 93(P), Suppl. 1994, p. 140.

U.S. Air Force (1951).

Valentino, D.J., Mazziotta, J.C., and Huang, H.K. Volume Rendering of Multi-modal Images. *IEEE Trans. Med. Imaging,* Vol. MI-10, 1991, pp. 554–562.

van der Heiden, G.H., Brauninger, U., Grandjean, E. Ergonomic studies on computer-aided design. In: Grandjean E., Ed. *Ergonomics and Health in Modern Offices.* London: Taylor and Francis, 1984, pp. 119–128.

Van Syckle, D.E., Sipple-Schmidt, T., and Parisot, C.R. Buying Imaging Products with DICOM Interface—Made Easy. In *SCAR '94,* J.M., Boehme, A.H., Rowberg, N.T., Wolfman, Eds. Carlsbad, CA: Symposia Foundation, 1994, pp. 529–536.

Verhoeven, L. Design Considerations of Digital Fluoroscopy/Fluorography Equipment. In *Specification, Acceptance Testing and Quality Control of Diagnostic X-ray Imaging Equipment, Proceedings of the 1991 AAPM Summer School,* J.A. Seibert, G.T. Barnes, R.G. Gould, Eds., Vol. II, 1991, pp. 734–789.

Vetterli, M., and Herley, C. Wavelets and Filter Banks: Theory and Design. *IEEE Trans. Signal Process.,* Vol. SP-40, 1992, pp. 2207–2232.

Villasenor, J.D., Belzer, B., and Liao, J. Wavelet Filter Evaluation for Image Compression. *IEEE Trans. Image Process.,* Vol. 4, N8:1053–1060.

Wang, J. Three-Dimensional Wavelet Compression. Ph.D. dissertation, UCLA, 1996.

Wang, J., and Huang, H.K. Film Digitization Aliasing Artifacts Caused by Grid Line Patterns. *IEEE Trans. Med. Imaging,* MI-Vol. 13, 1994, pp. 375–385.

Wang, J., and Huang, H.K. Medical Image Compression by Using 3-D Wavelet Transformation. *IEEE Trans. Med. Imaging.* Vol MI-15, No. 4, 1996, pp. 547–554.

Weinberg, W.S., Loloyan, M., and Chan, K.K. On-Line Acquisition of CT and MRI Studies from Multiple Scanners. *Proc SPIE,* Vol. 1446, 1991, pp. 430–435.

Wells, P.N.T. *Advances in Ultrasound Techniques and Instrumentation.* Ed., Churchill Livingstone, New York, 1993.

William, H., et al. *Numerical Recipes in C,* 2nd ed. New York: Cambridge University Press, 1992, pp. 661–666.

Wilson, A.J., and West, O.C. Single-Exposure Conventional and Computed Radiography: The Hybrid Cassette Revisited. *Invest. Radiol.,* Vol. 28, 1993, pp. 409–412.

Wintz, P.A. Transform Picture Coding. *Proc. IEEE,* 1972, pp. 809–820.

Wong, A.W.K., Huang, H.K., Arenson, R.L., and Lee, J.K. Multimedia Archive System for Radiologic Images. *Radiographics,* Vol. 14, 1994, pp. 1119–1126.

Wong, A.W.K., Huang, H.K., Bazzill, T.M., et al. Performance Characteristics of a Digital Imaging Network with Asynchronous Transfer Mode Technology. *Radiology,* Vol. 1978, 1995, p. 259.

Wong, A.W.K., Huang, H.K., Lee, J.K. Bassill, T.M., and Zhu, X. High-Performance Image Communication Network with Asynchronous Mode Technology. *SPIE Proc. Med. Imaging,* Vol. 2711, 1996, pp. 44–52.

Wong, A.W.K, and Huang, H.K. Integration of DICOM into an Operational PACS. *SPIE Proc. Med. Imaging,* Vol 3035, 1997, pp. 153–158.

Wong, C.K., and Huang, H.K. Calibration Procedure in Dual-Energy Scanning Using the Basis Function Technique. *Med. Phys.* Vol. 10, No. 5, 1983.

Wong, S., Zaremba, L., Gooden, D., and Huang, H.K. Radiologic Image Compression—A Review. *Proc. IEEE,* Vol. 83, 1995, pp. 194–219.

Wong, S.T.C., Abundo, M., and Huang, H.K. Authenticity Techniques for PACS Images and Records. *SPIE,* Vol. 2435, 1995, pp. 68–79.

Wong, S.T.C., and Huang, H.K. A Hospital Integrated Framework for Multimodality Image Base Management. *IEEE Trans. Syst., Man Cybernetics,* Vol. SMC-26, No 4, 1996, pp. 455–469.

Wong, S.T.C., and Huang, H.K. Design Methods and Architectural Issues of Integrated Medical Image Database Systems. *J. Comput. Med. Imaging Graphics,* Vol. 20, No. 4, 1996, pp. 285–299.

Wong, S.T.C., and Huang, H.K. Medical Image Databases. Special Issue. Editorial. *J. Comput. Med. Imaging Graphics,* Vol. 20, No. 4, 1996, pp. 187–188.

Wong, S.T.C., Soo Hoo, K., and Knowlton, R.C. Use of Image Coregistration and Visualization Techniques to Study Relationships Between MEG Neurophysiology and FDG-PET Metabolism in Epilepsy Imaging. *SPIE Proc. Med. Imaging,* Vol. 2709, 1996, pp. 280–289.

Wong, S.T.C., and Huang, H.K. Networked Multimedia for Medical Imaging. *IEEE Multimedia,* Special Issue: Multimedia in Medicine, Vol 4, No. 2, 1997, pp. 24–35.

Wong, W.K., Stewart, B.K., Lou, S.L., et al. Multiple Communiaction Networks for a Radiology PACS. *Proc. SPIE,* Vol. 1446, 1991, pp. 73–80.

Wong, W.K., Taira, R.K., and Huang, H.K. Digital Archive Center: Implementation for a Radiology Department. *Am. J. Roentgenol.,* Vol. 159, 1992, pp. 1101–1105.

Wong, W.K., and Huang, H.K. Subsystem Throughputs of a Clinical Picture Archiving and Communications Systems. J. Digital Imaging, Vol. 5, 1993, pp. 252—261.

Wong, W.K., Huang, H.K., Arenson, R.L., and Lee, J.K. Multimedia Archive System for Radiologic Images. *Radiographics,* Vol. 14, 1994, pp. 1119–1126.

Yin, L., Ramaswamy, M.R., Wong, A.W.K., et al. Access of Medical Information and Radiological Images Through a Local Area Network. *Proc SPIE,* Vol. 2165, pp. 21–26.

Yuste, M., Taurel, L., Rahmani, M., and Lemoye, D. Optical Absorption and ESR Study of F Centers in BaFCl and SrClF Crystals. *J. Phys. Chem. Solids,* Vol. 37, 1976, pp. 961–966.

Zeman, R.K., Fox, S.H., Silverman, P.M., et al. Helical (Spiral) CT of the Abdomen. *Am. J. Roentgenol.,* Vol. 160, 1993, pp. 719–725.

Zhang, J., and Huang, H.K. Background Recognition and Removal of Computed Radiography Images. *Radiology,* Vol. 201(P), 1996, p. 220.

Zhang, J., Wong, S.T.C., Andriole, K.P., et al. Real Time Mulilevel Process Monitoring and Control of CR Image Acquisition and Preprocessing for PACS and ICU. *SPIE Proc.,* Vol. 2711, 1996, pp. 290–296.

Zhang, J., Andriole, K., and Huang, H.K. Computed Radiographic Image Post-Processing in Picture Archiving and Communication System. *SPIE Proc.* Vol. 3035, 1997, pp. 310–320.

Zhang, J., and Huang, H.K. Automatic Background Recognition and Removal (ABRR) of Computed Radiography Images. *IEEE Trans. Med. Imaging,* Vol MI-16, No. 6, 1997, pp. 762–771.

Zhang, Y.-Q., Loew, H., and Pickholtz, R.L. A Combined-Transform Coding (CTC) Scheme for Medical Images. *IEEE Trans. Med. Imaging,* Vol. MI-11, No. 2, 1992, pp. 196–202.

Zhu, X.M., Lee, K.N., and Levin, D.L. Temporal Image Database Design for Outcome Analysis. *J. Comput. Med. Imaging Graphics,* Vol. 20, 1996, pp. 347–356.

Index

Absorption coefficient, 41
Acoustic noise, 319–320
Acquisition process recovery
 from dowmtime, 208–209
 from errors, 207
 from traps, 207–208
Acquisition residence time, 410
Acquisition systems, description of, 177–178
Adaptive block quantization technique, 141
Adaptive processing control, multilevel, 224–227
Admission, discharge, or transfers (ADT), 184, 276
Advanced Study Institute (ASI), 2
Air-blown fibers, 252
Air conditioning, 395–396
Algebraic reconstruction method, 94–95
Aliasing, artifacts, 50, 57–62
Ambient illuminence, 319
American College of Radiology (ACR), 383–384
American College of Radiology—National Electrical Manufacturers Association (ACR-NEMA), 131, 172, 175, 177, 181, 183–186, 188
American Standard Code for Information Interchange (ASCII), 181
Amplitude, 31, 60
Analog communications, 233. *See also* Video
Analog-to-digital (A/D) conversion, 112, 124–125, 149
Archive library, 272
Archive management, 344–348
Archive server, 271–272
Area scan, video and CCD camera, 50, 124
Asynchronous communication, 233
Asynchronous transfer mode (ATM), 180, 233, 238–249, 264, 376, 378

Atomic number, 41
Authenticity, for PACS images and records, 461–464
Automatic focusing, 120–121
Automatic orientation, 220, 222
Average gradient, film characteristic curve, 47
Average gray level, 330
Averaging mode, 112

Back-projection, 95, 101, 105
Background removing unexposed, 70–80, 220
Backup archive, 272
Bandpass/bandwidth, 112
Barrel effects, 311
Between hospital systems, communications, 242–249
Bidirectional model, 258
Bit allocation table, 140–141, 145
Bone age assessment, with digital hand atlas, 471–475
Boundary detection, 320–323
Bridge, 250
Broadband digital, 256
Broadband video, 253, 256, 259–260
Bromine, 45
Bucky, Gustave, 42. *See also* Scatter
Building distribution frame (BDF), 253

Cabling
 digital, 251
 planning for, 251–255
 video, 395
CAD/CAM, 72, 465–468
Calcium tungsten phosphor, 44
Carrier Sense Multiple Access with Collision Detection (CSMA/CD), 237
CD-ROM, 282
Central network authority (CNA), 264

511

512 INDEX

Central processing units, 271
Central Test Node (CTN), 205
Charge-coupled device (CCD), 50, 124
Chemical shift, 116
Chrominance coordinates, 171
Cine loop, ultrasound imaging, 113
Cine XCT, 99–101
Clerical staff, training of, 397
Clipping and bit truncation, 131–132
Cluster helical, spiral XCT, 98
Color Doppler ultrasound imaging, 113, 171–172
Color CRT, 313–314
Color image compression, 169–172
Color spaces, YCbCr and YIQ, 171
Commission Internationale de L'Eclairage (CIE), 170–171
Communication
  ACR-NEMA, digital image standard, 177–178
  between hospital systems, 242–249. *See also* Teleradiology; WAN; LAN
  network, 272–273
Composite video control, 125
Compressed image file, 129
Compression
  acceptable ratio, 152, 154–155
  block, 164–166
  clinical image, 130
  color image, 169–172
  composite, 149
  full-frame, 143–150
  irreversible, 130, 138–143, 172–173
  legal standards for, 174
  lossless, 130
  reversible, 130
  ratio, 130, 138
  teleradiology, 378
  3-D, 160–168
Compton scattering, 42
Computation, node in PACS, 457
Computed radiography (CR)
  advantages of, 67
  background removal, 70–80
  clinical applications of, 69–70
  image processing, 219–223
  operating characteristics, 67–68
Computerized tomography (CT), transmission X-ray
  introduction of, 64
  number, CT or Hounsfield, 101, 103
  cine XCT, 99–101
  spiral XCT, 98–99
Connectivity system, 3, 182
Contrast frequency response (CFR), 55–57
Contrast, MRI, 219–223
Contrast ratio (Cr), 312
Controller system
  configuration, 270–273
  software, 273–278
Conventional projection radiography
  characteristic curve of X-ray film, 46–48
  description of procedure used in, 39–41
  digitization, 52–62
  effect of kVp, mA, and mAs settings on radiographs, 41–42
  film optical density, 46
  how to reduce scatter, 42–43
  image intensifier tube, 48–50
  image receptor, 43–50
  setup of procedure and diagnostic area, 40
  x-ray film scanner, 50–52
Convolution, image reconstruction, 101
Convolution back-projection method, 105
CORROC2, 418
Cosine transform, using the fast Fourier transform, 129, 140
Cryptographic algorithms, key-based, 462–464
Cutoff gray level, 320

Daemon process, 181
Data access rights, 359
Database management, 210–211, 363
Database system, 272
Database-to-database transfer, 293
Deblurring, 323
Decoding, 142–143
Density resolution, 17–20
Detector circle radius, CT, 101
Detector fan, CT, 101
Detector specifications, CT, 101
Developer, X-ray film, 45
Difference image, 129–130, 152
Digital-based operation, 395–398
Digital chain, 82

Digital communications, 262–264
Digital dictaphone system, 302
Digital fingerprint, 462
Digital fluorography
 advantage of, 80
 components of, 80–82
 definition of, 80
 operational procedure for, 82–83
Digital image
 definition of, 15
 of an X-Ray film from video scanning, 50
Digital Imaging and Communication in Medicine (DICOM) standard
 compliance, 284–288
 composite commands, 191
 generally, 175, 181, 183, 188–196
 incompatibility in conformance statement, 447
 interface using, 209–213
 object classes, 189–192
 service classes, 189–192
Digital Imaging Network and Picture Acrchiving and Communication System (DIN/PACS), 2
Digitally generated patterns, 20, 23
Digital optical cartridge tapes, 282
Digital optical disk
 hierarchical system for, 278
 optical disk library/jukebox, 271
 physical description of, 278
Digital radiological image, definition of, 16
Digital radiology, 2
Digital subtraction angiography (DSA), 160–161
Digital subtraction arteriography (DSA), 160, 263
Digital-to-analog (D/A) conversion, 17, 51
Digital video angiography (DVA), 80
Digital video subtraction angiography (DVSA), 80
Digital voice, 301–303
Digitization
 definition of, 16
 quality of, 52–57
Digitizing artifact, 57
Digital mammography, 84–89, 223–224
Direct image capture, 89–90
Direct interface model, 202

Discrete cosine transform, 2-D, 140–142
Discrete Fourier transform, 25
Display-server management, 350–351
Display systems
 display monitors, 308–314
 distance and gray level measurements, 329–330
 examples of, 314–317
 histogram modification function, 329
 image reverse function, 329
 window and level function, 327–329
 zoom and scroll functions, 327
Display workstations
 basic software, 334–335
 networks, 265
 soft copy, 305
Distance calibration, 329–330
Distributed computing, in a PACS environment, 457–461
DR11-W interface, 178
Drying, X-ray film developer, 45
DSA mask subtraction, 160–161
DVD-ROM, 282–283

Edge spread function (ESF), 27–29, 32
Electronic Industries Association (EIA), 309
Electronic medical record (EMR), 303–304
Electronic noise, 33
Electronic patient record (EPR), 303
Emergency room module, PACS, 399–401
Emission computed tomography (ECT)
 description of, 103
 positron, 105–106
 single photon, 103–105
Entropy coding, 141–142, 168–169
Erasable magneto-optical disks, 278
Error-free compression
 background removal, 131–132
 clipping and bit truncation, 131–132
 Huffman coding, 134–138
 run-length coding, 132–134
Ethernet, communication system, 180, 237–238, 249–250. *See also* LAN
eV, 43
Event-driven multilevel adaptive process control, 229–230
Expert center, 370, 384

514 INDEX

External networks, 264–267
False positive (FP), ROC analysis, 157
Fan beam X-ray technique, large fan beam, 97
Fast Fourier transform (FFT)
  1-D FFT, 92–93
  2-D FFT, 116
Fault tolerance
  algorithm, 228–229
  design, 263
  methods, 206–209
Fibert distributed data interface (FDDI), 236, 238–264
Fiber-optic broadband video communication system, 258–262
Fiber-optic cables, 252
Field nonuniformity, laser imager, 55–56
Field size, X-rays, 42
Field uniformity, laser scanner, 55
File transfer protocol (FTP), 391
Film-based operation, 391–394
Film contrast, 41
Film fog level, 41–42
Film gamma, 47–48
Film grain, 33
Film latitude, 47
Film optical density, 46
Film/screen combination, 43–48
Film speed, 47–48
Filtered (convolution) back-projection method, 95–96
Filtering, digital image, 324–327
Five-point average, 323
Fixing, X-ray film developer, 45
Flagging, video monitor, 311
Flow velocity, 116
Fluorographic procedure, 80. *See also* Digital fluorography
Flux gain, image intensifier, 49
Flying-spot scan technique, 83–84
Food and drug administration, U.S., 131, 172–173, 176
Foot-lamberts (ft-L), 312
Fourier projection theorem, 91–94
Fourier spectrum, 23–24
Fourier transform, 21, 23–25
  discrete, 25
  fast, 92–93

inverse, 24, 93, 116
series, 31
Free induction decay (FID), 114–115
Frequency
  components, 20–21
  spatial, 20
Frequency domain, 20–25, 325–327
Frequency emphasis, 327
Frequency response of a scanner, 56
Fuji Photo Film Co., Ltd., 64
Full-field direct digital mammography (FFDDM), 86–89, 384–385
Full-frame bit allocation (FFBA) algorithm, 143–149
Full width at half-maximum (FWHM), 56

γ-ray emission profiles, 94
Gateway, network, 177–178, 251
Gaussian distribution, filter, 323
Geometric distortion, 311–312
Geometric mean modification, 104
Gigabit Ethernet, 249–250
Gray level value
  definition of, 16
  optical density versus, 53–54
Glare, video monitor, 310, 317–319
Gradient, image processing, 320
  fields, MR imaging, 115
Graphic user interface (GUI), 364, 482
Grid ratio, 43
Gurney-Mott theory, 44–45

H and D curve, 46
Hadamard transform, 138
Half-angle subtended, 121
Hammersmith Hospital, 8–9
Health Level 7 (HL7), health care database information exchange, 183–185, 276
Helical scanning, 98–99
Heterogenous databases
  distributed database system, 301
  integration of, 301
High contrast response, 29
High-pass filtering, 163, 167
Histogram, 17, 137, 152
  definition of, 17
  modification, 329
Hooks, video monitor, 311

INDEX **515**

Hospital information system (HIS), common data in, 1, 39, 178- 272, 289–296
Hospital-integrated PACS (HI-PACS), 1
Host computer, connection of film scanner to, 338
Hounsfield number, 101, 103
Hub room, 252–253
Huffman coding, 134–139
Huffman tree, 137
Hydrogen density, 114

IAG, *see* Image acquisition gateway.
ICU modules, PACS intensive care unit, 398–399, 419–423
ID card writer, 66
ID terminal, 66
IMAC, 1–2
Image
  archive manager, 344
  collection, 415–416
  compression, 129–176
  content indexing, 455–457
  contrast, 41
  delivery performance, PACS, 412–414
  display board, 305–308
  display measurement functions, 327–330
  distribution, 254–255
  enhancement, 320–327
  erasing, CR imaging plate, 64–65
  format, MRI, 116
  intensifier tube, 48–50
  memory, 50, 125, 127
  postprocessing, 173–174
  prefetching, 277–278, 346–347, 446
  preprocessing, 219–224
  processing, 320–335
  processing controller, CR,
  quality, measurement of noise, 33–38, 116–117
  reader and recorder, 64, 68–69
  unsharpness, 25, 27
Image acquisition, automated interface methods, 200–206
Image acquisition gateway, 285
  automated image acquisition interface methods, 200–206
  DICOM-compliant, 285–287

multilevel adaptive processing control, 224–231
software modules, 286–287
types of, defined, 199
Image database query support, 454–455
Image file server, distributed, 351–359
Image quality
  evaluation of, 415–418
  measurement of, 25–38
Image receptor
  characteristic curve of X-ray film, 46–48
  development of X-ray film, 45
  digital fluorography, 70, 80–83
  film optical density, 46
  film/screen combination, 43–48
  formation of latent image, 44–45
  image intensifier tube, 48–50
Image reconstruction
  algebraic reconstruction method, 94–95
  filtered back-projection method, 95–96
  Fourier projection theorem and, 91–94
  irreversible compression, 130
Image receiving, 274
Image recorder, 64, 68–69
Image recovery scheme
  basis for, 213–214
  design, 214–215
  results and extension of, 215–216
Image retrieving, 277
Image reverse, 329
Image routing, 275
Image series, 211–213
Image size, definition of, 16
Image stacking, 270, 274–275
Imaginary components, Fourier transform, 21
Imaging plate technology, laser-stimulated luminescence phosphor, 63–70. *See also* CR
Imaging system, handling shutdown of, 209
Implementation strategies, 389–398
Inbound, broadband system, 256
Industry standards, 181–182
Information retrieval, 343
Input image, 31
Installation, 389–398

Integrated Diagnostics Network (IDNET)
    IDNET-2, 201
    version 1 (IDNET-1), 201
Integrated Services Digital Network (ISDN),
    368
Integration
    of modules, 402–406
    multiple PACs, 464–465
Intensifying screen, 43
Interconnected network model, 204–206
Interfacing, 395
    HIS, 276–277, 292–295
    RIS, 276–277, 292–295
Intermediate distribution frame (IDF),
    253
Internal networks, 265–267
International Society for Optical
    Engineering (ISOE), 2
International Standards Organization (ISO),
    183–184, 234
Internet, 265, 388
Intravenous video arteriography (IVA), 80.
    See also DSA
Inverse Fourier transform, 24, 116
Inverse transform, 142–143
Irreversible compression, 130, 138–142,
    172–173
    description of, 130, 138, 140
    examples of, 138, 143
    measurement of differences between
        original and reconstructed image,
        151–160
    methodology for, 138
    quality of the reconstructed image, 155
    theory of, 130
Iteration algebraic method, image
    reconstruction, 94
Iterative modification, SPECT, 104–105

Japan Association of Medical Imaging
    Technology (JAMIT), 2
Joint photographic experts group (JPEG),
    140, 143, 171
Jukebox/optical disk library, 271
Just noticeable differences (JND), 312–
    313
Karhunen-Loeve, image compression
    method, 138
kVp, X-ray generation, 41–42

LAN (local area network), 238–249, 371,
    387
Laplacian operator, 323
Large-latitute film, 48
Laser film imager, 335–338
Laser printer, 57, 69
Laser scanner, 51–52
    accuracy of, 55–56
    specifications, 53
Laser-stimulated luminescence phosphor
    plate, operating characteristics of, 64–67.
    See also CR
Latent image
    center, 45
    formation of, 44–45
Latent-imaging center film, 45
Library search index, 432
Linear motion, CCD camera, 50
Line pairs, 311
Line pairing, video monitor, 311
Line scan, CCD camera technique, low-
    scattering imaging system, 83
Line spread function (LSF), 27, 29
Lookup table, 222–223, 226, 328–331
Low contrast response, 29
Low-pass filtering, 163, 327
Low-scattering digital radiographic system,
    83–84
LRI Research Network, 266
Luminance, 312
Lung nodule with temporal CT image
    database, 475–478

mA and mAs, 41–42
Magnetic disk, 269, 278
    advantages of, 271
    real-time disk, 278. *See also* RAID
Magnetic resonance imaging
    block diagram of, 115
    description of, 113–116
    fundamentals of, 113–114
    image format, resolution contrast,
        116–117
    introduction of, 113
    production, 114–116
    pulsing sequences and relaxation, 114
    tissue characterization, 116
Mammography, 479–484
Managed care organizations, 367, 369

INDEX   517

Manufacturers' implementation strategy, 406–407
Master/slave device, 178
Maximum absolute partial difference, image processing, 320. *See also* Gradient operator
Medical diagnostic imaging support (MDIS), 2, 402
Medical image database management, 457
Medical image database server (MIDS), 457
Medical image informatics infrastructure (MIII), 361–365, 449–454
Memory access model, 202–204
Microscopic imaging, 117–121
  real color, 125
Minification gain, image intensifier tube, 49
MITRE, 2
Modulation transfer function (MTF), 28–29, 31, 33–34, 57, 124
Moire patterns, 50, 58–59
Montage, 332–335
Motorized stage, 120
MUMPS, 185
Multiformat camera, 57
Multilevel adaptive processing control, 224–231
Multimedia
  medical data, 299–300
  in the radiology department, 300
Multiplexed, 259
Multiresolution analysis, wavelet transform, 163–164

National Electrical Manufacturers Association (NEMA) standard, 181, 186
National Television System Committee (NTSC), 171
NATO ASI, 2
Nearest integer function, 141, 168
Network distribution center (NDC), 253
Networking, 180–181, 234
Network interfaces
  master/slave, 178
  peer-to-peer, 178
Network management, 348–351
Network models, 201–206
Network residence time, 411

Network standards, 234
Neuroradiology, 426–436
NIH image, 357
Noise
  cleaning, 323–324
  measurement of, 33–38
Nonlinearity, video monitor, 311
Normalized mean-square error (NMSE), 151, 173
NT/PC display workstation, 338–342, 407
Nuclear medicine scanning
  gamma camera and components for, 107–109
  image format for, 108
  principles of, 106–107
Nuclear medicine module, 402
Nuclei, 113
Numerical aperture, 121
Nyquist frequency, 50, 57, 62

Observer testing, 416–417
Oil immersion lens, 121
One-dimensional projection, 91
  1-D FFT, 92–93
  1K monitors, 311
Open architecture, PACS), 182
Open Systems Interconnect (OSI), 183, 234, 236
  four-layer DOD, 236
  seven-layer OSI, 236
Operating systems, IAG hardware platforms, 285–2986
Optical carrier level 1 (OC1), 239
Optical carrier level 3 (OC3), 241
Optical density (OD)
  of film, 46–47
  versus gray level value, 53–54
Optical disk library/jukebox, 271
Original image, 129
Outbound, broadband system, 256
Outlining, image processing, 320
Output image, 31

Paradoxical enhancement, MR,
Parallel data transmission, 233
Patient folder manager concept, 340–351
Patient thickness, 42
PC/AT computer, 127

518 INDEX

Peak signal-to-noise ratio (PNSR), 169
Perception, 312–313
Perception coding, 176
Periodic function, 31
Personal health data (PHD), 2
Phantoms, physical, 20
Phase angle, 24
PHD, personal health data, 2
Phosphor, 309–310
Photocathode, 48
Photoelectric effect, 48
Photomultiplier tube, 64, 104
Physician desktop access, 424–426
Picture archiving and communication system (PACS)
   bottlenecks, 441–446
   communication, 233–267
   controller, 178–179
   database, 272
   display, 179–180
   evaluation, 6–7
   history of, 2
   ICU, intensive care unit modules, 398–399, 419–423
   implementation, 4–10
   infrastructure, 3–4, 181–183
   interface with other PACS modules, 216–219
   large scale, 7–10, 398
   modules, 398–402
   multimodality acquisition and review system, 300–301
   pitfalls, 436–441
Pincushion effect, video monitor, 311
Pitch, helical XCT, 98
Pixel, 15, 50
Plane selection, MRI, 116
Planning to install a PACS
   air conditioning, 395–396
   cabling, 395
   cost estimates of a film-based operation, 389–394
   digital-based operations, 395–397
   staffing, 396
   training, 396–397
Platter management, 275–276, 348
Point defects, X-ray film, 45
Point spread function, (PSF), 26–27

Positron emission computed tomography (PET), 105–106
Power spectrum, 33
Prefetch algorithm, 347–348
Prioritizing, 411
Process control theory, 227–228
Processing mode, DSA, 160
Processing image
   boundary detection, 320–323
   deblurring, 323
   filtering, 324–325, 327
   noise cleaning, 323–324
   outlining, 320
Pulse repetition frequency (PRF), US imaging, 111
Pulsing sequences, MR imaging, 114

Quantization, 140–141, 168
Quantum statistics, 33
Query protocol, 195–196, 297–299

Radio frequency (RF), 113–114
Radiographic grid, 42–43
Radiographs, effects of kVp, mA, and mAs settings on, 41–42
Radiological contrast, 33
Radiology information system (RIS), common data in, 1, 39, 178, 276–277, 291–296
Radiology reports, online, 343
Radiology Workshop, 355
Random access memory (RAM), 203, 307
Rare earth phosphors, 44
Real component, Fourier transform, 21
Real-time teleconsultation, 484–489
Receiver operating characteristic analysis (ROC), 156–158, 173, 415
   area A_z under, 157–158
Reconstructed image, 129, 151–156
Reconstruction matrix, size and time, 103
Recording, laser printer, 335
Redundant array of inexpensive disks (RAID), 279–282, 419
Reformatting, image, 219–220, 225
Refractive index of the medium, 121
Reliability, 182

Repeater, 250, 252
Residence time
  archive, 410
  distribution, 411
  display (1K), 411
  display (2K), 411
  image acquisition, 410
  image retrieval, 411
  network, 411
  total image, 411
Residents' training, 396
Resolution
  display screen, 310–311
  MRI, 121–123
Retrieval
  image, 355–358
Ringing, video monitor, 311
Rose model, 313
Rotation mode, 96–97
Router, 250
Run-length coding, 132, 134, 168–169

Salt and pepper noise, 323–324
Sampling, 50, 57, 60–62
Sampling frequency, 57
Samsung Medical Center, 9
S-bus, 240
Scan circle radius, 101
Scanners/ing
  area scan, video and CCD cameras, 124, 309
  laser, 51–53
  linearity, 55
  line scan, CCD camera, 124
  specifications of laser, 53
Scan speed, CT, 101
Scatter, how to reduce, 42–43
Scintillation crystal, 97
Sectional images, 224
Security, 182–183, 264, 364
Segmentation, 320
Sensitivity speck, 45
Sequential chain model, 201–202
Serial data transmission, 91
Server system operations, 283–284
Shared disk model, 204
Sharpness, measurement of, 26–33
Signal-to-noise ratio
  defined, 17–20, 33, 34
  peak, 151–152, 169
Silver, 45
Single helical, mode, 98
Single photon, 103
Single photon emission CT (SPECT), 103–105
Slice thickness, 101
Small computers system interface (SCSI), 271
SMPTE phantom, 149, 312
Snow, noise, 323–324
Source circle radius, 101
Source fan, 101
Spatial domain, 20–25, 324–325
Spatial linearity, laser imager, 338
Spatial resolution, 17–20
Spin-lattice relaxation time (T_1), 114
Spin-spin relaxation time (T_2), 114
Spiral (helical) XCT, 98–99
Standardization, 3, 263
Static magnetic field H_0, MR, 114
Static mode, 112
Stationary scintillation detector array, 97
Statistical analysis, ROC, 418
Statistical power, 158
Stepping motors, 120
Storage of image data
  computed radiography, 69–80
  digitial optical disk, 271, 374
  magnetic disk, 271
  media, 278–279
  random access memory (RAM), 305
  VRAM, 305
Structured query language (SQL), 272
Studies grouping, 275
Subject contrast, 41
Subsystem throughput analysis, 408–411
Sun SPARC, 240, 242, 425
Survey mode, 112
Synchronous communication, 233
System availability, 414–415
System connectivity, 3, 182
System efficiency analysis, 412–414
Systems integration, 364
System storage disk, CT, 103

TCP/IP, 180, 181, 192, 205, 210, 292
Technologist, training of, 396–397

520 INDEX

Telemammography, 384–386
Telemicroscopy, 386–388
Teleradiology, 369–384, 388
Television camera, description of, 124. *See also* Video camera
Templates, RFPs, 407
Temporal mask subtraction, 83
10 Base, network cable
 5, 252
 T, 252
 2, 252
 X, 251
Test objects and patterns, 20
3-D rendering node, 454–455
Threshold contrast, 312
Thumbnail sketch, 352
Tilt of angle, 121
T1, WAN, 374
Transform coding, 138
Transformed image, 129
Translation and rotation mode, 93, 96
Transmission, speed of, 262–263
Transmittance, 76
Transmitter-receiver pair, 259
Transverse (cross) section, 96
Trigger mechanism, between two databases, 296
True, ROC analysis, determination of, 416
True positive (TP), 157
 2-D FFT, 116
2K monitors, 311, 385
Two-way broadband communication, 256–258

UCLA, 2, 425
UCSF, 9–10, 78, 185
Ultrasound imaging
 cine loop, 113
 color Doppler, 113, 171–172
 components and procedures for, 109
 principles of B-mode, 109–112
 sampling modes and image display, 112–113
Uniformity, laser imager, 55
UNIX, operating system, 197–198, 273
Unsharpness, image modulation transfer function, 25

Unshielded twisted pair (UTP), 252
User acceptance, PACS, 415

Veterans Administration (VA), 8
VICOM, 321
Video broadband communication system, 255–262, 395
Video cables, 252
Video camera, 31, 81
Video image display, definition of, 17
Video/image conferencing, 460
Video monitor, 48, 113, 308–309
Video RAM (VRAM), 307
Video scanning
 analog/digital (A/D) conversion, 124–125
 digital image of an X-ray film from, 50–51
Vidicon camera, 119, 124
Viewing environments, 416–418
Voxel, 15, 101

Washing, X-ray film developer, 45
Wavelet, transform
 theory, 161–163
 3-D, 166–168
Weber-Fechner law, 313
Web server, 359–361
Weighted factor, 116
Whole-body PET image, 106
Wide are network (WAN), 238–249, 266, 371–372, 374, 376, 378, 387
Wiener spectrum, 33
Window and level, 327–329
Within-hospital systems, communications, *see* LAN
 digital cabling, 376–378, 395
 examples of, 251
 video cabling, 255
Workstation
 analysis, 315
 desktop, 316–317
 diagnostic, 314
 digitizing, 315–316
 display, 179–180, 265, 305–342
 ergonomics of, 317–320
 interactive teaching, 316
 printing, 315–316

review, 314–315
utilization index, 431
Write once, read many (WORM), 272

X-ray attenuation
  coefficient, 103
  profiles, 93
X-ray computerized tomography (XCT)
  block diagram of, 102
  gray level value, 16
  operating principles for, 101–103
  scanning mode, 98
  translation and rotation mode, 96
X-ray film

characteristic curve, 46–48
development of, 45
X-ray film, digitization of
  laser scanner and, 51–52
  sampling, 57–58
  specifications of film scanners, 53
  video scanning system for, 50–51
X-ray photon energy, 42
X-ray source, 40, 80
X-rays, scattered, 41–42
X-ray transmission profiles, 93
X-windows, user interface, 181

Z dimension, 112
Zoom and scroll, 327